MW00965104

HANDBOOK OF ADULT PSYCHOPATHOLOGY IN ASIANS

Handbook of Adult Psychopathology in Asians

Theory, Diagnosis, and Treatment

Edited by Edward C. Chang

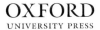

OXFORD
UNIVERSITY PRESS

OXFORD
UNIVERSITY PRESS

Oxford University Press, Inc., publishes works that further
Oxford University's objective of excellence in research,
scholarship, and education.

Oxford   New York
Auckland   Cape Town   Dar es Salaam   Hong Kong   Karachi
Kuala Lumpur   Madrid   Melbourne   Mexico City   Nairobi
New Delhi   Shanghai   Taipei   Toronto

With offices in
Argentina   Austria   Brazil   Chile   Czech Republic   France   Greece
Guatemala   Hungary   Italy   Japan   Poland   Portugal   Singapore
South Korea   Switzerland   Thailand   Turkey   Ukraine   Vietnam

Copyright © 2012 by Oxford University Press, Inc.

Published by Oxford University Press, Inc.
198 Madison Avenue, New York, New York 10016
www.oup.com

Library of Congress Cataloging-in-Publication Data
Handbook of adult psychopathology in Asians : theory, diagnosis,
and treatment / edited by Edward C. Chang.
p. ; cm.
Includes bibliographical references.
ISBN 978–0–19–517906–4 (alk. paper)
I. Chang, Edward C. (Edward Chin-Ho)
[DNLM: 1. Asian Continental Ancestry Group—psychology—Asia
2. Mental Disorders—ethnology—Asia. WA 305 JA1]
LC classificatiion not assigned
362.196'89008995—dc23
2011031966

1 3 5 7 9 8 6 4 2
Printed in the United States of America
on acid-free paper

First and foremost, this volume is dedicated to my courageous and loving parents, Tae Myung-Sook and Chang Suk-Choon. Beyond being a consequence of a historically significant moment in their interpersonal lives, it took many, many dedicated years filled with purposeful practice, patience, and great sacrifice on their part to teach me as a young immigrant boy growing up in Greenpoint, Brooklyn, why I should be aware and proud of my Asian heritage even if it embodied habits and sensibilities different from, and perhaps even undervalued by, those of the strange new society we dearly hoped to make our own one day. I will forever be indebted to both of you for helping me appreciate the rich complexities and ways of being Korean American (감사합니다) and, of course, providing me a middle name (Chin-Ho) that made me wonder as a young child how some American kids knew me without ever being formally introduced. To my dear wife, I would like to thank her for always being understanding and there to support my efforts no matter where they took me or us. And to my G12 Midwest ranked eleven-year-old Kapalua Princess, Olivia, I would like to thank her for inspiring my hopes and dreams of what an even brighter future we may all help to build if we sometimes just remember that living life is about finding unexpected opportunities, rather than dealing with predictable limitations. I hope to keep this wise lesson in mind as time passes. Finally, I would like to thank my dear colleagues, the wonderful contributors of this work, who have devoted their personal and professional lives in order to enrich our global understanding and treatment of mental illness in Asian adults. Without their passion and persistence, this critical work could not have been made possible.

CONTENTS

SECTION III
PSYCHOPATHOLOGY AND TREATMENT
MODELS INDIGENOUS TO ASIA

SECTION IV
CONCLUSION

FOREWORD

The significance and value of *Handbook of Adult Psychopathology in Asians: Theory, Diagnosis, and Treatment*, edited by Dr. Edward Chang, are highlighted by three facts. First, *National Geographic* researchers determined that the world's most typical person is a Han Chinese man. Second, Asians represent over 60% of the world's population. Asians include persons having origins in peoples of the Far East, Southeast Asia, or the Indian subcontinent, including, for example, China, India, Japan, Korea, Cambodia, Malaysia, Pakistan, the Philippines, Thailand, and Vietnam. Third, most of our knowledge of mental health is derived from studies of Americans or Western rather than Asian cultures. Given the population dominance of Asians in the world, and the relative lack of mental health knowledge concerning Asians, the Handbook is an important, refreshing, and much needed contribution.

A wide range of topics is actually covered in the Handbook, such as Asian psychology, nosology and disorders, culture, assessment, diagnosis, and treatment. The primary emphasis of the book is the presentation of mental disorders. The various chapters largely focus on disorders from the *Diagnostic and Statistical Manual* of the American Psychiatric Association. Consequently, mood disorders, anxiety disorders, schizophrenia, substance abuse, eating disorders, dissociative disorders, adjustment disorders, personality disorders, sleep disorders, somatoform disorders, and culture-bound syndromes are presented. In general, the chapters cover symptom expression and assessment, etiological factors in the disorders, and treatment. The contributors are distinguished researchers and scholars on Asians from various parts of the world.

A focus on Asians that is based on disorders from the *Diagnostic and Statistical Manual* is not an easy task. Asians are quite diverse in terms of cultural milieu, political orientation, geographic locations, socioeconomic status, and so forth. Furthermore, it is impossible to cover all Asian groups and all topics related to psychopathology, assessment, and treatment. And, as discussed by several chapter contributors, the use of the American Psychiatric Association's *Diagnostic and Statistical Manual* for various Asian groups may be problematic in terms of definition of disorders, diagnostic criteria, and symptom manifestations. But raising these issues allows the thoughtful examination of the adequacy of what we do as scientists and practitioners. What Dr. Chang and the various contributors have accomplished in the Handbook is a meaningful sampling of Asian populations and mental health issues.

At the core of this book is the principle that culture in general and Asian cultures in particular affect all of mental health. This is apparent in descriptions of how Asian cultural influences affect symptom expression and illness behaviors. Indeed, various contributors point to the need to consider indigenous conceptions of mental disorders, indigenous psychotherapies, and new ways of defining mental disorders. The principle of culture is most clearly revealed in three ways. First, the popular belief is that psychotherapies were first developed and articulated in the West. Yet, we find that Asians also utilized different forms of psychotherapies that either paralleled or predated those in the West. Second, the contributors succeed in demonstrating how those in the mental health field have often considered practices, concepts, and theories as being valid, etic, or universal phenomena applicable to all populations, when the practices and theories are actually emic or culturally limited in nature. For example, in the West, somatic disorders are diagnosed largely on the basis of symptoms that show strong psychological features; yet, in the East, these disorders are expressed with psychological and somatic symptoms because of a stronger holistic integration of mind and body features. While mental health research and conceptualizations are most advanced in Western societies, particularly the United States, there is the danger that these conceptualizations and attendant cultural biases become the norms and standards to use throughout the world. Third, it is always intriguing to compare the rate and distribution of mental disorders in various countries or societies—for example, is schizophrenia more prevalent in the United States than China, or do Asian Americans have a higher rate of mental disorders than non-Hispanic white Americans? These questions are important to raise. However, the answers are complex. Is the *Diagnostic and Statistical Manual* applicable to different cultural groups? Are symptoms of disorders and diagnostic categories valid for different cultural populations? Are measures of disorders invariant across different groups? How do we deal with so-called culture-bound syndromes in our estimates of prevalence of mental disorders?

These questions and issues point to the importance of understanding not only the mental health status of Asians, which is an important goal per se, but also the broader implications concerning the mental health field, its concepts, practices, assessment assumptions, treatment approaches, and limitations. *Handbook of Adult Psychopathology in Asians: Theory, Diagnosis, and Treatment* represents a significant advance in our understanding of Asians and the broader issues in mental health.

Stanley Sue
Palo Alto University
2011

PREFACE

The conceptual and practical impetus for the present work emerged from my early clinical experiences working with Asian adult patients as part of my year-long training as a clinical intern at a major New York City hospital. I can still recall the unexpected mix of excitement and calm I felt when I realized that I could connect with these patients in ways that went beyond the formalized conventions and alliance-seeking strategies I was trained to express and establish with all my adult patients. Indeed, as an immigrant and a son of traditional Korean parents, I quickly and easily found myself thrown into discourses with these patients involving contexts and themes that were often all too personally familiar. Yet, at the same time, I also felt tremendous challenge and frustration in trying to convey my understanding and appreciation of mental illness as culturally embodied among these diverse Asian adults to my non-Asian clinical supervisors. The source of that frustration was not due to my supervisors being unwilling to consider my contextualized clinical formulations of my patients' presenting problems, but it had more to do with my inability to find substantive resources to ground my formulations beyond my personal experiences and the very limited research on Asian adult mental health that existed at that time. Interestingly, the clinical internship I attended was world-renowned for their emphasis on appreciating the cultural context of Hispanics, and even included an in-house bilingual treatment program for Hispanic and Spanish-speaking patients. Ironically, however, an appreciation for culture and context in grappling with clinical issues was often difficult to find beyond the doors of that unique program. Nonetheless, I was fortunate in that my supervisors were willing to entertain and bet on my loosely justified thoughts, offering me sufficient time and space to incorporate culture in working with my Asian adult patients. Yet, within this generous opening, I continued to feel intellectually stunted and therapeutically lost because of the lack of empirical, scholarly, and clinical resources present and available to me and my supervisors for understanding mental illness among Asian adults. Needless to say, the world has changed in many unimaginable ways over the past decade or so since my year on internship. Works involving theory, research, and practice on Asian adult mental health have grown considerably, albeit at levels that still remain far behind those involving Caucasian or European adults. Nonetheless, we do have more information available than ever before, and the fruits of these emerging points of knowledge are highlighted in and by the existence of this volume. Accordingly, and I say with a sense of contentment, the present work is meant to represent a central resource for all current and future professionals who are involved or interested in the study and treatment of mental illness among Asian adults. No doubt, I am deeply indebted to the stellar group of contributors who have dedicated a great deal of their valuable time, energy, and expertise during the progress of this work to ultimately produce a volume that I know will help all of us ground and expand our global notions of what it means to consider culture and mental health in our efforts to understand and improve the lives of Asian adults.

Edward C. Chang
Ann Arbor, MI
2011

CONTRIBUTORS

Phillip D. Akutsu, PhD
Department of Psychology
California State University, Sacramento
Sacramento, CA

Sopagna Eap Braje, PhD
Clinical PhD Program
CSPP at Alliant International
University-San Diego
San Diego, CA

Allison V. Chan, DO
Palo Alto Medical Foundation
Sleep Medicine Center
Sunnyvale, CA

Doris Chang, PhD
Department of Psychology
New School for Social Research
New York, NY

Edward C. Chang, PhD
Department of Psychology
University of Michigan
Ann Arbor, MI

Fanny M. Cheung, PhD
Department of Psychology
The Chinese University of Hong Kong
Shatin, New Territories,
Hong Kong

Joyce P. Chu, PhD
Palo Alto University
Palo Alto, CA

Kevin M. Chun, PhD
Department of Psychology
University of San Francisco
San Francisco, CA

Lillian Huang Cummins, PhD
California School of Professional
Psychology at Alliant International
University, San Francisco Campus
San Francisco, CA

Jessica Dere, MSc
Department of Psychology
Concordia University
Montreal, Quebec, Canada

Cathryn G. Fabian, MS, MSW
School of Social Work
University of Michigan
Ann Arbor, MI

Kenneth Fung, MD, MSc
Toronto Western Hospital
University of Toronto
Toronto, Ontario, Canada

Xiaojia Ge, PhD
Institute for Child Development
University of Minnesota
Minneapolis, MN

Gordon C. Nagayama Hall, PhD
Department of Psychology
University of Oregon
Eugene, OR

Janie J. Hong, PhD
San Francisco Bay Area Center
for Cognitive Therapy
Oakland, CA

Jeanette Hsu, PhD
VA Palo Alto Health Care System
Palo Alto, CA

Hai-Gwo Hwu, MD
Department of Psychiatry
National Taiwan University
Hospital and School of Medicine
Taipei, Taiwan

Shuichi Katsuragawa, MD
Department of Psychiatry
Toho University Sakura Medical Center
Chiba, Japan

Kenji Kitanishi, MD
Department of Social Welfare
Japan Women's University
Kanagawa, Japan

Clete A. Kushida, MD, PhD, RPSGT
Stanford University School of Medicine
Stanford Sleep Medicine Center
Redwood City, CA

Janice Delgado Lehman, PsyD
The Permanente Medical Group
Department of Psychiatry
Fremont Medical Center
Fremont, CA

Freedom Leung, PhD
Department of Psychology
The Chinese University of Hong Kong
Shatin, New Territories, Hong Kong

Keh-Ming Lin, MD, MPH
Division of Mental Health and
Substance Abuse Research
National Health Research Institutes
and Center for Advanced Study in the
Behavioral Science

Rebecca Chun Liu, PsyD
San Francisco VA Medical Center
San Francisco, CA

Teruaki Maeshiro, PhD
Yamato Naikan Institute
Nara, Japan

Winnie W. S. Mak, PhD
Department of Psychology
The Chinese University of Hong Kong
Shatin, NT, Hong Kong

Sung Kil Min, MD
Seoul Metropolitan Eunpyeong Hospital
Seoul, Korea

Jessica Murakami-Brundage, MS
Department of Psychology
University of Oregon
Eugene, OR

Kei Nakamura, MD
Department of Psychiatry
Jikei University
Director of the Center for Morita Therapy
Jikei University Daisan Hospital
Tokyo, Japan

Sumie Okazaki, PhD
Department of Applied Psychology
Steinhardt School of Culture,
Education, and Human Development
New York University
New York, NY

Karen Chan Osilla, PhD
RAND Corporation
Santa Monica, CA

Andrew G. Ryder, PhD
Department of Psychology
Concordia University
Montreal, Canada

Anne Saw, PhD
Department of Psychology
Asian American Center on Disparities Research
University of California, Davis
Davis, CA

Donald M. Sesso, DO
Stanford University Medical Center
California Sleep Institute
East Palo Alto, CA

Wen-Shing Tseng, MD
Department of Psychiatry
University of Hawaii School
of Medicine
Honolulu, HI

Ming T. Tsuang, MD, PhD, DSc
Department of Psychiatry
University of California at San Diego
La Jolla, CA

Vivian Ota Wang, PhD
National Institutes of Health
Bethesda, MD

Eunice C. Wong, PhD
RAND Corporation
Santa Monica, CA

Jian Yang, MD, PhD
Toronto Western Hospital
Toronto, Canada

Albert Yeung, MD, DSc
Depression Clinical and
Research Program
Massachusetts General Hospital
Boston, MA

Cong Zhong, MD
Institute of Mental Health
Peking University
Beijing, China

Jinfu Zhu, MD
Department of Psychology
Xin Xiang Medical University
Xin Xiang, China

| 1 |

INTRODUCTION: FROM NOMOTHETIC TO IDIOGRAPHIC APPROACHES

Edward C. Chang and Cathryn G. Fabian

In teaching the rest of the world to think like us, we have been, for better and worse, homogenizing the way the world goes mad.

—from *Crazy Like Us,* Ethan Watters

Science is believed to involve a rational process in which trained individuals make careful observations, generate logical ideas, develop coherent theoretical models that account for their observations, and then submit their theory to empirical hypothesis testing in order to confirm or disconfirm their model (Ayer, 1959; Carnap, 1934; Popper, 1969; Whewell, 1858). Following in the tradition of the Enlightenment in Europe, modern philosophers of science believed that by engaging in this sort of objective process, scientists could help eliminate social ills and generate information and findings that would be beneficial to all members of society (Ayer, 1946). Indeed, in talking about the psychology of scientists, Holton (1978) noted that those who engaged in doing science often endorsed "scientific optimism," the idea that through science they were at the dawn of being able to solve something very important and useful to all. Without a doubt, the power of science has led to many social benefits and advances, and this is no less apparent when one looks at the evolution associated with the study of mental illness or psychopathology.

THE DIAGNOSTIC AND STATISTICAL MANUALS (DSMs) OF MENTAL DISORDERS: FROM CORE NEUROSES TO AN EXPANSIVE NOSOLOGY OF CLINICALLY SIGNIFICANT DYSFUNCTIONS

In 1948, the World Health Organization published the *Manual of the International Statistical Classification of Disease (ICD), Injuries, and Causes of Death* to classify disease and disorders around the world. In response to this global effort, the American Psychiatric Association (1952) produced the *Diagnostic and Statistical Manual of Mental Disorders* (DSM) to offer mental health professionals working in the United States a more situated tool for assessing, diagnosing, and eventually treating individuals with mental illnesses. The development of the *DSM* was particularly important for the armed forces, given that nomenclature found in existing systems at the time, like the Standard Nomenclature of Diseases and Operations (National Conference on Medical Nomenclature, 1952), failed to account for the wide range of behavioral dysfunctions observed in those involved in World War II.

The first and second editions of the *DSM* (American Psychiatric Association, 1954, 1968) were relatively short in length, and involved a classification of mental disorders largely limited to those disorders believed to be associated with brain injury and those believed to have psychogenic origins. By the 1980s, the American Psychiatric Association took a strong and decisive step forward in developing the third edition of the *DSM* (American Psychiatric Association, 1980, 1987). Unlike previous editions, the American Psychiatric Association took careful steps to use data from clinical field trails to help inform the development of the third edition of the *DSM*. Indeed, the development of the *DSM-III* (American Psychiatric Association, 1980) was distinctly predicated on improving the reliability of diagnoses. Several years later, a revision was made that incorporated an emphasis on concurrent and descriptive validity of the diagnoses provided, resulting in the *DSM-III-R* (American Psychiatric Association, 1987). Finally, more than a decade after the publication of the third edition, the *DSM-IV* (American Psychiatric Association, 1994) was produced. Unlike previous editions, the development of the *DSM-IV* was driven by concerted efforts to improve the clinical utility of the *DSM* and provide a more scientific and objective foundation for classifying mental disorders, ranging from reviews of the extant empirical literature, data reanalyses, to field trials (Widiger et al., 1991). It was also notable for including explicit references to culture-bound syndromes (Kleinman, 1997). Given that more than 15 years would pass before the next edition of the *DSM* was scheduled for publication (*DSM-5* is due in 2013), and updated edition of the *DSM-IV* was introduced, namely the *DSM-IV-Text Revision* (American Psychiatric Association, 2000). Three key objectives were sought in updating the *DSM-IV*, namely, updating information to be current with existing literature, correcting for errors and ambiguities that have become apparent in the *DSM-IV*, and updating the diagnostic codes to correspond with current *ICD* codes (First & Pincus, 2002). Currently, the *DSM* has become one of the most widely and frequently used tools in studying, assessing, diagnosing, and treating mental disorders around the world (Watters, 2010).

The DSM as a Tool Used by Scientists and Practitioners to Describe, Maintain, and Prescribe American Culture to the Rest of the World

According to Prilleltensky (1989), scientists often believe that by engaging in scientific activity to solve problems, they can achieve solutions with objectivity and without bias. Yet, the idea that science exclusively involves an objective process has been one that has been frequently questioned by others (Bronowski, 1956; Scarr, 1985). Increasingly, philosophers and scientists alike are becoming aware that the question to ask is not whether values are present in science, but rather what values are present (Fulford, 2005; Giorgi, 1975; Prilleltensky, 1997; Wakefield, 1992). In that regard, the *DSM* needs to not only be situated historically, but also situated within a multicultural context.

The DSM as a Core American Brand

In talking about American culture, Brandt (1970) pointed out that the American way of life is one of doing, and thus, it is not surprising that American scientists focus so heavily on seeking " 'law and order' in nature so that they could 'predict and control' it" (p. 1091). But, perhaps more importantly, Brandt also noted how Americans typically achieve "objectivity":

> Objectivity in American terms was to be achieved not by taking different viewpoints but by describing "how to do" something (operationism). Taking different viewpoints toward a problem was considered confusing and uneconomical. Americans need "consistency" and "parsimony" to make life simple instead of complex. (p. 1091)

Compounding this problem is a form of nationalism that often leads Americans to believe they are better than other people (Albee, 1986), and that American standards should be exported and prescribed to the rest of the world (Watters, 2010). And, as a result, it is not surprising to find that American scientists often devalue, and sometimes even disregard, research done in other countries, especially those done in other languages (Brandt, 1963). It is the confluence of these two factors (viz., seeking "objectivity" and devaluing non-American research), among others (e.g., emphasis on internal validity, public policy goals; Sadler, 2005; Sue, 1999), that has helped shape and maintains the common belief that the *DSM* is not just an artifact of American culture, but rather a rigorously detailed documentation on mental disorders generated from the fruits of many decades of unbiased scientific research and innovation.

Yet, it is clear that culture does matter in doing science, from the questions asked to the answers obtained (Basic Behavioral Science Task Force of the National Advisory Mental Health Council, 1996). In that regard, the inclusion of culture-bound syndromes in the *DSM-IV* may have suggested to some that the American Psychiatric Association was moving closer to appreciating the importance of culture in the context of mental disorders. Yet, as noted by Kleinman (1997), who served on the Taskforce on Culture and the DSM-IV, the editors of the *DSM-IV* eliminated or failed to incorporate a number of important suggestions for inclusion that would have helped make the *DSM* more culturally relevant and useful. Rather, the editors allowed for the inclusion of a limited number of syndromes (e.g., *koro, amok*) that was believed to be indicated in some cultural and ethnic groups. So if the goal was not to make the *DSM* more culturally useful, then what was the purpose of including any reference to culture in this edition? According to Kleinman (1997),

> The reason why culture appears at all in DSM…has all too little to do with the robust findings generated over the past several decades by cross-cultural and international research on mental illness and its treatment. This is research that relatively few academic psychiatrists or practitioners, save those with a special interest in culture, read. DSM-IV had to include something on culture for demographic, economic, and political reasons. (p. 343)

Thus, ironically, we again find an example of how values, rather than the impartial rigors of scientific activity, dictate what is and is not included in our fundamental understanding of the world around us. This consequence becomes particularly problematic when we appreciate the increasing global context and complexity of the world that we live in (Cohen, 2009; Mays, Rubin, Sabourin, & Walker, 1996), juxtaposed by the use of a popular diagnostic manual of mental disorders that has been derived largely from Western intellectual traditions and informed by studies of patients from mostly Western backgrounds (Alarcón et al., 2009; Lin & Lin, 2002; Mezzich, Ruiperez, & Villa, 2008), and typically applied in top-down fashion to individuals of all cultural backgrounds (Betancourt & López, 1993). As an American product that was historically derived from and designed to account for the behaviors of most Westerners (i.e., individuals of European descent), it is likely that the *DSM* may not be as useful a tool for understanding the behaviors, normal or abnormal, of most Easterners (i.e., individuals of Asian descent). Indeed, there are a number of reasons to consider a "bottom-up" approach to understanding mental disorders more indigenously, namely, emerging research pointing to fundamental differences in behavior between Easterners and Westerners, and research on the prevalence of mental disorders in Asians.

FUNDAMENTAL DIFFERENCES BETWEEN EASTERNERS AND WESTERNERS: AN ILLUSTRATION DRAWN FROM RESEARCH ON SELF-CRITICISM AND SELF-ENHANCEMENT MOTIVES

Despite the modern notion of self-criticism as bad and self-enhancement as good (Chang, 2007), this view may be more common in the West, but less common in the East (Kitayama, Markus, Matsumoto, & Norasakkunkit, 1997). Typically, Western cultures are considered to be individualistic given their emphasis on attending to the needs of the self over others (Greenwald, 1980; Weisz, Rothbaum, & Blackburn, 1984). Thus, for most Westerners, it is the attainment of personal happiness, rather than group happiness that is highly regarded and sought after, as codified and expressed in historical works such as the United States' Declaration of Independence. Therefore, it is not too surprising then that in Western cultures, maybe especially in the United States (Brandt, 1970), conditions associated with a lack of self-interest, such as anhedonia, an inability to experience personal pleasures, and dependency, a condition defined by a tendency to subordinate one's needs to those of others, are seen typically as signs of psychological dysfunction or mental illness. Accordingly, self-enhancement for Westerners is believed to represent a constructive process that allows them to maintain and support the independent self (Taylor & Brown, 1988).

Eastern cultures or cultures found in many Asian countries, have been considered collectivist, given their focus on fostering a view of the self as fundamentally interrelated with significant others (Doi, 1971/1973; Markus & Kitayama, 1991). Hence, attending to significant others, harmonious interdependence with them, and fitting in not only are valued, but also are often strongly expected among members living within these cultures. Thus, for example, in contrast to many Western psychological approaches that focus largely on treating and strengthening internal attributes of an independent self (Prilleltensky, 1989; Sarason, 1981), a key objective of some indigenous Japanese therapies is to help clients overcome and transcend a focus on the immediate and independent self (e.g., Morita, 1928/1998). One finds that the self fostered in Eastern cultures, as in Japan, is interdependent with significant others, such that important others "participate actively and continuously in the definition of the interdependent self" (Markus & Kitayama, 1991, p. 227). Accordingly, self-criticism for Easterners is believed to represent a constructive process that allows them to maintain and support the interdependent self or the group. Taken together, these culturally different patterns indicate a need to consider more inclusive models and a need to situate our understanding of self-criticism and self-enhancement motives in cultural context. Paralleling these culturally different patterns in fundamental dimensions of motivation between Easterners and Westerners, other researchers have also noted important cultural differences in styles of thinking, noting that Easterners are more inclined to appreciate and engage in dialectical reasoning, whereas Westerners are more inclined to appreciate and engage in logical reasoning (Peng & Nisbett, 1999).

PREVALENCE OF MENTAL DISORDERS IN ASIANS

Early researchers of psychopathology in Asia in the 1950s concluded that Asians were resilient and immune to even the more subtle mood disorders prevalent in Western societies (Kleinman, 1986). More contemporary data has supported this notion by revealing that East Asian countries generally have a lower prevalence of psychiatric disorders than Western countries (Simon et al., 2002; Weissman et al., 1996). Cho et al.'s (2007) review of the existing literature found that estimates of lifetime prevalence of major depressive disorder in East Asia countries (including South Korea, Japan, Taiwan, and Hong Kong) range from 1.1% to 3.4%, compared to 12.8% to 17.1% in Western countries. In a similar fashion, results from a cross-national study of psychiatric disorders conducted by the World Health Organization using the World Health-Composite International Diagnostic Interview (WMH-CIDI) also indicate substantially lower 12-month prevalence of mental disorders in Japan (8.8%), Beijing, (9.1%), and Shanghai (4.3%) compared to the United States (26.4%; WHO World Mental Health Survey Consortium, 2004). Among the Asian diasporas, epidemiological surveys have established similar findings of low prevalence rates of mental disorders, although data on Asian Americans is limited due to their exclusion from most major

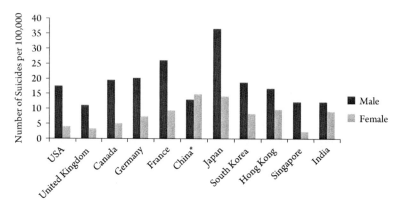

FIGURE 1.1: Suicide Rates Per Capita, by Country and Gender
select urban and rural areas only.

large-scale studies. Much of the existing data on the prevalence rates among Asian Americans is drawn from studies that focus on a single ethnic group, primarily Chinese, Japanese, and Filipinos. More recently, there has been a more concerted effort among researchers to include multiple Asian ethnic groups in such studies. Findings from the Collaborative Psychiatric Epidemiological Survey indicate that compared to African Americans, Caribbean blacks, and Latinos, Asian Americans have lower prevalence rates of mental disorders (Abe-Kim et al., 2007; Alegría et al., 2007; Williams et al., 2007). However, anecdotal evidence suggests that the rates of mental illness among Asians are trending upward, as evidenced by the finding that Asian nations have some of the highest per capita rates of suicide (World Health Organization, 2003). (See Figure 1.1.) These developments may be due in part to rapid social changes related to economic development, and to a more evolved understanding of mental health among Asian cultures that have ascribed to differ-ent notions of well-being (Dennis, 2004). Despite the appearance of low rates of mental illness in Asia, the true magnitude of the issue is likely much larger.

Perhaps, then the utilization of mental health services is as significant an issue of concern as the prevalence of mental disorders themselves. Researchers have identified numerous factors that may serve as barriers to accessing mental health services among Asians, including: use of social networks to provide informal support; use of spiritual leaders or indigenous healers; concerns about loss of face due to stigma of mental illness; lack of access to culturally appropriate services; and a "model minority" stereotype that views Asians as being less susceptible to mental health issues compared to other racial groups (Lin & Cheung, 1999; Herrick & Brown, 1998). Another possible explanation for the low prevalence rates of mental disorders in Asians may be due to underreporting. In Asia, a shortage of mental health professionals, including psychiatrists, psy-chologists, and social workers, leads many of those with mental disorders to go without formal diagnosis and treatment (World Health Organization, 2005). (See Figure 1.2.) Even when some services are available, Asians are less likely to utilize such services to address mental health issues. Cross-national data from the World Health Organization found that rates of service use in the past 12 months were lower in China (3.4%) and Japan (5.6%) than in most of the Western countries surveyed, including the United States (17.9%; Wang, Aguilar-Gaxiola, et al., 2007). Furthermore, among Asian Americans, service utilization rates vary according to nativity and generational

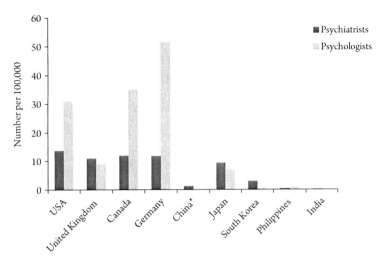

FIGURE 1.2: Number of Mental Health Professionals (Psychiatrists and Psychologists) Per Capita
no data available for number of psychologists in China.

status, suggesting that acculturation to Western culture also plays a role in accessing mental health services (Abe-Kim et al., 2007; Meyer, Zane, Cho, & Takeuchi, 2009). These lower mental health service utilization rates are further exacerbated by a tendency among Asians to delay seeking treatment after the onset of disorder (Alegría et al., 2002; Wang, Angermeyer, et al., 2007). Thus, the treatment of mental disorders among Asians necessitates a more holistic understanding of the role of culture in help-seeking behaviors, and of more structural barriers that prohibit those in need from seeking out services.

OVERVIEW OF THE PRESENT VOLUME

The present volume is broken down into three main sections. Section I focuses on broad conceptual and practical issues associated with the study of Asians. In Chapter 2, Saw and Okazaki provide an overview of Asian psychology that challenges the dominant mainstream Western paradigm. Through a review of several indigenous Asian psychologies, they call attention to salient values, relational concepts, and worldviews from a cultural perspective as they relate to psychopathology among Asians. In Chapter 3, Akutsu and Chu address the issue of the inadequacy of current research and assessment methods in informing clinical practice with Asian and Asian American clients. The authors identify common challenges faced by clinicians using currently available diagnostic tools with Asian clients, and provide a practical model for choosing appropriate assessment measures.

Section II focuses a critical appraisal on what we know about specific mental disorders in Asians. In Chapter 4, Wong and Osilla review the literature on substance use disorders among Asians, which is limited despite research that suggests prevalence rates may be rising. The authors also identify several key barriers to seeking treatment for substance use disorders that are particularly pertinent to Asians. In Chapter 5, Lin, Hwu, and Tsuang discuss the relevance and utility of current diagnostic criteria, etiological models, and treatment approaches for schizophrenia in

Asians, while also calling for further exploration into ethnic and cultural influences in diagnosis and treatment. In Chapter 6, Yeung and Chang explore the contradiction between the Western conceptualization of mood disorders and more holistic views of health and well-being in the East. This cultural dilemma not only leads to greater stigmatization of mental illness in general among Asians, but also leads those with mood disorders to delay or even avoid treatment. In Chapter 7, Hong provides an overview of the various anxiety disorders, highlighting unique cultural factors that limit the generalizability of current etiological theories and treatment approaches among Asians. In Chapter 8, Mak, Cheung, and Leung compare and critique diagnostic criteria for soma-toform disorders across different diagnostic systems. The authors also examine the rise and fall of neurasthenia as a distinct diagnosis in relation to other somatoform disorders. In Chapter 9, Tseng and Zhong review dissociation, conversion, and possession disorders as they occur in Asian societies. In addition, the authors expand on the current *DSM* classification to include some discussion of the closely related clinical phenomena of epidemic hysteria, possession psy-choses, and alternate-personality disorders. In Chapter 10, Cummins, Lehman, and Liu discuss the prevalence of eating disorders, and how cultural variations in their expression may contribute to the apparent lower rates among Asians and Asian Americans. While cultural influences on the etiology of eating disorders have not yet been established in the literature, the authors pro-vide suggestions for using existing treatment approaches in a culturally appropriate manner. In Chapter 11, Sesso, Chan, and Kushida discuss the diagnostic criteria, etiology, treatment, of sleep disorders. In Chapter 12, Chun and Hsu use a stress and coping framework to provide insight into the types of stressors that increase risk for adjustment disorders among Asians. More specifically, the authors identify stressors related to acculturation and to ethnic minority status as salient risk factors for the psychosocial dysfunction and psychological distress that are key characteristics of adjustment disorder. In Chapter 13, Ryder, Yang, Dere, and Fung supplement a review of the literature on personality disorders in Asians with culturally grounded lay theories or ideal and problematic personality attributes. The authors also call attention to issues with the applicability of predominant Western models of personality to Asians, and raise questions about the univer-sality of personality traits. On a related note, in Chapter 14, Braje, Murakami-Brundage, Hall, Wang, and Ge examine externalizing and antisocial behavior among Asians. Although these dis-orders are poorly understood in Asian populations due in part to the "model minority" stereo-type, the authors present a genocultural model of aggression that emphasizes cultural and social risk factors.

Section III introduces developments in Asian-specific indigenous models of psychopathology and treatment specific to Asia. In Chapter 15, Tseng, Min, Nakamura, and Katsuragawa describe various cultural-related specific psychiatric syndromes observed in Asian populations. Although occurrences of these disorders are rare, they are useful in highlighting the relationship between cul-ture and the manifestation of psychopathology. Finally, in Chapter 16, Tseng, Kitanishi, Maeshiro, and Zhu describe three unique culturally influenced psychotherapies developed in Asia, with particular emphasis on the philosophical thought and value systems underlying each treatment modality.

The present work then concludes with Section IV, which focuses on a broad and integrative discussion of the issues and challenges that remain in future efforts to study and treat mental disor-ders in Asians. Specifically, in Chapter 17, Fabian and Chang offer suggestions for future directions for research, intervention, training, and policy development as they pertain to psychopathology in Asians.

FINAL THOUGHTS

If there is a single collective point that the present volume seeks to make, it would be that culture does matter. It is not that in the human process of assessing, diagnosing, and treating others afflicted with mental illness that professionals should consider the patient's cultural context, but rather that we have no choice but to do so if we are to authentically respect the dignity and worth of the individuals we ultimately serve. No doubt, as scientists and practitioners, we too must always remain aware of how culture plays an intimate and powerful role in shaping the very questions we seek to answer and the range of solutions we arrive at. In our view, it is only by integrating culture as a dynamic framework for understanding human behavior that the science of psychopathology can truly advance for all.

REFERENCES

Abe-Kim, J., Takeuchi, D. T, Hong, S., Zane, N., Sue, S. Spencer, M. S., et al. (2007). Use of mental health related services among immigrant and U.S. born Asian Americans: Results from the National Latino and Asian American Study. *American Journal of Public Health, 97,* 91–98.

Albee, G. W. (1986). Toward a just society: Lessons from observations on the primary prevention of psychopathology. *American Psychologist, 41,* 891–898.

Alegría, M., Canino, G., Ríos, R., Vera, M., Calderón, J., Rusch, D., et al. (2002). Inequalities in use of specialty mental health services among Latinos, African Americans, and Non-Latino Whites. *Psychiatric Services, 53,* 1547–1555.

Alegría, M., Mulvaney-Day, N., Torres, M., Polo, A., Cao, Z., & Canino, G. (2007). Prevalence of psychiatric disorders across Latino subgroups in the United States. *American Journal of Public Health, 97*(1), 68–75.

Alarcón, R. D., Becker, A. E., Lewis-Fernández, R., Like, R. C., Desai, P., Foulks, E., et al. (2009). Issue for DSM-V: The role of culture in psychiatric diagnosis. *Journal of Nervous and Mental Disease, 197,* 559–560.

American Psychiatric Association. (1952). *Diagnostic and statistical manual of mental disorders.* Washington, DC: Author.

American Psychiatric Association. (1968). *Diagnostic and statistical manual of mental disorders* (2nd ed.). Washington, DC: Author.

American Psychiatric Association. (1980). *Diagnostic and statistical manual of mental disorders* (3rd ed.). Washington, DC: Author.

American Psychiatric Association. (1987). *Diagnostic and statistical manual of mental disorders* (Rev. 3rd ed.). Washington, DC: Author.

American Psychiatric Association. (1994). *Diagnostic and statistical manual of mental disorders* (4th ed.). Washington, DC: Author.

American Psychiatric Association. (2000). *Diagnostic and statistical manual of mental disorders-Text revision* (Rev. 4th ed.). Washington, DC: Author.

Ayer, A. J. (1946). *Language, truth, and logic.* New York: Dover.

Ayer, A. J. (1959). *Logical positivism.* Glencoe, IL: Free Press.

Basic Behavioral Science Task Force of the National Advisory Mental Health Council. (1996). Basic behavioral science research for mental health: Sociocultural and environmental processes. *American Psychologist, 51,* 722–731.

Betancourt, H., & López, S. R. (1993). The study of culture, ethnicity, and race in American psychology. *American Psychologist, 48,* 629–637.

Brandt, L. W. (1963). Linguistic isolation? *American Psychologist, 18,* 70.

Brandt, L. W. (1970). American psychology. *American Psychologist, 25,* 1091–1093.

Bronowski, J. (1956). *Science and human values.* New York: J. Messner.

Carnap, R. (1934). *The unity of science.* London: Kegan Paul.

Chang, E. C. (Ed.). (2007). *Self-criticism and self-enhancement: Theory, research, and clinical implications.* Washington, DC: American Psychological Association.

Cho, J. M., Kim, J.-K., Jeon, H. J., Suh, T., Chung, I.-W., Hong, J. P., et al. (2007). Lifetime and 12-month prevalence of DSM-IV psychiatric disorders among Korean adults. *Journal of Nervous and Mental Disease, 195,* 203–210.

Cohen, A. B. (2009). Many forms of culture. *American Psychologist, 64,* 194–204.

Dennis, C. (2004). Asia's tigers get the blues. *Nature, 429,* 696–698.

Doi, T. (1973). *The anatomy of dependence* (J. Bester, Trans.). Tokyo: Kodansha. (Original work published in 1971)

First, M. B., & Pincus, H. A. (2002). The DSM-IV Text Revision: Rationale and potential impact on clinical practice. *Psychiatric Services, 53,* 288–292.

Fulford, K. W. M. (2005). Values in psychiatric diagnosis: Developments in policy, training, and research. *Psychopathology, 38,* 171–176.

Giorgi, A. (1975). *Phenomenology as a human science.* Oxford, England: Harper & Row.

Greenwald, A. G. (1980). The totalitarian ego: Fabrication and revision of personal history. *American Psychologist, 35,* 603–618.

Herrick, C. A., & Brown, H. N. (1998). Underutilization of mental health services by Asian-Americans residing in the United States. *Issues in Mental Health Nursing, 19,* 225–240.

Holton, G. (1978). *The scientific imagination: Case studies.* Cambridge: Cambridge University Press.

Kitayama, S., Markus, H. R., Matsumoto, H., & Norasakkunkit, V. (1997). Individual and collective processes in the construction of the self: Self-enhancement in the United States and self-criticism in Japan. *Journal of Personality and Social Psychology, 72,* 1245–1267.

Kleinman, A. (1986). *Social origins of distress and disease: Depression, neurasthenia, and pain in modern China.* New Haven, CT: Yale University Press.

Kleinman, A. (1997). Triumph or pyrrhic victory? Inclusion of culture in the DSM-IV. *Harvard Review of Psychiatry, 4,* 343–344.

Lin, K.-M., & Cheung, F. (1999). Mentla health issues for Asian Americans. *Psychiatric Services, 50,* 774–780.

Lin, K.-M., & Lin, M. (2002). Challenging the myth of a culture free nosological system. In K. S. Kuraskai, S. Okazaki, & S. Sue (Eds.), *Asian American mental health: Assessment theories and methods* (pp. 67–73). New York: Kluwer Academic.

Markus, H. R., & Kitayama, S. (1991). Culture and the self: Implications for cognition, emotion, and motivation. *Psychological Review, 98,* 224–253.

Mays, V. M., Rubin, J., Sabourin, M., & Walker, L. (1996). Moving toward a global psychology: Changing theories and practice to meet the needs of a changing world. *American Psychologist, 51,* 485–487.

Mezzich, J. E., Ruiperez, M. A., & Villa, H. (2008). Culture and psychopathology. In C. H. Ng, K.-M. Lin, B. S. Singh, & E. Y. K. Chiu (Eds.), *Ethno-psychopharmacology: Advances in current practice* (pp. 5–26). New York: Cambridge University Press.

Morita, S. (1998). *Morita therapy and the true nature of anxiety-based disorders (shinkeishitsu)* (A. Kondo, Trans.). New York: State University of New York Press. (Original work published in 1928)

Meyer, O. L., Zane, N., Cho, Y. I., & Takeuchi, D. T. (2009). Use of specialty mental health services by Asian Americans with psychiatric disorders. *Journal of Consulting and Clinical Psychology, 77,* 1000–1005.

National Conference on Medical Nomenclature (U.S.). (1952). *Standard nomenclature of diseases and operations* (4th ed.). Philadelphia: Blakistone.

Peng, K., & Nisbett, R. E. (1999). Culture, dialectics, and reasoning about contradiction. *American Psychologist, 54,* 741–754.

Popper, K. R. (1969). *Conjectures and refutations: The growth of scientific knowledge.* London: Routledge & Kegan Paul.

Prilleltensky, I. (1989). Psychology and the status quo. *American Psychologist, 44,* 795–802.

Prilleltensky, I. (1997). Values, assumptions, and practices: Assessing the moral implications of psychological discourse and action. *American Psychologist, 52,* 517–535.

Sadler, J. Z. (2005). Social context and stakeholders' values in building diagnostic systems. *Psychopathology, 38,* 197–200.

Sarason, S. B. (1981). An asocial psychology and a misdirected clinical psychology. *American Psychologist, 36,* 827–836.

Scarr, S. (1985). Constructive psychology: Making facts and fables for our times. *American Psychologist, 40,* 499–512.

Simon, G. E., Goldbert, D. P., Von Koff, M., & Ustun, T. B. (2002). Understanding crossnational differences in depression prevalence. *Psychological Medicine, 32,* 585–594.

Taylor, S. E., & Brown, J. D. (1988). Illusion and well being: A social psychological perspective on mental health. *Psychological Bulletin, 103,* 193–210.

Wakefield, J. C. (1992). The concept of mental disorder: On the boundary between biological factors and social values. *American Psychologist, 47,* 373–388.

Wang, P. S., Aguilar-Gaxiola, E., Alonso, J., Angermeyer, M. A., Borges, G., Bromet, E. J., et al. (2007). Worldwide use of mental health services for anxiety, mood, and substance disorders: Results from 17 countries in the WHO World Mental Health (WMH) Surveys. *Lancet, 370,* 841–850.

Wang, P. S., Angermeyer, M., Borges, G., Bruffaerts, R., Chiu, W. T., de Girolamo, G., et al. (2007). Delay and failure in treatment seeking after first onset of mental disorders in the WHO World Mental Health (WMH) Survey Initiative. *World Psychiatry, 6,* 177–185.

Watters, E. (2010). *Crazy like us: The globalization of the American psyche.* New York: Free Press.

Weissman, M. M., Bland, G. C., Canino, G. J., Faravelli, C., Greenwald, S., Hwu H.-G., et al. (1996). Cross-national epidemiology of major depression and bipolar disorder. *Journal of the American Medical Association, 276,* 293–299.

Weisz, J. R., Rothbaum, F. M., & Blackburn, T. C. (1984). Standing out and standing in: The psychology of control in America and Japan. *American Psychologist, 39,* 955–969.

Whewell, W. (1858). *History of scientific ideas: Being the first part of the philosophy of the inductive sciences* (3rd ed.). London: Parker & Son.

Widiger, T. A., Frances, A. J., Pincus, H. A., Davis, W. W., & First, M. B. (1991). Toward an empirical classification for the DSM-IV. *Journal of Abnormal Psychology, 100,* 280–288.

WHO World Mental Health Survey Consortium. (2004). Prevalence, severity, and unmet need for treatment of mental disorders in the World Health Organization World Mental Health (WMH) Surveys. *Journal of the American Medical Association, 291,* 2581–2590.

Williams, D. R., Haile, R., Gonzalez, H. M., Neighbors, H. W., Baser, R. & Jackson, J. S. (2007). The mental health of black Caribbean immigrants: Results from the National Survey of American Life. *American Journal of Public Health, 97*(1), 52–59.

World Health Organization. (1948). *Manual of the international statistical classification of disease, injuries, and causes of death* (6th ed.). Geneva: World Health Organization.

World Health Organization (2003). Suicide rates (per 100,000), by country, year, and gender. Retrieved February 15, 2011 from http://www.who.idt/mental_health/prevention/suicide/suiciderates/en/.

World Health Organization (2005). *Mental Health Atlas 2005.* Geneva: Author.

INTRODUCTION TO THE PSYCHOLOGY OF ASIANS

| 2 |

WHAT IS THE PSYCHOLOGY
OF ASIANS?

ANNE SAW AND SUMIE OKAZAKI

Scholars both within and outside the continent of Asia have marked Asian psychology as unique from other psychologies. For example, the editors of the book *Progress in Asian Social Psychology* argue that "Asian psychologists think and do their research in ways different from their colleagues from other parts of the world, especially the West" (K.-S. Yang, Hwang, Pedersen, & Daibo, 2003, p. ix). These so-called differences extend beyond research practices to include ways in which individuals of Asian descent differ from those from other parts of the world with regard to how they think, feel, and behave, and the motivations for such psychological processes. Such an approach toward defining Asian psychology in contrast to Western psychology arises from the tradition of cross-cultural research conducted by scholars trained primarily in North America. However, the question "What is the psychology of Asians?" requires a complex answer because rather than there being a single Asian psychology, there are—in fact—psychologies that represent the many distinct cultural, ethnic, and national groups within and originating from the continent of Asia. To draw attention to the productive possibility that Asian psychologies can also be defined from a non-cross-cultural perspective, we primarily draw on scholarship informed by indigenous psychology scholars. As suggested by the pioneering Asian indigenous social psychologist, David Y. F. Ho (1998), Asian psychology is the study of psychological phenomena from an Asian perspective that is rooted in systems of thought based in or gleaned from Asian cultures. To this end, the histories, languages, and sociocultural practices of peoples from Asia all represent sources of data from which the field has developed and grown.

This chapter on the psychology of Asians provides a critical foundation to a volume devoted to understanding psychopathology among Asians. Culture shapes how individuals conceptualize and express psychological distress, thus culturally based explanatory models that take into account

Asian beliefs, values, and relational and personality styles greatly enhance the understanding of psychopathology among Asians from an Asian perspective. In addition, Asian psychological concepts are useful to an understanding of the impact of mental illness. For example, Lawrence Yang and colleagues (2007) recently explored the influence of moral experience, or what matters most for individuals in their everyday living, on stigma about schizophrenia among Chinese. Because social ties are central to the moral experience for many Chinese, the stigma of schizophrenia can place individuals with schizophrenia and their families at great social risk for losing invaluable social connections. Within this cultural context, schizophrenia signifies more than an individual affliction, and family members must conceal the individual's mental illness or shun him or her in order to maintain the social network. Yang et al. argued that through considering the relational aspect of Chinese families, we can better understand the cost of schizophrenia for Chinese with this mental illness.

In this chapter, we describe the history of Asian psychology and the core developments in this field as they relate to the study of psychopathology among Asians. We then discuss challenges posed by the globalization of psychology and psychopathology. As the field of Asian psychology is vast and growing rapidly, we provide selective coverage of the issues most salient to psychopathology and mental health.

ASIAN INDIGENOUS PSYCHOLOGY

Indigenous psychology provides a framework for understanding the psychology of Asians from an Asian perspective. Indigenous psychology has been described as "the study of human behavior and mental processes within a cultural context that relies on the values, concepts, belief systems, methodologies, and other resources indigenous to the specific ethnic or cultural group under investigation" (Ho, 1998, p. 94). Yang (2000) defined it as "an evolving system of psychological knowledge based on scientific research that is sufficiently compatible with the studied phenomena and their ecological, economic, social, cultural, and historical contexts" (p. 245). As a field of study, it has emerged out of intellectual movements in countries such as the Philippines, India, Korea, Japan, Hong Kong, mainland China, and Taiwan. In fact, because its development can be traced to multiple sites, Kim and Berry (1993) referred to the movement in the plural, as indigenous psychologies, which they defined as "the scientific study of human behavior (or the mind) that is native, that is not transported from other regions, and that is designed for its people" (p. 2). Furthermore, they cited six fundamental assumptions and research strategies that are shared by indigenous psychologies: (1) they emphasize understanding that is rooted in the ecological context, (2) they are not studies of "exotic people in faraway places" but are applicable to studies of both developed and developing countries, (3) they recognize cultural diversity within any particular society, (4) they do not favor any particular scientific method over another and encourage the use of multiple methods, (5) they do not hold a priori that a particular perspective is inherently superior to another, and (6) they seek to discover universal facts, principles, and laws but do not assume a priori the existence of psychological universals.

Indigenous psychology is often discussed as one of three culture-related psychologies—the other two being cross-cultural psychology and cultural psychology—that have arisen within the past several decades to counter the hegemonic assumption that psychology developed in the developed Western nations represents universal psychology. Cross-cultural psychology is generally interested in generating a universal psychology. Its hallmark features include its conception of culture and behavior (or mind) as distinguishable from one another (and often cast them as independent and dependent variables, respectively) and its methodological dominance of quantitative cross-cultural comparisons. Cultural psychology is generally interested in generating a culture-bound knowledge system, thus it considers culture and behavior (or the mind) to be mutually constitutive and inseparable. Consequently, its methodology of choice tends to be qualitative and interpretive. In a comparative conceptual analysis of the three psychologies, Kuo-Shu Yang (2000) concluded that indigenous psychology can be considered to be the broadest approach that can subsume both cross-cultural and cultural psychologies as special cases of indigenous psychology. (However, see Triandis, 2000, for a different perspective on the relationship among the three psychologies.)

The birth of indigenous psychology arose from a strong resistance to colonial influences on the field of psychology in Asia and a desire to clarify misrepresentations of Asians by Westerners (e.g., Bhatia, 2002; Ho, Peng, Lai, & Chen, 2001; J. B. P. Sinha, 2003). Some scholars have argued that blindly and wholeheartedly importing Western psychology to Asia "is a form of cultural imperialism that perpetuates the colonization of the mind" (Ho et al., 2001, p. 927). Okazaki, David, and Abelmann (2007) have noted that in many Asian countries, psychology as a discipline developed during colonial occupations and within prevailing cultural narratives of Orientalism (e.g., the inferiority of non-Westerners).

Ho and colleagues (2001) trace the academic origins of indigenous psychology back to Filipino psychologist Virgilio Enriquez, who introduced the field of *Sikolohiyang Pilipino* (Filipino psychology) to the Philippines in the 1970s. Indigenous movements in India, Korea, Japan, and Taiwan took hold a decade or so later. In the Philippines, José Rizal and other Filipino intellectuals voiced their unhappiness with colonial (both American and Spanish) portrayals of Filipinos and characterizations of Filipino behavior. They expressed their dissatisfaction with images of Filipinos as backward, primitive people in need of salvation through colonization (Pe-Pua & Protacio-Marcelino, 2000). Similar sentiments were voiced by scholars in India, who felt that Western characterizations of Indians were inaccurate and insulting (J. B. P. Sinha, 2003). Okazaki et al. (2007) point out that unlike the indigenous movements in countries like the Philippines and India, later indigenous movements in nations such as Korea, Japan, and Taiwan seem to be less explicit about indigenous psychology as a form of protest against colonial hegemony and instead have framed their movements as resistance to intellectual hegemony of the West. Differences in the momentum of indigenous psychology movements across Asian societies likely reflect the vast differences in the social and political contexts (particularly in relation to the Western colonial powers) within the past half-century. For example, *Sikolohiyang Pilipino* developed at the time of massive political upheaval and the emerging national pride in the Philippines in the 1970s.

The inability of Western psychology to accurately represent Asian psychological experiences in its research topics, methods, and ideology has been another major source of criticism among Asian indigenous psychologists. Many have argued that Western psychology's claims of universality, freedom from bias, and objectivity are false and that as a field it has promoted logical-positivistic, Western-centric research paradigms that place inordinate emphasis on quantitative data (e.g., Enriquez, 1994; Kim & Berry, 1993; Kim, Park, & Park, 1999; D. Sinha, 1997; K. S. Yang, 2000). Instead, proponents of indigenous psychology believe that the field should have indigenous compatibility as its goal, "such that the researcher's concepts, theory, methods, tools, and results adequately represent, reflect, or reveal the natural elements, structure, mechanism, or process of the studied phenomenon embedded in its context" (K. S. Yang, 2000, p. 250).

Although they problematize Western psychology's research paradigms, Asian indigenous psychologists seek to contribute to universal psychology rather than maintain an autochthonous discipline. There appears to be somewhat of a consensus among Asian psychologists that indigenous psychology should be complementary to rather than independent from universal psychology (e.g., Enriquez, 1993; Ho, 1998; D. Sinha, 1993; K. S. Yang, 2000). Ho (1998) has argued that one can fall into the pitfall of culturocentrism if one relies entirely on the native concepts of culture. Instead, the goal of indigenous psychology should be "cultural cross-fertilization"—indigenous psychology informing a universal psychology, and "mainstream" psychology also informing indigenous psychology (Ho, 1998; K. S. Yang, 2000).

ADVANCES IN ASIAN PSYCHOLOGY

The field of Asian psychology has seen exceptional growth in Asia and around the world. Beginning with Kim and Berry's (1993) seminal volume, *Indigenous Psychologies: Research and Experience in Cultural Context*, Asian indigenous psychology has received significant mainstream attention from and contributed extensively to diverse subfields of psychology (e.g., applied, clinical, cross-cultural, cultural, and social psychology; Kim, Yang, & Hwang, 2006). Two areas of advancement in Asian indigenous psychology that are particularly relevant to Asian psychopathology and mental health are core Asian values and research methods.

Core Values

Values shared by Asians are often described in psychological literature in contrast to Western values and beliefs using binaries such as collectivism versus individualism or interdependent versus independent. These cross-cultural comparisons have been criticized as essentializing and uninformative, and Asian indigenous psychology has attempted to move beyond these simplistic explanations and provide analyses of key values held by Asians from an Asian perspective. Advances along this line of scholarship have drawn from analyses of historical and political movements as well as philosophies and religions. A thorough review of Asian core values and value systems is beyond the scope of this section. Instead, we focus on three value systems rooted in Filipino and East Asian cultures as illustrative cases: *kapwa*, Confucianism, and Taoism.

Kapwa

Kapwa, loosely translated as shared identity between self and others, forms the basis of Filipino values (Enriquez, 1994). *Kapwa*, which eludes a simple acontextual description, represents a set of moral, personal, and social values that influence behavior on intrapersonal, interpersonal, and societal levels within Filipino relational contexts. The study of *kapwa* is viewed as an advancement of the concept of smooth interpersonal relations, which Frank Lynch (as cited in Enriquez, 1994; Pe-Pua, 2006; and Pe-Pua & Protacio-Marcelino, 2000) purported was the core value that could be used to understand social interactions among Filipinos. Enriquez argued that smooth interpersonal relations only represents a small part of a larger value system (*kapwa*) and that one must understand *kapwa* to fully understand Filipino social psychology.

SHARED HUMANITY

At its core, *kapwa* dictates that individuals are bound to one another by *pakikipagkapwa* ("humanness at its highest level," Enriquez, 1994, p. 45). It is through holding this core value that one comes to view himself or herself as no better than another person. *Kapwa* defines and sanctions what is appropriate for interpersonal relationships on all levels, including the relationship between a person and his or her government. In Filipino culture, individuals are either identified as *ibang-tao* ("outsider") or *hindi ibang-tao* ("one-of-us"). Within these categories, individuals are prescribed different levels of interaction. For example, when interacting with an outsider, a person can, at the most superficial level, maintain a level of civility, and at the deepest levels, conform and adjust to the other person's needs. When interacting with an insider, levels of interaction can range from mutual trust and rapport to full trust and unity of needs. Regardless of whether one is interacting with an insider or an outsider, the value of *pakikipagkapwa* must be upheld. Concepts related to *kapwa* have been identified as influential to Filipino conceptions of the development and treatment of psychopathology. For example, a study by Edman and Johnson (1999) examining Filipino American and European American beliefs about causes and treatment of mental health problems found that Filipino Americans were more likely than European Americans to believe that self-conceit (which can be viewed as lacking *kapwa*) is a cause of schizophrenia and that restoring social harmony is one way of treating depression and schizophrenia. Sanchez and Gaw (2007) suggest that the distinction between *ibang-tao* and *hindi ibang-tao* can influence how a patient interacts with his or her clinician.

Confucianism

Confucianism has been the most studied among all the philosophical and religious traditions in Asia (Ho et al., 2001). It is a philosophy over 2,000 years old that originated in China and was adopted in Japan, Korea, and several other Asian countries. Confucianism is a social code of ethics that emphasizes personal and social harmony through the virtues of propriety (i.e., acting according to rules of conduct) and sincerity (i.e., striving to do what is good).

BENEVOLENCE AND SOCIAL HARMONY

The highest attainment of personal and moral growth, when the self is in union with heaven, occurs as one is able to make his or her personal desires harmonious with the needs of others (Ho, 1995).

To achieve this goal, a person must perform the duties and obligations of his or her given role (e.g., a father must protect and provide for his family; a child must obey his or her parents and submit to their authority) while remaining within the bounds of his or her position in the social hierarchy (Bond & Hwang, 1986). Sincerity is valued as the driving force behind a person's behaviors. People are motivated to behave according to their roles because they feel compassion and duty for others and shame or guilt if they do not act properly (Huang & Charter, 1996). Ho (1995) suggests that role obligation supersedes a person's personality and goes further to argue that a person's identity is defined by his or her roles. Confucian values of benevolence and social harmony have been shown to have both negative and positive impacts on mental health. Huang and Charter (1996) argue that Confucianism "promotes the ideas that any personal pursuit without regard for the group is inappropriate and selfish, and implies that any form of psychological difficulty may be seen as a lack of self-discipline or character weakness" (p. 39). In contrast, several studies have found that maintenance of interpersonal harmony is positively related to psychological well-being and self-esteem (e.g., Chuang, 2005; Kwan, Bond, & Singelis, 1997).

Taoism

Described as the counterculture to Confucianism, Taoism has exerted its influence primarily in Chinese culture (Ho, 1995; Ho et al., 2001; Zhang et al., 2002). Scholars trace its origins over 2,000 years to the writings of Laozi (also spelled Lao Tsu or Lao Tzu). Although Confucianism and Taoism stand as opposites, Chinese people behave according to Confucian principles but use Taoist principles as psychological processes (e.g., to reason or cope; Peng, Spencer-Rodgers, & Nian, 2006; Zhang et al., 2002). Taoism emphasizes conforming to natural laws, dialecticism, and transcending beyond the self (Lee, 2003; Yip, 2005; Zhang et al., 2002).

FLEXIBILITY AND ADAPTABILITY

Taoist teachings advocate that individuals should have a "water personality," because water is flexible and accommodating (Lee, 2003). Individuals are taught to conform to natural laws, to "go with the flow" of life without attempting to exercise excessive control (Zhang et al., 2002). This concept of conforming to natural laws is referred to as *wei wu-wei*. It is often misunderstood as passivity, but, as Yip (2005) clarifies, it is actually "passive progressivity" that allows one to be in harmony with the natural world and to act or refrain from action depending on the situation.

DIALECTICISM

The ability to hold two seemingly oppositional views as complementary rather than contradictory is a key value in Taoism. In fact, the symbol of Taoism, the yin and yang, represent opposites that are connected and dependent on one another. There are several implications for having a dialectical perspective. For instance, because suffering and happiness are part of the natural world and occur in complement, one can accept suffering just as readily as one can welcome happiness (Yip, 2005). Furthermore, an individual who thinks dialectically can take a middle-road approach to conflict and problems because he or she is able to see both sides of an argument (Peng & Nisbett, 1999).

SELF-TRANSCENDENCE

The ultimate goal of Taoism is to transcend beyond the self. To this end, Taoists view secular pursuits such as wealth and egocentrism as impermanent and useless, and instead strive to move toward a higher level of enlightenment that has an infinite frame of reference (Yip, 2005). When an individual is able to reach transcendence, he or she has moved beyond his or her own needs, emotions, and thoughts, as well as the influence of others.

Flexibility, adaptability, conforming to natural laws, dialecticism, and self-transcendence have all been implicated as Taoist coping styles that may serve as potential barriers to Western modes of help-seeking (Yip, 2004). Taoism advocates accepting, adapting to, and transcending above psychological problems, whereas Western-influenced mental health professionals advocate self-improvement through tackling problems head-on. Although Taoism provides challenges to treating psychopathology through psychotherapy, Zhang et al. (2002) provide an example of integrating Taoist beliefs into more traditional, Westernized psychotherapy as a treatment for generalized anxiety disorder.

The Self in Relation to Others

Perhaps one of the most important advances in Asian psychology has been the theorizing of the self in relation to others. Although key differences exist in how Asian philosophies (e.g., Confucianism, Taoism, Buddhism, Hinduism) conceptualize the self, one critical similarity is the view that the most important aspect of the self is its relationship to others. Markus and Kitayama (1991) termed this the *interdependent self* and argue that individuals with this orientation see themselves "as part of an encompassing social relationship and recogniz[e] that one's behavior is determined, contingent on, and, to a large extent, organized by what the actor perceives to be the thoughts, feelings and actions of *others* in the relationship" (p. 227). Kirmayer (2007) argues that patients' internalized self-concept influences the type of psychotherapy that may be most beneficial to them. Individuals with an interdependent, or sociocentric, self-concept may find Western psychotherapy goals of self-expression of emotions and needs, self-advancement, and individual mastery of one's environment contradictory to their own goals of social harmony. In this section, we review several Asian relational concepts and their influence on psychopathology and mental health among Asians.

Asian Relational Concepts

Ho (1982) has pinpointed several examples in Asian cultures that illustrate the relational nature of the self. The Chinese concept of *ren*, which directly translates to "person," refers to the necessity of interpersonal relationships in defining the individual. Pictographically, *ren* is represented by two strokes, one stroke leaning on the other. Each stroke represents a person, thus, a whole person is actually represented by his or her dependence on another. Another Asian concept that exemplifies the value of interdependence is the Japanese concept of *amae*, which Ho (1982) defines as a state of depending and being dependent on another. Although this dependence can be viewed as psychopathological from a Western-centric perspective, in many Asian cultures, dependence is construed positively and as a sign of psychological well-being.

Reciprocity is central to many Asian cultures and can be demonstrated by the Japanese term *on* and the Filipino term *utang na loob*. *On* refers to the transactional relationship between a benefactor, who has provided a social credit, and a receiver, who owes a social debt. It has been suggested that *on* actually represents an interlocking network of innumerous benefactors and receivers such that one is always in debt to others and simultaneously responsible for providing for others (Lebra, 1976, as cited in Ho, 1982). A similar concept in Filipino culture is *utang na loob*, which can be translated as "debt inside oneself" (Ho, 1982) or "debt of gratitude" (Kaut, 1961, as cited in Pe-Pua & Protacio-Marcelino, 2000). Like *on*, the sense of indebtedness one feels does not go away once the debt has been repaid, but instead remains throughout one's life (Ho, 1982). In summarizing the scholarship on *utang na loob*, Pe-Pua and Protacio-Marcelino (2000) suggest that it is a positive concept that might be better understood as "gratitude/solidarity" rather than burden (p. 55). Reciprocity and indebtedness are the building blocks of Naikan psychotherapy, an indigenous Japanese form of psychotherapy. Naikan psychotherapists aim to alleviate patients' psychological distress by inducing guilt and gratitude toward their parents and significant others (Hedstrom, 1994; Reynolds, 1983).

Face is one of the most widely discussed Asian relational concepts. Face refers to a complex set of socially sanctioned claims about an individual or group's character and integrity that influence how the person or group behaves. Face behaviors refer to those that prevent the loss of face or maintain or enhance existing face. The Chinese concept of face has been divided into two related terms: *lian* and *mianzi*, both of which can be translated as "face" in English. Lau and Wong (2008) summarize the distinction between the two terms in this way: "*lian* is related to the protection of one's public image and the need to avoid losing face in public, while *mianzi* is concerned with the projection and the claiming of one's public image" (p. 52). Gong and colleagues (Gong, Gage, & Tacata, 2003) suggest that Filipino culture has four relational concepts—*hiya* (shame), *amor propio* (self-esteem), *pakikisama* (social belongingness), and *utang na loob* (indebtedness), that, when considered together, are similar to the Chinese concept of face. Comparable constructs have been identified in Japanese (Morisaki & Gudykunst, 1994) and Korean (Lim & Choi, 1996) cultures. L. H. Yang and colleagues (2007) propose that face loss is a complex experience with affective, somatic, social, and moral consequences. Concern for face impacts help-seeking behaviors and choice of intervention for Asians with mental illness. For example, Wong and colleagues (Lau & Wong, 2008; Tam & Wong, 2007) found that saving face is a concern among Hong Kong Chinese with depression. Concern for face has also been found to impact the types of help (i.e., lay, medical, folk, or mental health) Filipino Americans with mental health problems seek (Gong et al., 2003). These negative consequences of culturally rooted face concerns present significant challenges for mental health practitioners. One proposed approach for addressing face concerns is to provide mental health education for individuals, their families, and communities impacted by mental illness (e.g., Lau & Wong, 2008; L. H. Yang et al., 2007). Others have suggested that mental health practitioners must be more sensitive to the cultural value systems of their patients and provide culturally appropriate interventions (e.g., Gong et al. 2003; Kirmayer, 2007; Lau & Wong, 2008; Sanchez & Gaw, 2007).

Asian Philosophies of the Body and the Mind

Although medical anthropology traditions have traveled separate paths from those of indigenous psychology within Asian psychology, it has played a significant role in the understanding of the idioms of distress in Asia. Foremost in this tradition is the notion of the mind-body connection within Asian philosophy, which is often portrayed in contrast to the Cartesian notion of the body and the mind as dichotomous entities. A debate regarding whether or not the predominantly somatic presentation of distress among Asian clients constitutes a cultural variation of depression (Cheung, 1995; Kleinman, 1982; Ryder et al., 2008) has dominated the literature on culture-bound syndromes in Asia.

Another important Asian cultural phenomenon relevant to mental health is the philosophy and the practice of traditional Chinese medicine (TCM). Central in the TCM is the notion of qi, or the vital energy flowing throughout the body. Any loss or the disequilibrium of qi is thought to result in various health consequences, including those that affect mental and psychological functioning. Qi-gong (or exercise of vital energy) promoted by TCM, which dates back to the Shang Dynasty (16th to 11th centuries BC), has gained popularity in mainland China after the Cultural Revolution. Significantly, qi-gong induced mental disorders have been documented in Chinese-language literature (Ng, 1999) as well as in a case report of a Chinese immigrant woman in the United States (Hwang, 2007). L. H. Yang, Phelan, and Link (2008) found in a survey of 90 Chinese American community residents that although Western mental health services were perceived to be more efficacious for psychiatric conditions than TCM (e.g., herbal medicine, acupuncture, qi-gong, etc.), seeking Western services was also perceived as more shameful than seeking TCM services.

In another variant of Asian belief systems regarding vital body energy, Hinton and his colleagues (e.g., Hinton & Otto, 2006) delineated an ethnophysiological model of somatic sensations and symptom-generated catastrophic cognitions among traumatized Cambodian refugees, based on the Cambodian notions of "Wind" (khyâl)—a sort of "inner air." Notably, Hinton and colleagues situate the cultural meanings of the particular trauma-related symptoms (e.g., panic and fear induced by tinnitus and orthostatic dysfunctions) among Cambodian refugees within the context of specific historical trauma induced by the brutal Khmer Rouge rule. Hinton and Otto (2006) based their cultural modification of cognitive behavioral therapy to specifically address the meanings attached to panic and post-traumatic stress disorder (PTSD) symptoms experienced by Cambodian refugees. These selected examples illustrate that Asian cultural beliefs regarding health can be critically important to expressions of symptomatology, help-seeking, and treatment.

Innovations in Research Methods

Many Asian indigenous psychologists rely on local, ground-up, emic approaches or combinations of etic and emic approaches to conduct indigenously compatible research. Gabrenya and colleagues (2006) suggest that the turn away from Western research paradigms has almost universally led to a turn toward qualitative methods in indigenous psychology movements across Asia. For some scholars, the practice of indigenous psychology necessarily involves eschewing the use of self-report tests, scales, and questionnaires imported from the West; however, even indigenously developed surveys, tests, and interviews may fail to yield valid data, because participants may be culturally conditioned to comply with authorities and not reveal their true attitudes or feelings (Ho, Ho, & Ng, 2006). However, other scholars have adopted combined etic-emic approaches that are designed to build on and adapt Western scholarship for use in local Asian contexts.

Filipino scholars are credited with refining and advancing qualitative methodologies for indigenous psychology purposes. *Pagtatanung-tanong*, literally translated as "asking questions," is a process of data collection whereby the researcher asks questions and allows questioning from the research participant (Enriquez, 1993; Ho, 1998; Pe-Pua, 2006; Pe-Pua & Protacio-Marcelino, 2000). The process of *pagtatanung-tanong* is rooted in Filipino interactional styles, and data collection should flow as naturally as an everyday, casual conversation. Research participants are given control over the data collection process, from the allocation of time given to a particular topic to the direction of the interviewing process. Pe-Pua (2006) gives multiple examples in which various Filipino researchers used this method to study various indigenous concepts such as time, *pagkalalaki* (malehood or masculinity), and migration and return migration among Ilocanos who have lived in Hawaii for extended time before returning to the Philippines. Furthermore, Pe-Pua and colleagues (1996) used this approach to study the "astronaut" families and "parachute" children (in this case, Chinese families in which the child is sent to Australia for education while one or both parents reside primarily in Hong Kong but shuttle back and forth between Hong Kong and Australia). *Pagtatanung-tanong* can be very useful for members of many Asian communities for whom traditional paper-and-pencil survey or structured interview techniques may be foreign (e.g., those with less access to education) or in cases where collaborative, participatory approach to research is culturally consonant with the local population. However, the method can also be extremely time-consuming, and gathering a large enough pool of participants for consensus checks can be difficult unless research is conducted in intact, stable communities (Ho, 1998).

Another Filipino psychological research innovation is the *pakapa-kapa*, or "groping," research paradigm. Torres defined *pakapa-kapa* as "a suppositionless approach to social scientific investigations. As implied by the term itself, *pakapa-kapa* is an approach characterized by groping, searching and probing into an unsystematized mass of social data to obtain order, meaning and directions for research" (in Pe-Pua, 2006, p. 109). Because of its inductive and ground-up nature, the researcher often starts without a review of relevant literature or a well-defined research design (Ho, 1998; Pe-Pua, 2006; Pe-Pua & Protacio-Marcelino, 2000). Instead, the data are collected and "groped" until the researcher is able to make conceptual sense of them. Ho (1998) outlines several requirements for using *pakapa-kapa*, such as focusing on the research data without preconceptions and using the research participants' labels and categories rather than existing categories. Pe-Pua (2006) cautions that though *pakapa-kapa* entails using working with "unsystematized" sets of data, the process must itself be systematized and follow rigorous scientific research standards. However, she and others fail to describe exactly how *pakapa-kapa* can be used in non-Filipino contexts, thus, as Ho (1998) describes, for researchers untrained in Filipino indigenous research methods, carrying out *pakapa-kapa* may best be thought of as a first step in the research process or as a general attitude toward research. Ho and colleagues (2006) note that *pakapa-kapa* bears a strong resemblance to the grounded theory approach that had developed within Western qualitative methodological tradition. Both approaches eschew going into research with prior assumptions about hypothesis, research questions, or relevant literature, and both approaches are committed to discovery oriented, in-depth data collection methods. However, *pakapa-kapa* differs from grounded theory in one significant aspect. Whereas grounded research holds some theoretical position and requires its practitioners to have an adequate level of background knowledge regarding the area of inquiry, *pakapa-kapa* insists on the intellectual attitude of "as-if total ignorance" (Ho et al., 2006).

There has been a trend toward combining etic and emic approaches, especially in the area of personality assessment (Cheung, 2004). The Chinese Personality Assessment Inventory (CPAI) assesses indigenous and universal personality traits in clinical and nonclinical populations (Cheung et al., 1996). Cheung and her colleagues followed Western standards of test development but derived their culturally relevant personality constructs from Chinese popular literature (i.e., novels and proverbs), research literature, professional opinions, and pilot data of self- and other- personality descriptions to develop their inventory of 21 normal personality scales, 12 clinical scales, and 2 validity scales. In the revised version of the CPAI (i.e., Cross-Cultural Personality Inventory—2; Cheung, Cheung, Wada, & Zhang, 2003), Cheung and colleagues derived four factors from the normal personality scales (i.e., Dependability, Interpersonal Relatedness, Social Potency, Accommodation). Of particular note is that the Interpersonal Relatedness factor is composed of several relational constructs described in this chapter, including face and harmony. Cheung and colleagues (2001) suggest that the Interpersonal Relatedness factor may be unique to Chinese cultures or tap into universally relevant interpersonal aspects of personality not currently assessed by other personality inventories.

FUTURE CHALLENGES

Through reviews and examples of key Asian indigenous psychological concepts and approaches, we have suggested that psychopathology among Asians can be better understood and treated through a more relational and contextualized framework. Taking cues from the indigenous Asian psychology research methods that are not bound by a clear demarcation between the researcher and the subject, a more flexible ethnographic stance toward assessment and treatment of individuals of Asian descent may, in some cases, enhance the quality of data gathered in practice and research settings. However, there remain significant challenges to the incorporation of Asian indigenous psychology to the research and practice with Asian individuals.

It should be noted that indigenous psychology as an intellectual movement has also met with some criticism and debate among scholars. For example, Triandis (2000) noted that epistemological and empirical approaches that are often employed by indigenous psychologists are not always valued as scientific or relevant to Western-trained psychologists. And whereas Poortinga (1999) acknowledged that indigenization movement in psychology has shed light on the Western ethnocentric bias in psychology, he argued that the heavy reliance on "subjective" methods (e.g., hermeneutic and holistic analyses of narratives and opinions of informants) by some forms of indigenous psychologies have produced culture-specific knowledge at the cost of overstating the differences.

And in reviewing the progress of *Sikolohiyang Pilipino* (Filipino indigenous psychology), Church and Katigbak (2002) noted that the movement has not been as successful in formulating indigenous theories and that the questions about the objectivity and cultural uniqueness of its methods remain. Writing from an indigenous perspective, Pe-Pua (2006) argued that a method need not be unique to indigenous psychology but must be culturally appropriate and relevant to the local population. Pe-Pua further suggested that questions of investigator objectivity in indigenous methods can be addressed by having multiple researchers to represent various viewpoints and through repeated sampling from as many participants as possible. The debates not withstanding, the indigenous psychology movement reminds scholars and practitioners alike to consider Asian concepts, worldviews, and behavior as not only viable but also valid perspectives for understanding the psychological experiences of Asians.

One challenge to the incorporation of indigenous Asian psychological concepts in research and treatment of psychopathology is the increasing globalization of psychopharmacology. Kirmayer (2002) traced the wider acceptance of mild depression as a legitimate target of pharmacological intervention in Japan to the decisions of pharmaceutical companies to introduce and market antidepressant medications. According to a 2004 *New York Times Magazine* report, one pharmaceutical company coined the term *kokoro no kaze* (soul catching a cold) to relabel mild depressive state as pathological and requiring intervention (Schulz, 2004). This was in contrast to the prior Japanese cultural aesthetic that viewed melancholy and mild sadness an inevitable states of life that, consistent with the Buddhist percept of acceptance of life's suffering, was viewed as a sign of sensitivity. From this illustrative case of the effects of antidepressant medications' introduction in Japan, Kirmayer (2002) cautioned against a "global monoculture of happiness" (p. 316) that threatens to transform not only local-cultural modes of recognizing and reacting to individual and societal problems but also the local-cultural notions of selfhood and desirable psychological state.

Certainly, the movements toward cultural psychology, indigenous psychology, and multicultural psychology have helped to shed light on the possibility that psychological experiences of Asians must encompass viewpoints not always found within mainstream American psychology. However, even as the diversification of psychology continues to unfold, geopolitical events and movements in Asia also shape the evolving cultures in Asia. For example, with the transformation of psychiatry in various Asian nations under modernizing and globalizing influences (e.g., the widespread use of the *Diagnostic and Statistical Manual*, or *DSM*, system; pharmaceutical marketing), the diagnosis of neurasthenia in China and other Asian nations is becoming obsolete (Lee & Kleinman, 2007). In another example, anthropologist Vanessa Fong (2007) has documented a new variant of parent-child communication problems between Chinese singletons (i.e., only children born under China's one-child policy) and their parents. Fong found that, with the rapid social changes that accompanied China's rapid modernization and new ethos of independence and competitive excellence in pursuit of upward mobility, contemporary Chinese parents find it difficult to articulate their complex Chinese cultural models of desirable personhood that are rooted in their own upbringing.

There are many global trends affecting the Pacific Rim countries that ultimately impact how we as psychologists consider the psychologies of Asians. China has emerged as a major economical power in the past two decades, as symbolized by the 2008 Beijing Olympics. There is increasing hybridization of cultures that accompanies rampant transnationalism among many Asian families.

Migration and immigration between Asia and North America continue at a rapid rate. Psychologies of Asians must be responsive to these—and many other—dynamic shifts that are shaped by sociocultural forces within and outside of mental health disciplines.

REFERENCES

Bond, M. H., & Hwang, K. K. (1986). The social psychology of Chinese people. In M. H. Bond (Ed.), *The psychology of the Chinese people* (pp. 213–264). New York: Oxford University Press.

Cheung, F. M. (1995). Facts and myths about somatization among the Chinese. In T.-Y. Lin, W. S. Tseng, & E. K. Yeh (Eds.), *Chinese societies and mental health* (pp. 156–180). Hong Kong: Oxford University Press.

Cheung, F. M. (2004). Use of Western and indigenously developed personality tests in Asia. *Applied Psychology: An International Review, 53,* 173–191.

Cheung, F. M., Cheung, S. F., Wada, S., & Zhang, J. X. (2003). Indigenous measures of personality assessment in Asian countries: A review. *Psychological Assessment, 15,* 280–289.

Cheung, F. M., Leung, K., Fan, R. M., Song, W. Z., Zhang, J. X., & Zhang, J. Y. (1996). Development of the Chinese Personality Assessment Inventory. *Journal of Cross-Cultural Psychology, 27,* 181–199.

Cheung, F. M., Leung, K., Zhang, J. X., Sun, H. F., Gan, Y. G., Song, W. Z., & Xie, D. (2001). Indigenous Chinese personality constructs: Is the five-factor model complete? *Journal of Cross-Cultural Psychology, 32,* 407–433.

Chuang, Y. C. (2005). Effects of interaction pattern on family harmony and well-being: Test of interpersonal theory, relational-models theory, and Confucian ethics. *Asian Journal of Social Psychology, 8,* 272–291.

Church, A. T., & Katigbak, M. S. (2002). Indigenization of psychology in the Philippines. *International Journal of Psychology, 37,* 129–148.

Edman, J. L., & Johnson, R. C. (1999). Filipino American and Caucasian American beliefs about the causes and treatment of mental illness. *Cultural Diversity and Ethnic Minority Psychology, 5,* 380–386.

Enriquez, V. G. (1993). Developing a Filipino psychology. In U. Kim & J. W. Berry (Eds.), *Indigenous psychologies: Research and experience in cultural context* (pp. 152–169). Newbury Park, CA: Sage.

Enriquez, V. G. (1994). *From colonial to liberation psychology: The Philippine experience.* Manila, Philippines: De La Salle University Press.

Fong, V. L. (2007). Parent-child communication problems and the perceived inadequacies of Chinese only children. *Ethos, 35,* 85–127.

Gabrenya, W. K., Kung, M. C., & Chen, L. Y. (2006). Understanding the Taiwan indigenous psychology movement: A sociology of science approach. *Journal of Cross-Cultural Psychology, 37,* 597–622.

Gong, F., Gage, S. L., & Tacata, L. A., Jr. (2003). Helpseeking behavior among Filipino Americans: A cultural analysis of face and language. *Journal of Community Psychology, 31,* 469–488.

Hedstrom, L. J. (1994). Morita and Naikan therapies: American applications. *Psychotherapy, 31,* 154–160.

Hinton, D. E., & Otto, M. W. (2006). Symptom presentation and symptom meaning among traumatized Cambodian refugees: Relevance to a somatically focused cognitive-behavioral therapy. *Cognitive and Behavioral Practice, 13,* 249–260.

Ho, D. Y. F. (1982). Asian concepts in behavioral science. *Psychologia, 25,* 228–235.

Ho, D. Y. F. (1995). Selfhood and identity in Confucianism, Taoism, Buddhism, and Hinduism: Contrasts with the West. *Journal for the Theory of Social Behaviour, 25,* 115–139.

Ho, D. Y. F. (1998). Interpersonal relationships and relationship dominance: An analysis based on methodological relationalism. *Asian Journal of Social Psychology, 1,* 1–16.

Ho, D. Y. F., Ho, R. T. H., & Ng, S. M. (2006). Investigative research as a knowledge-generation method: Discovering and uncovering. *Journal for the Theory of Social Behavior, 36,* 17–38.

Ho, D. Y. F., Peng, S., Lai, A. C., & Chan, S. F. (2001). Indigenization and beyond: Methodological relationalism in the study of personality across cultural traditions. *Journal of Personality, 69,* 925–953.

Huang, D. D., & Charter, R. A. (1996). The origin and formulation of Chinese character: An introduction to Confucianism and its influence on Chinese behavior patterns. *Cultural Diversity and Mental Health, 2,* 35–42.

Hwang, W. (2007). Qi-gong psychotic reaction in a Chinese American woman. *Culture, Medicine, and Psychiatry, 31*, 547–560.

Kaut, C. R. (1961). *Utang-na-loob:* A system of contractual obligation. *Southwestern Journal of Anthropology, 17*, 256–272.

Kim, U., & Berry, J. W. (1993). *Indigenous psychologies: Research and experience in cultural context.* Newbury Park, CA: Sage.

Kim, U., Park, Y. S., & Park, D. H. (1999). The Korean indigenous psychology approach: Theoretical considerations and empirical applications. *Applied Psychology: An International Review, 48*, 55–73.

Kim, U., Yang, K. S., & Hwang, K. K. (2006). Preface. In *Indigenous and cultural psychology: Understanding people in context* (pp. xv–xviii). New York: Springer.

Kirmayer, L. J. (2002). Psychopharmacology in a globalizing world: The use of antidepressants in Japan. *Transcultural Psychiatry, 39*, 295–322.

Kirmayer, L. J. (2007). Psychotherapy and the cultural concept of the person. *Transcultural Psychiatry, 44*, 232–257.

Kleinman, A. (1982). Neurasthenia and depression: A study of somatization and culture in China. *Culture, Medicine, and Psychiatry, 6*, 117–190.

Kwan, V. S. Y., Bond, M. H., & Singelis, T. M. (1997). Pancultural explanations for life satisfaction: Adding relationship harmony to self-esteem. *Journal of Personality and Social Psychology, 73*, 1038–1051.

Lau, Y., & Wong, D. F. K. (2008). Are concern for face and willingness to seek help correlated to early postnatal depressive symptoms among Hong Kong Chinese women? A cross-sectional questionnaire survey. *International Journal of Nursing Studies, 45*, 51–64.

Lebra, T. S. (1976). *Japanese patterns of behavior.* Honolulu: The University Press of Hawaii.

Lee, Y. T. (2003). Daoistic humanism in ancient China: Broadening personality and counseling theories in the 21st century. *Journal of Humanistic Psychology, 43*, 64–85.

Lee, S. & Kleinman, A. (2007). Are somatoform disorders changing with time? The case of neurasthenia in China. *Psychosomatic Medicine, 69*, 846–849.

Lim, T., & Choi, S. (1996). Interpersonal relationships in Korea. In W. B. Gudykunst, S. Ting-Toomey, & T. Nishida, *Communication in personal relationships across cultures* (pp. 122–136). Thousand Oaks, CA: Sage.

Markus, H. R., & Kitayama, S. (1991). Culture and the self: Implications for cognition, emotion, and motivation. *Psychological Review, 98*, 224–253.

Morisaki, S., & Gudykunst, W. B. (1994). Face in Japan and the United States. In S. Ting-Toomey (Ed.), *The challenge of facework: Cross-cultural and interpersonal issues. SUNY series in human communication processes* (pp. 47–93). Albany: State University of New York Press.

Ng, B. (1999). Qigong-induced, mental disorders: A review. *Australian and New Zealand Journal of Psychiatry, 33*, 197–206.

Okazaki, S., David, E. J. R., & Abelmann, N. (2007). Colonialism and the psychology of culture. *Social and Personality Compass, 2*(1), 90–106. DOI: 10.1111/j.1751-9004.2007.00046.x

Peng, K., & Nisbett, R. E. (1999). Culture, dialectics, and reasoning about contradiction. *American Psychologist, 54*, 741–754.

Peng, K., Spencer-Rodgers, J., Nian, Z. (2006). Naïve dialecticism and the Tao of Chinese thought. In U. Kim, K. S. Yang, & K. K. Hwang (Eds.), *Indigenous and cultural psychology: Understanding people in context* (pp. 247–262). New York: Springer.

Pe-Pua, R. (2006). From decolonizing psychology to the development of a cross-indigenous perspective in methodology: The Philippine experience. In U. Kim, K. S. Yang, & K. K. Hwang (Eds.), *Indigenous and cultural psychology: Understanding people in context* (pp. 109–137). New York: Springer.

Pe-Pua, R., Mitchell, C., Iredale, R., & Castles, S. (1996). *Astronaut families and parachute children: The cycle of migration between Hong Kong and Australia.* Canberra, Australia: Australian Government Publishing Service.

Pe-Pua, R., & Protacio-Marcelino, E. (2000). Sikolohiyang Pilipino (Filipino psychology): A legacy of Virgilio G. Enriquez. *Asian Journal of Social Psychology, 3*, 49–71.

Poortinga, Y. H. (1999). Different psychologies? *Applied Psychology: An International Review, 48*, 419–432.

Reynolds, D. K. (1983). *Naikan psychotherapy: Meditation for self-development.* Chicago: University of Chicago Press.

Ryder, A. G., Yang, J., Zhu, X., Yao, S., Yi, J., & Heine, S. J. (2008). The cultural shaping of depression: Somatic symptoms in China, psychological symptoms in North America? *Journal of Abnormal Psychology, 117,* 300–313.

Sanchez, F., & Gaw, A. (2007). Mental health care of Filipino Americans. *Psychiatric Services, 6,* 810–815.

Schulz, K. (2004, August 22). Did antidepressants depress Japan? *New York Times Magazine.*

Sinha, D. (1997). Indigenizing psychology. In J. W. Berry, Y. H. Poortinga, & J. Pandey (Eds.), *Handbook of cross-cultural psychology: Vol. 1. Theory and method* (2nd ed., pp. 129–169). Needham Heights, MA: Allyn & Bacon.

Sinha, J. B. P. (2003). Trends toward indigenization of psychology in India. In K.-S. Yang, K.-K. Hwang, P. B. Pedersen, & I. Daibo (Eds.), *Progress in Asian social psychology: Conceptual and empirical contributions* (pp. 11–28). Westport, CT: Praeger.

Tam, P. W. C., & Wong, D. F. K. (2007). Qualitative analysis of dysfunctional attitudes in Chinese persons suffering from depression. *Hong Kong Journal of Psychiatry, 17,* 109–114.

Triandis, H. C. (2000). Dialectics between cultural and cross-cultural psychology. *Asian Journal of Social Psychology, 3,* 185–195.

Yang, K.-S., Hwang, K.-K., Pedersen, P. B., & Daibo, I. (2003). Preface. In K.-S. Yang, K.-K. Hwang, P. B. Pedersen, & I. Daibo (Eds.), *Progress in Asian social psychology: Conceptual and empirical contributions* (pp. ix–xi).Westport, CT: Praeger.

Yang, K. S. (2000). Monocultural and cross-cultural indigenous approaches: The royal road to the development of a balanced global psychology. *Asian Journal of Social Psychology, 3,* 241–263.

Yang, L. H., Kleinman, A., Link, B. G., Phelan, J. C., Lee, S., & Good, B. (2007). Culture and stigma: Adding moral experience to stigma theory. *Social Science and Medicine, 64,* 1524–1535.

Yang, L. H., Phelan, J. C., & Link, B. G. (2008). Stigma and beliefs of efficacy towards traditional Chinese medicine and Western psychiatric treatment among Chinese Americans. *Cultural Diversity and Ethnic Minority Psychology, 14,* 10–18.

Yip, K. (2004). Taoism and its impact on mental health of the Chinese communities. *International Journal of Social Psychiatry, 50,* 25–42.

Yip, K. (2005). Taoist concepts of mental health: Implications for social work practice with Chinese communities. *Families in Society: The Journal of Contemporary Social Sciences, 86,* 35–45.

Zhang, Y., Young, D., Lee, S., Li, L., Zhang, H., Xiao, Z., et al. (2002). Chinese Taoist cognitive psychotherapy in the treatment of generalized anxiety disorder in contemporary China. *Transcultural Psychiatry, 39,* 115–129.

| 3 |

ISSUES IN THE RESEARCH AND ASSESSMENT OF PSYCHOPATHOLOGY IN ASIANS

PHILLIP D. AKUTSU AND JOYCE P. CHU

INTRODUCTION

A Need for Accurate Psychopathology Assessment

People of Asian ethnic heritage are a culturally rich and diverse population that represent more than 43 distinct Asian and Asian American subgroups and speak over 100 Asian languages and dialects (U.S. Census Bureau, 2007; U.S. Department of Health and Human Services [DHHS], 2001). Specific concerns about disparities in access to mental health care for Asian and Asian American communities have given rise to research aimed at improving our basic understanding, identification, prevention, and treatment of psychopathology in this diverse ethnic population. In the past two decades, there has been a steady growth in research efforts that have targeted the special psychological needs of Asian and Asian American groups. Yet, inconsistencies in these findings regarding clinical diagnosis and psychopathology have illuminated inadequacies in available research methods and assessment tools used to examine psychopathology constructs in these populations.

Previous large-scale studies of clinical disorders and psychopathology have provided somewhat inconsistent findings about the mental health status of Asian and Asian American groups. For example, several epidemiological surveys such as the Epidemiological Catchment Area survey (ECA; Robins & Regier, 1991) and the National Comorbidity Survey (NCS; Kessler et al.,

1994) in the United States included a limited number of English-speaking Asian Americans in their studies. However, these small sample sizes did not allow for definitive conclusions to be drawn about the levels of psychopathology in this culturally diverse group. In comparison, a number of recent epidemiological studies—the Filipino American Community Epidemiological Study (FACES; Abe-Kim, Gong, & Takeuchi, 2004; Gong, Gage, & Tacata, 2003), the Chinese American Psychiatric Epidemiological Study (CAPES; Takeuchi et al., 1998; Zheng et al., 1997), and the National Latino and Asian American Survey (NLAAS; Alegria et al., 2004; Takeuchi et al., 2007); have found that Asian Americans consistently report with lower rates of mental illness than other ethnic groups. Cross-cultural assessment of mental illness has also reported that Asian groups in their native countries have been found with lower prevalence rates of psychopathology in comparison to people in the United States. For example, a cross-cultural study of over 60,000 adults in 14 countries using the World Mental Health-Composite International Diagnostic Interview (WMH-CIDI) in a face-to-face format showed the prevalence of mental disorders in Japan and China was far less than in the United States (Demyttenaere et al., 2004). These results are supportive of earlier clinical studies that found similar low rates of prevalence of psychological disorders in Asian countries (Parker, Gladstone, & Chee, 2001; Simon, Goldberg, Von Korff, & Ustun, 2002; Weissman et al., 1996, 1997). Although it is possible that Asian Americans and Asians in their native countries may report with lower rates of mental illness, scientists have raised the important concern that such epidemiological surveys are using diagnostic measures that may be culturally inadequate to assess true rates of mental illness in these Asian populations.

Indeed, it is essential that accurate information about psychopathology in Asians and Asian Americans be collected to establish base rates of clinical psychopathology, to develop clinical/community outreach and education efforts, and to create culturally effective mental health programs. The first step in establishing more culturally effective treatment for clients of Asian descent begins with the development of diagnostic measures and tools that ensure the clinical diagnosis and the assessment of psychopathology for these ethnic groups are valid, reliable, and accurate.

Goals of the Chapter

The purpose of this chapter is to present an overview of debates, issues, and advancements in the research and assessment of psychopathology in Asian and Asian American communities. We start by reviewing common methods of assessing psychopathology along with the specific cultural considerations that are associated with applying such methods with Asian and Asian American clients. We also highlight the limitations and challenges associated with existing assessment methods when used with Asian and Asian American populations to familiarize clinicians and researchers about important issues to be aware of in applying available diagnostic tools. Finally, we draw from the reported strengths and limitations of assessment methods to present a three-step model—a practical guide—for clinicians and scientists to minimize cultural barriers when choosing an appropriate assessment approach for Asian and Asian American clients. The chapter concludes with a brief summary of future research directions that may help to advance our knowledge and practice of clinical diagnosis with such populations.

ASSESSMENT METHODS FOR
PSYCHOPATHOLOGY

A number of well-known diagnostic instruments and methods have been used for the clinical assessment of psychopathology in Asians and Asian Americans. The majority of these diagnostic tools were adapted from commonly used instruments and methods developed on Western English-speaking populations, and some were translated into certain Asian languages or dialects (Butcher, Nezami, & Exner, 1998). However, there are also some diagnostic tools that have been developed specifically for clinical use with particular Asian or Asian American groups (Leung & Wong, 2003; S. Sue & Chang, 2003).

These assessment tools are used for many different purposes and contexts in working with individuals of Asian descent. For example, some assessment techniques have been used for research purposes to identify cultural differences in symptom expression among Asians or Asian Americans and other ethnic groups, while others have enlisted these tools to make diagnostic decisions or severity determinations in clinical work settings. Given the critical importance of accurate diagnostic assessment, both clinicians and researchers must use caution in making culturally appropriate decisions about which diagnostic approaches and measures are the best suited for the specific purpose of their scientific or clinical endeavors when working with Asians and Asian Americans.

In this section, we review different types of diagnostic methods that are available for assessing psychopathology in Asians and Asian Americans and highlight specific cultural factors that should be considered when evaluating the cultural relevance of using a particular assessment method. In particular, we will review the viability of self-report questionnaires, clinical interviews, and behavioral assessments in determining the level and severity of psychopathology with groups of Asian descent. Invariably, many of these assessment methods, particularly those developed with Western English-speaking samples, hold the potential for cultural bias or misuse with Asian and Asian American individuals. In some cases, these commonly used questionnaires have not been properly validated, normed, or translated for use with various Asian or Asian American subgroups. In other cases, some cultural adjustments and modifications have been applied to these diagnostic tools (e.g., the inclusion of culturally stems) to improve their use with different Asian or Asian American groups (Yang & WonPat-Borja, 2007). However, these culturally responsive changes to standard assessment measures may still not be sufficient to ensure accuracy in the determination of psychopathology in Asian ethnic clients. For example, some Asian Americans have been found to present with mental health symptoms that are culturally specific or culturally bound (American Psychiatric Association, 2000), and this would then require culturally different assessment strategies than those steeped or grounded in mainstream Western cultures. It is the intention of this chapter to introduce the clinician and researcher to pertinent cultural issues and the possible limitations that may be associated with each of the reported methods of assessment that have been previously applied to Asian and Asian American populations. With this given perspective, we hope this cogent discussion of several assessment approaches will foster a more culturally appropriate and competent approach in future efforts of assessing psychopathology among Asian and Asian American groups.

Self-Report: Symptom Scale Questionnaires

Self-report questionnaires are perhaps the most common tool used by clinicians and researchers to collect valuable clinical data to assess for various types of psychopathology. These standardized assessment tools are uniquely designed to measure specific constructs and require the least amount of time and investment on the part of clinicians and researchers. Self-report questionnaires that assess different types of psychopathology may be used for two main purposes: (1) to identify the presence and severity of certain symptoms to create a clinical profile or (2) to assess for a specific clinical diagnosis based on *DSM-IV* criteria.

Common symptom scales that have been used to assess the clinical profile or severity of depression symptoms, for example, have included the Center for Epidemiologic Studies Depression Scale (CES-D; Radloff, 1977), the Beck Depression Inventory II (BDI; Beck, Brown, & Steer, 1996), the Geriatric Depression Scale (GDS-15; Sheikh & Yesavage, 1986), and the Zung Self-Rating Depression Scale (Zung, 1965). Symptom scales that focused on the assessment of anxiety, on the other hand, have included the Beck Anxiety Inventory (BAI; Beck & Steer, 1993), the Fear of Negative Evaluation (Watson & Friend, 1969), the State Trait Anxiety Inventory (STAI; Spielberger, 1983), and the Social Avoidance and Distress Scale (Watson & Friend, 1969). A review of the mental health literature has shown use of these measures with various Asian and Asian American populations in both their standard English formats and in versions translated into specific Asian languages and dialects. In contrast to self-report measures that focus on a single diagnostic category like depression or generalized anxiety, there are also other general symptom scales including the Symptom Checklist 90 (SCL-90, also available in a 60- and 15-item form; Derogatis, 1977), the Brief Symptom Inventory (BSI; Derogatis & Melisaratos, 1983), and the Hopkins Symptom Checklist (HSCL; Derogatis et al., 1974), which provide a broader assessment of clinical symptoms that contribute to multiple diagnostic considerations. For example, the BSI assesses not only depression, but also other constructs such as anxiety, paranoia, or hostility. The Minnesota Multiphasic Personality Inventory (MMPI-2; Greene, 1991) and the Personality Assessment Inventory (PAI; Morey, 2007) are additional examples of personality self-report inventories that assess multiple symptom categories of psychopathology. These personality measures have been used in previous research with Asians and Asian Americans as several translated versions have been developed for specific Asian subgroups including the MMPI in Chinese, Japanese, Korean, and Thai (Butcher, Cheung, & Lim, 2003).

While many of these symptom scales assess for the severity of certain symptoms or present a general clinical profile, there are some self-report questionnaires specifically designed to provide a clinician or researcher with *DSM* diagnostic categories. For example, the Patient Health Questionnaire-9 (PHQ-9; Kroenke, Spitzer, & Williams, 2001) assesses the nine major symptoms of depression clearly described in the *Diagnostic and Statistical Manual of Mental Disorders* (*DSM-IV-TR*; American Psychiatric Association, 2000). The PHQ-9 is most commonly used in medical settings, where the patient is instructed to report the occurrence of each of the nine symptoms of depression in the last two weeks. The DSM Scale for Depression (DSD) was also specifically designed and constructed to use existing *DSM* diagnostic criteria and can be used to assess depressive symptoms indicating satisfaction of *DSM* criteria for depression among adolescents (Roberts, Roberts, & Chen, 1997).

While other self-report scales also measure adult psychopathology symptoms associated with other diagnostic categories, a comprehensive review of all such self-report scales is beyond the scope of this chapter. The reader should refer to Section II of this book for a more detailed discussion of each category of clinical disorders and the assessment measures that have been used to determine severity level and symptom profile with Asian and Asian American populations. It is important that clinicians and researchers alike carefully examine the literature to understand the psychometric properties and limitations of self-report questionnaires that assess for symptom profile or severity and those that map onto *DSM* criteria to make an informed decision about which type of questionnaire is well matched for their desired purpose. It is also important to recognize that despite the relative value and expediency of self-reported measures, these tools still require the skill and experience of a well-trained clinician or researcher to avoid any cultural mistakes or misunderstandings in the interpretation of the collected data to make an accurate diagnosis.

Cultural Considerations

Mental health professionals should exercise caution when choosing, administering, and interpreting a self-report questionnaire with Asian or Asian American clients, as cultural factors may serve as possible barriers to the cross-cultural validity of using many of these self-report questionnaires to accurately assess psychopathology for these ethnic populations. There are several methodology inconsistencies and concerns that present problems for the cross-cultural validity of self-report rating scales.

First, research has shown that Asians and Asian Americans exhibit a unique response style—a central tendency bias—when selecting a response on a Likert-type scale (Chen, Lee, & Stevenson, 1995; Hamamura, Heine, & Paulhus, 2008; Zax & Takahashi, 1967). This central tendency bias stems from choosing neutral or moderate responses rather than more extreme responses on the lower or higher ends of a rating scale. It is unknown whether such a response style represents true moderate responses to items by Asians and Asian Americans or is a socialized behavior based on cultural factors. This response bias can present a problem in determining the presence and severity of specific psychopathology symptoms to determine an accurate diagnosis.

Despite a tendency to report moderate responses, many of the previous studies using symptom scale questionnaires report that Asian Americans have higher levels of severity for depressive and anxiety symptoms than White Americans (Lam, Pepper, & Ryabchenko, 2004; Yang & WonPat-Borja, 2007). These higher levels of symptom severity for Asian Americans are remarkable given previous reports of lower rates of mood disorders and other psychopathology for Asian Americans when compared to White Americans (Alegria et al., 2004; Takeuchi et al., 1998; Takeuchi et al., 2007; Zhang & Snowden, 1999). It is unknown whether the elevated levels of severity in some studies are due to true ethnic differences in psychopathology in subclinical populations or whether the discrepancy is representative of different cultural styles of reporting mental health symptoms. Regardless, such discrepancies in response styles can present cause for concern about the criterion validity used to establish recommended clinical cutoff scores to determine psychopathology for different sample populations. For example, the manual for the BDI-II recommends the use of clear cutoff points to identify mild, moderate, and severe depression (Beck et al., 1996). However, higher cutoff scores may be strongly indicated when using this diagnostic measure for Asian American populations because BDI scores using these standards developed with Western populations were found to overestimate mood disorders in this ethnic group (Lam, Pepper, & Ryabchenko, 2004).

It is also possible that culture plays an important role in determining which types of symptoms are more likely to be endorsed by Asian Americans. For example, past research has determined that Asians and Asian Americans are more prone to report somatic or physical complaints than psychological or mood-related symptoms when discussing issues of mental health disorders (Leong et al., 2006; Ryder et al., 2008; U.S. DHHS, 2001). Given this perspective, it is possible that Asians and Asian Americans may endorse high levels of somatic complaints on certain self-report scales and inflate the severity of their reported clinical disorder.

Another response style issue that may threaten the cross-cultural validity of self-report questionnaires to assess psychopathology involves the format of questionnaire items. Research examining how to adapt evidence-based treatments for Asian American groups have espoused modification of worksheets and therapy materials to include more culturally congruent images and common language so this information is less likely to be misunderstood by less acculturated Asian Americans (e.g., Hwang, 2009). Similarly, some elderly Asians or Asian Americans with limited English proficiency may have greater difficulty differentiating between specific response options on a Likert-type scale (Chu, Huynh, & Arean, 2011). For example, many of these scales use anchoring points such as "somewhat true" and "moderately true" and these fine points of distinction are often indiscernible and confusing for individuals who have learned English as a second language. Some alternative recommendations for such materials include the use of binary rating scales when possible (e.g., yes/no or true/false) or the inclusion of a distinct descriptor (linguistic or even pictorial) above each Likert-type response option.

For Asians and Asian Americans, another major cultural consideration with self-report questionnaires is language proficiency, linguistic differences in words used on the questionnaire, and reading level. For Asian Americans who are first-generation immigrants or present with limited English proficiency, or Asians who are completing self-report questionnaires translated from English to an Asian dialect, there are specific mood- or emotion-related terms and words that may be difficult to fully understand because of a general lack of an equivalent emotional term in certain Asian languages. For example, an Asian American client completing an English questionnaire may not fully comprehend the subtle, yet important differences in the mood-related terms, "sadness," "despair," and "depression." Language and communication structure may also differ between English and many Asian languages, resulting in questions that translate poorly from one language to the next (Westermeyer & Janca, 1997). Specifically, many of these self-report scales use cultural idioms in their items and such culture-specific terms often lose their meaning in translation. For instance, the CES-D scale asks respondents to report the frequency of "feeling blue" and this has no cultural equivalence in most Asian languages.

In response, some clinicians and researchers have sought feedback to replace these items with cultural equivalent words or terms. In one example, it was suggested the word, "blue," might be substituted with the word "black" for Korean populations as this ethnic group in known to use this color term to discuss feelings of depression (Yang & WonPat-Borja, 2007). Because of these language equivalence and structural format issues, many Asians or Asian Americans with limited English proficiency may experience Western-derived self-report questionnaires as confusing, lengthy, and difficult to understand. As such, some Asian or Asian American clients may be arbitrary and selective in their responses to self-report scales because they may not fully comprehend the clinical meaning of specific items and their relevance to possible diagnosis and treatment planning. To overcome cultural misunderstandings and improve the accuracy of diagnostic assessment, many clinicians and researchers may need to hire and train bicultural and bilingual staff who can administer these questionnaires in person to provide explanations when there is confusion about a test item or format and to provide follow-up questions to specific standard items that are difficult to comprehend or understand from a cultural standpoint.

Interviews: General Intake Interviews and Diagnostic or Semistructured Interviews

The predominant method used by clinicians to assess for psychopathology is the clinical interview. The clinical interview must include a number of complex tasks, goals, and areas of inquiry and determining a working diagnosis is just one of the many objectives of such a clinical procedure. As such, clinicians typically approach the task of psychopathology assessment in one of two formats: a general unstructured clinical interview or a more formal semistructured diagnostic clinical interview.

The first type, the general unstructured clinical interview, often focuses on a comprehensive review and collection of clinical information and other relevant data (e.g., childhood, family, and work histories) to formulate a working clinical diagnosis and treatment plan (Morrison, 2007). In a general clinical interview, the clinician will typically focus on an exploration phase of clinical issues and treatment options where critical information is carefully gathered, therapeutic rapport is built, and clinical impressions are developed (Hill, 2004). For many Asian and Asian American clients with high levels of stigma and ambivalence about treatment-seeking, the most important objective in the general interview for the clinician may be to establish treatment engagement and a strong commitment for the client to return for further treatment after the first interview.

The multiple tasks and format of a general intake interview pose many hazards for assessment of psychopathology. In an attempt to build rapport, demonstrate empathy, and convey cultural sensitivity to reluctant Asian and Asian American clients, a thorough assessment of clinical symptoms may not be possible, and a more informal exploration of general clinical impressions may be prudent until greater client trust can been established. When working with ambivalent clients, it can be difficult to attend to and manage the therapeutic relationship while still completing a detailed review of clinical symptoms that is essential for developing a comprehensive clinical symptom profile. Given this perspective, any initial clinical impressions may be prone to cultural bias and misinterpretation of Asian or Asian American clients because they may be more guarded in their responses, speak more to somatic issues, and provide a more favorable picture of their clinical issues to the therapist. Many clinical experts have recommended the use of integrated assessment and guided inquiry to overcome these possible cultural barriers to a more comprehensive diagnostic assessment in the general intake interview. Using such a strategy, clinicians can cue themselves in the clinical interview about the types of information needed for diagnostic symptom inquiry and to encourage elaboration and redirection with the client to obtain needed information, while maintaining the common factors in the interview that are necessary for building a solid therapeutic relationship.

As opposed to general intake interviews, formal diagnostic interviews provide more direct inquiry about the presence and severity of certain mental health symptoms and test hypotheses about specific clinical disorders and their alternatives. To facilitate a more accurate gathering of information, many of these diagnostic interviews are semistructured to ensure a comprehensive review of symptoms associated with multiple clinical disorders. The semistructured diagnostic interview provides a set of structured questions that are related to specific symptoms which are asked verbatim by the clinician. To elicit a more complete picture of the client's experience, clinicians also present follow-up questions to initial inquiries for further clarification. Specific examples of such structured and semistructured interviews include the Structured Clinical Interview for DSM-IV Diagnoses (SCID; First, Spitzer, Gibbon, & Williams, 2002), the Composite International Diagnostic Interview (CIDI; Kessler & Ustun, 2004), the Hamilton Rating Scale for Depression (HRSD; Hamilton, 1960), and the Diagnostic Interview Schedule for Adults (DIS; Robins, 1989). The advantage of the semistructured interview is that clinicians are provided with a detailed and comprehensive assessment of clinical symptoms that can contribute to the identification of multiple clinical disorders. With this formal structure in place, clinicians are less likely to misdiagnose, make an incomplete clinical diagnosis, or diagnose based on clinical intuition alone. Though semistructured interviews are used often by clinical researchers, clinicians and therapists often find the rigid and structured nature of these interviews somewhat prohibitive, and many do not have easy access to formal training for using these instruments in their clinical practice. Yet, many recent efforts have been directed toward bridging the gap between academic and clinical settings in order to improve the integration of evidence-based practices and instruments like semistructured diagnostic interviews in clinical settings. For future research, the increased use of these formal types of diagnostic interviews can help to increase the early detection of clinical issues and decrease the possible misdiagnosis of Asian and Asian American populations.

Cultural Considerations

Despite efforts to develop sound guidelines for working with culturally diverse populations (e.g., American Psychological Association, 2003), the mental health field has still not agreed on uniform standards of "cultural competence." However, there are common elements that are consistent across the multiple models of cultural competence in the psychology literature: (1) greater awareness of therapist and patient biases, identities, and privileges; (2) increased knowledge about individual and cultural differences; and (3) improved skill and experience in the clinical encounter, including the development of culturally responsive formulations and treatment plans. When assessing for psychopathology in the context of a clinical interview, it is important to apply these specific aspects of cultural competence to increase the likelihood that culturally different clients may become more comfortable and increase the likelihood of accurate clinical understandings and exchanges between the therapist and client.

Of particular importance for conducting a culturally competent interview is to generate a working relationship and mutual understanding between the client and therapist to develop a "cultural explanation for the individual's illness." In 1991, a task force called the Group on Culture and Diagnosis was formed to develop specific guidelines to help incorporate cultural considerations and issues for the *DSM-IV*. This task force outlined five components important for a sound cultural formulation when making decisions about clinical diagnosis (Lewis-Fernandez & Diaz, 2002). One of these five components, "cultural explanations of the individual's illness," included the critical investigation of cultural idioms of psychological distress and explanatory models of illness. These two elements, described below, are culturally variant and particularly important for the task of assessing psychopathology in a clinical interview when working with Asians and Asian Americans.

Cultural idioms of distress refer to the specific manner or way that mental health symptoms are communicated about by different ethnic groups. Asians and Asian Americans, who report with high levels of stigma and shame toward professional help-seeking and engage in cultural practices of emotion inhibition, are less likely to openly talk about mental illness and thus may have unique cultural idioms of distress. Research, for example, has shown that people from Western cultures more often psychologize or emphasize negative moods or clinical symptoms than Asians who are more prone to somatize or express psychopathology in physical manifestations like a headache or stomach ache (Ryder et al., 2008). When Asians or Asian Americans experience certain types of psychopathology, they may present such problems in somatic terms to avoid the cultural shame or a loss of face that could be associated with reporting a mental illness. As such, clients of Asian descent may not express symptoms of depression in terms of "sadness" or "depression," but may be more inclined to report physical fatigue and lethargy or interpersonal frustration or stress. Clinicians and researchers unaware of these cultural variations in cultural idioms of mental health distress may thus misinterpret or misdetect a client's expression of their symptom experience and types of psychopathology.

When interviewing Asian or Asian American clients, it will also be important to evaluate and identify possible explanatory models of illness that may be associated with their cultural background. Specifically, explanatory models of illness can significantly influence one's cultural understanding of the causes of psychopathology, the cultural meaning that is ascribed to the mental health experience, and the cultural expectations about clinical treatment. An early pioneer in cultural psychiatry and medical anthropology, Kleinman (1978) developed eight questions to improve the general and cultural understanding of a client's explanatory model of illness: (1) What do you call your problem? (2) What do you think has caused your problem? (3) Why do you think it started when it did? (4) What do you think your sickness does? How does it work? (5) How severe is your sickness? Will it have a short or long course? (6) What kind of treatment do you think you should receive? What are the most important results you hope to receive from this treatment? (7) What are the chief problems your sickness has caused for you? and (8) What do you fear most about your sickness? Although these questions do not relate specifically to clinical symptoms or *DSM*-related diagnostic categories per se, the collection of such culturally relevant data is critically important in assisting the clinician to consider whether cultural matters will play a crucial role in the development of an accurate diagnosis of psychopathology. Within a clinical interview, clinicians can select some of these culturally related questions or modify certain questions to better fit their particular setting or client in order to determine the importance of culture to their particular situation. It is also possible for clinicians to only ask themselves these questions about a particular case to achieve a better cultural understanding of their client rather than asking the questions directly.

Cultural competency in clinical and semistructured interviews is a complex concept and skill to master, particularly for clinicians who have had limited exposure to culturally diverse populations. As previously mentioned, it is important for clinicians and researchers to familiarize themselves with the strengths and weaknesses of clinical interviews in the process of developing an accurate assessment of psychopathology for Asians and Asian Americans. The chances for cultural misunderstandings and misinterpretations will increase when the clinician or researcher conducting the diagnostic interview has limited experience in working with clients of Asian descent and/or an Asian American client has limited English capacity and knowledge about Western cultural practices associated with mental health. However, there are a growing number of training resources that are now available to clinicians and researchers who seek to increase their competence in the area of culture, and these training methods may be very salient for conducting culturally appropriate clinical interviews with Asian and Asian American clients.

Non-Self-Report: Behavioral Assessment

Self-report methods like questionnaires and interviews may be supported with another critical method of clinical observation, the behaviorally based assessment. In fact, multimethod approaches to assessment are often recommended, and one of the benefits of such strategies is the possible decrease of false negatives or the failed detection of certain types of psychopathology. Beyond the possible self-censoring or underreporting of certain clinical symptoms due to high levels of stigma and shame associated with mental illness, self-report methods of assessment may be problematic if the Asian or Asian American client is clearly unaware or does not recognize certain symptoms of mental illness because of a lack of cultural familiarity with psychopathology.

The most common clinical tool used for behavioral assessment is the formal mental status exam. A comprehensive mental status exam is a very detailed assessment by the clinician that focuses on the overall quality of the client's physical appearance, observed demeanor and attitudes, psychomotor state, speech use and patterns, cognition and perception, mood and affect, thought content and process, insight, and judgment. Specific observations in the formal mental status exam are recorded by the clinician to provide a clear detailed description of the client and the observed behavioral manifestations of the client that may support certain types of psychopathology. For example, a client with an anxiety disorder may present with fidgeting, pacing around the room, or seek repeated reassurances from the clinician during the interview, while a client with schizophrenia may show extreme suspiciousness and agitation toward the clinician, appear physically disheveled and unkempt, and report with many cognitive disturbances. Any incongruence between self-report measures and behaviors observed by the well-trained clinician can signal the presence of unreported or underreported psychopathology.

Although the mental status exam is often discussed in clinical training, its general use and application for determining clinical diagnosis or psychopathology is somewhat limited and has not been validated or recommended by researchers. Instead, to improve the accuracy of determining psychopathology, specific instruments are available to aid the clinician in conducting a comprehensive and/or structured behavioral assessment. The Mini-Mental State Exam (MMSE; Folstein, Folstein, & McHugh, 1975), for example, is a standardized assessment instrument that rates a client's cognitive status on a scale of 1 to 30. The clinician administers a series of tasks that require the client to demonstrate specific aspects of cognitive orientation, memory, recall, reading, writing, and fine motor functioning. Scores on the MMSE of 27 and above are considered normal, 20–26 reflect mild dementia, 10–19 support moderate dementia, and scores below 10 suggest severe dementia. In contrast, behaviorally anchored rating scales are clinician-rated instruments based on direct observations that provide a general description of the client on a graduated rating scale for certain behavioral constructs such as overall psychological functioning or psychiatric status. Axis V in the *DSM-IV*, for example, represents the Global Assessment of Functioning (GAF) Scale and provides a single score as a description of a client's level of functioning in a number of life domains. Clinicians must make a general assessment of their client's overall functioning and provide a score on a scale of 1 to 100, where scores of 1 to 10 indicate "persistent danger of severely hurting self or others OR persistent inability to maintain minimum personal hygiene OR serious suicidal act with clear expectation of death," and scores of 91 to 100 indicate "superior functioning in a wide range of activities, life's problems never seem to get out of hand, is sought out by others because of his or her many qualities. No symptoms" (American Psychiatric Association, 2000).

Cultural Considerations

In considering the use of behavioral assessment as a vehicle for improving the determination of certain types of psychopathology, several cultural issues must be taken in account by clinicians working with Asians and Asian Americans. For instance, traditional Asian values emphasize that direct eye contact is a sign of disrespect to another person, particularly one of higher authority or status. Without such cultural knowledge, it would be possible for a clinician to overpathologize this culturally related behavior and report in clinical observation that an Asian or Asian American client was engaging in an extremely distrustful, suspicious, and socially withdrawn manner by Western standards.

In another example, social cognition psychology research has found that many Asian and Asian American groups are more likely to be associated with a high-context culture than Americans, who are more associated with a low-context culture. This cross-cultural difference will be strongly reflected in the communication styles of high- versus low-context cultures. That is, people from low-context cultures like North Americans and other Western cultures tend to express themselves more verbally and explicitly in their communication, while Asians and Asian Americans from high-context cultures will rely more heavily on implicit or behavioral, nonverbal modes of communication (Hall, 1976; Triandis, 1995). Given this cultural difference, it will be important for clinicians to consider that the integration of behavioral assessments may be particularly critical for capturing these nonverbally communicated symptoms and facilitating a more accurate measurement of psychopathology of Asians and Asian Americans.

Past research also indicates that Asian cultures traditionally encourage the practice of emotional suppression or control more so than Western cultures (D. W. Sue & Sue, 2003). These cultural scripts concerning emotional control, in turn, may have a profound impact on behavioral and mood expression. Chentsova-Dutton et al. (2007), for example, found signs of emotional dampening via less crying behavior in response to a sad film for Asian Americans in a control group without depression compared to White Americans without depression, but greater crying behavior for clinically depressed Asian Americans compared to White Americans who were also clinically depressed. Another study found differences in the autonomic physiology of less variable cardiac interbeat intervals in response to a conversation about conflict for Asian Americans compared to White Americans (Tsai & Levenson, 1997). Overall, however, there is limited research in this field of study and this prevents a better understanding about how the practice of emotional control can manifest in behavioral signs of psychopathology. At minimum, clinicians should be aware that behavioral signs of psychopathology, like self-reported information, are also influenced by cultural factors.

CURRENT ISSUES AND LIMITATIONS WITH ASSESSMENT METHODS

The current literature presents a mixed review of the types of clinical assessment approaches that can provide clear diagnostic trends and patterns about Asian and Asian American groups. Given the inconsistent findings in the literature about the adequacy of certain assessment measures, it will be important for clinicians and researchers working with Asian and Asian American clients to familiarize themselves with some of the major issues and limitations in the assessment and diagnostic fields, as such knowledge can facilitate more informed diagnostic decision-making. The following section provides a discussion on the four main challenges that are faced when clinicians select, administer, or interpret a diagnostic tool for use with Asian and Asian American clients: the debate over etic versus emic approaches to assessment, issues of conceptual equivalence, translation procedures, and technical equivalence.

The Etic Versus Emic Debate

One of the central issues related to the need for valid and reliable assessment instruments in working with Asian and Asian American populations is the debate regarding etic versus emic approaches (Butcher, Nezami, & Exner, 1998). The etic approach to assessment assumes that psychiatric disorders are universal across different cultures with the same fundamental constellation of symptoms, while the emic approach states that clinical expressions of mental illness are culturally bound or linked to a specific cultural group. Alternatively, a particular Asian or Asian American group may present with a well-known mental illness such as major depression, yet report different clinical symptoms or emphasize less common symptoms due to culturally related influences.

The emic and etic approaches to assessment can have a profound impact on the clinical diagnosis of Asians and Asian Americans. If a clinician assumes that clinical disorders are culturally universal or etic in nature, the use and/or language translation of diagnostic tools developed in Western populations may be culturally appropriate and work effectively with Asians or Asian Americans. These measures can therefore be imported and/or translated, or applied with its original content without modification, for use with Asians and Asian Americans. However, if certain clinical disorders are culturally specific or emic in nature, the translation of diagnostic measures developed with

Western populations may provide false or inaccurate identification of psychopathology for clients of Asian descent. Based on the emic approach, clinicians and researchers have often argued that it may be necessary to develop indigenous measures—new diagnostic measures or tools that can incorporate the unique types of clinical symptoms, phrases or words, and cultural idioms native to a particular Asian or Asian American group (Zheng, Wei, Goa, Zhang, & Wong, 1988).

An alternative strategy that draws from both the etic and emic approaches to cross-cultural diagnosis of Asians and Asian Americans is a mixed etic-emic approach. Several investigators have examined the cultural applicability of different measures by soliciting qualitative feedback from mental health consumers, and found items to be generally relevant and applicable, but in need of some cultural modification. In such cases, these researchers have added cultural stems to standard questions on self-report measures. These cultural stems include follow-up items that clarify the meaning of an item or assess for additional information that may be applicable to an Asian or Asian American group, but were possibly missed by the items in the original measure (Yang & WonPat-Borja, 2007). As such, this mixed etic-emic approach is used in situations where a standard scale is deemed fairly appropriate for use with Asians or Asian Americans (etic approach), but also requires specific modifications (e.g., semantic equivalence) and additions (e.g., cultural idioms, culture-bound symptoms) to the diagnostic instrument to increase the cross-cultural validity for this cultural group (emic approach).

A major challenge in the issue of etic versus emic approaches is the lack of evidence-based recommendations that point toward the appropriate conditions for importing or creating an indigenous measure versus modifying an original measure with culturally appropriate stems or additions. In reviewing the literature, the majority of research on clinical diagnosis with Asian Americans has relied on the etic approach and focused on the translation of English-language assessment methods for determining rates of psychopathology for Asian American populations (e.g., Leong, Okazaki, & Tak, 2003). Some of this research has been applied to immigrant Asian American groups in the United States and other cross-cultural efforts have focused on collecting data with clinical and nonclinical Asian populations in China, Hong Kong, Japan, and other Asian countries. Invariably, there has been a tendency to use English-translated measures for several reasons. First, many clinicians and researchers have been trained with these well-known measures and have greater familiarity and confidence with these diagnostic tools despite the limited evidence of their psychometric validity and reliability with a particular Asian American population. Second, even clinicians and researchers who are aware of the cultural limitations of translated diagnostic measures are often forced to use these Western-based instruments due to a lack of viable alternatives that have been empirically tested and validated with Asian and Asian American groups.

At this time, there are several common translated measures of psychopathology, such as the Beck Depression Inventory or the MMPI-2, that have been shown to have empirically valid and reliable psychometric properties with individuals of Asian descent (Butcher, Cheung, & Lim, 2003; Leung, Okazaki, & Tak, 2003). However, a cursory review of these more well known clinical measures on psychopathology with Asians and Asian Americans provides a somewhat inconsistent picture, with certain measures such as the MMPI-2 showing fairly strong support for its translations into different Asian languages (Butcher, Cheung, & Lim, 2003) versus other measures that provide less than stellar performance in clinically diagnosing clients of Asian descent. Even with clinical measures such as the Beck Depression Inventory and MMPI-2 that were translated and found to provide supportive results in the diagnosis of Asian and Asian American popula- tions, there have been reports of elevations in the scores for certain categories or subscales, thus raising concerns that different norms or standards may be warranted. For example, the MMPI-2 has consistently shown that Asian Americans have higher elevations on the depression subscale, yet it is not clear if this result is demonstrating a certain response set or greater honesty in respond- ing to these items or if this result is a "true" reflection of higher rates of depressive symptomatology (Yang & WonPat-Borja, 2007).

In response to these continued issues of validity and reliability in the equivalence of these trans- lated diagnostic tools, a number of clinicians and researchers have turned to the emic approach, developing new culturally specific assessment measures specifically designed and developed with Asian samples. For example, a recent study found that the Chinese Depression Inventory (CDI), which was developed in China, proved to be a more accurate and culturally sensitive measure of the severity of depression for Chinese clients than a translated Chinese version of the Beck Depression Inventory (Zheng & Lin, 2007). In addition, studies have examined the Chinese Personality Assessment Inventory (Cheung et al., 1996) as a substitute for the MMPI-2 for Chinese popu- lations. It will be important to promote more research in this field of study and to assess if such measures can be more widely adopted and tested with other Asian and Asian American groups by the psychiatric and psychological communities.

Conceptual and Construct Equivalence Across Cultures

The critical issue of test equivalence plays a strong role in reinforcing confidence in an assess- ment measure used with Asian American and Asian clients. Several researchers have highlighted a number of the key conditions that should be considered when attempting to examine the cultural equivalence of an assessment measure for culturally different populations (Brislin, 1986; Van de Vijver, 2001; Van de Vijver & Leung, 1997). Specifically, several types of cultural equivalence such as linguistic, conceptual, functional, and psychometric equivalence have been proposed to deter- mine the validity and reliability of using English versions or translated, Asian-language versions of standard assessment instruments with Asian and Asian American groups. A comprehensive review of these equivalence subtypes linked to clinical assessment is beyond the scope of this chapter, and the reader is referred to Kwan, Gong, and Maestas (2010) and Kinoshita and Hsu (2006) for more in-depth analysis and discussion of these equivalence issues with Asian Americans. In this chapter, we highlight two types of test equivalence that are particularly important for clinicians who are seeking to assess psychopathology in Asian and Asian American clients: conceptual equivalence and technical equivalence.

Conceptual equivalence is strongly associated with the etic versus emic approaches and focuses on the possible cultural misunderstanding or misinterpretation of certain psychopathological constructs and concepts across different cultures. Specifically, conceptual equivalence refers to a high level of consistency between two cultures in defining a particular theoretical construct such as a symptom profile of a mental disorder and this type of equivalence should focus on the facto- rial, discriminant, convergent, and construct validity of clinical symptoms of psychopathology. If it is culturally determined that mental disorders are conceptually equivalent in definition between

Asian and White Americans or Asian and non-Asian individuals, this would yield a situation that would be more conducive to using etic approaches for the assessment, or importation and/or translation of a psychological measure that was validated with Western populations. If there is some evidence that clinical disorders or various types of psychopathology have little or limited conceptual equivalence, this would support the need for the creation of a culturally specific or indigenous culture–based measure.

A review of the literature shows conceptual equivalence varies and depends on the specific mental disorder in question. For example, previous studies identified various forms of clinical syndromes or psychopathologies that are "culturally specific" to certain cultures and countries. The fourth edition, text revision, of the *Diagnostic and Statistical Manual of Mental Disorders* (*DSM-TR-IV*) includes several culturally bound disorders (e.g., amok, hwabyung, koro, Taijin-Kyofu-Sho) present only in specific countries and world regions including Asian countries (American Psychiatric Association, 2000). This recognition of culturally bound disorders reflects the concept of cultural relativism, or an emic approach supporting that lifestyles, cultural values, and worldviews can affect the expression and determination of certain types of psychopathology (D. Sue, Sue, & Sue, 2006). Previous research also suggests there may be culturally specific behavioral responses that are associated with certain types of psychopathology for Asians and Asian Americans. For example, Asians in their native countries and Asians Americans were found to report lower rates of acting-out symptoms that are often linked to psychopathology in the United States (Asian American Federation of New York, 2003; Chun, Eastman, Wang, & Sue, 1998; Hong & Domokos-Cheng Ham, 2001).

When considering the specific conditions relating to culture-bound syndromes, mental health professionals have often questioned whether these so-called syndromes may be a culturally modified representation of common mental disorders found in Western cultures. For example, Kleinman and Kleinman (1985) investigated the culturally specific psychopathology associated with high levels of reported neurasthenia in China, a mental health condition that is no longer a diagnostic category in the *DSM-IV*. They found that Chinese individuals who were diagnosed with neurasthenia reported with more somatic complaints than typical symptoms associated with major depression including diminished enjoyment and sadness. However, when these Chinese clients were prescribed antidepressants, they reported with improved psychological functioning and a reduction of somatic complaints, supporting the idea that neurasthenia may be a more culturally accepted method for reporting symptoms of major depression for Chinese clients. Given this example, it is clear that the critical issues of assessment concerning culturally specific versus universal psychopathology can be very complex and requires more empirical cross-cultural investigations.

In fact, some clinicians and researchers have cautioned that it is imperative for diagnostic approaches with Asians and Asian Americans to make the clear distinction between culturally bound syndromes and cultural variations of DSM diagnostic categories. In the former case, there are certain types of culturally bound mental health conditions (e.g., hwa-byung for Koreans, Kyol goeu for Cambodian Khmer refugees) that have been clearly identified with clients in specific regions in Asia (Hinton, Um, & Ba, 2001; Lin, 1983). The latter case speaks to minor or slight cultural variations in the symptoms that are associated with specific categories in the *DSM-IV-TR*. For example, a client of Asian descent might present with a clinical profile that is relatively consistent with major depression, but exhibit some ethnic differences in the presentation of specific symptoms such as irritable mood, somatic, or concentration complaints rather than emotional symptoms like sadness.

Overall, research has supported the idea that culture plays a critical role in the determination of specific types of psychopathology. The skilled clinician or researcher must take cultural variation in psychopathology (including the issue of conceptual equivalence) into consideration when examining certain types of clinical disorders for Asian and Asian American groups.

Translation of Imported Measures

With the determination that conceptual equivalence in a particular psychopathology construct is culturally adequate, one may choose to utilize a standard questionnaire, interview, or behavioral assessment that has been validated with Western populations with Asian American clients. However, this choice to import a standard measure for assessment purposes still may require the need for translation into the client's primary Asian language or dialect.

Despite the importance of proper translation of assessment instruments, many clinicians and researchers have often used translated versions of commonly used diagnostic instruments without further investigations of the psychometric properties for use with Asian or Asian American populations. Social scientists have repeatedly pointed to clear inadequacies of current translation methodologies in the field of diagnostic assessment (Leung & Wong, 2003; S. Sue & Chang, 2003). Though many translation protocols have been proposed over the last several decades (Brislin, 1986; Westermeyer & Janca, 1997), there is large variation in choice and utilization of such protocols. One of the most common approaches to translation involves the techniques of translation and back-translation, followed by evaluation of linguistic/semantic equivalence. Linguistic equivalence is achieved when the perceived meaning of questionnaire items in the original and translated versions of a measure is the same. Other translation recommendations include the addition of a pilot study examining the translated measure with diverse representatives from the population of interest, followed by a reevaluation of pilot data and interviews with consumers regarding test item content (e.g., Sartorius & Janca, 1996; Westermeyer & Janca, 1997).

Unfortunately, few studies report details of their translation protocols, presenting uncertainty about the adequacy of linguistic equivalence in their measures. In the absence of uniform guidelines or standard reporting requirements regarding translation, translation methodologies have largely varied from one study to the next. As a result, some questionnaires have multiple translated versions, each with their own linguistic variations. For clinicians and researchers looking to utilize translated measures, it is often unclear which of these translated versions is most appropriate.

In response to these limitations in the uniformity of translation guidelines, some researchers have proposed a standardized translation methodology for imported questionnaires: continual translation and back-translation until linguistic equivalence is achieved, followed with an evaluation by a bilingual committee and field trials to validate this translated instrument with the population of interest (e.g., Leung & Wong, 2003). Researchers and clinicians should avail themselves of such recommended protocols when evaluating or creating translated measures, and report results of their translation methodologies when disseminating information.

Technical Equivalence

Regardless of one's choice to use an imported, translated, or indigenous measure, cultural differences in clinical diagnosis among Asians and Asian Americans can also arise from differences in test-taking behavior. Technical equivalence refers to matters of test administration that can affect an individual's reporting of mental health symptoms such as test format (e.g., Likert-type versus True/False questions, or self-report versus interview or behavioral assessments), response style, or test environment. Essentially, these cultural concerns arise from method bias rather than any cultural differences in the content or psychometric properties of a test.

As previously discussed, research has shown conflicting findings in severity and/or prevalence of mental disorders like depression, depending on the assessment format that is being used. For example, use of self-report inventories like the CES-D or the BDI have yielded higher levels of depression severity in some Asian and Asian American groups compared to White Americans (e.g., Lam, Pepper, & Ryabchenko, 2004; Yen, Robins, & Lin, 2000), whereas interview protocols like the SCID have yielded no ethnic differences in depression prevalence (Lam et al., 2004). The inherent difficulty of studying and quantifying reporting biases has hindered efforts to examine possible differences in the endorsement of certain symptoms due to method bias within the same sample. However, one recent study found that Asians were more likely to report somatic symptoms in a spontaneous manner or in response to clinical interview questions than report such somatic complaints in a self-administered symptom questionnaire (Ryder et al., 2008). This study is one of the first to illuminate cultural differences in the reporting of psychopathology due to test format within the same sample of Asian individuals.

Other factors may also affect the technical equivalence of a diagnostic tool and create differences in test-taking behaviors. Different response styles and response sets, for example, have been reported in different Asian and Asian American groups such as the tendency to report more moderate scores (Chen, Lee, & Stevenson, 1995; Hamamura, Heine, & Paulhus, 2008; Zax & Takahashi, 1967) or the tendency to report based on cultural sanctions and the need for social approval (Middleton & Jones, 2000). Such response styles can affect the validity of a particular diagnostic measure. In addition, qualities of the test environment can also influence test-taking behavior. For Asians and Asian Americans in particular, when issues of stigma or shame about mental illness are salient, a client may feel more comfortable and open to revealing their true experiences on an assessment measure while in a more private compared to a public space.

Ultimately, depending on the nature of the information requested, it will be important for clinicians and researchers to consider which format is best suited to gather information on culturally sensitive and taboo subjects for Asians and Asian Americans. It is possible that certain types of clinical data collection may work well with some Asian or Asian American groups, while other diagnostic forms or procedures may be a better fit given the unique circumstances or specifics of the inquiry. How to decide which procedure to use in assessing psychopathology with Asians and Asian Americans will require greater investment of time and knowledge, and consultation with cultural experts may be helpful.

Invariably, it would seem the best approach for conducting a culturally appropriate assessment of psychopathology among Asians and Asian Americans would be a multimethod strategy.

Although a multimethod strategy may require more time and resources, such a strategy may lead to more accurate diagnostic decisions. For example, information that is gained from self-reported surveys can be supplemented with semistructured or structured interviews and behavioral observations. Certain measures utilizing a Likert-type scale can be supplemented with a free-response qualitative inquiry or a binary True/False response option. Clinicians may also consider requesting information from family or other collateral sources to gain an alternative perspective from multiple sources of information.

PRACTICAL GUIDE FOR CLINICIANS AND RESEARCHERS

How to Choose an Assessment Method

Cultural barriers to assessment can be minimized through careful consideration of a combination of three factors or steps: individual difference factors, assessment goals, and choice of assessment method and instrument. In this section, we review these steps and provide a brief summary that is intended as a practical guide for choosing appropriate assessment methods for Asian and Asian American clients.

Individual Difference Factors

Individual differences such as personality, coping style, or perceived stigma about mental illness may affect the likelihood to report psychopathology experience. Asians or Asian Americans who typically utilize an avoidance coping style or practice emotion inhibition (Chang, 2001) or hold a high level of stigma regarding mental illness may be less likely to be aware of and/or openly report their psychopathology experience (D. W. Sue & Sue, 2003). An emphasis on relational or interdependent ways of being among Asian and Asian American groups (e.g., Gong, Gage, & Tacata, 2003; Markus & Kitayama, 1991; Morisaki & Gudykunst, 1994) may also result in altered or diminished reporting of psychological symptoms due to concerns about loss of face and social expectations. It would be important with such clients to utilize strategies that can compensate for possible reticence in reporting about mental health problems. For example, a clinician working with an Asian client may make an extra effort to ensure the client feels comfortable with the clinical assessment situation, consider the possible need to interpret assessment results as an underestimation of psychopathology, or combine self-report with face-to-face interviews and using questions less likely to activate shame about mental illness.

Some particularly important individual differences to consider in clinical assessment include the critical need to consider the client's acculturation level, linguistic ability, and reading level. Level of acculturation among Asian Americans can indicate whether measures validated with mainstream populations and imported measures from Western cultures will present equivalence problems such as linguistic, criterion, and conceptual equivalence. Asian American clients with limited English proficiency or Asian Americans who are proficient in English, but prefer their native Asian language, may have difficulty understanding many English questions and respond inaccurately based on such linguistic misunderstanding. Reading level or linguistic differences in word choice between different dialects of Asian languages can affect the conceptual equivalence of an instrument for Asian or Asian American clients. Some assessment instruments have been specifically designed or written at a lower reading level, which may help to mitigate such literacy and linguistic concerns.

One individual difference of particular relevance to Asian American clients is that of client-therapist ethnic match. Some Asian Americans are more comfortable and more likely to stay in treatment when talking with an ethnically matched clinician (Gamst, Dana, Der-Karabetian, & Kramer, 2001); this preference for a clinician is often dependent on the individual's stage of ethnic identity development. For example, Asian Americans who are in the Immersion-Emersion stage of the Minority Identity Development Model (Atkinson, Morten, & Sue, 1989) are more likely to affiliate with others of their Asian minority culture rather than the American majority culture. These Asian American clients may be more likely to report accurate symptoms of psychopathology when talking with an Asian American clinician.

At a minimum, clinicians should fully understand the level of acculturation, reading level, relational style, and linguistic preferences of their Asian and Asian American clients and the strengths and weaknesses of certain assessment instruments in order to find an assessment measure and administration style with appropriate fit for the specific client and situation. In fact, psychotherapy research has supported the idea that cultural *fit* is particularly important in treatment outcome and therapeutic relationships with culturally diverse populations (Beutler & Harwood, 2000). This concept of fit should be applied to situations of assessment as well, with clinicians being advised to individually tailor their choice of assessment to the special needs of the client.

Assessment Goals

Once a clinician assesses for individual difference factors such as stigma, reporting bias, acculturation, or linguistic and reading ability that may affect the appropriateness of a particular assessment method, the next step is to choose an appropriate assessment method and instrument. The purpose or goal of the psychopathology assessment must be carefully considered. A goal of differential diagnosis may indicate a need for a clinical interview using guided questioning, a semistructured clinical interview, or a self-report questionnaire that maps directly onto *DSM-IV* diagnostic criteria. The goal of severity tracking for assessment of symptom progression or treatment effectiveness may indicate the need to use a questionnaire that is sensitive to small changes in symptom experience over shorter time periods or the use of mood tracking or mental status behavioral assessment on a regular basis. On the other hand, a goal of simply understanding a client's experience of psychopathology—the meaning attributed to their experience—may call for an unstructured clinical interview or generalized symptom assessment scales.

In some instances, it may be useful to compare the assessment results with other indicators. For example, comparison of current results with previous symptom assessment may provide an indicator of disease progression. Alternatively, assessment may be part of a research effort or a clinic-wide effort, in which case choosing assessment instruments that have been previously administered will allow for symptom tracking, comparisons, and consistency.

Choice of Assessment Method and Instrument

After developing an understanding of possible individual differences and establishing the intended goals of assessment, there are several technical considerations that one must consider when choosing an assessment tool. First, the choice of assessment *method*—self-administered self-report, clinician-administered self-report, behavioral assessment, or clinical interview—can be important in overcoming cultural reporting barriers. As previously discussed, different assessment methods do not report with similar levels of technical equivalence; each can yield disparate test-taking behaviors and a different likelihood for the client to openly reporting true experiences. An Asian or Asian American client that is sensitive to issues of shame about mental illness, for example, may feel reluctant to reveal his experiences to another person and may be more likely to accurately report symptoms via a self-report measure rather than in a clinical interview.

Psychometric properties must also be considered when choosing an appropriate instrument. The clinician should ensure that whenever possible, assessment instruments have been appropriately normed and validated with the population of interest. Clinicians and researchers should evaluate and choose instruments that have the highest level of equivalence for the population of interest with regard to content, linguistic/semantic, conceptual, criterion, and normative equivalence (see Kinoshita & Hsu, 2006, or Kwan, Gong, & Maestas, 2010, for a more detailed review).

Not only must one look for a psychometrically sound instrument, but it is especially important when working with Asian and Asian American clients to make a decision about whether to use an instrument that is indigenously created (emic approach), imported but modified with cultural stems (mixed etic-emic approach), or imported and, if needed, translated (etic approach). Such a decision must be informed by understanding how well a psychopathology construct applies cross-culturally to one's client (conceptual equivalence), the availability of existing measures, and the language ability of the client. When one is uncertain about how a measure will apply with a particular client population, it is advisable to pilot-test an instrument and to obtain feedback from consumers about the wording, meaning, and clarity of the instrument items.

Finally, specific considerations about technical test-taking administration must be considered. Older Asian or Asian American adults, for example, may have difficulty sustaining attention for long periods of time and completing longer assessment instruments so shorter instruments may be more age-appropriate for these clients. These elderly clients may also prefer questionnaire items with fewer Likert-type scale points (e.g., four instead of seven), binary ratings (e.g., yes/no or true/false), or distinct descriptors (linguistic or even pictorial) above each response option. The type of assessment environment or setting is also important when working with Asian and Asian American clients. As mentioned previously, Asians and Asian Americans with major concerns about shame and stigma attached to mental illness, for example, may prefer to complete a self-report questionnaire in the context of a private room rather than completing this measure in a public waiting room with other clients present.

Practical Guide: Summary

The following is a summary of guidelines and questions to consider when choosing an appropriate psychopathology assessment method for an Asian or Asian American client:

1. Identify and understand individual differences or cultural considerations that are relevant for your client. What is the client's level of acculturation, reading level, linguistic ability, relational style, and coping preferences? What do these individual/cultural factors suggest for the selection of specific assessment instruments and administration style?
2. Know the specific purpose for your assessment: Are you focusing on differential diagnosis, severity tracking, understanding of illness experience or meaning, or general symptom assessment? Do you need to compare the assessment results of your client to other groups, research findings, or clinic clients?
3. Review the literature on assessment issues with your targeted group. Which assessment instruments have appropriate psychometric validation, norms, and equivalence for your specific client group?
4. Determine which assessment instrument is the most culturally appropriate. Do you need to choose an instrument that is created indigenously (the emic approach), imported with cultural stems or modifications (the mixed etic-emic approach), or imported and/or translated (the etic approach)?
5. Consider the cultural concerns of the test-taking format and setting. What are your test-administration limitations? Does the client have a need for privacy? How long do you have with the person? Will your client respond better to items with binary or multiple Likert-type point scales, or longer versus shorter administration times?

CLOSING REMARKS

A review of the mental health literature on clinical diagnosis and psychopathology with Asian and Asian American groups provides several key conclusions. First, there have been limited attempts to study the clinical assessment of psychopathology of Asian American and Asian groups in the mental health literature and the majority of available research on psychopathology and mental illness on such populations has been collected in the past several decades. In general, the relatively small population of Asian Americans in the United States and the stereotype of Asian Americans as a "model minority" have significantly hampered more focused efforts to study such issues on clinical diagnosis and psychopathology for Asian American populations. In the past, limited efforts were made to study or include Asian Americans in epidemiological studies of mental illness in the United States. When Asian Americans were included in such diagnostic studies, they were usually placed in aggregate with other ethnic minority groups and specific considerations of their diagnostic needs and prevalence/incidence rates of mental illness were difficult to determine using such gross measures or procedures.

Second, the specific assessment methods that have been applied to determine rates of mental illness for Asian American and Asian populations have been varied, but most of these procedures have been based on evaluation methods developed for White Americans or Western populations.

For example, clinical diagnoses of Asian and Asian American populations have focused on varied procedures including self-reported inventories by the client, structured diagnostic interviews by clinicians, and behavioral assessments or observations by clinical staff. Inherently, most of these common assessment scales or interviews were developed first in English and subsequently translated into other non-English languages including specific Asian languages and dialects (Ægisdóttir, Grestein, & Cinarbas, 2008; van de Vijver & Leung, 1997, Westermeyer & Janca, 1997;). However, the research literature to support the reliability and validity of such translated diagnostic measures with Asian and Asian American populations is only recently growing, and such concerns raise issues of legitimacy and accuracy in the results of such assessment tools (Kinoshita & Hsu, 2006; Kwan, Gong, & Maestas, 2010; Okazaki & S. Sue, 2000).

Third, many of the current studies of psychopathology focus on a small fraction of the diagnostic categories in the *DSM-IV-TR*. In a review of the literature, it is clear that most of the empirical research on Asians and Asian Americans tends to focus on a small cluster of diagnostic categories, which include mood disorders, especially major depression, and anxiety disorders, particularly post-traumatic stress disorders. While these are important diagnostic categories, which require greater attention when considering the diagnosis of Asian and Asian American populations, it is important to note that such an approach does not allow for a greater understanding of other types of psychopathology.

Fourth, compounding the issue of the narrow scope of current diagnostic studies with Asians and Asian Americans is the tendency for many of the present investigations to collect data with nonclinical samples. For the most part, many existing studies focus on student or nonclinical community populations and a broad assessment of symptoms that may be related to a diagnosable clinical disorder. As such, to move the field of psychopathology assessment and research to the next level, there is a need to consider the assessment of both clinical and nonclinical populations of Asian descent. Studies that involve clinical populations will allow for cross-cultural comparisons with clearly identifiable clients, the direct testing of the cultural appropriateness of certain diagnostic tools, and the determination of prevalence rates in the general public.

Fifth, most of the research in the field of clinical assessment uses a cross-sectional method for studying clinical disorders and psychopathology of Asians or Asian Americans and other cultural groups. This cross-sectional approach not only provides a simple snapshot of psychopathology at only one time point, but it can be particularly prone to cultural biases in over- or underreporting symptoms among Asians and Asian Americans. For future research, it may be prudent for investigators to consider a longitudinal design to assess reported symptoms at various stages of clinical progression to determine a more accurate presentation of a client's clinical profile. This longitudinal approach to clinical diagnosis may also provide more valuable information about the progression of a particular mental disorder, the increase or decrease of certain types of symptoms in treatment, and so forth, when working with Asian and Asian American client populations.

Finally, it is important to note that given the limited body of psychopathology research among individuals of Asian descent, clear distinctions cannot yet be made about recommendations for the research and assessment of psychopathology among Asians compared to Asian Americans. In fact, research has been relatively more abundant on Asian American populations in the United States than Asian groups in their native countries. Much of the research reviewed in this chapter is reflective of this bias in a larger number of studies conducted with Asian American populations.

Yet, there is some indication that knowledge about Asian individuals may be informed by Asian American literature and vice versa. Asian Americans who immigrate from Asian countries bring their beliefs and practices from their country of origin about mental health constructs such as suicide (e.g., Corin, 1995). As such, a strict demarcation may not apply between findings and trends in Asians versus Asian Americans. It will be prudent for future research to further investigate critical differences in the research and assessment of psychopathology among Asian versus Asian American clients.

SUGGESTIONS FOR FUTURE RESEARCH

Currently, valid and reliable diagnosis of psychopathology for the purposes of practice or research among Asians and Asian Americans is at a nascent point in its development. As discussed in this chapter, several advancements exist in the field of cross-cultural assessment of psychopathology: (1) the creation of indigenous measures in cases where conceptual equivalence of a mental disorder is low, (2) the modification of mainstream measures with cultural stems or additions when only minor changes are needed for cross-cultural validity, and (3) the increasing availability of translated measures. Despite these advancements, larger problems prevail, including little consistency in and reporting of translation methods, inadequate cross-cultural knowledge about different psychopathology constructs, and few standard guidelines to direct the choice of diagnostic method or tool.

Intuitively, a major solution for the problem of validity and reliability of diagnostic tools with Asians and Asian Americans is the increase of more culturally competent investigations for establishing possible norms and standards with these samples. Without further research in this area, there will continue to be questions about the appropriateness of using well-known assessment measures with Asian and Asian American groups. Specifically, if more research can be completed to establish the range of normal responses to certain subscales or scales that are being used to diagnose Asians and Asian Americans, this would help to reduce the likelihood for false positives and negatives regarding certain forms of psychopathology. At such a nascent point in this field of cross-cultural assessment, research methods conducive to exploratory efforts such as case studies, qualitative methods, or mixed method research will be particularly useful in advancing knowledge. Such methods can be used to gather feedback from Asian and Asian American clients about the cross-cultural applicability of any given measure or to determine when cultural stems or additions to certain test items are needed to provide greater clarification and validity in an existing measure.

These research endeavors will require an influx of finances and resources, but these concerted efforts will be critical for current and future generations of culturally diverse client populations. Until this research effort can be completed, many clinicians and researchers have suggested the continued use of standard diagnostic tools with the cautionary suggestion that cultural considerations should be included in the selection, administration, scoring, and interpretation of results from the diagnostic tools used and in the development of the final report or diagnosis for a particular Asian or Asian American client. Others suggest the creation of indigenous measures appropriate to Asian or Asian American populations in cases where conceptual equivalence is low and mainstream measures are of questionable cross-cultural application. Given the stated ethical principles by the American Psychological Association (2002) that support focused efforts from psychologists to provide culturally appropriate assessment of Asian Americans and other ethnic groups, it will be important for graduate training programs and continuing education workshops to educate providers and researchers about culture-specific diagnostic tools and culturally modified tools as possible supplements or alternatives to standard diagnostic measures based on U.S. and Western cultural populations.

REFERENCES

Abe-Kim, J., Gong, F., & Takeuchi, D. (2004). Religiosity, spirituality, and help-seeking among Filipino Americans: Religious clergy or mental health professionals? *Journal of Community Psychology, 32,* 675–689.

Ægisdóttir, S., Grestein, L., & Cinarbas, D. C. (2008). Methodological issues in cross-cultural counseling research: Test equivalence, bias, and translations. *Counseling Psychologist, 36,* 188–219.

Alegria, M., Takeuchi, D., Canino, G., Duan, N., Shrout, P., Meng, X., et al. (2004). Considering context, place and culture: The National Latino and Asian American Study. *International Journal of Methods in Psychiatric Research, 13*(4), 208–220.

American Counseling Association. (2006). ACA code of ethics. *Journal of Counseling and Development, 94,* 235–254.

American Psychological Association. (2002). Ethical principles of psychologists and code of conduct. *American Psychologist, 57,* 1060–1073.

American Psychological Association. (2003). Guidelines on multicultural education, training, research, practice, and organizational change for psychologists. *American Psychologist, 58*(5), 377–402.

American Psychiatric Association. (2000). *Diagnostic and statistical manual of mental disorders* (4th ed., text rev.). Washington, DC: Author. (*DSM-IV-TR*)

Asian American Federation of New York. (2003). *Asian American mental health; A post-September 11th needs assessment.* New York: Author.

Atkinson, D. R., Morten, G., & Sue, D. W. (1989). A minority identity development model. In Dr. Atkinson, G. Morten, & D. W. Sue (Eds.), *Counseling American Minorities* (pp. 35–52). Dubuque, IA: Brown.

Beck, A. T., Brown, G., & Steer, R. A. (1996). *Beck Depression Inventory II manual.* San Antonio, TX: The Psychological Corporation.

Beck, Aaron T., & Robert A. Steer. *Beck Anxiety Inventory manual.* San Antonio, TX: The Psychological Corporation, Harcourt Brace & Company, 1993.

Beutler, L.E., & Harwood, T.M. (2000). Prescriptive psychotherapy: A practical guide to systematic treatment selection. New York: Oxford University Press.

Brislin, R. W. (1986). The wording and translation of research instruments. In W. J. Lonner & J. W. Berry (eds.), *Field methods in cross-cultural research* (pp. 137–164). Beverly Hills, CA: Sage.

Butcher, J.N., Cheung, F.M., & Lim, J. (2003). Use of the MMPI-2 with Asian populations. *Psychological Assessment, 15* (3), 248–256.

Butcher, J. N., Nezami, E., & Exner, J. (1998). Psychological assessment of people in diverse cultures. In S. S. Kazarian & D. R. Evans (Eds.), *Cultural clinical psychology: Theory, research, and practice* (pp. 61–105). New York: Oxford University Press.

Chang, E. C. (2001). A look at the coping strategies and styles of Asian Americans: Similar and different? In C. R. Snyder (Ed.), *Coping with stress: Effective people and processes* (pp. 222–239). London: Oxford University Press.

Chen, C., Lee, S.-Y., & Stevenson, H. W. (1995). Response style and cross-cultural comparisons of rating scales among East Asian and North Americans students. *Psychological Science, 6,* 170–175.

Chentsova-Dutton, Y. E., Chu, J. P., Tsai, J. L., Rottenberg, J., Gross, J. J., & Gotlib, I. H. (2007). Depression and emotional reactivity: Variation among Asian Americans of East Asian descent and European Americans. *Journal of Abnormal Psychology, 116*(4), 776–785.

Cheung, F. M., Leung, K., Fan, R. M., Song, W.-Z., Zhang, J.-X., & Zhang, J.-P. (1996). Assessment of the Chinese Personality Assessment Inventory. *Journal of Cross-Cultural Psychology, 27*(2), 181–199.

Cheung, F. M. (1995). *The Chinese Minnesota Multiphasic Personality Inventory manual.* Shatin, Hong Kong: Chinese University Press.

Chu, J. P., Huynh, L., & Arean, P. A. (2011). Cultural adaptation of evidence-based practice utilizing an iterative stakeholder process and theoretical framework: Problem solving therapy for Chinese older adults. Manuscript submitted for publication.

Chun, K. M., Eastman, K. L., Wang, G. C. S., & Sue, S. (1998). Psychopathology. In N. W. S. Zane & L. C. Lee (Eds.), *Handbook of Asian American psychology* (pp. 457–483). Thousand Oaks, CA: Sage.

Corin, E. (1995). From a cultural stance: Suicide and aging in a changing world. *International Psychogeriatrics, 7*(2), 335–355.

Demyttenaere, K., Bruffaerts, R., Posada-Villa, J., Gasquet, I., Kovess, V., Lepine J. P., et al. and WHO World Mental Health Survey Consortium (2004). Prevalence, severity, and unmet need for treatment of mental disorders in the World Health Organization World Mental Health Surveys. *Journal of the Medical Association of America, 291*(21), 2581–2590.

Derogatis, L. R. (1977). *The SCL-90 manual I: Scoring, administration, and procedures for the SCL-90.* Baltimore: Clinical Psychometric Research.

Derogatis, L. R., Lipman, R. S., Rickels, K., Uhlenbuth, E. H., & Covi, L. (1974). The Hopkins Symptom Checklist (HSCL): A self-report symptoms inventory. *Behavioural Science, 19*(1), 1–15.

Derogatis, L. R., & Melisaratos, N. (1983). The Brief Symptom Inventory: An introductory report. *Psychological Medicine, 13,* 595–605.

First, M. B., Spitzer, R. L., Gibbon, M., & Williams, J. B. W. (2002). *Structured clinical interview for DSM-IV-TR Axis I disorders: Research version, non-patient edition.* New York: Biometrics Research, New York State Psychiatric Institute. (SCID-I/NP)

Folstein, M. F., Folstein, S. E., & McHugh, P. R. (1975). Mini-mental state: A practical method for grading the cognitive state of patients for the clinician. *Journal of Psychiatric Research, 12,* 189–198.

Gamst, G., Dana, R. H., Der-Karabetian, A., & Kramer, T. (2001). Asian American mental health clients: Effects of ethnic match and age on global assessment and visitation. *Journal of Mental Health Counseling, 23*(1), 57–72.

Gong, F., Gage, S. J. L., & Tacata, L. A., Jr. (2003). Help-seeking behavior among Filipino Americans: A cultural analysis of face and language. *Journal of Community Psychology, 31,* 469–488.

Greene, R. L. (1991). *The MMPI-2/MMPI: An interpretive manual.* Boston: Allyn & Bacon.

Hall, E. (1976). *Beyond culture.* New York: Doubleday.

Hamamura, T., Heine, S. J., & Paulhus, D. L. (2008). Cultural differences in response styles: The role of dialectical thinking. *Personality and Individual Differences, 44*(4), 932–942.

Hamilton, M. (1960). A rating scale for depression. *Journal of Neurology, Neurosurgery, and Psychiatry, 23,* 56–62.

Hill, C. (2004). *Helping skills: Facilitating exploration, insight, and action* (2nd ed.). Washington, D.C.: American Psychological Association.

Hinton, D., Um, K., & Ba, P. (2001). *Kyol goeu* (wind overload): I. A cultural syndrome of orthostatic panic among Khmer refugees. *Transcultural Psychiatry, 38,* 403–432.

Hong G. K., & Domokos-Cheng Ham, M. (2001). *Psychotherapy and counseling with Asian American clients.* Thousand Oaks, CA: Sage.

Hwang, W. (2009). The formative method for adapting psychotherapy (FMAP): A community-based developmental approach to culturally adapting therapy. *Professional Psychology: Research and Practice, 40*(4), 369–377.

Kessler, R. C., McGonagle, K. A., Zhao, S., Nelson, C. B., Hughes, M., Eshleman, S., et al. (1994). Lifetime and 12-month prevalence of DSM–III–R psychiatric disorders in the United States. *Archives of General Psychiatry, 51,* 8–19.

Kessler, R. C., & Ustun, T. B. (2004). The World Mental Health (WMH) Survey Initiative Version of the World Health Organization (WHO) Composite International Diagnostic Interview (CIDI). *The International Journal of Methods in Psychiatric Research, 13*(2), 93–121.

Kinoshita, L. M., & Hsu, J. (2006). Assessment of Asian Americans: Fundamental issues and clinical applications. In F. T. L. Leong, A. G. Inman., A. Ebreo., L. H. Yang., L. M. Kinoshita., & M. Fu (Eds.), *Handbook of Asian American psychology* (2nd ed., pp. 409–428). Thousand Oaks, CA: Sage.

Kleinman A. (1978). Culture, illness and cure: Clinical lesions from anthropologic and cross-cultural research. *Annals of Internal Medicine, 88,* 251–258.

Kleinman, A., & Kleinman, J. (1985). Somatization: The interconnections in Chinese society among culture, depressive experiences, and the meaning of pain. In A. Kleinman & B. Good (Eds.), *Culture and depression* (pp. 429–490). Berkeley: University of California Press.

Kroenke, K., Spitzer R. L., & Williams J. B. (2001). The PHQ-9: Validity of a brief depression severity measure. *Journal of General Internal Medicine, 16*(9), 606–613.

Kwan, K.-L. K., Gong, Y., & Maestas, M. (2010). Language, translation, and validity in the adaptation of psychological tests for multicultural counseling. In J. G. Ponterotto, J. M. Casas, L. A. Suzuki, & C. M Alexander (eds.), *Handbook of multicultural counseling* (3rd ed., pp. 397–412). Thousand Oaks, CA: Sage.

Lam, C. Y., Pepper, C. M., & Ryabchenko, K. A. (2004). Case identification of mood disorders in Asian American and Caucasian American college students. *Psychiatric Quarterly, 75*(4), 361–373.

Leong, F. T. L., Inman, A. G., Ebreo, A., Yang, L. H., Kinoshita, L. M., & Fu, M. (Eds.). (2006). *Handbook of Asian American psychology* (2nd ed.) Thousand Oaks, CA: Sage.

Leong, F. T. L., Okazaki, S., & Tak, J. (2003). Assessment of depression and anxiety in East Asia. *Psychological Assessment, 15*(3), 290–305.

Leung, P. W. L., & Wong, M. T. (2003). Measures of child and adolescent psychopathology in Asia. *Psychological Assessment, 15*(3), 268–279.

Lewis-Fernandez, R., & Diaz, N. (2002). The cultural formulation: A method for assessing cultural factors affecting the clinical encounter. *Psychiatric Quarterly, 73*(4), 271–295.

Lin, K. M. (1983). *Hwa-Byung: A Korean culture-bound syndrome. American Journal of Psychiatry, 140,* 105–107.

Middleton, K. L., & Jones, J. L. (2000). Socially desirable response sets: The impact of country culture. *Psychology and Marketing, 17*(2), 149–163.

Morey, L. C. (2007). *The Personality Assessment Inventory professional manual.* Lutz, FL: Psychological Assessment Resources.

Morisaki, S., & Gudykunst, W. B. (1994). Face in Japan and the United States. In S. Ting-Toomey (Ed.), *The challenge of facework: Cross-cultural and interpersonal issues. SUNY series in human communication processes* (pp. 47–93). Albany: State University of New York Press.

Morrison, J. (2007). *The first interview* (3rd ed.). New York: Guilford.

Okazaki, S., & Sue, S. (2000). Implications of test revisions for assessment with Asian Americans. *Psychological Assessment, 12*(3), 272–280.

Parker G., Gladstone, G., & Chee, K. T. (2001). Depression in the planet's largest ethnic group: The Chinese. *American Journal of Psychiatry, 158*(6), 857–864.

Radloff, L. S. (1977). The CES-D scale: A self report depression scale for research in the general population. *Applied Psychological Measurement, 1,* 385–401.

Roberts, R. E., Roberts, C. R., & Chen, Y. R. (1997). Ethnocultural differences in prevalence of adolescent depression. *American Journal Community Psychology, 25,* 95–110.

Robins, L., et al. (1989). *NIMH diagnostic interview schedule, version III, revised (DIS-III-R).* St. Louis, MO: Washington University.

Robins, L. N., & Regier, D. A. (1991). *Psychiatric disorders in America: The epidemiologic catchment area study.* New York: Free Press.

Ryder, A. G., Yang, J., Zhu, X., Yaho, S., Yi, J., Heine, S. J., et al. (2008). The cultural shaping of depression: Somatic symptoms in China, psychological symptoms in North America? *Journal of Abnormal Psychology, 117*(2), 300–313.

Sartorius, N., & Janca, A. (1996). Psychiatric assessment instruments developed by the World Health Organization. *Social Psychiatry and Psychiatric Epidemiology, 31,* 55–69.

Sheikh, J. I., & Yesavage, J. A. (1986). Geriatric Depression Scale (GDS): Recent evidence and development of a shorter version. In T. L. Brink (Ed.), *Clinical gerontology: A guide to assessment and intervention* (pp. 165–173). New York: Haworth.

Simon, G. E., Goldberg, D. T., Von Korff, M., & Ustun, T. B. (2002). Understanding cross-national differences in depression prevalence. *Psychological Medicine, 32*, 585–594.

Spielberger, C. D. (1983). *Manual for the States–Trait Personality Inventory (STAI; Form Y)*. Palo Alto, CA: Consulting Psychologists Press.

Sue, D. W., & Sue, D. (2003). *Counseling the culturally different: Theory and practice* (4th ed.). New York: Wiley.

Sue, D., Sue, D. W., & Sue, S. (2006). *Understanding abnormal behavior* (8th ed.). Boston: Houghton Mifflin.

Sue, S., & Chang, J. (2003). The state of psychological assessment in Asia. *Psychological Assessment, 15*(3), 306–310.

Takeuchi, D. T., Chung, R. C., Lin, K. M., Shen, H., Kurasaki, K., Chun, C. A., et al. (1998). Lifetime and twelve-month prevalence rates of major depressive episodes and dysthymia among Chinese Americans in Los Angeles. *American Journal of Psychiatry, 155*(10), 1407–1414.

Takeuchi, D. T., Zane, N., Hong, S., Chae, D. H., Gong, F., Gee, G. C., et al. (2007). Immigration-related factors and mental disorders among Asian Americans. *American Journal of Public Health, 97*(1), 84–90.

Triandis, H. C. (1995). *Individualism and collectivism*. Boulder, CO: Westview.

Tsai, J. L., & Levenson, R. W. (1997). Cultural influences of emotional responding: Chinese American and European American dating couples during interpersonal conflict. *Journal of Cross-Cultural Psychology, 28*, 600–625.

U.S. Census Bureau. (2007). *Statistical abstract of the United States: 2007*. Washington, DC: United States Department of Commerce.

U.S. Department of Health and Human Services. (2001). *Mental health: Culture, race, and ethnicity—A supplement to "Mental health: A report of the surgeon general."* Rockville, MD: U.S. Department of Health and Human Services, Substance Abuse and Mental Health Services Administration, Center for Mental Health Services.

Van de Vijver, F. J. R., & Leung, K. (1997). *Methods and data analysis for cross-cultural research*. Thousand Oaks, CA: Sage.

Watson, D., & Friend, R. (1969). Measurement of social-evaluative anxiety. *Journal of Consulting and Clinical Psychology, 33*, 448–457.

Weissman, M. M., Bland, R. C., Canino, G. J., Faravelli, C., Greenwald, S., Hwu, H. -G., et al. (1996). Cross-national epidemiology of major depression and bipolar disorder. *Journal of the American Medical Association, 276*, 293–299.

Weissman, M. M., Bland, R. C., Canino, G. J., Faravelli, C., Greenwald, S., Hwu, H. -G., et al. (1997). The cross-national epidemiology of panic disorder. *Archives of General Psychiatry 54*, 305–309.

Westermeyer, J., & Janca. A. (1997). Language, culture and psychopathology: Conceptual and methodological issues. *Transcultural Psychiatry, 34*(4), 291–311.Yang, L. H., & WonPat-Borja, A. J. (2007). Psychopathology among Asian-Americans. In: F. T. L. Leong, A. G. Inman, A. Ebreo, L. H. Yang, L. M. Kinoshita, & M. Fu (Eds.), *Handbook of Asian American psychology* (2nd ed., pp. 379–405). Thousand Oaks, CA: Sage.

Yen, S., Robins, C. J., & Lin, N. (2000). A cross-cultural comparison of depressive symptom manifestation: China and the United States. *Journal of Consulting and Clinical Psychology, 68*(6), 993–999.

Zax, M., & Takahashi, S. (1967). Cultural influences on response style: Comparison of Japanese and American college students. *Journal of Social Psychology, 71*, 3–10.

Zhang, A. Y., & Snowden, L. R. (1999). Ethnic characteristics of mental disorders in five U.S. communities. *Cultural Diversity and Ethnic Minority Psychology, 5*(2), 134–146.

Zheng, Y. P., & Lin. K.-M. (2007). Comparison of the Chinese Depression Inventory and the Chinese version of the Beck Depression Inventory. *Acta Psychiatrica Scandinavica, 84*(6), 531–536.

Zheng, Y. P, Lin, K. M., Takeuchi, D., Kurasaki, K. S., Wang, Y. X., & Cheung, F. (1997). An epidemiological study of neurasthenia in Chinese-Americans in Los Angeles. *Comprehensive Psychiatry, 38*, 249–259.

Zheng, Y. P., Wei, L., Goa, L., Zhang, G., & Wong, C. (1988). Applicability of the Chinese Beck Depression Inventory. *Comprehensive Psychiatry, 29*, 484–489.

Zung, W. W. (1965). A self-rating depression scale. *Archives of General Psychiatry, 12*, 63–70.

DIAGNOSIS AND TREATMENT OF ADULT PSYCHOPATHOLOGY IN ASIANS

| 4 |

SUBSTANCE USE DISORDERS IN ASIANS

Eunice C. Wong and Karen Chan Osilla

The *Diagnostic and Statistical Manual of Mental Disorders-IV-TR* (*DSM IV-TR*) has been most widely used to classify substance use diagnoses (American Psychiatric Association, 2000). Table 4.1 illustrates the criteria for these diagnoses. To meet criteria for substance abuse, an individual's substance use has to lead to one or more of the following problems within a 12-month period: Failure to fulfill major responsibilities, use during hazardous situations (e.g., driving), legal problems, and/or continued use despite social or interpersonal consequences (American Psychiatric Association, 2000). In addition, the individual must not have had a previous diagnosis of substance dependence. The criteria for substance dependence is characterized by more physiological characteristics, including three or more of the following (see Table 4.1): Tolerance; withdrawal; use in larger amounts and over longer periods of time than intended; desire or unsuccessful efforts to control use; significant amount of time to obtain, use, and recover from the substance; important activities given up or reduced; and/or continued use despite problems (American Psychiatric Association, 2000).

There has been recent debate about updating these diagnostic classifications for the next iteration of the *DSM*. The main arguments include specificity of abuse with nonproblem use, specificity of symptoms to one disorder compared to symptoms common to several diagnoses (Widiger & Clark, 2000), withdrawal being an option versus a requirement for dependence (Langenbucher et al., 2000), and validity of the diagnoses with adolescents (Hasin et al., 2003). Therefore future iterations of the *DSM* are likely to evolve.

Substance use can be viewed along a continuum where factors that impact initiation may be different from factors leading to disorders. In fact, substance use has been increasingly conceptualized as a continuum of consumption patterns and associated problems (Institute of Medicine, 1990; U.S. Department of Health and Human Services, 2005). This continuum has been conceptualized more commonly for alcohol than drug use, where drinking patterns range from none to heavy and problem severity ranges from none to severe (Institute of Medicine, 1990). Understanding where an individual is located on the continuum based on the consumption levels and severity of problems is important for tailoring prevention, intervention, and treatment efforts. For example, in a stepped-care approach for alcohol problems, less intense and less costly services such as brief interventions may be conducted for an individual with at-risk drinking and nonsevere problems

---

TABLE 4.1: DSM-IV Criteria for Substance Abuse and Dependence (APA, 2000)[1]

Substance Abuse

- A maladaptive pattern of substance use leading to clinically significant impairment or distress, as manifested by one (or more) of the following, occurring within a 12-month period:

  1. recurrent substance use resulting in a failure to fulfill major role obligations at work, school, home (e.g., repeated absences or poor work performance related to substance use; substance-related absences, suspensions, or expulsions from school; neglect of children or household)
  2. recurrent substance use in situations in which it is physically hazardous (e.g., driving an automobile or operating a machine when impaired by substance use)
  3. recurrent substance-related legal problems (e.g., arrests for substance-related disorderly conduct)
  4. continued substance use despite having persistent or recurrent social or interpersonal problems caused or exacerbated by the effects of the substance (e.g., arguments with spouse about consequences of intoxication, physical fights)

- The symptoms have never met the criteria for Substance Dependence for this class of substances.

Substance Dependence

- A maladaptive pattern of substance use, leading to clinically significant impairment or distress, as manifested by three (or more) of the following, occurring at any time in the same 12-month period:

  1. tolerance, as defined by either of the following:
     - a need for markedly increased amounts of the substance to achieve intoxication or desired effect
     - markedly diminished effect with continued use of the same amount of substance
  2. withdrawal, as manifested by either of the following
     - the characteristic withdrawal syndrome for the substance
     - the same (or a closely related) substance is taken to relieve or avoid withdrawal symptoms
  3. the substance is often taken in larger amounts or over a longer period than was intended
  4. there is a persistent desire or unsuccessful efforts to cut down or control substance use
  5. a great deal of time is spent in activities to obtain the substance, use the substance, or recover from its effects
  6. important social, occupational or recreational activities are given up or reduced because of substance use
  7. the substance use is continued despite knowledge of having a persistent or recurrent physical or psychological problem that is likely to have been caused or exacerbated by the substance (e.g., continued drinking despite recognition that an ulcer was made worse by alcohol consumption)

---

[1] DSM-IV-TR, Diagnostic and Statistical Manual of Mental Disorders, ed. 4-TR. Washington DC: American Psychiatric Association (APA). 2000.

before more intensive outpatient and inpatient treatments (Sobell & Sobell, 1999). Understanding the factors that impact different points along the continuum of substance use may also help tailor prevention and intervention efforts. For the purposes of the present chapter, substance use disorders (SUDs) will be used to refer to alcohol and drug abuse and dependence problems.

Prevalence

Research on SUDs in Asian populations within the United States is expanding but continues to be rather limited. Few studies specifically address issues of substance abuse or dependence. The majority of existing research focus on patterns of substance use (N. W. S. Zane & Huh-Kim, 1998). The extent to which SUDs impact the Asian American population has not been fully understood. Most studies on problematic substance use within Asian American populations have been conducted with unrepresentative, small, or convenience-based samples (Nemoto et al., 1999; Sharma, 2004; Yi & Daniel, 2001). Recently, however, several large-scale epidemiological studies have been able to provide information on the prevalence of substance use disorders among Asian American and Pacific Islanders (AAPIs) (Sakai, Ho, Shore, Risk, & Price, 2005; Takeuchi et al., 2007; Wong, Klingle, & Price, 2004). In general, these studies suggest that AAPIs experience significantly lower levels of substance use disorders compared to the general U.S. population. For instance, the National Household Survey on Drug Abuse (NHSDA), a household interview survey conducted with a nationally representative U.S. sample of noninstitutionalized adults, found that 1.6% AAPIs met criteria for past year alcohol dependence compared to 2.7% of whites (Sakai et al., 2005). In terms of alcohol abuse, the National Epidemiologic Survey on Alcohol and Related Conditions (NESARC) yielded similar findings with AAPIs demonstrating the lowest rates (2.13%) compared to other ethnic groups such as whites (5.10%), Hispanics (3.97%) and blacks (3.29%) (Grant et al., 2004). Comparable findings for illicit drug use have been found with AAPIs exhibiting half the rate of past year drug dependence (0.6%) compared to whites (1.5%) (Sakai et al., 2005).

Despite the relatively low rates of SUDs, recent research indicates that SUDs may be on the rise for AAPIs. For example, between 1991 and 2001, rates of alcohol dependence more than doubled among AAPIs, increasing from 4% to 10% (Grant et al., 2004). Moreover, when rates of substance use are disaggregated by AAPI subgroups, a very different portrait is revealed (Price, Risk, Wong, & Klingle, 2002). When disaggregated, certain AAPI groups are shown to demonstrate substance use rates that are comparable to the general U.S. population. For instance, research on adolescent and adult alcohol, tobacco, and other drug use show that Native Hawaiians and other Pacific Islanders report lifetime and past month rates that are similar to, if not higher than, whites (U.S. Department of Health and Human Services, 2001a; Wong et al., 2004). Also, Korean and Japanese Americans have been shown to exhibit rates of illegal drug use that match those of the general U.S. population (U.S. Department of Health and Human Services, 2001a).

Further, findings suggest that AAPIs may face similar risk for SUDs as other ethnic groups in the United States once exposed to substances. For instance, Sakai et al. (2005) found that when individuals who had never tried alcohol or drugs were excluded, the prevalence of substance use disorders were similar between Asian and White Americans. Some evidence even indicateswhen

AAPIs do engage in substance use, they may use much more frequently and intensely. In a study involving seventh to twelve graders in New York, AAPIs who reported alcohol use tended to engage in heavy drinking (Barnes & Welte, 1986). Moreover, among binge drinkers, AAPIs consumed greater amounts of alcohol compared to European Americans.

Prevalence rates of substance use and SUDs have been primarily derived from self-report data. Some have posited that the low rates of substance use and SUDs may be partly due to underreporting because of stigma (N. W. S. Zane & Huh-Kim, 1998). In at least one instance, underreporting was shown in which smoking rates among Cambodian Americans were found to be lower when obtained via self-report than a salivary assay test (S. S. Kim, Ziedonis, & Chen, 2007). The discrepancy was especially large for Cambodian American women with 5.6% self-reporting smoking and 14.8% testing positive for smoking via the assay. Further research is needed to determine the degree to which prevalence estimates may be affected by underreporting. Prevalence rates of substance use and SUDs on Asian immigrants in countries other than the United States are scant. However, a recent study conducted in Canada indicated that rates of SUDs were higher among white than Asian Canadians (Tiwari & Jianli, 2006).

Information on SUDs is even more rare for many parts of Asia and the Pacific Islands (Devaney, Reid, & Baldwin, 2007). Limited data is collected on the prevalence of substance use, and SUDs can only be mostly inferred from information on drug treatment admission rates. Although the rates of substance and problem use vary across Asian countries, opiate and amphetamine-type stimulants (ATS) appear to the most prevalent substances affecting this region of the world. Globally, between 12.8 and 21.8 million people (0.3% to 0.5% of the world population aged 15–64) reported past year use of opiates, more than half of whom reside in Asia (United Nations Office on Drugs and Crime, 2010). It has been estimated that over 60% of treatment demand in Asia is due to opiate addiction (United Nations Office on Drugs and Crime, 2010). Recent estimates indicate that between 4.6 million and 20.6 million people in East and Southeast Asia report past year use of ATS (United Nations Office on Drugs and Crime, 2009). In some Asian countries, methamphetamine use is becoming more widespread and in many places ranks as the second most commonly used drug (Kozel, Lund, Douglas, & McKetin, 2007). Approximately 55% of the world's ATS users are in Asia (United Nations Office on Drugs and Crime, 2007), and there is an accompanying growing demand for treatment. For many substances, such as cannabis, there is a dearth of scientifically valid data to fully understand the impact of use and abuse of substances across many regions of Asia (United Nations Office on Drugs and Crime, 2010).

ETIOLOGY OF SUBSTANCE USE DISORDERS

Etiological models of substance use disorders have focused predominantly on biological, socio-contextual, and psychological factors (Miller & Carroll, 2006). A paucity of research has examined the generalizability of existing etiological models for Asians (Harachi, Catalano, Kim, & Choi, 2001). Moreover, few studies have investigated the role of specific cultural influences on the development or prevention of substance use disorders in Asian populations (Su, 1999). Of the available etiological studies conducted with Asians, the research has been predominantly limited to investigating risk and protective factors associated with patterns of substance *use* rather than *abuse*.

Nonetheless, research suggests that understanding factors related to substance use initiation may be particularly relevant for Asians. Although Asians have generally exhibited low rates of substance use disorders, findings suggest that once Asians are exposed to alcohol and drugs they may be at comparable risk for developing abuse and dependence problems (Sakai et al., 2005). Sakai and colleagues (2005) found that when individuals who had never tried alcohol or drugs were excluded, the prevalence of substance use disorders were similar between AAPIs and White Americans. Moreover, initiation of substance use is a necessary requisite to the development of SUDs.

The following section provides a review of etiological related studies focused on factors related to patterns of substance use and abuse for Asian populations. Available research will be reviewed according to four key domains: biological, sociocontextual, psychological, and cultural.

Biological Factors

Research on the biological factors associated with substance use has ranged from studies examining neurological pathways affected by drug use to genes affected by alcohol metabolism (Miller & Carroll, 2006). Among Asians, the biological research has mostly focused on genes that affect how alcohol is broken down in the body. These genes include aldehyde dehydrogenase (ALDH2) and alcohol dehydrogenase (ADH1B or AHD2). ALDH2 and ADH1B/AHD2. These genes vary in subtype number, and research shows that certain Asian groups have variants of these genes (i.e., ALDH2*2 and ADH1B*2). Asians have been shown to possess these gene variants at greater rates than whites (see Luczak et al., 2006, for a review). For example, possession of at least one ALDH2*2 allele has been found in approximately 30% of Chinese, 45% of Japanese, 28% of Koreans, 10% of Thais, and 1% of Filipinos, compared to 2–3% of Europeans. Possession of at least one ADH1B*2 allele has been found for 92% of Chinese, 84% of Japanese, 96% of Koreans, 81% Filipinos, and 54% of Thais, compared to 1–23% of Europeans (Goedde et al., 1992). These genetic variations are associated with decreased rates of alcohol metabolism and slower elimination of alcohol from the blood (Goedde et al., 1992). As a result, Asians with these genetic variations often experience physiological symptoms such as flushing (turning red), nausea, and increased heart rate and blood pressure upon ingesting alcohol (F. T. Nishimura et al., 2002).

Genetic variations in ALDH2 and ADH1B may lower the risk for alcohol dependence. A recent meta-analysis showed that Asians with one to two ADH1B*2 alleles and no ALDH2*2 alleles were four to five times less likely than individuals with no ADH1B*2 alleles to be alcohol dependent (Luczak, Glatt, & Wall, 2006). A similar protective effect was found among Asians with ALDH2*2 alleles such that Asians with one to two ALDH2*2 alleles were four to eight times less likely to be alcohol dependent (Luczak et al., 2006). These results suggest that biological factors may partially contribute to the lower rates of alcohol dependence evidenced among Asians.

These genetic variations may also be associated with lower likelihood of binge drinking among Asians with ALDH2*2 and ADH1B*2. Among Chinese, Korean, and white college students, students with ALDH2*2 were five times less likely than students without the variation to binge drink (Luczak, Wall, Shea, Byun, & Carr, 2001). The presence of ALDH2*2 appears to have more of a protective effect on heavier drinking than alcohol initiation or intoxication. Individuals with ALDH2*2 demonstrate similar rates of first-time alcohol use and intoxication compared to those without ALDH2*2 (T. L. Wall, Shea, Chan, & Carr, 2001). One potential mechanism that may explain this relationship is the increased acetaldehyde that results from not metabolizing alcohol, which in turn may lead to heightened responses to alcohol and decreased rates of heavy drinking (T. L. Wall, Shea, Luczak, Cook, & Carr, 2005). These genetic variations, however, are not likely to account entirely for ethnic group differences in alcohol use. In one study involving college students, ethnic group differences in binge drinking between Koreans and Chinese remained even after accounting for the differential presence of the ALDH2*2 (Luczak et al., 2001). Further research examining the interaction between these genetic variations and the environment is needed.

In addition, more research examining how these genetic variations impact rates of tobacco and drug use is warranted. While most studies have examined how these genetic variants protect from binge drinking and alcohol use disorders, these variants may partially protect individuals from drug use disorders. For example, Chinese, Korean, and Japanese college students with an ALDH2*2 allele were less likely to engage in regular tobacco use than students without this allele (T. L. Wall et al., 2001). It is also important to note that Asians are not the only group to have genetic variations in ALDH and ADH1B. For example, additional variations in ALDH1 and ADH1B have been shown to impact rates of alcohol dependence among Native Americans (Ehlers, Spence, Wall, Gilder, & Carr, 2004; T. L. Wall, Carr, & Ehlers, 2003) and Jewish Americans (Shea, Wall, Carr, & Li, 2001).

Social and Contextual Factors

Substantial research has focused on social and contextual influences on substance use and abuse (Hawkins, Catalano, & Miller, 1992; Miller & Carroll, 2006). Important social and contextual factors that have been linked to substance use and abuse can generally be categorized into the following broad categories: family, peer, neighborhood, and environment. Although there is still limited research investigating the impact of these social and contextual influences for Asians, a growing number of studies have examined the role of family and peer influences on substance use and abuse among Asians.

Family Influences

Characteristics of the family environment, such as the amount of family discord or family bonding, have been significantly associated with substance use and abuse (Hawkins et al., 1992). Generally, family discord or conflict has been linked to an increased risk in substance use, whereas family bonding has served as a protective factor in decreasing risk for substance use (Hawkins et al., 1992). Accumulating evidence suggests that family discord may be a relevant predictor of substance use and disorder for Asians (Guo, Hill, Hawkins, Catalano, & Abbott, 2002). In their review article, Harachi, Catalano, Kim, and Choi (2001) report on a number of studies showing that family discord was positively related to an increased risk for substance use among AAPIs (e.g., Zane, Park, & Aoki, 1999).

Other recent studies reveal a more complex relationship between family factors and patterns of substance use. Among Asians, family bonding (e.g., greater parent-youth communication) has been shown to exert indirect effects on substance use. In a study of at-risk Asian American youths with delinquency, poor academic performance, and parental drug use, high levels of parent-youth communication were related to less susceptibility to negative peer pressure, which in turn was associated with lower drug use (I. J. Kim, Zane, & Hong, 2002). Family bonding has also been shown to moderate the effects of risk factors associated with substance use. Using data from the National Longitudinal Study of Adolescent Health, a survey conducted with a nationally representative sample of adolescents, Hahm, Lahiff, and Guterman (2003) found that the degree of parent-child attachment mitigated the effects of youth acculturation on risk for substance use disorders. Higher levels of acculturation were associated with greater rates of alcohol use only for AAPI adolescents with low parental attachment. In contrast, AAPI adolescents with medium to high parental attachment did not demonstrate an increased risk for alcohol use even when highly acculturated. However, it is important to note that this effect was found only for the most highly acculturated AAPI adolescents (i.e., U.S.-born and residing within English-speaking households).

Contradictory findings showing no significant associations between family bonding and substance use have also been demonstrated among Asian Americans. In a longitudinal study following students from eleven Los Angeles Country schools into adulthood, family bonding or support was significantly associated with lower levels of drug use for European Americans but not for Asian Americans (Galaif & Newcomb, 1999). The authors noted that the null findings may have been due to insufficient power given the small sample size and low frequency of drug use among the Asian American sample. In addition, confirmatory factors analyses indicated that the constructs employed in the study may not have been equivalent across ethnic groups, suggesting the need for more culturally appropriate measures.

Family management practices such as parental styles and attitudes have also been documented to exert considerable risk and protective influences on substance use and disorders (Hawkins et al., 1992). For Asian American youth, a number of studies have found that parental disapproval of substance use appears to serve as a protective factor (Gillmore et al., 1990; Guo et al., 2002; Sasao, 1999). In the Seattle Social Development Project, a longitudinal study of 5th graders, Gillmore et al. (1990) examined predictors of substance use initiation among urban Asian American, White American, and African American students. Parental disapproval of substance use was significantly and negatively associated with alcohol use for Asian American students only. Using data from the same study, Guo et al. (2002) found that high levels of family monitoring and rules were significantly related to a decreased risk of substance use initiation for both Asian and White Americans. Similar findings with Vietnamese and Chinese high school students were found, in which parents' disapproval of substance use was related to lower lifetime reports of substance use (Sasao, 1994, 1999). In a study conducted with urban middle school students in Seattle, variations across Asian American subgroups were found with respect to family influences on substance use initiation (Harachi et al., 2001). Although higher levels of family management were related to a decreased risk in substance use initiation for all Asian American subgroups, greater levels of household rules were significantly associated with substance use only for Filipino families. Moreover, greater parental-child involvement served as a significant protective factor against substance use initiation for Chinese and Southeast Asian groups but not for Filipinos.

There is also evidence that certain types of family management practices may not exert significant influences on Asian American youth substance use. For example, Catalano et al. (1992)

found that parental oversight into a child's peer associations and the revoking of privileges were not related to substance use initiation among AAPI youth.

Peer Influences

Increasing evidence suggests that peer substance use is a significant predictor of substance use for Asian American youths. In a study of Los Angeles County high school students, Asian American youth reported knowing the least number of peers and adults engaged in substance use compared to other European American, African American, and Hispanic American students (Newcomb & Bentler, 1986). Nevertheless, perceptions of peer substance use were significantly related to self-reported use for all ethnic groups including Asian Americans. Moreover, with the exception of African Americans, peer substance use exerted a greater influence on substance use initiation than adult substance use. In the Seattle Social Development Project described previously (Gillmore et al., 1990), peer use of alcohol was significantly associated with drug use for urban 5th graders across various ethnic groups (i.e., Asian Americans, European Americans, and African Americans).

In a statewide California survey of high school students, Nakashima & Wong (2000) examined predictors of alcohol misuse between Korean and European Americans. Common predictors of alcohol misuse for both groups included peer encouragement to get drunk, grade level, and school adjustment. Interestingly, peer encouragement to get drunk exhibited a larger effect on alcohol misuse for Korean Americans than European Americans. The odds of reporting alcohol misuse among Korean Americans who reported having friends who encouraged them to get drunk was 17.94 compared to 7.16 for European Americans. In addition, European Americans had a host of other factors related to alcohol misuse that were not significant for Korean Americans, such as peer encouragement to drink, school adjustment, depression, self-esteem, and family stopping you from getting drunk. Otsuki (2003) examined peer and other psychosocial influences on substance use among Asian American female high school students. Perception of friends' substance use was significantly associated with past month alcohol use, current cigarette use, and past month marijuana use. Perception of friends' substance use exerted the largest effect on self-reported marijuana use.

Consistent with existing research, peers have been found to exert protective influences for Asian Americans as well. Peers' disapproval of substance use has been linked to a decreased risk for Asian American youth (Sasao, 1999; Unger et al., 2001). In a study conducted with a representative sample of 5,870 eighth grade students in California, friends' smoking was significantly associated with reports of past 30-day smoking for several ethnic groups, even after controlling for a number of potential covariates (e.g., age, gender, acculturation, tobacco-related knowledge, perceived positive and negative consequences of smoking, and perceived access to cigarettes) (Unger et al., 2001). However, compared to European Americans, the effect of friends' smoking was weaker for Asian Americans, African Americans, and Hispanic Americans. Unger and colleagues (2001) attributed the ethnic group variations in peer influences on smoking to differences in collectivism (i.e., valuing needs of in-group over one's own needs). They hypothesize that adolescents from collectivistic cultures may be more likely to conform to the roles and social norms prescribed by their parents and society, which in turn render them less susceptible to peer influences. Finally, Guo et al. (2002) found that peers' involvement in prosocial activities were associated with a decreased risk in substance use initiation across several ethnic groups including Asian Americans. Moreover, no differential effects in peers' involvement in prosocial activities were found across the ethnic groups.

Access

There is some evidence that suggests that substance use may be related to the degree of availability of substances (Hawkins et al., 1992). Some have posited that the lower prevalence of substance use and disorders among Asian Americans may partly be due to differential access to substances. In a 5-year longitudinal study of adolescents, Maddahian, Newcomb, and Bentler (1988) found that ethnic differences in substance use paralleled patterns of access to substances. For example, European Americans reported the greatest ease of access to alcohol compared to Asian Americans and African Americans. Correspondingly, rates of alcohol use were significantly greater among European Americans than Asian Americans and African Americans. Moreover, subsequent analyses revealed that ethnic group differences in cannabis use were greatly diminished after accounting for access related variables such as availability from friends and ease of acquisition. Gillmore et al. (1990) found that among urban 5th graders, Asian American reported the least availability of marijuana. However, availability of marijuana was positively associated with increased substance use across all ethnic groups including Asian Americans.

Unfair Treatment

A number of recent studies have examined the role of everyday unfair treatment on risk for substance use and disorders among Asian Americans. Using data from the Filipino American Community Epidemiological Survey (FACES), which involved 2,217 adult Filipino Americans residing in San Francisco or Honolulu, Gee, Delva, and Takeuchi (2007) found a significant positive association between reports of everyday unfair treatment (e.g., discrimination, disrespect) and alcohol dependence. Even after controlling for a number of factors (e.g., age, gender, location of residence, employment status, educational level, ethnic identity, nativity, language spoken, marital status, and several health conditions), unfair treatment continued to be significantly associated with alcohol dependence, prescription drug use, and illicit drug use. Similar findings have been demonstrated using data drawn from the National Latino and Asian American Study, the first study conducted with a nationally representative sample of AAPIs. Specifically, endorsement of any incidents of unfair treatment was positively related to a lifetime history of alcohol abuse or dependence (Chae, Takeuchi, Barbeau, Bennett, Lindsey, Stoddard et al., 2008). In addition, smoking was also shown to be connected to reports of unfair treatment. The odds of being a current smoker was four times higher among those who reported high levels of unfair treatment compared to those who reported no unfair treatment (Chae, Takeuchi, Barbeau, Bennett, Lindsey, & Krieger, 2008; Chae, Takeuchi, Barbeau, Bennett, Lindsey, Stoddard et al., 2008).

Psychological Factors

A host of psychological factors have been associated with the development of substance use and disorders. For example, temperament traits (e.g., impulsivity, sensation-seeking, negative affect), poor coping (e.g., cognitive or behavioral deficits), expectancies (e.g., positive expectancies of substance's effects), and motivation are psychological influences that have been connected to substance use and disorders (Marlatt & Gordon, 1985; Miller & Carroll, 2006). Only a handful of studies have involved an examination of psychological factors in the etiology of substance use and substance disorders for Asians.

A few studies have explored whether self-esteem is linked to substance use among Asian American youths. Maddahian et al. (1988) found that low self-esteem was a significant correlate of substance use across various ethnic groups but particularly for Asian American adolescents. Findings indicated that low self-esteem was a significant risk factor for alcohol and drug use and abuse for 38% of Asian Americans compared to only 25% of European Americans. However, Nakashima and Wong (2000) found no significant effects for self-esteem when examining risk for alcohol misuse or problem drinking among Korean American youth. Self-esteem has been shown to be significantly associated with cigarette smoking across various Asian American subgroups with some evidence of differential effects across gender (Otsuki, 2003). For instance, low self esteem was significantly associated with cigarette smoking for females of Chinese, Korean, and Filipino descent and for males of Japanese descent only. Finally, substance use and disorders have been found to frequently co-occur with depression (Grant et al., 2004; Kessler et al., 1997). Among adolescent youths, depression has been positively associated with increased use of alcohol and other drugs among youths of various ethnic backgrounds including Asian Americans (Maddahian et al., 1988).

Cultural Factors

Nativity Status and Age at Immigration

The National Latino and Asian American Study (NLAAS) provides one of the most comprehensive examinations of the relationship between acculturation and substance use disorders (Alegria et al., 2004). NLAAS is the first study conducted with a nationally representative sample of AAPIs in the United States. Findings from NLAAS indicate that nativity or birth origin is significantly associated with lifetime SUD for both AAPI men and women (Takeuchi et al., 2007). AAPIs born in the United States were more likely to experience a lifetime SUD than AAPIs who were born in another country. Moreover, the odds of experiencing any substance abuse disorder increased sharply with each successive generation. For example, compared to first-generation AAPI women (i.e., non-U.S.-born), the odds of any lifetime SUD were nearly eight times greater for second-generation (i.e., first family to be born in the United States) and nearly 10 times greater for third-generation women.

Further, there is some evidence that the age at time of immigration may contribute to risk for SUDs. Based on the NLAAS, AAPI men who immigrated to the United States between ages 18 and 34 had a significantly lower risk for SUDs than AAPI men born in the United States. Among

Filipino Americans specifically, as the age at the time of immigration decreased, the risk for alcohol dependence increased (Gong, Takeuchi, Agbayani-Siewert, & Tacata, 2003).

Ethnic Identity

Ethnic identity has been defined as the degree to which an individual identifies with his/her own ethnic cultural group or group of origin (Castro & Garfinkle, 2003; Phinney, 1992). Though ethnic identity has typically been heralded as a protective factor against substance use (Zickler, 2003), available empirical evidence has been somewhat mixed. For example, higher levels of ethnic identity have been positively associated with heavy drug use and an earlier onset of drug initiation (James, Kim, & Armijo, 2000; Marsiglia, Kulis, & Hecht, 2001). Ethnic identity has been shown to exert protective (Felix-Ortiz & Newcomb, 1995), risk (James et al., 2000), and nonsignificant influences on substance use (Trimble, 1995). Some have noted that a direct link between ethnic identification and drug use has not been sufficiently established (Beauvais, 1998) and that this may be due to the fact that ethnic identity may play more of a moderating role (Brook, Whiteman, Balka, Win, & Gursen, 1998). For instance, among Hispanic Americans, the effects of ethnic pride on alcohol use varied depending on the degree of traditional family norms (Castro & Alarcon, 2002). Individuals with a high level of ethnic pride *and* nontraditional family norms (i.e., liberal home environment) had the highest probability of lifetime alcohol use. In contrast, individuals with ethnic pride *and* traditional family norms (i.e., conservative home environment) had the lowest probability of lifetime alcohol use. Thus, the effects of ethnic identity may depend on the particular set of attitudes and values held by one's cultural group concerning drug use.

Among Asian Americans, ethnic identity has demonstrated more consistent effects. Higher levels of ethnic identity have been associated with lower levels of mental health problems (R. M. Lee, 2003; Mossakowski, 2003), decreased risk-taking behaviors (Beadnell et al., 2003), and diminished risk for substance use disorders (Chi, Kitano, & Lubben, 1988; Gong et al., 2003; Scheier, Botvin, Diaz, & Ifill-Williams, 1997). A small pilot study involving Asian American youth found that stronger ethnic identification was significantly related to lower rates of alcohol use (James, Kim, & Moore, 1997). Based on data from the NLAAS, AAPIs with lower levels of ethnic identify were significantly more likely to report having a history of an alcohol use disorder than AAPIs with high levels of ethnic identity (Chae, Takeuchi, Barbeau, Bennett, Lindsey, & Krieger, 2008; Chae, Takeuchi, Barbeau, Bennett, Lindsey, Stoddard, et al., 2008). Further, ethnic identification was found to moderate the effects of racial/ethnic discrimination on problematic alcohol use and nicotine use. Specifically, racial/ethnic discrimination was associated with an increased risk of an alcohol disorder and of being a current smoker for individuals with low levels of ethnic identification, but not for individuals with high levels of ethnic identification.

Cultural Norms and Attitudes

Cultural norms and attitudes have been associated with increased risk for substance use. For instance, alcohol is often a natural part of social gatherings and events within Asian communities

(O'Hare, 1995). Offering alcoholic beverages to guests may be considered a gesture of hospitality (Kwon-Ahn, 2001). Among Asian Indians, drinking may be considered a status symbol of one's standing in the community (Sandhu & Malik, 2001). In upper socioeconomic classes of Asian Indians, alcohol is often central to personal and professional interactions. Among Korean males, after-work social gatherings are commonplace, where coworkers may offer one another drinks and refusal of drinks may be seen as impolite, unsociable, or effeminate (Kwon-Ahn, 2001; C. K. Lee et al., 1990). Similarly, heavy drinking is often associated with social gatherings among Chinese and Japanese American men (Chi, Kitano, & Lubben, 1988). In such contexts, drunken behavior may be tolerated to a greater extent, and recognition of problematic use may be more difficult to identify. Among some Asian groups, alcohol may be used for medicinal purposes. For instance, Southeast Asians have been reported to view alcohol as possessing healing properties (Makimoto, 1998). In a sample of college students, Asians held stronger expectations for alcohol to provide tension relief than whites (O'Hare, 1995). However, no ethnic group differences in patterns of alcohol use were found. Few, if any, studies have examined the relationship between cultural norms and attitudes toward substance use and the development of SUDS.

Summary

Knowledge on the etiology of SUDs for Asians has been gradually accruing. Existing research lends some support for the generalizability of existing etiological models of substance use and SUDs for Asians, but most of the research has been conducted among Asian American populations. Still, findings have not always been consistent or uniform. For example, Maddahian et al. (1988) found that certain risk factors were related to increased drug use for European and Hispanic Americans but not for Asian Americans and Hispanic Americans. Moreover, even when common factors associated with substance use and SUDs have been established across ethnic groups, the strength of associations can vary. Newcomb et al. (1987) devised a risk factor index that was significantly related to cocaine and cannabis use across European American, Hispanic American, African American, Native American, and AAPI adolescents, but the relationship was weakest for Asian Americans.

The lack of consistency in findings may be due to several factors. Asians are a considerably heterogeneous group. Thus, when treated as an aggregate group, the characteristics of Asians in one study may differ widely from the characteristics of Asians in another study. For example, Asians in one study may differ from another study in acculturation levels, ethnic group composition, or psychopathology (e.g., refugee vs. nonrefugee group). Such variations may lead to differential findings with respect to factors that are associated with the etiology of substance use and SUDs. In addition, findings may vary depending on the type of substance examined (e.g., alcohol vs. illicit substances). Moreover, not all studies account for factors that may be confounded with ethnicity (e.g., socioeconomic status, demographics), which may lead to discrepant findings. Addressing these inconsistencies will be important for future research. Additional research is also needed to distinguish between factors that are linked to substance use versus SUDs. Finally, more research conducted with young adults and older individuals is warranted given that existing research with Asian populations has primarily focused on adolescent student samples.

TREATMENT FOR SUBSTANCE USE DISORDERS

Service Utilization

Asian Americans generally have been characterized as underutilizing SUD treatment services (Uba, 1994; N. W. S. Zane & Huh-Kim, 1998). This has been primarily based on AAPIs' low utilization rates of SUD treatment, their relative underrepresentation in treatment centers compared to their proportion in the population, and clinical observations (Sakai et al., 2005). Although suggestive of underutilization, such patterns of service use may also be indicative of low treatment need. However, two recent studies provide evidence that appear to confirm that AAPIs significantly underutilize SUD services relative to White Americans (Sakai et al., 2005; Wu, Ringwalt, & Williams, 2003). In the 1997 NHSDA, after controlling for a host of demographic related factors (e.g., age, gender, education, employment), AAPIs were the only ethnic minority group that were significantly less likely to use needed SUD services relative to White Americans among respondents meeting at least one of the *DSM-IV* criteria for alcohol or drug dependence (Sakai et al., 2005; Wu et al., 2003).

Based on data compiled from the years 2000 to 2003 from the National Household Survey on Drug Abuse, when looking at respondents with demonstrated treatment need (i.e., past year substance dependence), AAPIs were significantly less likely to have obtained SUD treatment compared to White Americans (Sakai et al., 2005). These ethnic group differences in service utilization were greatly diminished after accounting for nativity status and education. Thus, AAPIs' underutilization of SUD services may be attributable to AAPIs' lower acculturation levels. In addition, AAPIs' higher education levels may be related to greater access to other resources to deal with SUDs, greater stigma, or lower levels of functional impairment, which may inhibit service-seeking. Further research is needed to better understand possible explanatory factors for the observed ethnic group differences in SUD treatment utilization.

Recent statistics indicate that need for SUD treatment is rapidly growing among AAPIs. According to the 1999 Treatment Episode Data Set (TEDS), which contains information on admissions to publicly funded SUD facilities, treatment demand increased dramatically for AAPIs. Between 1994 and 1999, substance abuse treatment admissions increased by 37% for AAPIs (Substance Abuse and Mental Health Services Administration [SAMHSA], 2002b). The rate of increase in treatment admission was even greater when considering AAPI adolescents aged 12 to 17 during the same time period. AAPI adolescent admissions increased by 52% compared to only 20% by the general youth treatment population (SAMHSA, 2002a). Despite the increasing rates of treatment admissions, AAPIs still only made up 1% of all treatment admissions even though they made up nearly 4% of the U.S. population in 1999 (SAMHSA, 2002b).

In terms of the primary substance of abuse for all AAPI admissions, alcohol was the most highly endorsed (34%) followed by marijuana (19%), stimulants (19%), opiates (15%), and cocaine (11%) (SAMHSA, 2002b). When restricted to AAPI adolescent admissions, marijuana was the leading primary substance of abuse (59%) followed by alcohol (25%), stimulants (9%), cocaine (2%) and opiates (1%). AAPI adult and adolescents were admitted for stimulant abuse nearly three to four times more often compared to the total treatment population. Approximately 40% of AAPIs were referred to treatment through the criminal justice system, and the next largest referral source was via self- or individual referral (27–30%) (SAMHSA, 2002b).

Preliminary findings on AAPI SUD treatment outcomes provide a mixed picture. In a multi-site randomized clinical trial of brief interventions for marijuana-dependent adults, the odds of pretreatment dropout were three times higher for Asian Americans and Native Americans than European Americans even after controlling for a number of covariates (e.g., employment, education, age, other drug use) (Vendetti, McRee, Miller, Christiansen, & Herrell, 2002). However, Asian Americans and Native Americans were combined as a single group under "other," which may have masked important group differences. In contrast, no ethnic group differences in either treatment retention or duration were found between AAPIs and non-AAPIs enrolled in publicly funded treatment centers in California (Niv, Wong, & Hser, 2007). Moreover, with the exception of alcohol outcomes, no significant ethnic group differences in drug, employment, legal, medical, or psychiatric outcomes were found. AAPIs exhibited significantly lower alcohol problem severity at the nine-month follow-up interview relative to non-AAPIs. Findings should be viewed in light of the fact that the non-AAPI comparison group may have contained a great degree of heterogeneity, given that it was an aggregate of many different ethnic groups.

Treatment Barriers

A variety of cultural and practical barriers have been attributed to the low rates of treatment utilization by Asians (Leong & Lau, 2001; U.S. Department of Health and Human Services, 2001b; Uba, 1994). Practical barriers include lack of transportation, high cost of services, lack of insurance, and unavailability of treatment (U.S. Department of Health and Human Services, 2001b). Cultural barriers such as problem recognition, stigma, and lack of credibility of available treatments may also serve as significant obstacles to accessing services (D. W. Sue, Sue, & Sue, 2003). Though much of the literature on treatment barriers for AAPIs have been based on mental health services research (N. Zane, Hall, Sue, Young, & Nunez, 2004), many of the same barriers are likely to be relevant for SUD treatment. A more detailed discussion of areas where cultural disconnects may occur between Asians and standard SUD treatment is provided below.

Problem Recognition

Some have posited that Asians may not seek SUD treatment because of the lack of recognition of problematic substance use (Sakai et al., 2005). Failure to recognize and self-monitor problematic substance use has been attributed to cultural influences on how SUD is defined, cultural attitudes toward alcohol and substance use, and stigma associated with SUDs. According to the *DSM-IV*, substance dependence is defined by symptoms of physiological dependence (i.e., tolerance or withdrawal), loss of control over use, substantial time spent on supporting addiction, interference in social, occupational, or recreational activities, and failure to discontinue use even in light of harmful physical or psychological effects. When defining problematic use, Asians may place greater emphasis on the degree to which substance use impairs one's functioning than on the physiological symptoms that define dependence according to *DSM-IV* criteria (James et al., 1997). For instance, even if physiological signs of substance dependence may be present, Asians may not consider such use problematic as long as family obligations such as maintaining employment are met. There is also some evidence that Asians may associate alcoholism more with the negative physiological consequences of chronic alcohol use (e.g., liver damage) than with the inability to control one's drinking (Cho & Faulkner, 1993).

Others have posited that the stigma associated with substance abuse in Asian communities may be so great that individuals may not recognize problematic use out of sheer denial. Denial of substance abuse has been identified as the primary barrier to substance abuse treatment for Asian Americans (Ja & Aoki, 1993; James et al., 1997; Yen, 1992). Many AAPIs may enter treatment involuntarily through the legal system, child protective agencies, physicians, or employer mandates (Amodeo, Robb, Peou, & Tran, 1996). As described earlier, the largest source of referral for AAPI treatment admissions occurred via the criminal justice system (SAMHSA, 2000a).

Evidence confirming that AAPIs may experience problems recognizing SUDs has been documented. Among 10th-grade respondents in the HSAD, the proportion meeting criteria for a *DSM-III-R* SUD was consistently greater than the proportion perceiving a need for treatment across AAPI groups (e.g., 9.5% vs. 4% Chinese; 20% vs. 6% Filipino, 30% vs. 7% Native Hawaiian) (Wong et al., 2004). Interestingly, findings were similar for White Americans, with 28% meeting criteria for a SUD, but only 4% perceiving a need for treatment. Based on data compiled from the 2000 to 2003 NHSDA, among respondents with a SUD, AAPIs were six times less likely to perceive a need for treatment compared to European Americans (Sakai et al., 2005). Nevertheless, at an absolute level, only a small proportion of AAPIs (1.4%) and White Americans (9.3%) with an SUD reported needing treatment.

Stigma

Even upon recognition of problematic substance use, Asians may still be reluctant to seek treatment because of the stigma associated with SUDs and the use of drug treatment services (James et al., 1997; Shon & Ja, 1982). Asians may view SUDs as a lapse in willpower, moral weakness, or a medical problem (Fong & Tsuang, 2007; E. Lee, 2000; M. Y. Lee, Law, & Eo, 2003), which can compromise not only the reputation of the individual involved in problematic use but incur "loss of face" to the immediate and extended family for subsequent generations (Gong et al., 2003; Shon & Ja, 1982). Individuals with SUD problems may be seen as overly self-indulgent, nonproductive, and lacking in "good moral character." Consequently, Asians may make extended efforts to manage the SUD within the family and avoid outside professional help unless absolutely necessary (Ja & Aoki, 1993). Among Asian youth, reliance on oneself and friends may be the preferred coping strategy before turning to the family for help (M. Y. Lee, Law, Eo, & Oliver, 2002).

Lack of Credibility of Treatment

Standard treatments, which have been typically developed within a Western cultural framework, may not be viewed as a credible approach to SUDs by many Asians (S. Sue, 1999; S. Sue & Zane, 1989). Lack of familiarity and cultural mismatches with the treatment process and interventions have been cited as factors that may lessen the credibility of existing treatments among Asians (Kwon-Ahn, 2001; S. Sue, 1999). One aspect of treatment that may be unfamiliar and a cause of discomfort for Asians is talking about one's problems, particularly with an outside professional (Nguyen, 1982; D. W. Sue et al., 2003; Yamamoto & Acosta, 1982). Essentially, for many Asians, it may be unclear on how "talk therapy" can alleviate one's problem with SUDs. Compared to White Americans, AAPIs have been found to be significantly less likely to discuss mental health problems with friends, relatives, physicians, or mental health specialists (Zhang, Snowden, & Sue, 1998). AAPIs may be less likely to talk about personal problems to professionals or even family members because of cultural values that encourage self-reliance or because of stigma (Nemoto et al., 1999). Yet, a core feature of most SUD treatments involves discussing problematic substance use and related risk factors. Given the lack of familiarity with SUD treatment, many Asians may not understand why talking about one's problems is an important part of the treatment process. Moreover, treatment often focuses on examining negative thoughts or emotions, which may be directly opposed to culturally normative ways of coping. For instance, when faced with mental health problems, AAPIs have been described as relying on the avoidance of morbid thoughts and the suppression of negative emotions as an appropriate coping method (Butler, Lee, & Gross, 2007; Lam & Zane, 2004; Leong & Lau, 2001).

Asians' perceptions of SUD problems as a lapse in willpower or self-discipline can also lessen the credibility of existing treatments (Uba, 1994). For instance, Asians may believe that increased willpower or determination is all that is needed to overcome addictive behaviors and may not see the relevance of professional treatment. In addition, the perceived credibility of treatments may vary depending on the extent to which treatments align with beliefs about the role of willpower and addictive behaviors. For example, a core principle of Alcoholics Anonymous is acknowledging one's powerlessness over addiction, which may run counter to Asians' conceptualizations of coping with SUDs.

Although many Asians may lack familiarity with standard Western treatments, this does not mean that Asians enter treatment devoid of expectations. Studies suggest that Asians may expect, and be most responsive to, treatment that is brief, structured, and directive (Hwang, 2006; Lin & Cheung, 1999). Many Asians may enter treatment only as a last resort after their SUDs have caused significant impairment (Bui & Takeuchi, 1992; Durvasula & Sue, 1996). The main focus for many Asians may be on how to quickly return to previous functioning and on the restoration of roles and responsibilities (Murase & Johnson, 1974). However, the connection between core components of treatment and the resumption of responsibilities may not be readily apparent. For example, the twelve steps in Alcoholics Anonymous have no explicit mention of functional outcomes that may be particularly salient for Asians. Similarly, treatment programs that focus on thoughts or emotions associated with addictive behaviors without making explicit the connection to the restoration of roles and responsibilities may fail to garner credibility in the eyes of Asians. Interestingly, even though no significant ethnic group differences in treatment outcomes were found among respondents enrolled in California publicly funded treatment centers, AAPIs still rated alcohol and drug treatment as significantly less important compared to non-AAPIs (Niv et al., 2007).

Evidence-Based Practices

Although various research and professional organizations have developed guidelines and criteria for identifying evidence-based practices (EBPs) for SUDs (Miller, Zweben, & Johnson, 2005; Oregon Department of Human Services, 2009; SAMHSA, 2008), there has been no study on the effectiveness of such interventions with Asian populations (Alcohol and Drug Abuse Institute, 2010). EBPs for SUDs include interventions such as contingency management, cognitive behavioral approaches, 12-step facilitation, brief interventions, strategic family therapy, behavioral couples therapy, and a variety of pharmacological therapies (Alcohol and Drug Abuse Institute, 2010; Chambless & Ollendick, 2001; SAMHSA, 2008).

Nonetheless, the identification of EBPs remains controversial (Chambless & Ollendick, 2001; Glasner-Edwards & Rawson, 2010). There is a lack of consensus on the criteria and types of evidence used to classify EBPs, concern about the emphasis on manualized treatments versus therapist-client factors, and apprehension about the transferability of interventions developed in tightly controlled scientific conditions to real-world clinical settings (Glasner-Edwards & Rawson, 2010). Consequently, some have advocated for the dissemination of evidence-based skills or the use of a practice-based evidence approach (Glasner-Edwards & Rawson, 2010). Based on existing empirical support, Glasner-Edwards and Rawson (2010) recommended that efforts should be focused on the dissemination of evidence-based skills such as contingency management, motivational interviewing, cognitive behavioral–based coping skills and relapse prevention strategies, and family and couples counseling approaches that create social environments supportive of recovery. A practice-based evidence approach relies on continuous and real-time assessment of client outcomes, which is used to provide feedback to therapists with the aims of improving treatment quality and outcomes (Lambert & Burlingame, 2007; Lucock et al., 2003). A practice-based approach may be a viable means to track potential structural or cultural barriers to positive treatment engagement, process, or outcomes among Asian populations. Further research, however, is still needed to understand appropriate and effective approaches to addressing such barriers with Asians.

Given the many culturally based barriers that have been posited to impede Asians utilization of substance abuse treatment, the need for culturally competent services has been underscored (Andrade et al., 2006; S. T. Nishimura, Goebert, Ramisetty-Mikler, & Caetano, 2005; N. W. S. Zane & Huh-Kim, 1998). No studies to the authors' knowledge have examined the effectiveness of evidence-based substance abuse treatments among Asian populations. Thus, it is unclear whether available evidence-based substance abuse treatments would yield comparable outcomes for Asian populations or whether they would benefit from cultural tailoring. One study adapted a generic early intervention model consisting of screening, assessment, brief intervention, full intervention with a referral, and follow-up for substance abuse clinics serving Asian American communities in New York (Yu, Clark, Chandra, Dias, & Lai, 2009). Cultural adaptations included translating materials into seven major Asian languages, conducting screenings in community events outside of formal health settings, the provision of culturally competent bilingual counselors, and the targeting of cultural barriers to treatment. In addition, motivational interviewing and case management services were offered throughout the intervention and were posited to aid in keeping Asian clients engaged in treatment. At 6-month follow-up, positive outcomes were found with improvements on a number of domains including past 30-day alcohol or illicit drug use and reduced involvement in the criminal justice system (Yu et al., 2009).

Another study examined the effectiveness of a Hawaiian culture-based adolescent substance abuse treatment program (R. Kim & Jackson, 2009). The program involved multisystemic, culturally tailored services that included family therapy, nontraditional residential adventure-based experiential therapy (e.g., working in the *lo'I kalo* or taro field, canoe paddling), and a spiritual component to foster Hawaiian cultural concepts of kuliana (responsibility) and pono (righteousness). At 12-month follow-up, substantial gains were found on multiple domains including decreased substance use and criminal justice involvement and more positive mental health and social functioning (R. Kim & Jackson, 2009). Although these initial studies on culturally tailored substance abuse interventions yield promising findings, further research is needed to establish whether such practices are warranted as evidence-based treatments. Moreover, additional research (including randomized controlled study designs, comparisons to standard evidence-based treatments) will be better able to inform the importance and impact of culturally modified substance abuse treatment programs for Asians.

CONCLUSIONS

SUDs appear to be on the rise for Asians. Available estimates indicate that a substantial proportion of the substance-using population reside within Asia. However, research on the etiology and treatment of SUDs for Asians may not be accelerating at a sufficient pace to meet this growing concern. Currently, little is known about the effectiveness of standard SUD treatments for Asians. Further, empirical investigations on culturally appropriate SUD treatments are virtually nonexistent. Knowledge on potential barriers to treatment as well as guidance on strategies to improve access to services for Asians has been largely inferred from mental health services research. More research is needed to understand the unique factors related to SUD services that may affect treatment access, process, and outcomes when working with Asians. Finally, the successful treatment of SUDs will likely require addressing the wide heterogeneity between and within Asian groups as well as variations across types of substances. Responding to these complexities will greatly add to our knowledge base on how to tailor substance abuse treatments to diverse populations.

REFERENCES

Alcohol and Drug Abuse Institute. (2010). *Evidence based practices for treating substance use disorders.* Retrieved August 30, 2010, from http://adai.washington.edu/ebp/matrix.pdf.

Alegria, M., Vila, D., Woo, M., Canino, G., Takeuchi, D., Vera, M., et al. (2004). Cultural relevance and equivalence in the NLAAS instrument: Integrating etic and emic in the development of cross-cultural measures for a psychiatric epidemiology and services study of Latinos. *International Journal of Methods in Psychiatric Research, 13*(4), 270–288.

American Psychiatric Association. (2000). *Diagnostic and statistical manual of mental disorders* (4th ed., text revision). Washington, DC: Author. (*DSM-IV-TR*)

Amodeo, M., Robb, N., Peou, S., & Tran, H. (1996). Adapting mainstream substance-abuse interventions for Southeast Asian clients. *Families in Society, 77*(7), 403–413.

Andrade, N. N., Hishinuma, E. S., McDermott, J. F., Jr., Johnson, R. C., Goebert, D. A., Makini, G. K., Jr., et al. (2006). The National Center on Indigenous Hawaiian Behavioral Health study of prevalence of psychiatric disorders in native Hawaiian adolescents. *Journal of the American Academy of Child and Adolescent Psychiatry, 45*(1), 26–36.

Barnes, G. M., & Welte, J. W. (1986). Patterns and predictors of alcohol use among 7–12th grade students in New York State. *Journal of Studies on Alcohol, 47*(1), 53–62.

Beadnell, B., Stielstra, S., Baker, S., Morrison, D., Knox, K., Gutierrez, L., et al. (2003). Ethnic identity and sexual risk-taking among African-American women enrolled in an HIV/STD prevention intervention. *Psychology, Health, and Medicine, 8*(2), 187–198.

Beauvais, F. (1998). Cultural identification and substance use in North America: An annotated bibliography. *Substance Use and Misuse, 33*(6), 1315–1336.

Brook, J. S., Whiteman, M., Balka, E. B., Win, P. T., & Gursen, M. D. (1998). Drug use among Puerto Ricans: Ethnic identity as a protective factor. *Hispanic Journal of Behavioral Sciences, 20*(2), 241.

Bui, K. V. T., & Takeuchi, D. T. (1992). Ethnic minority adolescents and the use of community mental health care services. *American Journal of Community Psychology, 20*(4), 403–417.

Butler, E. A., Lee, T. L., & Gross, J. J. (2007). Emotion regulation and culture: Are the social consequences of emotion suppression culture-specific? *Emotion, 7*(1), 30–48.

Castro, F. G., & Alarcon, E. H. (2002). Integrating cultural variables into drug abuse prevention and treatment with racial/ethnic minorities. *Journal of Drug Issues, 32*(3), 783–810.

Castro, F. G., & Garfinkle, J. (2003). Critical issues in the development of culturally relevant substance abuse treatments for specific minority groups. *Alcoholism: Clinical and Experimental Research, 27*(8), 1381.

Catalano, R. F., Morrison, D. M., Wells, E. A., Gillmore, M. R., Iritani, B., & Hawkins, J. D. (1992). Ethnic differences in family factors related to early drug initiation. *Journal of Studies on Alcohol, 53*(3), 208.

Chae, D. H., Takeuchi, D. T., Barbeau, E. M., Bennett, G. G., Lindsey, J., & Krieger, N. (2008). Unfair treatment, racial/ethnic discrimination, ethnic identification, and smoking among Asian Americans in the National Latino and Asian American Study. *American Journal of Public Health, 98*(3), 485–492.

Chae, D. H., Takeuchi, D. T., Barbeau, E. M., Bennett, G. G., Lindsey, J. C., Stoddard, A. M., et al. (2008). Alcohol disorders among Asian Americans: Associations with unfair treatment, racial/ethnic discrimination, and ethnic identification (the National Latino and Asian Americans Study, 2002–2003). *Journal of Epidemiology and Community Health, 62*(11), 973–979.

Chambless, D. L., & Ollendick, T. H. (2001). Empirically supported psychological interventions: Controversies and evidence. *Annual Review of Psychology, 52*, 685–716.

Chi, I., Kitano, H. H. L., & Lubben, J. E. (1988). Male Chinese drinking behavior in Los Angeles. *Journal of Studies on Alcohol, 49*(1), 21–25.

Cho, Y. I., & Faulkner, W. R. (1993). Conceptions of alcoholism among Koreans and Americans. *International Journal of the Addictions, 28*(8), 681.

Devaney, D. M. L., Reid, G., & Baldwin, S. (2007). Prevalence of illicit drug use in Asia and the Pacific. *Drug and Alcohol Review, 26*(1), 97–102.

Durvasula, R., & Sue, S. (1996). Severity of disturbance among Asian American outpatients. *Cultural Diversity and Mental Health, 2*(1), 43.

Ehlers, C. L., Spence, J. P., Wall, T. L., Gilder, D. A., & Carr, L. G. (2004). Association of ALDH1 promoter polymorphisms with alcohol-related phenotypes in Southwest California Indians. *Alcoholism: Clinical and Experimental Research, 28*(10), 1481.

Felix-Ortiz, M., & Newcomb, M. D. (1995). Cultural identity and drug use among Latino and Latina adolescents. In G. J. Botvin, S. P. Schinke, & M. A. Orlandi (Eds.), *Drug abuse prevention with multiethnic youth* (pp. 147–165). Thousand Oaks, CA: Sage.

Fong, T., & Tsuang, J. (2007). Asian-Americans, Addictions, and Barriers to Treatment. *Psychiatry (Edgmont) 4*(11), 51–59.

Galaif, E. R., & Newcomb, M. D. (1999). Predictors of polydrug use among four ethnic groups A 12-year longitudinal study. *Addictive Behaviors, 24*(5), 607–631.

Gee, G. C., Delva, J., & Takeuchi, D. T. (2007). Relationships between self-reported unfair treatment and prescription medication use, illicit drug use, and alcohol dependence among Filipino Americans. *American Journal of Public Health, 97*(5), 933–940.

Gillmore, M. R., Catalano, R. F., Morrison, D. M., Wells, E. A., Iritani, B., & Hawkins, J. D. (1990). Racial differences in acceptability and availability of drugs and early initiation of substance use. *American Journal of Drug and Alcohol Abuse, 16*(3–4), 185–206.

Glasner-Edwards, S., & Rawson, R. (2010). Evidence-based practices in addiction treatment: Review and recommendations for public policy. *Health Policy, 97*, 93–104.

Goedde, HW, Agarwal, DP, Fritze, G., Meier-Tackmann, D., Singh, S., Beckmann, G., et al. (1992). Distribution of ADH 2 and ALDH2 genotypes in different populations. *Human Genetics, 88*(3), 344–346.

Gong, F., Takeuchi, D. T., Agbayani-Siewert, P., & Tacata, L. (2003). Acculturation, psychological distress, and alcohol use: Investigating the effects of ethnic identity and religiosity. In K. M. Chun, P. B. Organista, & G. Marín (Eds.), *Acculturation: Advances in theory, measurement, and applied research*, 109–206. Washington, DC: American Psychological Association.

Grant, B. F., Dawson, D. A., Stinson, F. S., Chou, S. P., Dufour, M. C., & Pickering, R. P. (2004). The 12-month prevalence and trends in DSM-IV alcohol abuse and dependence: United States, 1991–1992 and 2001–2002. *Drug and Alcohol Dependence, 74*(3), 223–234.

Guo, J., Hill, K. G., Hawkins, J. D., Catalano, R. F., & Abbott, R. D. (2002). A developmental analysis of sociodemographic, family, and peer effects on adolescent illicit drug initiation. *Journal of the American Academy of Child and Adolescent Psychiatry, 41*(7), 838–845.

Hahm, H. C., Lahiff, M., & Guterman, N. B. (2003). Acculturation and parental attachment in Asian-American adolescents' alcohol use. *Journal of Adolescent Health, 33*(2), 119–129.

Harachi, T. W., Catalano, R. F., Kim, S., & Choi, Y. (2001). Etiology and prevention of substance use among Asian American youth. *Prevention Science, 2*(1), 57–65.

Hasin, D. S., Schuckit, M. A., Martin, C. S., Grant, B. F., Bucholz, K. K., & Helzer, J. E. (2003). The validity of DSM-IV alcohol dependence: what do we know and what do we need to know? *Alcoholism: Clinical and Experimental Research, 27*(2), 244.

Hawkins, J. D., Catalano, R. F., & Miller, J. Y. (1992). Risk and protective factors for alcohol and other drug problems in adolescence and early adulthood: Implications for substance abuse prevention. *Psychological Bulletin, 112*(1), 64–105.

Hwang, W. C. (2006). The psychotherapy adaptation and modification framework: application to Asian Americans. *American Psychologist, 61*(7), 702.

Institute of Medicine. (1990). *Broadening the base of treatment for alcohol problems: Report of a study by a committee of the Institute of Medicine, Division of Mental Health and Behavioral Medicine.* Washington, DC: National Academy Press.

Ja, D. Y., & Aoki, B. (1993). Substance abuse treatment: Cultural barriers in the Asian-American community. *Journal of Psychoactive Drugs, 25*(1), 61–71.

James, W. H., Kim, G. K., & Armijo, E. (2000). The influence of ethnic identity on drug use among ethnic minority adolescents. *Journal of Drug Education, 30*(3), 265–280.

James, W. H., Kim, G. K., & Moore, D. D. (1997). Examining racial and ethnic differences in Asian adolescent drug use: The contributions of culture, background, and lifestyle. *Drugs: Education, Prevention, and Policy, 4*(1), 39–51.

Kessler, R. C., Crum, R. M., Warner, L. A., Nelson, C. B., Schulenberg, J., & Anthony, J. C. (1997). Lifetime co-occurrence of DSM-III-R alcohol abuse and dependence with other psychiatric disorders in the National Comorbidity Survey. *Archives of General Psychiatry, 54*(4), 313.

Kim, I. J., Zane, N. W. S., & Hong, S. (2002). Protective factors against substance use among Asian American youth: A test of the peer cluster theory. *Journal of Community Psychology, 30*(5), 565–584.

Kim, R., & Jackson, D. (2009). Outcome evaluation findings of a Hawaiian culture-based adolescent substance abuse treatment program. *Psychological Services, 6*(1), 43–55.

Kim, S. S., Ziedonis, D., & Chen, K. W. (2007). Tobacco use and dependence in Asian Americans: A review of the literature. *Nicotine and Tobacco Research, 9*(2), 169–184.

Kozel, N. J., Lund, J., Douglas, J., & McKetin, R. (2007). *Patterns and trends of amphetamine-type stimulants (ATS) and other drugs of abuse in East Asia and the Pacific 2006.* Bangkok: United Nations Office on Drugs and Crime, Regional Center for East Asia and the Pacific.

Kwon-Ahn, Y. H. (2001). Substance abuse among Korean Americans: A sociocultural perspective and framework for intervention. In S. L. A. Straussner (Ed.), *Ethnocultural factors in substance abuse treatment*. New York: Guilford.

Lam, A. G., & Zane, N. W. S. (2004). Ethnic differences in coping with interpersonal stressors: A test of self-construals as cultural mediators. *Journal of Cross-Cultural Psychology, 35*(4), 446.

Lambert, M. J., & Burlingame, G. M. (2007). Uniting practice-based evidence with evidence-based practice. *Behavioral Healthcare, 27*(10), 16–20.

Langenbucher, J., Martin, C. S., Labouvie, E., Sanjuan, P. M., Bavly, L., & Pollock, N. K. (2000). Toward the DSM-V: The withdrawal-gate model versus the DSM-IV in the diagnosis of alcohol abuse and dependence. *Journal of Consulting and clinical Psychology, 68*(5), 799–809.

Lee, C. K., Kwak, Y. S., Yamamoto, J. O. E., Rhee, H. E. E., Kim, Y., Han, J., et al. (1990). Psychiatric epidemiology in Korea: Part II. Urban and rural differences. *Journal of Nervous and Mental Disease, 178*(4), 247.

Lee, E. (2000). *Working with Asian Americans: A Guide for Clinicians*. New York: Guilford.

Lee, M. Y., Law, F. M., Eo, E., & Oliver, E. (2002). Perception of substance use problems in Asian American communities by Chinese, Indian, and Vietnamese American youth. *Journal of Ethnic and Cultural Diversity in Social Work, 11*(3–4), 159–189.

Lee, M. Y., Law, P., & Eo, E. (2003). Perception of substance use problems in Asian American Communities by Chinese, Indian, Korean, and Vietnamese Populations. *Journal of Ethnicity in Substance Abuse, 2*(3), 1–29.

Lee, R. M. (2003). Do ethnic identity and other-group orientation protect against discrimination for Asian Americans? *Journal of Counseling Psychology, 50*(2), 9.

Leong, F. T. L., & Lau, A. S. L. (2001). Barriers to providing effective mental health services to Asian Americans. *Mental Health Services Research, 3*(4), 201–214.

Lin, K. M., & Cheung, F. (1999). Mental health issues for Asian Americans. *Psychiatric Services, 50*(6), 774.

Lucock, M., Leach, C., Iveson, S., Lynch, K., Horsefield, C., & Hall, P. (2003). A systematic approach to practice-based evidence in a psychological therapies service. *Clinical Psychology and Psychotherapy, 10*(6), 389–399.

Luczak, S. E., Glatt, S. J., & Wall, T. J. (2006). Meta-Analyses of ALDH2 and ADH1B with alcohol dependence in Asians. *Psychological Bulletin, 132*(4), 607–621.

Luczak, S. E., Wall, T. L., Shea, S. H., Byun, S. M., & Carr, L. G. (2001). Binge drinking in Chinese, Korean, and white college students: Genetic and ethnic group differences. *Psychology of Addictive Behaviors, 15*(4), 306–309.

Maddahian, E., Newcomb, M. D., & Bentler, P. M. (1988). Risk factors for substance use: Ethnic differences among adolescents. *Journal of Substance Abuse, 1*(1), 11–23.

Makimoto, K. (1998). Drinking patterns and drinking problems among Asian-Americans and Pacific Islanders. *Alcohol Health and Research World, 22*(4), 270–275.

Marlatt, G. A., & Gordon, J. R. (1985). *Relapse prevention*. New York: Guilford.

Marsiglia, F. F., Kulis, S., & Hecht, M. L. (2001). Ethnic labels and ethnic identity as predictors of drug use among middle school students in the Southwest. *Journal of Research on Adolescence, 11*(1), 21–48.

Miller, W. R., & Carroll, K. (2006). *Rethinking substance abuse: what the science shows, and what we should do about it*. New York: Guilford.

Miller, W. R., Zweben, J., & Johnson, W. R. (2005). Evidence-based treatment: Why, what, where, when, and how? *Journal of Substance Abuse Treatment, 29*(4), 267–276.

Mossakowski, K. N. (2003). Coping with perceived discrimination: Does ethnic identity protect mental health? *Journal of Health and Social Behavior*, 318–331.

Murase, T., & Johnson, F. (1974). Naikan, Morita, and Western psychotherapy. *Archives of General Psychiatry, 31*(1), 121–128.

Nakashima, J., & Wong, M. M. (2000). Characteristics of alcohol consumption, correlates of alcohol misuse among Korean American adolescents. *Journal of Drug Education, 30*(3), 343–359.

Nemoto, T., Aoki, B., Huang, K., Morris, A., Nguyen, H., & Wong, W. (1999). Drug use behaviors among Asian drug users in San Francisco. *Addictive Behaviors, 24*(6), 823–838.

Newcomb, M. D., & Bentler, P. M. (1986). Frequency and sequence of drug use: A longitudinal study from early adolescence to young adulthood. *Journal of Drug Education, 16*(2), 101–120.

Newcomb M. D., Maddahian E., Skager R., & Bentler P. M. (1987). Substance abuse and psychosocial risk factors among teenagers: Associations with sex, age, ethnicity, and type of school. *The American Journal of Drug and Alcohol Abuse,13*(4), 413–433.

Nguyen, S. D. (1982). Psychiatric and psychosomatic problems among Southeast Asian refugees. *Psychiatric Journal of the University of Ottawa, 7*(3), 163–172.

Nishimura, F. T., Fukunaga, T., Kajiura, H., Umeno, K., Takakura, H., Ono, T., et al. (2002). Effects of aldehyde dehydrogenase-2 genotype on cardiovascular and endocrine responses to alcohol in young Japanese subjects. *Autonomic Neuroscience: Basic and Clinical, 102*(1–2), 60.

Nishimura, S. T., Goebert, D. A., Ramisetty-Mikler, S., & Caetano, R. (2005). Adolescent alcohol use and suicide indicators among adolescents in Hawaii. *Cultural Diversity and Ethnic Minority Psychology, 11*(4), 309–320.

Niv, N., Wong, E. C., & Hser, Y.-I. (2007). Asian Americans in community-based substance abuse treatment: Service needs, utilization, and outcomes. *Journal of Substance Abuse Treatment, 33*(3), 313–319.

O'Hare, T. (1995). Differences in Asian and white drinking: Consumption level, drinking contexts, and expectancies. *Addictive Behaviors, 20*(2), 261–266.

Oregon Department of Human Services. (2009). *Addiction and mental health services approved practices and processes.* Retrieved August 30, 2010, from http://www.oregon.gov/DHS/mentalhealth/ebp/practices.shtml.

Otsuki, T. A. (2003). Substance use, self-esteem, and depression among Asian American adolescents. *Journal of Drug Education, 33*(4), 369–390.

Phinney, J. S. (1992). The multigroup ethnic identity measure: A new scale for use with diverse groups. *Journal of Adolescent Research, 7*(2), 156.

Price, R. K., Risk, N. K., Wong, M. M., & Klingle, R. S. (2002). Substance use and abuse by Asian Americans and Pacific Islanders: Preliminary results from four national epidemiologic studies. *Public Health Reports, 117*(Suppl 1), S39.

Sakai, J. T., Ho, P. M., Shore, J. H., Risk, N. K., & Price, R. K. (2005). Asians in the United States: Substance dependence and use of substance-dependence treatment. *Journal of Substance Abuse Treatment, 29*(2), 75–84.

Sandhu, D. S., & Malik, R. (2001). Ethnocultural background and substance abuse treatment of Asian Indian Americans. In S. L. A. Straussner (Ed.), *Ethnocultural factors in substance abuse treatment,* 368–392. New York: Guilford.

Sasao, T. (1999). Identifying at-risk Asian American adolescents in multiethnic schools: Implications for substance abuse prevention interventions and program evaluation. In *Identifying at-risk Asian American adolescents in multiethnic schools: Implications for substance abuse prevention interventions and program evaluation* (pp. 143–167): DHHS Publication No. SMA 98–3193.

Scheier, L. M., Botvin, G. J., Diaz, T., & Ifill-Williams, M. (1997). Ethnic identity as a moderator of psychosocial risk and adolescent alcohol and marijuana use: Concurrent and longitudinal analyses. *Journal of Child and Adolescent Substance Abuse, 6,* 21–47.

Sharma, M. (2004). Substance abuse and Asian Americans: Need for more research. *Journal of Alcohol and Drug Education, 47*(3), 1–3.

Shea, S., Wall, T., Carr, L., & Li, T.-K. (2001). ADH2 and alcohol-related phenotypes in Ashkenazic Jewish American college students. *Behavior Genetics, 31*(2), 231–239.

Shon, S. P., & Ja, D. Y. (1982). Asian families. In M. McGoldrick, J. K. Pearce, & J. Giordano (Eds.), *Ethnicity and family therapy* (pp. 208–228). New York: Guilford.

Sobell, M. B., & Sobell, L. C. (1999). Stepped care for alcohol problems: An efficient method for planning and delivering clinical services. In *Changing addictive behavior: Bridging clinical and public health strategies* (pp. 331–343). New York: Guilford.

Su, S. S. (1999). Stress and coping as a conceptual framework for studying alcohol and drug use among Asian American adolescents. *Drugs and Society, 14*(1–2), 37–56.

Substance Abuse and Mental Health Services Administration (SAMHSA). (2002a, July 5). *The DASIS Report. Asian and Pacific Islander Adolescents in Substance Abuse Treatment: 1999.* Rockville, MD: Office of Applied Studies, Substance Abuse and Mental Health Services Administration, Department of Health and Human Services.

Substance Abuse and Mental Health Services Administration. (2002b, August 16). *The DASIS Report. Asians and Pacific Islanders in Substance Abuse Treatment: 1999.* Rockville, MD: Office of Applied Studies, Substance Abuse and Mental Health Services Administration, Department of Health and Human Services.

Substance Abuse and Mental Health Services Administration. (2008). *National registry of evidence-based programs and practices.* Retrieved August 30, 2010, from http://www.nrepp.samhsa.gov.

Sue, D. W., Sue, D., & Sue, D. (2003). *Counseling the culturally diverse: Theory and practice*. Hoboken, NJ: Wiley.

Sue, S. (1999). Science, ethnicity, and bias: Where have we gone wrong? *American Psychologist, 54*(12), 1070–1077.

Sue, S., & Zane, N. (1989). The role of culture and cultural techniques in psychotherapy. *American Psychologist, 42*, 37–45.

Takeuchi, D. T., Zane, N., Hong, S., Chae, D. H., Gong, F., Gee, G. C., et al. (2007). Immigration-related factors and mental disorders among Asian Americans. *American Journal of Public Health, 97*(1), 84–90.

Tiwari, S. K., & Jianli, W. (2006). The epidemiology of mental and substance use-related disorders among white, Chinese, and other Asian populations in Canada. *Canadian Journal of Psychiatry, 51*(14), 904–912.

Trimble, J. E. (1995). Toward an understanding of ethnicity and ethnic identity, and their relationship with drug use research. In G. J. Botvin, S. P. Schinke, & M. A. Orlandi (Eds.), *Drug abuse prevention with multi-ethnic youth* (pp. 3–27). Thousand Oaks, CA: Sage.

Uba, L. (1994). *Asian Americans: Personality patterns, identity, and mental health*. New York: Guilford.

Unger, J. B., Rohrbach, L. A., Cruz, T. B., Baezconde-Garbanati, L., Howard, K. A., Palmer, P. H., et al. (2001). Ethnic variation in peer influences on adolescent smoking. *Nicotine and Tobacco Research, 3*(2), 167–176.

United Nations Office on Drugs and Crime. (2007). *World Drug Report 2007*. Retrieved on August 26, 2010, from http://www.unodc.org/unodc/en/data-and-analysis/WDR-2007html.

United Nations Office on Drugs and Crime. (2009). *World Drug Report 2009*. Retrieved on August 23, 2010, from http://www.unodc.org/unodc/en/data-and-analysis/WDR-2009.html.

United Nations Office on Drugs and Crime. (2010). *World Drug Report 2010*. Retrieved on August 26, 2010, from http://www.unodc.org/unodc/en/data-and-analysis/WDR-2010.html.

U.S. Department of Health and Human Services. (2001a). *Drug use among racial/ethnic minorities*. U.S. Department of Health and Human Services, National Institute on Drug Abuse.

U.S. Department of Health and Human Services. (2001b). *Mental health: Culture, race, and ethnicity: A supplement to "Mental Health: A Report of the Surgeon General."* Rockville, MD: U.S. Department of Health and Human Services.

U.S. Department of Health and Human Services. (2005). *Helping patients who drink too much: A clinician's guide*. Rockville, MD: National Institutes of Health, National Institute on Alcohol Abuse and Alcoholism.

Vendetti, J., McRee, B., Miller, M., Christiansen, K., & Herrell, J. (2002). Correlates of pre-treatment drop-out among persons with marijuana dependence. *Addiction, 97*(Suppl 1), 125–134.

Wall, T. L., Carr, L. G., & Ehlers, C. L. (2003). Protective association of genetic variation in alcohol dehydrogenase with alcohol dependence in Native American mission Indians. *American Journal of Psychiatry, 160*(1), 41–46.

Wall, T. L., Shea, S. H., Chan, K. K., & Carr, L. G. (2001). A genetic association with the development of alcohol and other substance use behavior in Asian Americans. *Journal of Abnormal Psychology, 110*(1), 173–178.

Wall, T. L., Shea, S. H., Luczak, S. E., Cook, T. A., & Carr, L. G. (2005). Genetic associations of alcohol dehydrogenase with alcohol use disorders and endophenotypes in white college students. *Journal of Abnormal Psychology, 114*(3), 456–465.

Widiger, T. A., & Clark, L. A. (2000). Toward DSM-V and the classification of psychopathology. *Psychological Bulletin, 126*(6), 946–963.

Wong, M. M., Klingle, R. S., & Price, R. K. (2004). Alcohol, tobacco, and other drug use among Asian American and Pacific Islander adolescents in California and Hawaii. *Addictive Behaviors, 29*(1), 127–141.

Wu, L.-T., Ringwalt, C. L., & Williams, C. E. (2003). Use of substance abuse treatment services by persons with mental health and substance use problems. *Psychiatric Services, 54*(3), 363–369.

Yamamoto, J., & Acosta, F. X. (1982). Treatment of Asian Americans and Hispanic Americans: similarities and differences. *Journal of the American Academy of Psychoanalysis, 10*(4), 585–607.

Yen, S. (1992). Cultural competence for evaluators working with Asian/Pacific Island-American communities; some common themes and important implications. In M. Orlandi, R. Weston & L. Epstein (Eds.), *Cultural competence for evaluators* (pp. 236–291). Rockville, MD: U.S. Department of Health and Human Services.

Yi, J. K., & Daniel, A. M. (2001). Substance use among Vietnamese American college students. *College Student Journal, 35*(1), 13–23.

Yu, J., Clark, L. P., Chandra, L., Dias, A., & Lai, T. F. M. (2009). Reducing cultural barriers to substance abuse treatment among Asian Americans: A case study in New York City. *Journal of Substance Abuse Treatment, 37*(4), 398–406.

Zane, N., Hall, G. C. N., Sue, S., Young, K., & Nunez, J. (2004). Research on psychotherapy with culturally diverse populations. In M. J. Lambert (Ed.), *Bergin and Garfield's handbook of psychotherapy and behavior change* (5th ed., pp. 767–804). New York: Wiley.

Zane, N. W. S., & Huh-Kim, J. (1998). Addictive behaviors. In L. C. Lee & N. W. S. Zane (Eds.), *Handbook of Asian American Psychology* (pp. 527–554). Thousand Oaks, CA: Sage.

Zhang, A. Y., Snowden, L. R., & Sue, S. (1998). Differences between Asian and white Americans' help seeking and utilization patterns in the Los Angeles area. *Journal of Community Psychology, 26*(4), 317–326.

Zickler, P. (2003). *Ethnic identification and cultural ties may help prevent drug use.* Bethesda, MD: NIDA Notes. Retrieved July 25, 2007, from www.drugabuse.gov/NIDA_notes/NNVol14N3/Ethnic.html.

| 5 |

SCHIZOPHRENIA AND OTHER PSYCHOSIS IN ASIANS AND ASIAN AMERICANS

Keh-Ming Lin, Hai-Gwo Hwu, and Ming T. Tsuang

INTRODUCTION

Are schizophrenia, and psychotic disorders in general, universal? Do schizophrenia and other psychosis exist in all societies, or might they have been the product of modern civilizations (Evans, McGrath, & Milns, 2003), particularly those influenced by European cultures (Fabrega, 2001)? To what extent are they biologically based, and in what ways might they be culturally shaped (Desjarlais et al., 1995; Jablensky & Sartorius, 1988; Jablensky, Sartorius & Ernberg, 1992; Kleinman, 1988; Tsuang, 1982; Tsuang, 2000)? More specifically, do they exist in Asia? Are they common in populations with Asian roots? These are the questions that have confronted scholars and clinicians ever since the concept of "dementia praecox," the term preceding "schizophrenia," was coined by Emil Kraepelin, one of the founding fathers of modern psychiatry. Partially for the reason of addressing such a question, Kraepelin made a historical journey to East Asia around the turn of the century, reaching Java in 1904 (Jilek, 1995). He found to his satisfaction, that there indeed were patients, not necessarily confined in the hospital, as tended to be the case in Germany and other European countries at the time, who showed symptoms and clinical courses very similar to those he had seen in Europe. This has been regarded by some as the starting point of a field termed "comparative psychiatry" (Jilek, 1995; H. B. Murphy, 1982). In subsequent decades, medical anthropologists, psychiatric clinicians and researchers have continued to provide evidences indicating that phenomena similar to what had been classified as schizophrenia and other types of psychoses could be found in practically all human groups, including those in Asia (Leff, 1981; Mezzich, Kleinman, Fabrega, & Parron 1996; Mezzich et al.,

1999; Westermeyer, 1985). However, questions remain in regard to whether there are ethnic, cultural, regional, and even temporal variations in terms of the prevalence and incidence of these atrocious problems, whether, to what extent, and in what manner their symptomatology, "natural" course, and outcomes might be influenced by sociocultural factors, how such factors might affect diagnostic practices, and how the labeling might affect those inflicted with such disorders as well as their loved ones.

This chapter is focused on the Asian and Asian American populations. But Asians (and Asian Americans) represent a huge and extremely divergent group, easily encompassing more than half of the total world population at this point, with people speaking divergent languages, adhering to practically all religions on the earth, and ranging widely in their worldviews, from the traditional to the postmodern. Some of the societies suffer from extreme poverty, while others are some of the most industrialized and most prosperous (L. C. Lee & Zane, 1998; Lin & Cheung, 1999; T. Y. Lin, Tseng, & Yeh, 1995). Any simplistic conclusions would thus be extremely dangerous and could be misleading and harmful. Instead, what the authors would like to strive at achieving with this chapter is a general picture highlighting issues and trends that are particularly worth noting, providing readers with guides and directions that maybe useful for more detailed and in-depth understanding of related issues.

ISSUES RELATED TO NOSOLOGY AND MANIFESTATIONS

Coined a century earlier by Eugene Bleuler, one of the pioneers in psychopathology, the term and concept of "schizophrenia" remained ambiguous with fluid boundaries until the rise of Neo-Krapaelinian movement in the 1950s (Mayes & Horwitz, 2005; Feighner et al., 1972), leading to the development of specific criteria for the diagnosis as reflected in *DSM-III* published in 1980 (American Psychiatric Association [APA], 1980). The diagnostic scheme has since remained similar in subsequent *DSM* editions, reflecting only relatively minor changes. Briefly, in *DSM-IV-TR* (APA, 1994), major criteria include characteristic symptoms (two of five symptoms including delusions, hallucinations, disorganized speech, gross disorders, or catatonic behavior, and negative symptoms), presence of dysfunction, and continuous signs of disturbance for at lease six months. Disorders with prominent psychotic symptoms not qualified for the diagnosis are classified as schizophreniform disorder, schizoaffective disorder, delusional disorder, brief psychotic disorder, shared psychotic disorder, psychotic disorder due to a general medical condition, substance-induced psychotic disorder, and psychotic disorder not otherwise specified. Psychotic symptoms also are often seen in patients suffering from mood disorders, especially bipolar I disorder and major depressive disorder (with psychotic features). *DSM-III* and its latter versions have been extensively applied across ethnic/cultural groups and across nations with surprising ease. By improving specificity and interrater reliability, these criterion-based diagnostic systems also represent a methodological breakthrough for cross-cultural and cross-national comparative studies (Mezzich, Kleinman, Fabrega & Parron, 1996). However, as discussed later in this chapter, misdiagnosis remains a major concern for cross-cultural research and practice (Alarcon et al., 2002; Mezzich et al., 1999).

Epidemiology

Although psychoses and phenomena similar to those that would be regarded as schizophrenia and other psychotic disorders have been well documented in Ancient Asian texts since antiquity (Lin, Kleinman, & Lin, 1981; Lin, 1981), until the last century, psychotic patients had rarely been isolated from their families and the communities in Asian societies as in the West (Foucault, 1965; Bivins & Pickstone, 2007). Thus, although references pointing to psychotic behaviors abound in historical records and other written materials, and medical texts refer to their classification, etiology, and treatment (K. M. Lin 1981), little is documented regarding the magnitude of these problems in Asian societies. However, starting in the late nineteenth century, a number of forces, including missionary and colonial influences, and the ascendancy of the organized modern medical care systems, led to the mushrooming of mental institutions largely modeled after those in the West. Such developments supported the thesis that there had been a previously unmet need for the care of patients largely characterized by bizarre and odd behaviors and often chronic deteriorating course. However, since the initiation and maintenance of such institutions depend on complex factors including the level of affluence, the policy of the societies, and the degree of stigma associated with mental illnesses, it would be grossly misleading to use hospitalization data as proxies for estimating the prevalence and incidence of psychotic problems in different societies.

Large-scale, systematic, community-based surveys using increasingly standardized and sophisticated methodologies have been attempted in different Asian countries since the end of World War II. For example, in Taiwan, Tsung-yi Lin and his colleagues conducted a groundbreaking study including three communities encompassing urban, suburban, and rural regions, and found an overall rate of psychosis of 0.38%, including 0.21% schizophrenia (Lin, Kleinman, & Lin, 1981; T. Y. Lin, et al., 1995). Fifteen years later, when a survey with a similar design was conducted by the same group in the same communities, rates for psychoses remained essentially the same, although those for "minor" mental health problems had increased dramatically in the meantime.

In the early 1980s, modeling after the Epidemiological Catchment Area Project, and using a detailed and structured instrument, the Diagnostic Interview Schedule (DIS), researchers in Taiwan found rates for psychotic disorders still in the range of those reported earlier (Hwu, Yeh, & Chang, 1989; W. M. Compton et al., 1991). Similar surveys in China during this period also in general reported similar results, finding prevalence of various psychotic disorders mostly at the lower range of what had been reported in the West, but with even lower rates of other types of psychiatric disorders (Lin & Kleinman, 1981; Xiang et al., 2008). Around the same time, studies with similar designs using comparable structured interview tools (i.e., DIS) in Korea also revealed similar findings regarding psychotic disorders, although reporting much higher rates of "minor psychiatric disorders," including depression and particularly alcohol use disorders, than those coming from Chinese communities (Lee, 1988; C. K. Lee et al., 1990a, 1990b; L. C. Lee & Zane, 1998).

Based on the experiences with the DIS, a new research tool named the Composite International Diagnostic Interview (CIDI) was developed and initially employed for a nationally representative study in the United States (the National Comorbidity Study), which was subsequently adopted by the World Health Organization (WHO) for a new wave of epidemiological surveys conducted in many countries from practically all continents, including sites in many Asian countries (China, Hong Kong, India, Japan, Taiwan). The results, as reviewed by a number of authors (e.g., Goldner et al., 2002; Isaac, Chand, & Murthy, 2007; Jablensky & Sartorius, 1988), showed remarkable consistency across time and research methodology, generally reporting that the lifetime prevalence of schizophrenia ranged between 0.5% and 2% of the general population. However, data derived from the Asian sites showed substantially lower rates (less than .05%). The reason for such discrepancy remains unclear, and methodological problems including under-reporting could not be completely ruled out. In this regard, a recent study conducted in Taiwan estimating the prevalence of schizophrenia by analyzing the National Health Insurance claim data is illuminating (Chien et al., 2004). It showed that in 1996, when the universal coverage first started, the estimated treated prevalence was 0.334%. Five years later, as services became more widely available, the proportion nearly doubled, reaching 0.664%. Since treated prevalence is significantly lower than the "real" prevalence" (in any society, a large portion of those who would have been classified as schizophrenic continue to manage to evade the mental health care system, the so-called walking schizophrenics), the actual prevalence is expected to be much higher, and probably would fall in the ranges of those reported from other developed countries.

Although at least two large-scale, community-based epidemiological surveys have been conducted among Asian Americans in the United States in the past decade (the Chinese American *Psychiatric Epidemiological* Study [*CAPES*] and the National Latino and Asian American Study [NLAAS]) (Takeuchi et al., 1998, 2007), methodological and sample size considerations precluded the systematic examination of the epidemiology of psychotic disorders. However, responding to the demands and needs from Asian American communities, multicultural/multilingual mental health services have been established in a number of major metropolitan areas in the North America, including Los Angeles, New York, San Francisco, and Vancouver, BC. The majority of the patients receiving treatment from these clinics are severely mentally ill, and many of them suffer from schizophrenia or related conditions, testifying to the fact that Asian Americans are far from immune from these devastating disorders (Cheung & Snowden, 1990; H. Chen, Kramer, Chen, & Chung, 2005; Chow 2002; Lu, Du, Gaw, & Lin, 2002; Sue et al., 1991; Yamamoto, 1978).

To summarize, there is little doubt that schizophrenia and related psychotic conditions exist in all societies, including all Asian communities. Epidemiological data have been available for these conditions only from some of the Asian groups, which have tended to show rates that fall within the lower range as compared to those reported from the West. To what extent such differences reflected methodological, including sampling, problems, remain to be further elucidated.

Symptomatology

As the concept of schizophrenia, diagnostic classifications, and assessment tools evolve over time, data also have emerged suggesting substantial variations, both across ethnic/cultural lines and over time, in symptom manifestations and the distribution of subtypes of schizophrenia, as well as boundaries between schizophrenia, bipolar disorder, and other related conditions (Kupfer, First, & Regier, 2002; K. M. Lin, 1996a, 1996b; Maslowski et al., 1998; Tsuang & Simpson, 1984). For example, whereas earlier literature reported high prevalence of schizophrenic patients characterized by symptoms patterns compatible with the catatonic and hebephrenic subtypes, these forms of clinical presentation have become rare in recent decades (Ungvari et al., 2007; Stompe et al, 2003).

Instead, the majority of the patients seen in the clinical settings in recent years tend to be classified as either with disorganized or paranoid types. Such temporal trends have been observed in various cultural groups including those from Asian countries (Rin, Schooler, & Caudill, 1973; Tateyama et al., 1999). It is not entirely clear to what extent such temporal changes reflect shifts in the diagnostic system and patient population characteristics. For example, in the past, behaviorally less disturbing patients might have been less likely to reach the mental health system. As services became gradually more widely available, those who had been less disturbing to the society or less easily persuaded to receive psychiatric care started to enter the system. Similar problems exist in terms of the explanation for the observation of higher rates of acute psychosis, typically with fulminant clinical course in patients from less developed countries as well as those residing in rural areas who have been less exposed to modern lifestyles and worldviews (e.g., recent migrants or immigrants from the countryside to the city). It is debatable whether "selection biases" also plays a role here, meaning that cases with abrupt onset and severe symptoms more likely to be seen by mental health professionals than those whose conditions were more insidious. However, results from recent studies including the WHO international, multisite Determinants of Outcome project support the view that this form of psychotic manifestation is indeed more frequently seen in less modernized non-Western populations (Jablensky, Sartorius, & Emberg, 1992; Isaac, 2007).

Studies on the psychopathology of schizophrenia have traditionally focused on two dimensions, forms and contents. It has long been assumed that whereas the contents of patients' psychotic manifestations and symptom patterns are largely influenced by their sociocultural backgrounds, the underlying form or structure remains cross-culturally similar and may be regarded as universal. For example, while the propensity for paranoia and delusional thinking exists in all populations, the content or type of delusions and hallucinations may vary dramatically across ethnic/cultural groups (Bhavsar & Bhugra, 2008; Charney et al., 2002; Stompe, Ortwein-Swoboda, Ritter, & Schanda, 2003; Thomas et al., 2007). Religious affiliations, political milieus, family and social ties, and prevailing beliefs and life experiences significantly determine the nature and targets of one's delusion or paranoia. In communities where religious and spiritual traditions still hold strong sway, delusions with religious contents often outweigh other types of delusions: while those with traditional Chinese backgrounds maybe more likely to be in communication with their deceased ancestors or local deities (Tseng & McDermott, 1981; Lin, 1981; al-Issa, 1995), devout Catholics would more likely talk about divine interventions coming from Jesus or Maria (or being their incarnation). In politically oppressed countries, patients often form delusions of being persecuted by the government, by the army, or by the secret police. In a parallel fashion, American schizophrenic patients during the Cold War years not infrequently would believe that the KGB or the CIA were after them. In addition, one of this chapter's authors was quite surprised by the high prevalence of American schizophrenic patients being constantly preoccupied with the thoughts and delusions (as well as hallucinations accompanying these delusions) of people calling them homosexuals ("faggots"), whether they actually had homosexual inclinations or not. This is despite the fact that homosexuals were not necessarily less discriminated against in Asian countries, and might have to do with a higher level of "homophobia" associated with a greater emphasis of American culture in general on individualism and personal identity, leading schizophrenic patients already suffering from identify confusion to be even more preoccupied on any salient feature in this regard.

Conversion and dissociative phenomena often represent significant challenges for clinicians working in cross-cultural settings (Tseng & McDermott, 1981). In more traditional societies where members are much more immersed in traditional or local religious/spiritual beliefs, such problems often are presented in the form of "possession," which might be transient or persistent, reversible or irreversible, ego-syntonic or ego-alien. There appears to be a general consensus that possession phenomena are much more common in non-Western societies, including Asian societies, for reasons that will not be belabored here (Tseng & McDermott, 1981; Lewis-Fernandez, 1992; Mezzich & Lin, 1995; Mezzich, Lin, & Hughes, 1999). Suffice it to say that, along with its salience in the general populations, possession or possession-like symptoms also are more frequently observed among patients with schizophrenic and other psychosis, representing additional challenges for mental health professionals working in the cultural situations.

Somatization represents another major domain deserving careful attention when clinicians work with patients with Asian and other "non-Western" populations. Although the meaning and implication of "somatization" in Asians has been debated (Kleinman & Singer, 1977; Kendell, 1975; Kleinman, 1980, 1982; Kleinman & Kleinman, 1985; Kirmayer & Robbins, 1996; Kirmayer & Young, 1998; see also Chapter 8 in this volume), it is now clear that the somatic clinical presentations are reflections of "idiom of distress" rather than innate psychopathology (i.e., patients are not ignorant of their psychological states, but are accustomed to preferentially express their distress through physical terms), the fact remains that most patients, and their family members, might initially focus their complaints exclusively or largely on physical problems. Without deeper and more careful probing, such mode of presentation may camouflage the existence of psychotic symptoms (e.g., complaints of feeling "empty" or "heaviness" in the head might or might not be associated with experiences of thought poverty or thought insertion). On the other hand, for patients who have been more deeply imbued in the Asian medical systems, the meaning for their somatic symptoms may not be easily understood or may be misunderstood for clinicians not familiar with such traditions, leading to mislabeling somatizing patients as psychotic. For example, concerns about cold or hot sensations, or fear of a block or lump in the body, might appear less bizarre when seen in light of the traditional medical belief systems including the yin-yang balance and the importance of the circulation of Qi (vital energy) (Lim & Lin, 1996).

Culture-Bound Syndromes

The meaning and place of the term "culture-bound syndrome" have long been debated, especially since the inclusion of a list of such proposed syndromes in an appendix of the American Psychiatric Association's *Diagnostic and Statistical Manual* (4th ed.; APA, 1994). It appears reasonable to state that both "culture-bound" and "syndrome" are problematic terms (see Chapter 15 in this volume). Probably none of the phenomena included in the list are exactly culture-bound. For example, koro, a condition that has been reported from Southern Chinese for over two centuries, involving an observation that one's penis is shrinking. This at times leads to extreme panic, typically in those with the age-old belief that if the shrinking continues, the penis would disappear completely, leading to death (Bernstein & Gaw, 1990; Mezzich & Lin, 1995; Mezzich, Lin, & Hughes, 1999; Rosca-Rebaudengo, Durst, & Minuchin-Itzigsohn, 1996). In communities laden with political or social tension, outbreaks of koro epidemics have been reported, leading to hundreds or thousands of patients being rushed to hospitals, holding on to their penises either with their own hands, with family member's help, or using specifically designed instruments. Such behaviors might appear extremely bizarre for those unfamiliar with the medical beliefs, but the majority of such cases recovered fully and showed no residual signs of psychosis. Since koro-like episodes, both in sporadic and in epidemic forms, have been reported in other sociocultural settings (Dzokoto & Adams, 2005; Buckle et al., 2007), it certainly is not "culturally specific." Nevertheless, clinicians confronted with situations like this will have to deal with the challenging task of discerning cultural phenomena from psychopathology, and the interaction between the two.

Other so-called culture-bound syndromes, such as the "Dhat syndrome" (Bhatia & Malik, 1991; Bottero, 1991) among Indians and "Taijin-Kyofu-Sho" (fear of people) in Japanese (Chang, 1997; Russell, 1989), represent similar challenges. For example, is taijin kyofusho just a severe form of social phobia? Are Japanese more likely to succumb to such an extreme form of social phobia that would render them totally incapacitated, at times accompanied with profound fear or beliefs that others in their proximity could easily detect their "defects," such as bodily odor, facial flushing (thus it is also called "erythrophobia"), or facial expressions that they fear would be offensive? Is the boundary between Taijin-Kyofu-Sho and schizophrenia perhaps similar to that between severe obsessive-compulsive disorders and psychosis? Although many similar questions await further clarification, it is important to note that the existence of these and other so-called culture-bound syndromes highlight the potency of culture in not only coloring, but actually shaping, the "lived" experiences of the patients, which need to be taken into consideration in order for the clinical assessment of such patients to be accurate and useful (K. M. Lin & Lin, 2002).

Differential Diagnosis and Misdiagnosis

The discussions and examples included in the previous several sections highlight the importance of culture in the assessment and differential diagnosis of psychotic patients, and point to the higher likelihood that patients with non-Western backgrounds, particularly those still imbued in their traditional cultures of origin, might be more likely misdiagnosed, particularly in cross-cultural clinical settings, where mental health professionals may not be sufficiently familiar with such "contextual" issues, or may possess biased or stereotypical views on the patients' cultural traits. That misdiagnosis is a particular hazard for patients with ethnic minority backgrounds, including many Asian Americans, has been amply demonstrated in the literature. A case in point is the issue of misclassifying patients with mood disorders as schizophrenic. A large body of literature has demonstrated that African Americans, and to a lesser extent, Hispanic Americans and Asian Americans, are much more likely to be labeled with schizophrenia even though objective and systematic assessment (often with standard instruments) would indicate otherwise (Adebimpe, 1981; B. E. Jones & Gray, 1986; Lawson, 1986; Strakowski et al., 2003). Most often this came at the expense of misidentifying bipolar disorder as schizophrenia. It is at present not completely clear what might be responsible for this trend that has persisted for over half a century, despite convincing research data showing the gap. Limited research evidence suggests that matching clinicians' and patients' ethnic and cultural backgrounds exerts no, or at most minimal, effects in mitigating this problem, suggesting that the "socializing" effects of professional training outweigh cultural affiliation or congruence.

Cultural distance, especially when coupled with language barrier and other socioeconomic limitations, might lead to mislabeling of patients with more severe diagnosis, at times leading to tragic consequences (Lin & Cheung, 1999; K. M. Lin, 1996a, 1996b). For example, earlier studies revealed that many Asian patients had been chronically incarcerated in the state hospital system in California for decades, with a diagnosis of schizophrenia in no way substantiated by the medical records. Investigations showed that they might have first been admitted after some behavioral disturbances probably secondary to the stress of maladjustment in a foreign land. After protesting the "incarceration" for a few months, they often settled down and became "professional" or even "model" patients in the institutions. Such tragedies might not be limited to times past, as in recent years we have waves of new immigrants and refugees who are often by themselves, devoid of significant family or social ties, and thus without adequate advocacy, possessing limited English-language skills, and typically suffering from a full array of psychological and behavioral problems, including post-traumatic stress disorder, that might be easily misconstrued as signs or prodromes of schizophrenia (K. M. Lin, 1990; Kinzie, 2006).

The Degree of Fit Between DSM Nosology/Diagnostic Schemes and Asian Populations

From what has been discussed in the previous sections, it is apparent that the concept of schizophrenia, as reflected in the current and recent *DSM* classification systems (dating from 1980), is relevant and useful for the Asian populations. It is less clear whether, and to what extent, individual diagnostic criteria might represent the best fit for separate Asian populations. The mere fact that "categories" (i.e., "disorders") as defined by a number of criteria or factors are able to sort members of a population into different groups does not by itself guarantee that these categories are useful or optimal for that particular population. Few empirical studies have specifically examined the magnitude and nature of issues related to such "categorical fallacy," which may be a major reason behind the observation regarding misdiagnosis and classification of patients with psychotic-like presentations in cross-cultural settings (K. M. Lin & Lin, 2002). As discussed in previous sections, this should be a major focus for future studies aiming at clarifying the applicability of *DSM* diagnostic systems in Asian populations.

ETIOLOGICAL MODELS

Throughout the last century, divergent etiological models have powerfully influenced mental health professionals' conceptualization of schizophrenia, and informed the development of their treatment approaches. Embedded in the term "schizophrenia," as well as its precursor, "dementia praecox," was the conviction held by the field's leading thinkers, regarding human behaviors, especially those labeled "deviant," as predominantly determined by heredity (Tsuang, Bar, Stone, & Faraone, 2004). With the ascendancy of psychoanalysis and dynamic psychiatry, a totally different view became dominant, essentially ignoring the "biological" aspect of psychiatric disorders, focusing instead on the "pathogenetic" role of social environments in causing mental disorders (Scheff, 1999, 2006), including schizophrenia. Although both traditions have made profound contributions in enriching our understanding of conditions such as schizophrenia, the tension and "schism" between the two schools remain visible, barely hidden under the veneer of the recent emphasis on the importance of gene-environmental interactions (Charney et al., 2002; Dick, Riley, & Kendler, 2010; Tsuang et al., 2004), and the call for a more integrated, "biopsychosocial" (or "biopsychosociocultural") approach (Corcoran et al., 2003; Day et al., 19887).

"Biological" Models

Genetic and Neurotransmitter Mechanisms

The imprint of the tradition of "descriptive psychiatry" on research and practices related to schizophrenia is readily visible. Evidences accumulated through a large number of twin studies, and more recently molecular genetic studies, demonstrate that hereditary factors explain approximately 50% of the risk for developing schizophrenia (Tsuang, 1982, 1984, 2000). Recent molecular genetic studies have led to significant progress in our understanding of the contribution of specific genes and/or genome regions in this regard (Owen, Craddock, & O'Donovan, 2005). However, as each proposed gene only explains a small portion of the variance for the risk for schizophrenia, the concept of a "candidate gene" for schizophrenia has remain elusive, leading to the common belief that schizophrenia is a "complex disease" that could only be explained by the combination of multiple risk genes, as well as gene-gene interactions (Dick, Riley, & Kendler, 2010; P. J. Harrison & Owen, 2003; Tsuang et al., 2004).

The biologically oriented etiological model has also led to major efforts in using various brain imaging methodologies (e.g., functional magnetic resonance imaging [fMRI], positron emission tomography [PET]), demonstrating that schizophrenia patients tend to have smaller brain volume, with larger ventricular sizes, and that they are more likely to show hypoactivity in the frontal and temporal lobes, as well as the hippocampus (Broyd et al., 2008). These altered activities have been linked to neurocognitive deficits commonly observed among schizophrenic patients (Kircher & Thienel, 2005).

The largely serendipitous finding of the antipsychotic effects of the phenothiazines and butyrophenones (as well as reserpine) in the 1950s served as the watershed for the ascendency of the movement of "biological psychiatry," and the emergence of the "dopamine hypothesis" (H. M. Jones & Pilowsky, 2002). Subsequent pharmacological and brain imaging studies have demonstrated the utility of such a hypothesis in explaining aspects of schizophrenia. However, in recent years, the finding that a number of "atypical" antipsychotics, typically with strong affinity to other neurotransmitter receptor pathways, especially serotonergic receptors, indicate that other mechanisms may be equally important for mediating the pathogenesis of schizophrenia as well as the antipsychotic effects of neuroleptics (Seeman, 2002). In addition, the psychotomimetic effects of glutamate blocking drugs, such as phencyclidine and ketamine, suggest that the neurotransmitter glutamate and the function of the NMDA (N-methyl D-aspartate) glutamate receptors also play important roles in the pathogenesis of schizophrenia (Coyle, 2006; Konradi & Heckers, 2003; Lane et al., 2006; Tsai, Lane, Yang, Chong, & Lange, 2004).

To the extent that schizophrenia and other psychotic disorders are genetically determined, questions arise as to what evolutionary purposes such genetic predilections might confer to those who suffer from such a condition, in order for it to survive evolutionary pressure. Theories abound, including balanced selection (e.g., traits associated with schizophrenia may also contribute to creativity) and imperfection of the mechanism(s) allowing for the emergence of the higher cortical functions believed to be unique to homo sapiens (e.g., language capability, "theory of mind," and the concept of the "self"). Progress not withstanding, overall these hypotheses remain speculative in nature and represent subjects of intense debates (Adriaens, 2007; Crow, 2008).

Environmental Effects Mediated Through "Biological" Mechanisms

Etiological models implicating "nongenetic" biological mechanisms also have been proposed. It is plausible that many kinds of assaults, including perinatal traumata, infection, altered immune functions, and exposure to neurotoxic substances, would lead to neurodevelopmental abnormalities, which then increase the risk for schizophrenia and other psychotic disorders. Extant literature indicates that perinatal traumata (e.g., trauma to the brain at birth) are significantly associated with the risk of schizophrenia (Brown, 2006). In addition, data showing effect of seasons at birth (Davies, Welham, Chant, Torrey, & McGrath, 2003) on the prevalence of schizophrenia suggest that prenatal or perinatal infection also is a risk factor. In comparison, support for other "physical" environmental etiological factors has not yet been substantive.

Although abuse of various substances is highly prevalent among schizophrenic patients, the cause-effect relationship remains unclear (C. Y. Chen & Lin, 2009; Gregg, Barrowclough, & Haddock, 2007). Recent data provide strong support for a causal relationship between the abuse of cannabis in adolescence and the subsequently development of schizophrenic disorder (M. T. Compton et al., 2009; McGrath et al., 2010). In addition, it is clear that psychostimulants have the capacity of inducing psychotic symptoms (C. K. Chen et al., 2003; Barr et al., 2006; Ujike, 2002), and a portion of these patients may continue to manifest both positive and negative symptoms of schizophrenia (Barr et al., 2006), even after they have abstained from the stimulants. However, methodological difficulties made it problematic to affirm such a claim.

Psychosocial Etiological Models

Reflecting the strong influence of the psychoanalytic movement dominant in the first half of the last century, mental health professionals as well as opinion leaders in Western societies commonly regarded all psychiatric disorders, including schizophrenia, as psychogenic, with deep roots in patients' familial and social environments (Hartwell, 1996). Taken to the extreme, such a model led to the development of the "double-bind" theory and the concept of "schizophrenogenic mother" (Bateson, 1972; Gibney, 2006; C. E. Harrison, 1996). At the same time, searching for links between social disruptions and mental/behavioral disturbances, prominent social scientists formulated "labeling" theories, leading to the extreme position that mental disorders including schizophrenia were not diseases but creations of the society to define and alienate those members whose behaviors deviated from the accepted norms (Goffman, 1961; Scheff, 2006). Although these theories, taken to the extreme, now might appear preposterous (Laing, 1965; Szasz, 1960), they have served to stimulate the thinking of the mental health field in regard to psychosocial influences on both the pathoetiology and pathogenesis of conditions such as schizophrenia (Fromm-Reichmann, 1950; Greenberg, 1964; Hornstein, 2000; Menninger, 1963).

More recently, progress in cognitive psychology and attribution theories has continued to enrich our understanding, not only with regard to the nature of neurocognitive deficits, but also psychosocial mechanisms that might contribute to onset and course of schizophrenia (Beck, 2004; Bell, Halligan, & Ellis, 2006; Bhugra, 2000; Cantor-Graae, 2007; Green & Nuechterlein, 1999; Kuipers et al., 2006). At the same time, findings linking poverty, urbanization, migration (Jarvis, 2007; Selten, Cantor-Graae, & Kahn, 2007), and familiar milieu to schizophrenia further substantiate the importance of psychosocial forces as risk factors for such a disorder.

Evolving from these advances, the stress-diathesis model has gained steadily more support from leaders in the field, purporting that both inherent vulnerability (genetic and hereditary in nature) and environmental stressors (biological as well as psychosocial) are necessary for precipitating the development of schizophrenia (Charney et al., 2002; Dick, Riley, & Kendler, 2010; Mueser & McGurk, 2004; Tsuang et al., 2004). Further, recent studies have shed lights on the nature and extent of neuroplasticity throughout different developmental stages (Frost et al., 2004), indicating that "psychosocial" stressors affect individuals not only at the psychological level, but could significantly change brain development and neurocircuit connections as well. Such a model points to the paramount import of elucidating mechanisms for interactions between genetic, environmental, and developmental processes, a quest that is conceptually straightforward but is in reality fraught with methodological challenges and pitfalls.

Etiological Models and the Asian Populations

As may be apparent from the discussions above, ethnicity and culture influence the vulnerability and pathogenesis of schizophrenia in the context of practically all of the models mentioned above. For example, in most, if not all, of the genetic polymorphisms (distribution of genotypes and allele types) that have been shown to be associated with schizophrenia, ethnic variation is the rule rather than exception (Hamer & Sirota, 2000; K. M. Lin, 2000, 2002). It is reasonable to expect that perinatal traumata and other biologically based environmental assaults on the brain vary widely across nations and ethnic/cultural groups (Cannon, Jones, & Murray, 2002; K. M. Lin & Kleinman, 1988). Psychosocial stressors vary and maybe profoundly influenced by cultural practices and psychosocial milieus of different populations (L. C. Lee & Zane, 1998; Uba, 1994). These are all fertile areas challenging cross-cultural researchers in the decades to come.

ISSUES RELATED TO TREATMENT, CLINICAL COURSE, AND OUTCOME

Evidence-Based Treatment for Schizophrenia

The serendipitous discovery of phenothiazines in the 1950s heralded a new era for the treatment and management of schizophrenia. In subsequent decades, a large body of literature has emerged, substantiating the effectiveness of a large family of "antipsychotics" in ameliorating "positive" psychotic symptoms (e.g., delusions; hallucinations; disorganized thinking, speech, and behavior). Their effects on "negative" symptoms (e.g., withdrawal, blunted affect, anhedonia, alogia) and neurocognitive deficits are much more limited (Bloom & Kupfer, 1995; Breier, Tran, Herrera, Tollefson, & Bymaster, 2001; B. P. Murphy, Chung, Park, McGorry, 2006). The second- and third-generation antipsychotics have been reported to be more effective for the latter, although the validity and extent of such distinctions are still under debate (Stip, 2000), with the possible exception of the superiority of clozapine as compared to the "first-generation antipsychotics," particularly in terms of negative symptoms (Wahlbeck, Cheine, & Essali, 2007).

As is true with the medication management of practically all chronic conditions, adherence (compliance) is a serious challenge. For schizophrenia, such challenges are further aggravated by problems with insight and the profundity of the associated dysfunction. Various studies indicated that commonly more than 50% of schizophrenic patients showed poor or partial adherence (Samalin, Blanc, & Llorca, 2010; Velligan et al., 2009, 2010). Confirming such observations, the Clinical Antipsychotic Trials of Intervention Effectiveness (CATIE), a National Institute of Mental Health (NIMH)-funded, large-scale comparative study of the long-term effectiveness of different classes of antipsychotics, revealed that only 26% of subjects completed the 18-month trial (Lieberman et al., 2005). Since discontinuation of antipsychotics is associated with alarmingly high rates of relapses, nonadherence remains a major challenge for the care of schizophrenic patients (Lysaker, Buck, Salvatore, Popolo, & Dimaggio, 2009; Masand, Roca, Turner, & Kane, 2009).

Even where medications are effective and adherence is not a hindrance, most patients with history of schizophrenia continue to be beleaguered with enormous obstacles in overcoming disruptions in many aspects of their lives, including employment, housing, and social and familial relationships. Unless these problems are simultaneously addressed, most patients will continue to suffer from dysfunctions in multiple dimensions, even if their schizophrenic symptoms are adequately controlled (Lewis et al., 2002; Sensky et al., 2000). Over the decades, professional efforts in these arenas have evolved from psychoeducation (Kopelowicz & Liberman, 2003), skill training, rehabilitation, and support (housing, vocational, academic, financial, social, recreational) to the creation of programs providing comprehensive and integrated services (Liberman & Kopelowicz, 2005; Miller, Brown, Pilon, Scheffler, & Davis, 2010; Ragins, 2002), and the recent development of assertive community treatment modalities. While these approaches make inherent sense and have been supported with empirical data, much room is left for additional research efforts (Chien & Chan, 2004; Chien, Chan, & Thompson, 2006; C. Lee, Wu, Habil, Dyachkova, & Lee 2006; Weng, Xiang, & Liberman, 2005).

More discreet and focused psychosocial treatment approaches, including cognitive behavioral therapy (CBT), neuropsychological rehabilitation, and cognitive enhancement therapy, also have been demonstrated to be effective in remedying aspects of schizophrenic pathologies, including alterations in self-esteem, social functioning, and insight (Schulze Mönking, Hornung, Stricker, & Buchkremer, 1997). In addition, based on findings showing that patients who are "trapped" in highly emotionally charged family settings are more likely to suffer from subsequent relapses despite compliance with antipsychotic medication management (Chien, Thompson, & Norman, 2008; Leff et al., 1987), specific family treatment approaches have been developed and proven efficacious (Gleeson et al., 2010). However, since most of these concepts are still evolving, evidence-based studies are still needed to determine what represent essential ingredients in these approaches, especially across divergent sociocultural strata (Karno et al., 1987; Lopez, Nelson, Snyder, & Mintz, 1999; Sota et al., 2008; Weisman, 1997).

The widespread use of antipsychotic medications in various Asian groups, bolstered further by small-scale studies demonstrating efficacy of some of these pharmaceuticals, suggests that these medications likely work equally well in these populations (K. M. Lin, Chen, & Chen, 2008; K. M, Lin, Smith, & Ortiz, 2001; Ng, Lin, Singh, & Chiu, 2008). Similarly, the rationale of integrated services and rehabilitation programs should hold true for most, if not all, cultural/ ethnic groups (Chan, Yip, Tso, Cheng, & Tam, 2009; Chien & Chan, 2004; Chien, Chan & Thompson, 2006; Li & Arthur, 2005; Oka et al., 2004; Shin & Lukens, 2002; Tang, Leung, & Lam, 2008; Weng, Xiang, & Liberman, 2005). However, since relatively little research has been done in these populations, much awaits further clarification, including how these programs should be structured and delivered, and what factors might importantly influence therapeutic outcomes. For example, antipsychotics as well as many medications have been demonstrated to be metabolized differently across ethnic groups, leading to differential dosing requirements and side-effect profiles (K. M. Lin, 2008; K. M. Lin, Yu, Chen, Lin & Poland, 1995; Lin, & Smith, 2008). Clinicians negligent of such difference might inadvertently expose patients unnecessarily to excessive risks, and worsen the problems with medication adherence. Similar cultural considerations most likely exist in term of psychosocial interventions. These represent some of the crucial research issues to be considered in promoting evidence-based treatment for Asian and Asian American populations.

Severity and Delay in Treatment

As elegantly demonstrated by Tsung-yi Lin and his associates in their original studies, subsequently replicated by others in different settings, Asian Americans tend to rely on family and informal social networks rather than professionals in coping with family members suffering from mental health problems (T. Y. Lin & Lin, 1978; T. Y. Lin, Tardiff, Donetz, & Goresky, 1978). Consequently, there is typically a significant delay in patients' contact with mental health professionals (K. M. Lin, Inui, Kleinman, & Womack, 1982; Okazaki, 2000). In one study, the delay between the onset of severe psychopathology and the first contact and treatment with mental health professionals is three years on average. Along with this apparent underutilization of mental health services, data clearly indicated that those who eventually reach the systems typically have more severe symptom profiles, and are more chronic in their disease course. Since it is clear now that earlier interventions lead to a higher probability of remission, less relapse, and less severe clinical course over all, this state of affairs is indeed exceedingly regrettable (Haas, Garratt, & Sweeney, 1998; Gunduz-Bruce et al., 2005; Marshall et al., 2005).

Based on this literature, and the advocacy of community activists, a number of multicultural and multilingual programs, both outpatient and inpatient, have been initiated in metropolitan areas with high concentration of Asian Americans, including Los Angeles, San Francisco, New York, Seattle, and Portland. Typically, congruent with the literature on the delay in contact and treatment, the initial cases treated in these programs tended to be those with severe and chronic psychotic conditions. Gradually, as the programs gained the trust of the community, patients with comparatively less severe conditions would start to emerge, and other activities including prevention, community education and outreach, and other programs such as case management, were then successfully introduced.

In retrospect, it appears that these programs have been successful, at least in part due to their ability to adapt their structure and function to the needs of the local Asian communities. Most if not all of them are either embedded in general health care and/or social services settings, and have strong ties with these sectors, as well as Asian community organizations including social, cultural, political, and religious ones. These approaches perhaps to a large degree reflect the programs' ability to adapt to Asians' general preferences of integration rather than overcompartmentalization, minimizing the artificial dichotomy of mental and physical health that currently exists in our health care systems, and intentionally bridging the gap between ours and other human and social services to the extent possible (Chow, 2002).

CLINICAL COURSE AND OUTCOME

As extensively reviewed by one of the authors of this chapter, there appear to be very substantial cross-national variations in the clinical course and outcome of schizophrenia and related psychosis (K. M. Lin & Kleinman, 1988; Patel et al., 2006). Earlier anecdotal reports, field observations, and data-based studies indicated that psychotic patients from "less developed" countries typically had comparatively better clinical outcome, in that a relatively higher proportion of these patients tended to remit, improve, or become less symptomatic and less disturbing over time. These surprising and perhaps counterintuitive findings were confirmed by a number of well designed, large-scale, multinational and multisite studies sponsored by the World Health Organization (WHO), including the International Pilot Study on Schizophrenia (IPSS) and the Determinant of Outcome study (Davidson & McGlashan, 1997; Edgerton & Cohen, 1994; Kulhara, 1994; Leff, Sartorius, Jablensky, Korten, & Ernberg, 1992; Sartorius, Gulbinat, Harrison, Laska, & Siegel, 1996). Study sites of these projects encompassed those from Europe and the Americas on the one hand, and Asia and Africa on the other. Since the "less developed" countries and sites also have been observed to be more likely to have psychotic patients who tend to have acute onset and a fulminant course (Das, Malhotra, & Basu, 1999), often leading to complete resolution of symptoms in a relatively short time span, the Determinant of Outcome study took this into consideration, and included all incident cases identified in the communities, not only those reaching the health care sectors. Interestingly, after controlling for acuteness, the inverse relationship between socioeconomic development of the sites and the outcome of the patients remain the same. Various explanations for such discrepancies, including the availability of social support and contact and differential survival rates of those with obstetrical complications, leading more of the infants with such complications and hence increased risks for mental illnesses to grow into adulthood and manifest psychopathologies. However, the fact that as societies became progressively more affluent (such as in Taiwan), the prognosis of schizophrenia seemed to deteriorate, appears to support the thesis that there are forces in the modern societies that render it more difficult for those suffering from schizophrenia to adapt (Hwu et al., 1981).

Reports in Mexican Americans suggest that such a differential also exists in the United States. Among Mexican Americans, it has been clear that those more acculturated tend to have worse health status in general, and suffer from more mental health and behavioral problems in particular. Schizophrenic patients from more acculturated families also appeared to have less favorable outcomes. One mechanism that has been explored has to do with the concept of "expressed emotion." Patients with caretakers who are highly critical of them are much more likely to relapse, even with adequate medication management (Kopelowicz et al., 2002). Studies demonstrated that parents who ascribe to the more traditional explanatory models for their children's misfortunes, such as the concept of "nervios" (nerves), were much less critical and more accepting of the patients (Jenkins, 1988), because the concept was much less stigmatizing. Similar findings on an increased risk in second-generation Caribbeans in the Great Britain, as compared to the first-generation immigrants, also have been replicated and widely discussed (Davidson & McGlashan, 1997). Ethnic identity and changes in social support systems have been hypothesized as possible causes for these seemingly paradoxical results (Cohen, Patel, Thara, & Gureje, 2008). To what extent such observations might also apply to Asian Americans remains a fascinating and important question deserving further investigation (S. Lee et al., 2009; Mossakowski, 2003; Takeuchi, Alegría, Jackson, & Williams, 2007).

FAMILY INVOLVEMENT

Reflecting our general understanding of the primacy of family in Asian societies, family plays a central role in the assessment and care of Asian American patients, especially those inflicted with severe, psychotic problems (Kleinman 1988; T. Y. Lin, Tseng, & Yeh, 1995). They are in a sense the primary "gatekeepers," making decisions on whether patients enter mental health care. They typically contact the clinics or the clinicians ahead of the patients' visit, and expect to be included in the consultation room as well as in participating in making all treatment decisions (K. M. Lin, Miller, Poland, Nuccio, & Yamaguchi, 1991). Since this is often at odds with the principles basic to the American health care systems and mental health practices, emphasizing individualism, privacy, and individual decisions, the family might be regarded as intrusive or controlling, resulting unfortunately too often in power struggle and misunderstanding. To be sure, family involvement may not always be good, a case in point is the consistent delay in treatment entry with Asian American patients. Interventions for such delays evidently need to take such tendency of more intensive family involvement into consideration.

STIGMA AND RENAMING

Remarkable progress notwithstanding, stigmata associated with any psychiatric disorders, particularly with schizophrenia, bipolar disorder, and other psychotic conditions, remain major challenges for the field and for the society. Although not yet supported with definitive research data, it is generally assumed by researchers and clinicians with extensive cross-cultural experiences that stigmata associated with mental disorders typically represent an even graver problem among most Asian and Asian American communities (Jorm et al., 2005; Ng, 1997). A large and sophisticated literature already exists in the social sciences, indicating that irrespective of one's view on the primary cause of "deviant behaviors," including those manifested by schizophrenic patients, what matters even more in the "fate" of these patients is the subsequent process of "social labeling," or the society's reaction and response to the person's "stigmata," be it physical defects, unusual behaviors, or race and gender (Goffman, 1961; Schulze, 2007). According to this view, one would expect that social factors play an even more important role in determining the course and outcome than biological forces, and researchers would do well to pay at least equal attention to the idea of the "social course" of illnesses, in addition to the concept of "natural course" that has been customarily the focus of researchers' attention (Kleinman, 1988).

It is true that any term, once associated with a group of patients that has been stigmatized, quickly become stigmatizing and even derogatory itself. Thus, while professionals might have been striving hard to make psychiatric labels value-neutral (e.g., from "dementia praecox" to "schizophrenia"), new labels quickly came to connote the perceived undesirable traits associated with the older ones. Based on this, there has long been reluctance in the change of the "labels" even though existing labels are often associated with deep-rooted stigmata that are difficult to mollify.

However, such a state of affairs may be even more problematic and more difficult to deal with in the Asian context, at least in those countries where the term "schizophrenia" in the native language clearly says that your mind is disintegrating or splitting. For example, while not many English users are conscious of the fact that "schizo" means splitting, and "phrenia" means the mind or the brain, when the term is translated into Chinese, Japanese, and Korean, the literal meaning and all the negative implications are right on the surface. A patient that in the old days was just regarded as "crazy," or "odd" now has a scientific term following him or her for life, certifying him/her that the person has a brain that is "fragmented." This is clearly misleading, demeaning, and is counterproductive of efforts for treatment and rehabilitation.

It is mostly for this reason that in Japan, as advocated by the patients and families' advocacy groups, the Japanese Psychiatric Society finally replaced the old term "Seishin Bunretsu Byo" ("mind-split-disease" translated from "schizophrenia") with a new diagnostic label called "Togo Shitcho Sho" ("integration disorder") in 2002. After some initial trepidation and hesitation, psychiatrists generally found that the term was much more easily accepted by patients and the general society, and was conducive to efforts in outreach and community education, as well as in promoting prevention and rehabilitation (Sato, 2006). Although similar proposals have been made in China, Korea, and Taiwan, such a move has not yet been adopted, and there remains no clear consensus among professionals regarding the wisdom of such a proposal. Clearly more research and consensus-building will be needed to decide on whether this is a worthwhile endeavor, at least in terms of our ongoing fights against the pernicious effects of stigmata. What is at issue, beside the practical implications indicated above, is the implied "ethnocentric" nature of the debate. When the term "schizophrenia" was coined, it was done in the European setting, and the term used archaic linguistic roots that should not stimulate stigmatizing associations by itself. When translated, the term typically loses this mantle of distance and ambiguity. Since it is true that now the term is widely used in all corners of the world, and the majority of patients affected by such labels are no longer of European or North American traditions, the label's (and in fact any diagnostic labels') appropriateness and usefulness do justify careful scrutiny in such a global context. Above and beyond these practical considerations, of course, whether an alternative term in English (and its counterparts in various European languages) might also help to mitigate stigmata associated with schizophrenia, also likely is a worthy question to at least deserve serious consideration among scholars working in these settings (Levin, 2006).

CONCLUSIONS

In this overview, the authors reviewed the literature relevant to schizophrenia in the Asian and Asian American populations. Topics reviewed include epidemiology, symptom manifestations, subtyping, severity, clinical course, differential diagnosis, misdiagnosis, family involvement, stigma, labeling, and finally the effect of conceptualization and naming itself. Although much awaits further research attention, it seems clear that in practically all issues involved, what is most prominent is the juxtapositioning of universality and cultural specificity that go hand in hand. Future work with these populations, who collectively represent over half of the world population, would not only lead to crucial information and insights important for professionals working with patients imbued or influenced by these cultures, but also contributes toward the generation and testing of new concepts and perspectives regarding phenomena related to schizophrenia, and thus represent a crucial aspect of schizophrenia research.

REFERENCES

Adriaens, P. R. (2007). Evolutionary psychiatry and the schizophrenia paradox: A critique. *Biology and Philosophy, 22,* 513–528.

Adebimpe, V. R. (1981). Overview: White norms and psychiatric diagnosis of black patients. *American Journal of Psychiatry, 138,* 279–285.

Alarcon, R. D., Bell, C. C., Kirmayer, L. J., Lin, KM, Ustun, B., & Wisner, K. L. (2002). Beyond the funhouse mirrors. In D. Kupfer, M. B. First, & D. A. Regier (Eds.), *A research agenda for DSM-V* (pp. 219–281). Washington, DC: American Psychiatric Association.

al-Issa, I. (1995). The illusion of reality or the reality of illusion: Hallucinations and culture. *British Journal of Psychiatry, 166,* 368–373.

American Psychiatric Association (APA). (1980). *Diagnostic and statistical manual of mental disorders* (3rd ed.). Washington, DC: Author.

American Psychiatric Association (APA). (1994). *Diagnostic and statistical manual of mental disorders* (4th ed., text revision). Washington, DC: Author. (*DSM-IV-TR*)

Barr, A. M., Panenka, W. J., MacEwan, G. W., Thornton, A. E., Lang, D. J., Honer, W. G., et al. (2006). The need for speed: An update on methamphetamine addiction. *Journal of Psychiatry and Neuroscience, 31,* 301–313.

Bateson, G. (1972). *Steps to an ecology of mind: Collected essays in anthropology, psychiatry, evolution, and epistemology.* Chicago, University of Chicago Press.

Beck, A. T. (2004). A cognitive model of schizophrenia. *Journal of Cognitive Psychotherapy, 18*(3), 281–288.

Bell, V., Halligan, P. W., & Ellis, H. D. (2006). Explaining delusions: A cognitive perspective. *Trends in Cognitive Science, 10*(5), 219–226.

Bernstein, R. L., & Gaw, A. C. (1990). Koro: Proposed classification for DSM-IV. *American Journal of Psychiatry, 147,* 1670–1674.

Bhatia, M. S., & Malik, S. C. (1991). Dhat syndrome: A useful diagnostic entity in Indian culture *British Journal of Psychiatry, 159,* 691–695.

Bhavsar, V., & Bhugra, D. (2008). Religious delusions: Finding meanings in psychosis. *Psychopathology, 41,* 165–172.

Bhugra, D. (2000). Migration and schizophrenia. *Acta Psychiatrica Scandinavica, 104*(Suppl 407), 68–73.

Bivins, R. & Pickstone, J.V. (eds) (2007). *Medicine, madness and social history: Essays in honour of Roy Porter.* Basingstoke, UK, and New York: Palgrave Macmillan.

Bloom, F. E., & Kupfer, D. J. (Eds.). (1995). *Psychopharmacology: The fourth generation of progress.* New York: Raven.

Bottero, A. (1991). Consumption by semen loss in India and elsewhere. *Culture, Medicine, and Psychiatry, 15,* 303–320.

Breier, A., Tran, P. V., Herrera, J. M, Tollefson, G. D., & Bymaster, F. P. (Eds.). (2001). *Current issues in the psychopharmacology of schizophrenia.* Philadelphia: Lippincott Williams and Wilkins.

Brown, A. S. (2006). Prenatal infection as a risk factor for schizophrenia. *Schizophrenia Bulletin, 32,* 200–202.

Broyd, S. J., Demanuele, C., Debener, S., Helps, S. K., James, C. J., & Sonuga-Barke, E. J. S. (2008). Default-mode brain dysfunction in mental disorders: A systematic review. *Neuroscience and Biobehavioral Reviews, 33,* 279–296.

Buckle, C., Chuah, Y. M., Fones, C. S., & Wong, A. H. (2007). A conceptual history of Koro. *Transcultural Psychiatry, 44,* 27–43.

Cannon, M., Jones, P. B., & Murray, R. M. (2002). Obstetric complications and schizophrenia: Historical and meta-analytic review. *American Journal of Psychiatry, 159,* 1080–1092.

Cantor-Graae, E. (2007). The contribution of social factors to the development of schizophrenia: A review of recent findings. *Canadian Journal of Psychiatry, 52,* 277–286.

Chan, S. W., Yip, B., Tso, S., Cheng, B. S., & Tam, W. (2009). Evaluation of a psychoeducation program for Chinese clients with schizophrenia and their family caregivers. *Patient Education and Counseling, 75,* 67–76.

Chang, S. C. (1997). Social anxiety (phobia) and east Asian culture. *Depression and Anxiety, 5,* 115–120.

Charney, S. D., Barlow, D. H., Botteron, K., Coben, J. D., Goldman, D., Gar, R. E., et al. (2002). Neuroscience research agenda to guide development of a pathophysiologically based classification system. In D. Kupfer, M. B. First, & D. A. Regier (Eds.), *A research agenda for DSM-V* (pp. 31–84). Washington, DC: American Psychiatric Association.

Chen, C. K., Lin, S. K., Sham, P. C., Ball, D., Loh, E. W., Hsiao, C. C., et al. (2003). Pre-morbid characteristics and co-morbidity of methamphetamine users with and without psychosis. *Psychological Medicine, 33,* 1407–1414.

Chen, C. Y., & Lin, K. M. (2009). Health consequences of illegal drugs use. *Current Opinion in Psychiatry, 22,* 287–292,

Chen, H., Kramer, E. J., Chen, T., & Chung, H. (2005). Engaging Asian Americans for mental health research: Challenges and solutions. *Journal of Immigrant Health, 7,* 109–116.

Cheung, F. K., & Snowden, L. R. (1990). Community mental health and ethnic minority populations. *Community Mental Health Journal, 26,* 277–291.

Chien, W. T., & Chan, S. W. (2004). One-year follow-up of a multiple-family-group intervention for Chinese families of patients with schizophrenia. *Psychiatric Services, 55,* 1276–1284.

Chien, W. T., Chan, S. W., & Thompson, D. R. (2006). Effects of a mutual support group for families of Chinese people with schizophrenia: Eighteen-month follow-up. *British Journal of Psychiatry, 189,* 41–49.

Chien, W. T., Thompson, D. R., & Norman, I. (2008). Evaluation of a peer-led mutual support group for Chinese families of people with schizophrenia. *American Journal of Community Psychology, 42,* 122–134.

Chow, J. (2002). Asian American and Pacific Islander mental health and substance abuse agencies: Organizational characteristics and service gaps. *Administration and Policy in Mental Health, 30,* 79–86.

Cohen, A., Patel, V., Thara, R., & Gureje, O. (2008). Questioning an axiom: Better prognosis for schizophrenia in the developing world? *Schizophrenia Bulletin, 34,* 229–244.

Compton, M. T., Kelley, M. E., Ramsay, C. E., Pringle, M., Goulding, S. M., Esterberg, M. L., et al. (2009). Association of pre-onset cannabis, alcohol, and tobacco use with age at onset of prodrome and age at onset of psychosis in first-episode patients. *American Journal of Psychiatry, 166,* 1251–1257.

Compton, W. M., III, Helzer, J. E., Hwu, H. G., Yeh, E. K., McEvoy, L., Tipp, J. E., et al. (1991). New methods in cross-cultural psychiatry: Psychiatric illness in Taiwan and the United States. *American Journal of Psychiatry, 148,* 1697–1704.

Corcoran, C. Walker, E., Huot, R., Mittal, V., Tessner, K., Kestler, L., & Malaspina, D. (2003). The stress cascade and schizophrenia: Etiology and onset. *Schizophrenia Bulletin, 29*(4), 671–692. http://en.wikipedia.org/wiki/PubMed_Identifier

Coyle, J. T. (2006). Substance use disorders and schizophrenia: A question of shared glutamatergic mechanisms. *Neurotoxicity Research, 10,* 221–233.

Crow, T. J. (2008). The "big bang" theory of the origin of psychosis and the faculty of language. *Schizophrenia Research, 102*(1–3), 31–52.

Davidson, L., & McGlashan, T. H. (1997). The varied outcomes of schizophrenia. *Canadian Journal of Psychiatry, 42,* 34–43.

Das, S. K., Malhotra, S., & Basu, D. (1999). Family study of acute and transient psychotic disorders: Comparison with schizophrenia. *Social Psychiatry and Psychiatric Epidemiology, 34,* 328–332.

Davies, G. Welham, J., Chant, D., Torrey, E. F., & McGrath, J. (2003). A systematic review and meta-analysis of Northern Hemisphere season of birth studies in schizophrenia. *Schizophrenia Bulletin, 29*(3), 587–593.

Day, R. Nielsen, J. A., Korten, A., Ernberg, G., Dube, K. C., Gebhart, J., et al. (1987). Stressful life events preceding the acute onset of schizophrenia: A cross-national study from the World Health Organization. *Culture, Medicine, and Psychiatry, 11*(2), 123–205.

Desjarlais, R., Eisenberg, L., Good, B., & Kleinman, A. (1995). *World mental health: Problems and priorities in low-income countries.* New York: Oxford University Press.

Dick, D. M., Riley, B., & Kendler, K. S. (2010). Nature and nurture in neuropsychiatric genetics: Where do we stand? *Dialogues in Clinical Neuroscience, 12,* 7–23.

Dzokoto, V. A., & Adams, G. (2005). Understanding genital-shrinking epidemics in West Africa: Koro, juju, or mass psychogenic illness? *Culture, Medicine, and Psychiatry, 29,* 53–78.

Edgerton, R. B., & Cohen, A. (1994). Culture and schizophrenia: The DOSMD challenge. *British Journal of Psychiatry, 164,* 222 231.

Evans, K., McGrath, J., & Milns, R. (2003). Searching for schizophrenia in ancient Greek and Roman literature: A systematic review. *Acta Psychiatrica Scandinavica, 107,* 323–330.

Fabrega, H., Jr. (2001). Culture and history in psychiatric diagnosis and practice. *Psychiatric Clinics of North America, 24,* 391–405.

Feighner, J. P., Robins, E., Guze, S. B., Woodruff, R. A., Jr., Winokur, G., & Munoz, R. (1972). Diagnostic criteria for use in psychiatric research. *Archives of General Psychiatry, 26*(1), 57–63.

Foucault, M. (1965). Madness and Civilization: A History of Insanity in the Age of Reason. New York: Random House.

Fromm-Reichmann, F. (1950). *Principles of intensive psychotherapy.* Chicago: University of Chicago Press.

Frost, D. O., Tamminga, C. A., Medoff, D. R., Caviness, V., Innocenti, G., & Carpenter, W. T. (2004). Neuroplasticity and schizophrenia. *Biological Psychiatry, 56,* 540–543.

Gibney, P. (2006) The double bind theory: Still crazy-making after all these years. *Psychotherapy in Australia, 12*(3), 48–55.

Gleeson, J. F., Cotton, S. M., Alvarez-Jimenez, M., Wade, D., Crisp, K., Newman, B., et al. (2010). Family outcomes from a randomized control trial of relapse prevention therapy in first-episode psychosis. *Journal of Clinical Psychiatry, 71,* 475–483.

Goffman, E. (1961). *Asylums: Essays on the social situation of mental patients and other inmates.* Garden City, NY, Anchor Books.

Goldner, E. M., Hsu, L., Waraich, P., & Somers, J. M. (2002). Prevalence and incidence studies of schizophrenic disorders: A systematic review of the literature. *Canadian Journal of Psychiatry, 47*, 833–843.

Green, M. F., & Nuechterlein, K. H. (1999). Should schizophrenia be treated as a neurocognitive disorder? *Schizophrenia Bulletin, 25*, 309–319.

Greenberg, J. (1964). *I never promised you a rose garden.* New York: Holt, Rinehart and Winston.

Gregg, L., Barrowclough, C., & Haddock, G. (2007). Reasons for increased substance use in psychosis. *Clinical Psychology Review, 27*, 494–510.

Gunduz-Bruce, H., McMeniman, M., Robinson, D. G., Woerner, M. G., Kane, J. M., Schooler, N. R., et al. (2005). Duration of untreated psychosis and time to treatment response for delusions and hallucinations. *American Journal of Psychiatry, 162*, 1966–1969.

Haas, G. L., Garratt, L. S. & Sweeney, J. A. (1998) Delay to first antipsychotic medication in schizophrenia: Impact on symptomatology and clinical course of illness. *Journal of Psychiatric Research, 32*, 51–159.

Hamer, D., & Sirota, L. (2000). Beware the chopsticks gene. *Molecular Psychiatry, 5*, 11–13.

Harrison, C. E. (1996). The schizophrenogenic mother concept in American psychiatry. *Psychiatry, 59*, 274–297.

Harrison, P. J., & Owen, M. J. (2003). Genes for schizophrenia? Recent findings and their pathophysiological implications. *The Lancet, 361*, 417.

Hartwell, C. E. (1996). The schizophrenogenic mother concept in American psychiatry. *Psychiatry, 58*, 274–297.

Hornstein, G. A. (2000). *To redeem one person is to redeem the world: The life of Frieda Fromm-Reichmann.* New York: Free Press.

Hwu, H. G., Chen, C. C., Tsuang, M. T., & Tseng, W. S. (1981). Derealization syndrome and the outcome of schizophrenia: A report from the international pilot study of schizophrenia. *British Journal of Psychiatry, 139*, 313–318.

Hwu, H. G., Yeh, E. K., & Chang, L. Y. (1989). Prevalence of psychiatric disorders in Taiwan defined by the Chinese Diagnostic Interview Schedule. *Acta Psychiatrica Scandinavica, 79*, 136–147.

Isaac, M., Chand, P., & Murthy, P. (2007). Schizophrenia outcome measures in the wider international community. *British Journal of Psychiatry, 50*(Suppl), s71–s77.

Jablensky, A., & Sartorius, N. (1988). Is schizophrenia universal? *Acta Psychiatrica Scandinavica, 344*(Suppl), 65–70.

Jablensky, A., Sartorius, N., & Ernberg, G. (1992). Schizophrenia: Manifestations, incidence, and course in different cultures: A World Health Organization ten-country study. *Psychological Medicine, 22*, 1–97.

Jarvis, G. E. (2007). The social causes of psychosis in North American psychiatry: A review of a disappearing literature. *Canadian Journal of Psychiatry, 52*, 287–294.

Jenkins, J. H. (1988). Ethnopsychiatric interpretations of schizophrenic illness: The problem of nervios within Mexican-American families. *Culture, Medicine, and Psychiatry, 12*, 301–329.

Jilek, W. G. (1995). Emil Kraepelin and comparative sociocultural psychiatry. *European Archives of Psychiatry and Clinical Neuroscience, 245*, 231–238.

Jones, B. E., & Gray, B. A. (1986). Problems in diagnosing schizophrenia and affective disorders among blacks. *Hospital and Community Psychiatry, 37*, 61–65.

Jones, H. M., & Pilowsky, L. S. (2002). Dopamine and antipsychotic drug action revisited. *British Journal of Psychiatry, 181*, 271–275.

Jorm, A. F., Nakane, Y., Christensen, H., Yoshioka, K., Griffiths, K. M., & Wata, Y. (2005). Public beliefs about treatment and outcome of mental disorders: A comparison of Australia and Japan. *BMC Medicine, 3*, 12.

Karno, M., Jenkins, J. H., de la Selva, A., Santana, F., Telles, C., Lopez, S., et al. (1987). Expressed emotion and schizophrenic outcome among Mexican-American families. *Journal of Nervous and Mental Disease, 175*, 143–151.

Kendell, R. E. (1975). Psychiatric diagnosis in Britain and the United States. *British Journal of Psychiatry, Spec No 9*, 453–461.

Kinzie, J. D. (2006). Immigrants and refugees: The psychiatric perspective. *Transcultural Psychiatry, 43*, 577–591.

Kircher, T. T., & Thienel, R. (2005). Functional brain imaging of symptoms and cognition in schizophrenia. *Progress in Brain Research, 150*, 299–308.

Kirmayer, L. J., & Robbins, J. M. (1996). Patients who somatize in primary care: A longitudinal study of cognitive and social characteristics. *Psychological Medicine, 26,* 937–951.

Kirmayer, L. J., & Young, A. (1998). Culture and somatization: Clinical, epidemiological, and ethnographic perspectives. *Psychosomatic Medicine, 60,* 420–430.

Kleinman, A. (1980). *Patients and healers in the context of culture.* Berkeley: University of California Press.

Kleinman, A. (1982). Neurasthenia and depression: A study of somatization and culture in China. *Culture, Medicine, and Psychiatry, 6,* 117–190.

Kleinman, A. (1988). *Rethinking psychiatry.* New York: Free Press.

Kleinman, A., & Kleinman, J. (1985). Somatization: The interconnections in Chinese society among culture, depressive experiences, and the meanings of pain. In A. Kleinman & B. J. Good (Eds.), *Culture and depression: Studies in the anthropology and cross-cultural psychiatry of affect and disorder* (Berkeley and Los Angeles: University of California Press).

Kleinman, A. M., & Singer, K. (1977). Depression, somatization, and the "New Cross-Cultural Psychiatry." *Social Science and Medicine, 11,* 3–10.

Konradi, C., Heckers, S. (2003). Molecular aspects of glutamate dysregulation: Implications for schizophrenia and its treatment. *Pharmacology and Therapeutics, 97*(2), 153–179.

Kopelowicz, A., & Liberman, R. P. (2003). Integrating treatment with rehabilitation for persons with major mental illnesses. *Psychiatric Services, 54,* 1491–1498.

Kopelowicz, A., Zarate, R., Gonzalez, V., Lopez, S. R., Ortega, P., Obregon, N., et al. (2002). Evaluation of expressed emotion in schizophrenia: A comparison of Caucasians and Mexican-Americans. *Schizophrenia Research, 55,* 179–186.

Kuipers, E., Garety, P., Fowler, D., Freeman, D., Dunn, G., & Bebbington, P. (2006). Cognitive, emotional, and social processes in psychosis: Refining cognitive behavioral therapy for persistent positive symptoms. *Schizophrenia Bulletin, 32*(Suppl 1), S24–S31.

Kulhara, P. (1994). Outcome of schizophrenia: Some transcultural observations with particular reference to developing countries. *European Archives of Psychiatry* and *Clinical Neuroscience, 244,* 227–235.

Kupfer, D. J., First, M. B., & Regier, D. A. (Eds.). (2002). *A Research Agenda for DSM-V.* Washington, DC: American Psychiatric Press.

Laing, R. D. (1965). *The divided self.* New York, Penguin Modern Classics.

Lane, H. Y., Liu, Y. C., Huang, C. L., Chang, Y. C., Wu, P. L., Lu, C. T., et al. (2006). Risperidone-related weight gain: Genetic and nongenetic predictors. *Journal of Clinical Psychopharmacology, 26,* 128–134.

Lawson, W. B. (1986). Racial and ethnic factors in psychiatric research. *Hospital and Community Psychiatry, 37,* 50–54.

Lee, C., Wu, K. H., Habil, H., Dyachkova, Y., & Lee, P. (2006). Treatment with olanzapine, risperidone, or typical antipsychotic drugs in Asian patients with schizophrenia. *Australian and New Zealand Journal of Psychiatry, 40,* 437–445.

Lee, C. K. (1998). A nationwide epidemiological study of mental disorders in Korea. *Psychiatry and Clinical Neurosciences, 52 Suppl,* S268–S274.

Lee, C. K., Kwak, Y. S., Yamamoto, J., Rhee, H., Kim, Y. S., Han, J. H., et al. (1990a). Psychiatric epidemiology in Korea: Part I. Gender and age differences in Seoul. *Journal of Nervous and Mental Disease, 178,* 242–246.

Lee, C. K., Kwak, Y. S., Yamamoto, J., Rhee, H., Kim, Y. S., Han, J. H., et al. (1990b). Psychiatric epidemiology in Korea: Part II. Urban and rural differences. *Journal of Nervous and Mental Disease, 178,* 247–252.

Lee, L. C., & Zane, N. W. S. (Eds.). (1998). *Handbook of Asian American psychology.* Thousand Oaks, CA: Sage.

Lee, S. Juon, H. S., Martinez, G., Hsu, C. E., Robinson, E. S. Bawa, J., et al. (2009). Model minority at risk: Expressed needs of mental health by Asian American young adults. *Journal of Community Health, 34*(2),144–152.

Leff, J., Sartorius, N., Jablensky, A., Korten, A., & Ernberg, G. (1992). The International Pilot Study of Schizophrenia: Five-year follow-up findings. *Psychological Medicine, 22*(1), 131–145.

Leff, J. (1981). *Psychiatry around the globe.* New York: Dekker.

Leff, J., Wig, N. N., Ghosh, A., Bedi, H., Menon, D. K., Kuipers, L., et al. (1987). Expressed emotion and schizophrenia in north India: III. Influence of relatives' expressed emotion on the course of schizophrenia in Chandigarh. *British Journal of Psychiatry, 151,* 166–173.

Levin, T. (2006). Schizophrenia should be renamed to help educate patients and the public. *International Journal of Social Psychiatry, 52,* 324–331.

Lewis, S., Tarrier, N., Haddock, G., Bentall, R., Kinderman, P., Kingdon, D., et al. (2002). Randomised controlled trial of cognitive-behavioural therapy in early schizophrenia: Acute-phase outcomes. *British Journal of Psychiatry, 43*(Suppl), s91–s97.

Lewis-Fernandez, R. (1992). The proposed DSM-IV trance and possession disorder category: Potential benefits and risks. *Transcultural Psychiatric Research Review, 29*(4), 301–317.

Li, Z., & Arthur, D. (2005). Family education for people with schizophrenia in Beijing, China: Randomised controlled trial. *British Journal of Psychiatry, 187,* 339–345.

Liberman, R. P., & Kopelowicz, A. (2005). Recovery from schizophrenia: A concept in search of research. *Psychiatric Services, 56,* 735–742.

Lieberman, J. A., Stroup, T. S., McEvoy, J. P., Swartz, M. S., Rosenheck, R. A., Perkins, D. O., et al. (2005). Effectiveness of antipsychotic drugs in patients with chronic schizophrenia. *New England Journal of Medicine, 353,* 1209–1223.

Lim, R. F., & Lin, K. M. (1996). Cultural formulation of psychiatric diagnosis. Case no. 03. Psychosis following Qi-gong in a Chinese immigrant. *Culture, Medicine, and Psychiatry, 20,* 369–378.

Lin, K. M. (1981). Traditional Chinese medical beliefs and their relevance for mental illness and psychiatry. In A. Kleinman & T. Y. Lin (Eds.), *Normal and Abnormal Behavior in Chinese Culture* (pp. 95–11). Dordrecht, Holland: Reidel.

Lin, K. M. (1990). Assessment and diagnostic issues in the psychiatric care of refugee patients. In W. Holzman & T. Bornemann (Eds.), *Mental Health of Immigrants and Refugees.* Austin, Texas: Hogg Foundation for Mental Health, The University of Texas.

Lin, K. M. (1996a). Culture and DSM-IV: Asian American perspectives. In J. Mezzich, A. Kleinman, H. Fabrega Jr., & D. Parron (Eds.), *Culture and psychiatric diagnosis.* Washington, DC: American Psychiatric Press.

Lin, K. M. (1996b). Cultural influences on the diagnosis of psychotic and organic disorders. In J. E. Mezzich, A. Kleinman, H. Fabrega Jr., & D. Parron (Eds.), *Culture and psychiatric diagnosis.* Washington, DC: American Psychiatric Press.

Lin, K. M. (2000). Human genome and diversity at the threshold of the millennium: Challenges and opportunities for Pacific Rim psychiatrists. *Column for the Cross-Cultural Psychiatry, Pacific Rim College of Psychiatrists Newsletter,* 3–4.

Lin, K. M. (2002). Foreword. In E. J. Frackiewicz, T. M. Shiovitz, & S. S. Hhee (Eds.), *Ethnicity in drug development and therapeutics* (pp. x–xii). London: Greenwich Medical Media.

Lin, K. M. (2008). Culture and ethnicity in psychopharmacotherapy. In C. Ng, K. M. Lin, B. Singh, & E. Chiu (Eds.), *Ethno-psychopharmacology: Advances in current practice* (pp. 27–37). Cambridge: Cambridge University Press.

Lin, K. M. & Cheung, F. (1999). Mental health issues for Asian Americans. *Psychiatric Services, 50*(6), 774–780.

Lin, K. M., Chen, C. H., & Chen, C. Y. (2008). Ethnopsychopharmacology. *International Review of Psychiatry, 20*(5), 452–459.

Lin, K. M., Inui, T. S., Kleinman, A. M., & Womack, W. M. (1982). Sociocultural determinants of the help-seeking behavior of patients with mental illness. *Journal of Nervous and Mental Disease, 170,* 78–85.

Lin, K. M., & Kleinman, A. (1981). Recent development of psychiatric epidemiology in China. *Culture, Medicine, and Psychiatry, 5,* 135–143.

Lin, K. M., & Kleinman, A. M. (1988). Psychopathology and clinical course of schizophrenia: A cross-cultural perspective. *Schizophrenia Bulletin, 14,* 555–567.

Lin, K.M., Kleinman, A. & Lin, T.Y.(1981). Overview of Mental Disorders in Chinese Cultures: Review of Epidemiological and Clinical Studies. In A. Kleinman and T. Y. Lin (Eds.): Normal and Abnormal Behavior in Chinese Culture. Dordrecht, Holland: D. Reidel Publishing Company, pp. 237–272.

Lin, K. M., & Lin, M. (2002). Challenging the myth of a culture-free nosological system. In K. Kurasaki, S. Okazaki, & S. Sue (Eds.), *Asian American mental health: Assessment theories and methods* (pp. 67–73). New York: Plenum.

Lin, K. M., Miller, M. H., Poland, R. E., Nuccio, I., & Yamaguchi, M. (1991). Ethnicity and family involvement in the treatment of schizophrenic patients. *Journal of Nervous and Mental Disease, 179,* 631–633.

Lin, K. M., & Poland, R. E. (1995). Ethnicity, culture, and psychopharmacology. In F. E. Bloom & D. J. Kupfer (Eds.), *Psychopharmacology: The fourth generation of progress* (ch. 162, pp. 1907–1917). New York: Raven.

Lin, K. M., Smith, M., & Ortiz, V. (2001). Culture and psychopharmacology. In J. E. Mezzich & H. Fabrega (Eds.), *Cultural psychiatry: International perspectives. Psychiatric Clinics of North America, 24,* 523–538.

Lin, K. M., Yu, S. H., Chen, C. H., Lin, M. T., & Smith, M. W. (2008). Psychopharmacology: Ethnic and cultural perspectives. In A. Tasman, J. Kay, J. Lieberman, M. First, & M. Maj (Eds.), *Psychiatry* (3rd ed., pp. 2012–2022). Chichester, UK: Wiley.

Lin, T. Y., & Lin, M. C. (1978). Service delivery issues in Asian-North American communities. *American Journal of Psychiatry, 135,* 454–456.

Lin, T. Y., Tardiff, K., Donetz, G., & Goresky, W. (1978). Ethnicity and patterns of help-seeking. *Culture, Medicine, and Psychiatry, 2,* 3–13.

Lin, T. Y., Tseng, W., & Yeh, E. K. (1995). *Chinese societies and mental health.* Hong Kong: Oxford University Press.

Lopez, S. R., Nelson, K. A., Snyder, K. S., & Mintz, J. (1999). Attributions and affective reactions of family members and course of schizophrenia. *Journal of Abnormal Psychology, 108,* 307–314.

Lu, F. G., Du, N., Gaw, A., & Lin, K. M. (2002). A psychiatric residency curriculum about Asian-American issues. *Academic Psychiatry, 26,* 225–236.

Lysaker, P. H., Buck, K. D., Salvatore, G., Popolo, R., & Dimaggio, G. (2009). Lack of awareness of illness in schizophrenia: Conceptualizations, correlates, and treatment approaches. *Expert Review of Neurotherapeutics, 9,* 1035–1043.

Marshall, M., Lewis, S., Lockwood, A., Drake, R., Jones, P., & Croudace, T. (2005). Association between duration of untreated psychosis and outcome in cohorts of first-episode patients: A systematic review. *Archives of General Psychiatry, 62,* 975–983.

Masand, P. S., Roca, M., Turner, M. S., & Kane, J. M. (2009). Partial adherence to antipsychotic medication impacts the course of illness in patients with schizophrenia: A review. *Primary Care Companion to The Journal of Clinical Psychiatry, 11,* 147–154.

Maslowski, J., Jansen van, R. D., & Mthoko, N. (1998). A polydiagnostic approach to the differences in the symptoms of schizophrenia in different cultural and ethnic populations. *Acta Psychiatrica Scandinavica, 98,* 41–46.

Mayes, R., & Horwitz, A. V. (2005). DSM-III and the revolution in the classification of mental illness. *Journal of the History of the Behavioral Sciences, 41,* 249–267.

McGrath, J., Welham, J., Scott, J., Varghese, D., Degenhardt, L., Hayatbakhsh, M. R., et al. (2010). Association between cannabis use and psychosis-related outcomes using sibling pair analysis in a cohort of young adults. *Archives of General Psychiatry, 67,* 440–447.

Menninger, K. A. (1963) *The vital balance: The life process in mental health and illness.* New York: Viking.

Mezzich, J. E., Kirmayer, L. J., Kleinman, A., Fabrega, H., Jr., Parron, D. L., Good, B. J., et al. (1999). The place of culture in DSM-IV. *Journal of Nervous and Mental Disease, 187,* 457–464.

Mezzich, J. E., Kleinman, A., Fabrega, H., Jr., & Parron, D. (Eds.). (1996). *Culture and psychiatric diagnosis.* Washington, DC: American Psychiatric Press.

Mezzich, J. E., Kleinman, A., Fabrega, H., Jr., Parron, D., Good, B. J., Lin, K. M., et al. (1997). Cultural issues for DSM-IV. In American Psychiatric Association (Ed.), *DSM-IV source book* (Vol. 3, pp. 861–866), Washington DC: American Psychiatric Press.

Mezzich, J. E., & Lin, K. M. (1995). Acute and transient psychotic disorders and culture-bound syndromes. In H. I. Kaplan & B. J. Sadock (Eds.), *Comprehensive textbook of psychiatry* (6th ed., pp. 1049–1059). Baltimore, MD: Williams and Wilkins.

Mezzich, J. E., Lin, K. M., & Hughes, C. C. (1999). Acute brief psychoses and culture-bound syndromes. In: H. I. Kaplan & B. J. Sadock (Eds.), *Comprehensive textbook of psychiatry,* (7th ed., pp. 1264–1276). Baltimore, MD: William and Wilkins.

Miller, L., Brown, T. T. Pilon, D., Scheffler, R. M., & Davis, M., (2010) Patterns of recovery from severe mental illness: A pilot study of outcomes. *Community Mental Health Journal, 46,* 177–187.

Mossakowski, K. N. (2003). Coping with perceived discrimination: Does ethnic identity protect mental health? *Journal of Health and Social Behavior, 44*(3), 318–331

Mueser, K. T., & McGurk, S. R. (2004). Schizophrenia. *Lancet, 363,* 2063–2072.

Murphy, H. B. (1982). Comparative psychiatry: The international and intercultural distribution of mental illness. *Monographien aus dem Gesamtgebiete der Psychiatrie, 28*, 1–327.

Murphy, B. P., Chung, Y. C., Park, T. W., & McGorry, P. D. (2006). Pharmacological treatment of primary negative symptoms in schizophrenia: A systematic review. *Schizophrenia Research, 88*, 5–25.

Ng, C. H. (1997). The stigma of mental illness in Asian cultures. *Australian and New Zealand Journal of Psychiatry, 31*, 382–390.

Ng, C. H., Lin, K. M., Singh, B., & Chiu, E. (Eds.). *Ethno-psychopharmacology: Advances in current practice.* Cambridge: Cambridge University Press, 2008.

Okazaki, S. (2000). Treatment delay among Asian-American patients with severe mental illness. *American Journal of Orthopsychiatry, 70*, 58–64.

Owen, M. J. Craddock, N., O'Donovan, M. C. (2005). Schizophrenia: Genes at last? *Trends in Genetics, 21*(9), 518–525.

Patel, V., Cohen, A., Thara, R., & Gureje, O. (2006). Is the outcome of schizophrenia really better in developing countries? *Revista Brasileira de Psiquiatria, 28*, 149–152.

Ragins, M. (2002) *A road to recovery.* Retrieved from http://www.mhavillage.org/writings.html.

Rin, H., Schooler, C., & Caudill, W. A. (1973). Symptomatology and hospitalization: Culture, social structure, and psychopathology in Taiwan and Japan. *Journal of Nervous and Mental Disease, 157*, 296–312.

Rosca-Rebaudengo, P., Durst, R., & Minuchin-Itzigsohn, S. (1996). Transculturation, psychosis, and koro symptoms. *Israel Journal of Psychiatry* and *Related Sciences, 33*, 54–62.

Russell, J. G. (1989). Anxiety disorders in Japan: A review of the Japanese literature on shinkeishitsu and taijin-kyofusho. *Culture, Medicine, and Psychiatry, 13*, 391–403.

Samalin, L., Blanc, O., & Llorca, P. M. (2010). Optimizing treatment of schizophrenia to minimize relapse. *Expert Review of Neurotherapeutics, 10*, 147–150.

Sato, M. (2006). Renaming schizophrenia: A Japanese perspective. *World Psychiatry, 5*, 53–55.

Sartorius, N., Gulbinat, W., Harrison, G., Laska, E., & Siegel, C. (1996). Long-term follow-up of schizophrenia in 16 countries: A description of the International Study of Schizophrenia conducted by the World Health Organization. *Social Psychiatry* and *Psychiatric Epidemiology, 31*, 249–258.

Scheff, T. J. (1999). *Being mentally ill: A sociological theory.* New York: Aldine de Gruyter.

Scheff, T. J., Jr. (2006). *Goffman unbound! A new paradigm for social science.* Boulder, CO, Paradigm.

Schulze, B. (2007). Stigma and mental health professionals: A review of the evidence on an intricate relationship. *International Review of Psychiatry, 19*, 137–155.

Schulze Mönking, H., Hornung, W. P., Stricker, K., & Buchkremer, G. (1997). Expressed-emotion development and course of schizophrenic illness: Considerations based on results of a CFI replication. *European archives of psychiatry and clinical neuroscience, 247*, 31–34.

Seeman, P. (2002). Atypical antipsychotics: Mechanism of action. *Canadian Journal of Psychiatry, 47*, 27–38.

Selten, J. P., Cantor-Graae, E., & Kahn, R. S. (2007). Migration and schizophrenia. *Current Opinion in Psychiatry, 20*, 111–115.

Sensky, T., Turkington, D., Kingdon, D., Scott, J. L., Scott, J., Siddle, R., et al. (2000). A randomized controlled trial of cognitive-behavioral therapy for persistent symptoms in schizophrenia resistant to medication. *Archives of General Psychiatry, 57*, 165–172.

Shin, S. K., & Lukens, E. P. (2002). Effects of psychoeducation for Korean Americans with chronic mental illness. *Psychiatric Services, 53*, 1125–1131.

Sota, S., Shimodera, S., Kii, M., Okamura, K., Suto, K., Suwaki, M., et al. (2008). Effect of a family psychoeducational program on relatives of schizophrenia patients. *Psychiatry and Clinical Neurosciences, 62*, 379–385.

Stip, E. (2000). Novel antipsychotics: Issues and controversies; Typicality of atypical antipsychotics. *Journal of Psychiatry and Neuroscience, 25*, 137–153.

Stompe, T., Ortwein-Swoboda, G., Ritter, K., & Schanda, H. (2003). Old wine in new bottles? Stability and plasticity of the contents of schizophrenic delusions. *Psychopathology, 36*, 6–12.

Strakowski, S. M., Keck, P. E., Jr., Arnold, L. M., Collins, J., Wilson, R. M., Fleck, D. E., et al. (2003). Ethnicity and diagnosis in patients with affective disorders. *Journal of Clinical Psychiatry, 64*, 747–754.

Sue, S., Fujino, D. C., Hu, L. T., Takeuchi, D. T., & Zane, N. W. (1991). Community mental health services for ethnic minority groups: A test of the cultural responsiveness hypothesis. *Journal of Consulting and Clinical Psychology, 59*, 533–540.

Szasz, T. (1960). The myth of mental illness. *American Psychologist, 15*, 113–118.

Takeuchi, D. T., Alegría, M., Jackson, J. S., & Williams, D. W. (2007). Immigration and mental health: Diverse findings in Asian, black, and Latino populations. *American Journal of Public Health, 97*(1), 12–13.

Takeuchi, D,T., Chung, R.C.Y., Lin, K.M., Shen, H., Kurasaki, K., Chun, C.A., & Sue, S. (1998). Lifetime and Twelve-Month Prevalence Rates of Major Depressive Episodes and Dysthymia Among Chinese Americans in Los Angeles. *American Journal of Psychiatry, 155*(10), 1407–1414.

Tang, V. W., Leung, S. K., & Lam, L. C. (2008). Clinical correlates of the caregiving experience for Chinese caregivers of patients with schizophrenia. *Social Psychiatry and Psychiatric Epidemiology, 43*, 720–726.

Tateyama, M., Kudo, I., Hashimoto, M., Abe, Y., Kainuma, A., Yoshimura, K., et al. (1999). Is paranoid schizophrenia the most common subtype? Comparison of subtype diagnoses by Japanese and European psychiatrists, using the summaries of the same patients. *Psychopathology, 32*, 98–106.

Thomas, P., Mathur, P., Gottesman, I. I., Nagpal, R., Nimgaonkar, V. L., & Deshpande, S. N. (2007). Correlates of hallucinations in schizophrenia: A cross-cultural evaluation. *Schizophrenia Research, 92*, 41–49.

Tsai, G., Lane, H. Y., Yang, P., Chong, M. Y., & Lange, N. (2004). Glycine transporter I inhibitor, N-methylglycine (sarcosine), added to antipsychotics for the treatment of schizophrenia. *Biological Psychiatry, 55*, 452–456.

Tseng, W. S., & McDermott, J. F., Jr. (1981). *Culture, mind, and therapy: An introduction to cultural psychiatry.* New York: Brunner/Mazel.

Tsuang, M. T. (1982). *Schizophrenia: The facts.* New York: Oxford University Press.

Tsuang, M. T., & Simpson, J. C. (1984). Schizoaffective disorder: Concept and reality. *Schizophrenia Bulletin, 10*, 14–25.

Tsuang, M. (2000). Schizophrenia: Genes and environment. *Biological Psychiatry, 47*, 210–220.

Tsuang, M. T., Bar, J. L., Stone, W. S., & Faraone, S. V. (2004). Gene-environment interactions in mental disorders. *World Psychiatry, 3*, 73–83.

Uba, L. (1994). *Asian Americans: Personality patterns, identity, and mental health.* New York: Guilford.

Ujike, H. (2002). Stimulant-induced psychosis and schizophrenia: The role of sensitization. *Current Psychiatry Reports, 4*, 177–184.

Ungvari, G. S., Goggins, W., Leung, S. K., & Gerevich, J. (2007). Schizophrenia with prominent catatonic features ("catatonic schizophrenia"): II. Factor analysis of the catatonic syndrome. *Progress in Neuropsychopharmacology and Biological Psychiatry, 31*, 462–468.

Velligan, D. I., Weiden, P. J., Sajatovic, M., Scott, J., Carpenter, D., Ross, R., et al. (2009). The expert consensus guideline series: Adherence problems in patients with serious and persistent mental illness. *Journal of Clinical Psychiatry, 70*(Suppl 4), 1–46.

Velligan, D. I., Weiden, P. J., Sajatovic, M., Scott, J., Carpenter, D., Ross, R., et al. (2010). Assessment of adherence problems in patients with serious and persistent mental illness: Recommendations from the Expert Consensus Guidelines. *Journal of Psychiatric Practice, 16*, 34–45.

Wahlbeck, K., Cheine, M. V., & Essali, A. (2007). Clozapine versus typical neuroleptic medication for schizophrenia. *The Cochrane Database of Systematic Reviews.* Hoboken, NJ: Wiley.

Weisman, A. G. (1997). Understanding cross-cultural prognostic variability for schizophrenia. *Cultural Diversity and Mental Health, 3*, 23–35.

Westermeyer, J. (1985). Psychiatric diagnosis across cultural boundaries. *American Journal of Psychiatry, 142*, 798–805.

World Health Organization (WHO). (1974). The international pilot study of schizophrenia. *Schizophrenia Bulletin,* 21–34.

Xiang, Y. T., Ma, X., Cai, Z. J., Li, S. R., Xiang, Y. Q., Guo, H. L., et al. (2008). Prevalence and socio-demographic correlates of schizophrenia in Beijing, China. *Schizophrenia Research, 102*, 270–277.

Yamamoto, J. (1978). Research priorities in Asian-American mental health delivery. *American Journal of Psychiatry, 135*, 457–458.

| 6 |

MOOD DISORDERS IN ASIANS

Albert Yeung and Doris Chang

CURRENT *DSM* NOSOLOGY AND CRITERIA FOR MOOD DISORDERS

According to the fourth edition of the *Diagnostic and Statistical Manual of Mental Disorders* (*DSM-IV*) (APA, 1994) and the tenth revision of the *International Classification of Diseases and Related Health Problems* (ICD-10)(WHO, 1992), mood disorders include unipolar depressive disorders and bipolar disorders. Patients are diagnosed with having Major Depressive Disorder (MDD) if they have one or more depressive episodes. A depressive episode is defined as having depressive mood or reduced interest/pleasure for at least two weeks, accompanied by vegetative, cognitive, and psychomotor symptoms for a total of at least five symptoms all together. The accompanying symptoms include insomnia or hypersomnia, loss of energy, loss or increase of appetite or weight, diminished ability to think or concentrate, psychomotor agitation or retardation, feelings of worthlessness or excessive guilt, and recurrent thoughts of death or suicide. To be diagnosed with MDD, the symptoms and impairment from the major depressive episode cannot be better accounted for by other major psychotic disorders and the patient must not have had a manic episode. A manic episode is defined as having a distinct period of persistently elevated, expansive, or irritable mood, lasting at least 1 week accompanied by three or more (four if the mood is only irritable) mania-associated symptoms. These symptoms cause marked impairment in functioning and are not due to substance use or a medical condition. The mania-associated symptoms include inflated self-esteem or grandiosity, decreased need for sleep, talkativeness or feeling pressured to keep talking, flight of ideas or racing thoughts, distractibility, increased goal-directed activity (at work, at school, or sexually) or psychomotor agitation, and excessive involvement in pleasurable activities that have a high potential for painful consequences. To be diagnosed with bipolar disorder, the patient needs to have a current or previous episode of mania that is not better accounted for by a major psychiatric disorder such as schizoaffective disorder, schizophreniform disorder, or delusional disorder.

STRENGTH, WEAKNESSES, AND ALTERNATIVES IN APPLYING CURRENT NOSOLOGY AND DIAGNOSTIC CRITERIA TO IDENTIFY MOOD DISORDERS IN ASIANS

Do the Concepts of Mood Disorders Fit Well for Asians?

In this chapter, we used a broad definition of Asians as those who identify themselves as being Asians or with Asian heritage. Since Asians are a heterogeneous group with diverse character-istics (Barreto & Segal, 2005), we specified the subgroup of Asians sampled (e.g., Vietnamese Americans or Chinese Americans) when we described the findings in specific studies. There are different viewpoints on whether the diagnoses of mood disorders apply well to Asians. One argu-ment is that mood disorders are medical disorders that can be found universally in all ethnic and racial groups. *DSM-IV* and ICD-10 diagnostic criteria were developed with the assumption that they will apply across different cultures and races. Yet, anthropologists contend that the concept of depressive disorder is rooted in Western cultures and may not apply well in other cultures. For example, many Asians tend to communicate their distress using somatic symptoms and concep-tualize their illnesses as physical, rather than mental ailments (Saint Arnault & Kim, 2008; D. T. S. Lee, Kleinman, & Kleinman, 2007; Karasz et al., 2007).

We will present existing data to show that both arguments may be valid. These arguments address different aspects of mood disorders, one from a more biological perspective and the other from a cultural perspective. It is important to point out that the demarcation of cultures as "Eastern" or "Asian" and "Western" is arbitrary, as cultures are rapidly being influenced and trans-formed, particularly in this era of rapid globalization.

The Prevalence of Depression Among Asians

There are various ways to examine whether the concepts of mood disorders as defined by *DSM-IV* and ICD-10 diagnostic criteria apply well to Asians. One way is to study whether they exist in Asian populations, and whether the prevalence of mood disorders among Asians are comparable to other populations. Due to the paucity of published data on the prevalence of mania among Asians, we will focus on the prevalence of depression among Asians, particularly among Chinese and Chinese Americans, for whom we have the most data. Takeuchi et al. (1998) conducted a large-scale community-based study of depression among Chinese Americans in Los Angeles County using the Composite International Diagnostic Interview (WHO, 1990) as the diagnostic instrument. They found the lifetime prevalence of major depression among Chinese Americans was 6.9%, much lower than the national estimate of 17.1% (Kessler et al, 1994). Two epidemio-logical studies in the 1980s reported low prevalence of depression among Chinese populations in

Asia. Hwu et al. (1989) reported a 1.5% lifetime prevalence of depression among ethnic Chinese in Taiwan, which is the lowest rate among the 10 countries surveyed in the Cross-National Collaborative Study on Depression (Weissman et al., 1996). C. N. Chen et al. (1993) conducted a survey in Hong Kong and reported that the lifetime prevalence of depression among Chinese was 1.29% to 2.4%. This rate is notably lower than the rates of lifetime depression among U.S. populations reported in the ECA study (5.8% in New Haven, Connecticut, 2.9% in Baltimore, 4.4% in St. Louis, and 5.6% in Los Angeles) (Paykel, 1992). In a more recent epidemiological survey, the Collaborative Psychiatric Epidemiology Surveys (CPES) sponsored by the U.S. National Institute of Mental Health showed that the prevalence of any depressive disorder in the past 12 months was lowest among Asian Americans (5.4%), which was less than half of the prevalence found among non-Latino whites (11.2%). Among Asian American populations, Vietnamese women were found to have significantly lower prevalence of any depressive disorder compared to Chinese women. Chinese, Filipino, and other Asian American groups, including Vietnamese men, showed no difference in their prevalence of lifetime depressive disorder (Alegria et al., 2008). These findings generated many academic discussions on whether depression is relatively uncommon among Asians.

Another international study has provided further data to this query. The WHO collaborative study *Mental Illness in General Healthcare* investigated the prevalence of depression in primary care settings in 14 countries worldwide (Usturn & Sartorius; 1995). In this study, the investigators used a 2-stage approach; the initial screening was performed with the General Health Questionnaire (GHQ-12), and it was followed by a standardized in-person interview using the Composite International Diagnostic Interview (CIDI-PHC) (Sartorius et al., 1993). Diagnosis was based on ICD-10 (WHO, 1990) and *DSM-III-R* criteria (American Psychiatric Association, 1987). The study found wide variations in the rates of depression among primary care patients, ranging from 2.6% (Nagasaki) to 29.5% (Santiago). The populations with the lowest prevalence of ICD-10 depression were Japanese in Nagasaki (2.6%) and Chinese in Shanghai (4.0%), compared to the average prevalence of 10% across all centers.

Other epidemiological studies, however, have demonstrated that depression is more common among Asians than previously thought. T. A. Cheng (1989) conducted a community survey in Taiwan and found the prevalence of depression was 8.5%. Chong et al. (2001) studied Taiwanese elders and reported the 1-month prevalence of major depression was 5.9%. D. T. S. Lee, Yip, Chiu, Leung, and Chung (2001) reported that the 3-month prevalence rate for postpartum depression in Hong Kong was 6.1%, and argued that depression is not rare in contemporary Hong Kong Chinese women. These studies suggest that the occurrence of depression among Chinese is comparable to the 5–10% prevalence rate in community populations in the United States and European countries (Katon & Schulberg, 1992). Our group at Massachusetts General Hospital performed a two-phase epidemiological survey in the primary care clinic of a community health center in Boston. In this study, the prevalence of MDD among immigrant Chinese Americans in a primary care setting was estimated to be 19.6%. Comparing this to the 5–10% prevalence rate in other similar settings, we concluded that MDD is common among immigrant Chinese Americans in urban primary care settings (Yeung, Chan, et al., 2004).

Interpreting the diverse findings across different epidemiological studies is complicated by the fact that prevalence statistics are influenced by a number of factors. These factors include choice of the research setting and the demographics of the studied population (e.g., subjects with different age or gender distributions, patients may be recruited from the community, specific institutions, or primary care clinics). Moreover, varied definitions and criteria for depression from the *DSM-II, DSM-III*, ICD-8, and ICD-9 were used in the studies. There were also an assortment of diagnostic procedures used (e.g., diagnosis from the clinician, researcher, or patient), and as well as varied instruments used (e.g., the Composite International Diagnostic Interview or the Structured Clinical Interview Dialogue). These studies support, to some extent, the universality of MDD while its prevalence may vary significantly across different cultural and ethnic groups. More importantly, results from these studies suggest that underrecognition and undertreatment of depression among Asians are widespread both in the United States and in Asian countries.

PRESENTING SYMPTOMS, ILLNESS BELIEFS, AND HELP-SEEKING OF ASIANS WITH DEPRESSION

A recent study of Chinese and Japanese American immigrants found a relationship between acculturation and the specific expression of depression in Asian Americans (such as affective, somatic, or interpersonal complaints), and that the relationship may be mediated by the focus of self-attention (H. Chen, Guarnaccia, & Cheung , 2003). Specifically, as Asian immigrants become more bicultural, their focus shifts to more affective aspects and less somatic aspects of experience. Unsurprisingly, this shift is associated with a trend toward more reports of affective symptoms of depression than somatic symptoms. Thus, the findings of the study suggest that culture may influence depression by imbuing certain kinds of subjective experiences with greater meaning and salience, which may directly or indirectly precipitate certain patterns of depressive symptom formation and/or reporting.

In an earlier study (Yeung, Chang, Gresham, Nierenberg, & Fava, 2004), our team studied 29 Chinese American patients with confirmed MDD using the Explanatory Model Interview Catalogue (EMIC) (Weiss, 1992) to systematically examine their illness beliefs. These beliefs included their chief complaints, labels of their illness, perceptions of stigma, causal attributions, and help-seeking patterns. We found that 93% of depressed subjects reported having depressed mood when they filled out the Beck Depression Inventory (BDI). Yet, their presenting complaints were very different. None of the subjects spontaneously reported depressed mood, and only four (14%) reported psychological symptoms such as irritability, rumination, and poor memory. Twenty-two depressed Chinese Americans (76%) complained about somatic symptoms (Table 6.1). When asked how they would label of their illness, 21 patients (72%) did not know the name of their illness or did not consider it a diagnosable medical illness, and 5 patients (17%) attributed their symptoms to pre-existing medical problems. Only three patients (10%) labeled their illness as a psychiatric condition (Table 6.2). Help-seeking for their depressive symptoms generally involved general hospitals (69%), lay help (62%), and alternative treatments such as acupuncture and Chinese herbs (55%), but rarely mental health services (3.5%) (Table 6.3) (Yeung, Chang, et al., 2004). The results of this study suggest that due to cultural differences, many Chinese do not consider depressed mood a symptom to report to their physicians. In addition, many Chinese are unfamiliar with depression as a treatable psychiatric disorder, and offer no explanatory model on depression.

TABLE 6.1: Chief Complaints of Chinese-Americans with Major Depressive Disorder (N = 29)

Chief complaints (%)	N (%)
Physical symptoms	12 (42)
Depressive neurovegetative s/s	10 (34)
Depressive psychological s/s	4 (14)
Irritability, Rumination,	
Poor memory	
Nervousness	2 (7)
Depressed Mood	0 (0)
No complaints	1 (3.5)

Source: Yeung et al., J Nerv & Ment Dis 192 (4): 324-327, 2004.

TABLE 6.2: Labels Used by Chinese-American Patients with Major Depressive Disorder to Describe Their Illness (N = 29)

Name of the Illness	N (%)
"Don't know"	16 (55)
"Not an illness"	5 (17)
Medical Illnesses	5 (17)
"hypertension"	1
"cold"	2
"poor health"	1
"injured arm"	1
"Post-Traumatic Stress Syndrome"	1 (3.5)
"Craziness"	2 (7)

Source: Yeung et al., J Nerv & Ment Dis 192 (4): 324-327, 2004.

TABLE 6.3: Methods of Help-Seeking by Depressed Chinese-American Patients (N = 29)

Methods	Frequency (%)
General Hospital	20 (69)
Lay Help	18 (62)
Alternative Treatment by Providers	16 (55)
Spiritual Treatment	4 (14)
Alternative Treatment by Self	3 (11)
Mental Health Professionals	1 (3.5)

Source: Yeung et al., J Nerv & Ment Dis 192 (4): 324-327, 2004.

The findings of the studies can be interpreted as evidence that many Chinese, in the process of rapid modernization in the past decades, have relinquished indigenous or traditional explanatory models, such as neurasthenia. However, they have not yet adopted or accepted the Western psychiatric concepts of mental disorders. Recent studies suggest that many Asians continue to embrace holistic conceptualizations of illness, and focus on the somatic symptoms (D. T. S. Lee, Kleinman, & Kleinman, 2007; Saint Arnault & Kim, 2008; Dinh et al., 2009).

THE UTILITY AND CHALLENGES OF IDENTIFYING DEPRESSION IN ASIANS

Professional Diagnoses Versus Indigenous Illness Beliefs

The development of a universal classification system for psychiatric disorders (e.g., the diagnostic criteria developed by the *DSM-IV* and the ICD-10) has greatly enhanced the sharing of knowledge on mental disorders across cultures. It has also increased the consistency of clinical diagnosis and treatment of mental disorders in different parts of the world. International epidemiological studies have shown that most psychiatric disorders can be identified among people from different races and cultures, even though the prevalence, meaning, and prognosis may vary significantly.

On the other hand, sometimes there are obstacles and problems when we diagnose Asians with mood disorders. The concepts of mood disorders, such as mania or depression, are rooted in Western culture. Many Asians with traditional illness beliefs are unfamiliar with these disease concepts. The discrepancy between professional and lay disease concepts may have contributed to the low health literacy (F. K. Wong, Lam, & Poon, 2010), high stigma toward mood symptoms (Hsu et al., 2008), and underutilization of mental health services among Asians. To overcome these obstacles, it would be beneficial to provide psychoeducation to Asian communities, particularly to those communities unfamiliar with depression. This will help demystify mood disorders and inform Asians that depression is a treatable condition that improves with professional interventions just like many other medical problems.

In addition, the label of "depression" may be stigmatizing for many Asians who try to avoid being associated with having any mental illnesses. As a result, many Asians with mood disorders are reluctant to seek treatment in order to avoid being labeled with a mental illness. In future *DSM* and ICD versions, it would be beneficial to use nosologies that incorporate both Western and Eastern conceptions so that they can be more readily accepted by patients from non-Western cultures. In the mean time, clinicians who serve Asians with traditional illness beliefs need training to understand and appreciate their patients' viewpoints about their illnesses, and effectively negotiate with their patients, who may have very different illness explanatory models. They need to serve as a bridge to link indigenous beliefs and professional concepts, and discuss mood disorders in a culturally sensitive way so that Asian patients will understand and accept treatment for them. When patients and their clinicians have compatible visions of illnesses and treatment goals, patients are more willing to engage in treatment.

In a recent study to improve recognition and engagement of depressed patients (Yeung, Yu, Fung, Vorono, & Fava, 2006), our team systematically screened for depression among Chinese immigrants in a primary care clinic using the bilingual Personal Health Questionniare-9, and encouraged people who screened positive for depression to receive a psychiatric assessment. In the assessment, an Engagement Interview Protocol (EIP) was specially designed to effectively discuss psychiatric diagnoses with cultural sensitivity. The EIP used the following approaches: (1) Elicit the patient's illness beliefs, (2) Understand and acknowledge multiple explanatory models, (3) Discuss depressive symptoms in the context of patients' physical health and social network, (4) Introduce Western psychiatric theories in ways that reflect common assumptions in traditional Chinese medicine, (5) Involve patients' families whenever possible, and (6) Use terminology that avoids unintended stigma (Yeung & Kam, 2008). In that study, our team was successful in engaging more than 90% of the depressed Chinese Americans who were assessed to receive treatment for depression. The study demonstrated that a combination of systematic depression screening and culturally sensitive interview may be an effective approach to successfully engage culturally diverse Asians with depression in treatment.

PERSPECTIVES ON THE CAUSES OF MOOD DISORDERS IN ASIANS

Critical Appraisal of Major Etiological Models of Mood Disorders

Biological Models

While the exact etiologies of mood disorders are still unclear, there are several dominant biological models that have been found useful to explain, at least in part, the etiologies of the mood disorders. These models include the biogenic amine hypotheses, neuroendocrine links, and genetic models (Kaplan & Sadock, 1995). Recent pharmacogenetic research has identified specific profiles of genetic polymorphism among Asian populations (H. Kim et al., 2006; Kau et al., 2008; Kishi et al., 2009), which may give rise to variations in treatment responses across racial and ethnic groups. Nevertheless, these biological hypotheses continue to be used across racial groups, including Asians who suffer from depression.

BIOGENIC AMINE HYPOTHESES

The biogenic amine hypotheses of depression were based on the observation that reserpine induces decreased blood pressure by depleting biogenic amine stores, and at the same time precipitates clinical depression in some patients. In addition, antidepressant medications that are effective in treating clinical depression raise the levels of biogenic amines in the brain. The biogenic amine hypotheses consider the depletion or imbalance of biogenic amines, particularly norepinephrine and serotonin, the cause of clinical depression. These hypotheses are compatible with findings from animal studies. Using neurobiological techniques to probe different areas of the brain involved with emotion, it has been shown that norepinephrine-containing neurons are involved with many functions that are profoundly disrupted in melancholia, including mood, arousal, appetite, reward, and drives. Other biogenic amine neurotransmitters that have similar functions are catecholamine dopamine, which is important for drive, pleasure, sex, and psychomotor activity, and serotonin, which is involved in the regulatory control of affects, aggression, sleep, and appetite. Based on the biogenic amine hypotheses, new classes of antidepressants have been developed and now play an important role for treatment of depression. Despite these exciting advances, the biochemistry of mood disorders remains unclear. There is no evidence to show that a deficiency or an excess of biogenic amines in specific brain structures leads to the occurrence of mood disorders. In addition, the new compounds that act on the serotonin system were found to be effective not only for depression, but also on obsessive-compulsive disorder (OCD), post-traumatic stress disorder (PTSD), panic disorder, social phobia, bulimia nervosa, and borderline personality disorder. This raises the question whether biogenic amines like serotonin are involved not just with depression, but with all reactions to social disruption and distress.

NEUROENDOCRINE HYPOTHESES

The link between stress, homeostatic failure, and depression has been widely studied as a possible mechanism of depressive illness. This proposed mechanism formulates that repeated stress leads to overproduction of steroidal hormone by the hypothalamic-pituitary-adrenal axis, which can be detected by the dexamethasone suppression test. It has been shown that there is an increase in the concentration of corticotrophin-releasing factor in the cerebrospinal fluid of patients with major depressive disorder. Similarly, patients with depression have blunted growth hormone response to clonidine (the α_2-adrenergic receptor agonist) and blunted thyroid-stimulating hormone upon thyrotropin stimulation. The neuroendocrine hypotheses are conceptually appealing since extensive medical studies have demonstrated that the impacts of stress on relevant brain areas are mediated by hormonal changes. The drawback of these hypotheses is the lack of specificity of such changes. In addition to patients with MDD, people who suffer from anxiety disorders such as panic disorder and PTSD also manifest dexamethasone nonsuppression and blunted response to clonidine and thyrotropin stimulation.

GENETIC MODELS

Numerous studies in the past decades, which use designs such as family studies, twin studies, and adoption studies, have all shown that mood disorders are heritable conditions. Based on family studies, the morbid rates of bipolar disorder in first-degree relatives of bipolar probands ranged between 3% and 8%, compared to the rate of 1% in the general population, suggesting a strong familiar risk. Similarly, the morbid risks of unipolar disorder among first-degree relatives of unipolar probands were 2- to 3-fold above the general population. These findings strongly support familial tendency of mood disorders. Furthermore, the rate of unipolar disorder in the families of bipolar probands and the rate of bipolar disorder in the families of unipolar probands are elevated, suggesting some common genetic connections between the two forms of mood disorder. Based on twin studies of mood disorders, the concordance rates are 2- to 4-fold for mood disorder in monozygotic (MZ) twins compared to dizygotic twins, with the concordance ratio for bipolar-bipolar pairs higher than that for unipolar-unipolar pairs. The data provide strong evidence for the role of genetic factors in mood disorders, particularly for bipolar disorder. For monozygotic twins, the concordance for mood disorder ranged from 58% to 93%, indicating that nonheritable environmental factors also play an important role in mood disorders (Kelsoe, 1995).

In adoption studies, the rates of psychiatric illness are determined in both the biological and adoptive parents of the probands who were adopted at birth and later found to have a mood disorder. Due to the difficulty in obtaining appropriate proband subjects, only a limited number of studies have been reported. One study on the biological relatives of bipolar probands found a 3-fold increase in the rate of bipolar disorder and a 2-fold increase in the rate of unipolar disorder. Another study in the biological relatives of affectively ill probands showed a 3-fold increase in the rate of unipolar disorder and a 6-fold increase in the rate of completed suicide. Yet, other adoption studies showed no increase in the rates of the illness among biological relatives of the probands of mood disorders, possibly due to small sample sizes.

GENETIC LINKAGE STUDIES

With the advent of molecular genetics technologies, researchers have, in recent years, focused on studying DNA markers in large pedigrees in which many family members have bipolar disorder. Linkage studies have now identified markers associated with major mental disorders, which have been replicated in more than one study. In a meta-analysis, Badner and Gershon (2002) combined the findings of individual studies that provided the strongest evidence for susceptibility loci on chromosome 13 and 22 for bipolar disorder. However, no single locus for bipolar disorder has been consistently replicated, and the contribution of any identified locus was small. It is likely that future studies will identify more genes with small hereditary effects and will have better understanding of the interactions of these genes.

LIMITATIONS OF THE BIOLOGICAL MODELS

The biological models such as the biogenic amine hypotheses and the neuroendocrine hypotheses lack specificity. These models most likely represent broader pathological responses toward stress, and not just mood disorders. Genetic studies have shown that mood disorders, and particularly bipolar disorder, are hereditary disorders. More research is needed to identify the genes that contribute to mood disorders, their modes of transmission, the interactions between genetic loadings and environmental factors for the occurrence of mood disorders, and the similarity and variations of genetic polymorphism among racial groups.

Psychological Models

Numerous psychological models have been developed to explain the origins of depression. Given space limitations, we will focus our discussion on psychodynamic, behavioral, cognitive/ cognitive-behavioral, and interpersonal models of depression, which constitute the most influential models in the field. We acknowledge however, that these are mainstream psychological models grounded in a Western biomedical perspective that conceptualizes depression as a psychiatric condition rather than as a bodily or spiritual problem. Whereas few indigenous alternatives to these mainstream professional theories have been described in the English-language literature, a growing number of studies have documented cultural differences in lay theories of depression. Though important in assessing the potential credibility of these principal etiological models with patients, such lay theories are beyond the scope of this chapter, although we provide a few illustrative examples in the discussion below.

PSYCHODYNAMIC MODELS

While psychodynamic formulations have been very influential in the field of psychology, the theories tend to emphasize personality development and structure over disorder-specific etiological models. Disorders are frequently linked to early conflicts and disruptions in relationships with primary attachment figures and the defensive patterns that arise in response; however, the specific form the pathology takes is assumed to vary across individuals (McWilliams, 1999). To complicate matters, there are a number of different psychodynamic models associated with different psychoanalytic thinkers, each of which identifies different predisposing factors and transactional processes that are thought to contribute to the development of depression. Nevertheless, in their review of the major psychoanalytic schools, namely traditional Freudian, object-relations, and self-psychology, Busch, Ruden, and Shapiro (2004) identified a number of core dynamics of depression that have been identified across etiological models.

According to these authors, almost all psychoanalytic theories emphasize sensitivity to narcissistic injury as predisposing individuals to experience shame and anger, which may serve as risk factors for later depressive episodes. Second, conflicted anger, for example, aggressive feelings accompanied by guilt, is also seen as contributing to the depressive's tendency toward self-denigration and self-punishment, and producing the self-defeating behaviors that serve to maintain depressive tendencies. Third, those aggressive feelings are ultimately directed toward the self via harsh and punitive self-judgments, although the specific processes underlying this dynamic varies across models. Fourth, some psychodynamic thinkers emphasize efforts to modulate self-esteem and aggression through idealizing and devaluing others, which may result in depression when individuals fail to meet their expectations. Others view low self-esteem and subsequent depression as resulting from individuals' inability to achieve their unrealistic narcissistic aspirations and expectations. Finally, defenses such as denial, projection, and passive aggression are also identified as immediate strategies for protecting one against emotional pain, but may result in further insults to one's self-esteem. In summary, psychodynamic models tend to emphasize two distinct pathways toward depression, one involving aggression toward others that is redirected toward the self, and the other emphasizing the role of low self-esteem among individuals whose unrealistic expectations of themselves produces inevitable achievement failures (Busch et al., 2004). It is important to note, however, that these models were primarily developed through clinical observation and case studies but do not enjoy the same degree of empirical support as do the other etiological models reviewed below.

BEHAVIORAL OR SOCIAL LEARNING MODELS

Classic behavioral models view depression as the result of operant conditioning. Specifically, depression may be caused by (1) a lack of positive reinforcement in response to one's behavior, and/or (2) the presence of punishment, or person-environment interactions with aversive consequences. These conditions may cause depression directly or indirectly by reducing the client's engagement with potentially rewarding experiences (Lewinsohn, Biglan, & Zeiss, 1976). The rate of reinforcement and/or punishment is seen as functionally related to the availability of such conditions in their immediate environments, individuals' skills in effectively eliciting positive reinforcement or coping with aversive events, and the variable impact of these specific events on the individual. Support for the behavioral perspective is provided by studies that show that depressed individuals exhibit a number of social skill deficits and behavioral withdrawal patterns that decrease the likelihood of experiencing positive reinforcement (Jacobson & Anderson, 1982, Lewinsohn & Libet, 1972). For example, Dykman et al. (1991) studied depressed and nondepressed subjects engaged in group discussions and found that the negative cognitions of depressed individuals are based in part on real observable deficits in depressed individuals' social skills. Another study found that the number of pleasant activities engaged in was correlated with mood for depressed, nondepressed psychiatric, and normal controls, as depressed subjects engaged in significantly fewer pleasant activities (Lewinsohn & Graf, 1973). Although the influence of purely behavioral models of depression declined in the 1960s and 1970s as a result of the cognitive revolution, aspects of behaviorism were reintegrated in later cognitive/cognitive behavioral models. In recent years, there has been renewed interest in behavioral models of depression as a result of clinical research suggesting that behavioral treatments alone may be as efficacious as more complex treatments for depression that integrate behavior and cognitive interventions (Jacobson et al., 1996).

COGNITIVE/COGNITIVE BEHAVIORAL MODELS

According to cognitive and cognitive behavioral models of depression, the ways in which individuals interpret and react to life experiences predict both the incidence and chronicity of depression. Depressogenic appraisal and response styles are thought to interact with negative life events (or the absence of positive life events) in a diathesis-stress relationship. Of all the cognitive vulnerability-stress models of depression, Beck's cognitive theory of depression (Beck et al., 1979; Clark, Beck, & Alford, 1999) is arguably the most influential psychological theory for explaining depressive phenomena. Beck and colleagues attribute depression to a dysfunctional cognitive structure characterized by inaccurate interpretations (cognitive distortions) of life situations; rigid and maladaptive assumptions, beliefs, and attitudes (negative schemas); and a global negative view of the self, the world, and the future (negative cognitive triad) (Young, Weinberger, & Beck, 2001). Cognitive distortions ("He doesn't care about me") are viewed as stemming from underlying negative schemas ("I am unlovable"), which are shaped by early life experiences and are thought to be relatively stable. These negative schemas predispose individuals to adopt a biased and inflexible view of the world and contribute to the maintenance of irrational expectations of the self and others ("There is no one I can count on."). This dysfunctional cognitive structure is thought to increase individuals' psychological vulnerability to depression, particularly when combined with environmental stressors that may overwhelm coping capabilities (Clark et al., 1999).

Beck's cognitive theory of depression is also sometimes referred to as a cognitive behavioral model in its acknowledgment of the important role that behaviors may play in the origin and maintenance of depressive states. Maladaptive behaviors, including decreases in activity level and dysfunctional coping styles, may stem from depression-related mechanisms while also actively generating the adverse interpersonal conditions that maintain depressive states (see also the "Interpersonal Models" section below). Substantial empirical research supports the cognitive model of depression (Clark et al., 1999); however, there remains some dispute as to the relative contributions of cognitive or behavioral mechanisms in the development and maintenance of depression.

Another influential cognitive theory is Abramson, Metalsky, and Alloy's (1989) hopelessness theory of depression. According to this theory, hopelessness, or the view that one cannot change one's life circumstances, is the central mediating factor that determines whether negative events will lead to depression. According to hopelessness theory, individuals who expect that desired outcomes will not occur or that aversive outcomes will occur, and that they are powerless to change the likelihood of these outcomes, are predisposed to develop a specific depressive subtype called *hopelessness depression.*

These two main cognitive models have spawned a substantial body of research as well as numerous other cognitive theories that propose alternative causal chains. Nolen-Hoeksema's (1991) response style theory of depression for example, emphasizes the role of rumination in prolonging depressive episodes. Empirical tests of response style theory have demonstrated that individuals who respond to their depression by focusing on their symptoms and the possible causes and consequences of their symptoms will experience longer depression compared to individuals who take action to distract themselves from their symptoms.

INTERPERSONAL MODELS

Whereas psychodynamic, behavioral, and cognitive models of depression emphasize internal, intraindividual processes, interpersonal models view depression as contextually embedded in the interpersonal arena. One of the earliest interpersonal theories was Coyne's (1976) interactional systems theory of depression, which identified an interactional sequence between spouses that appeared to increase vulnerability to depression. According to this theory, individuals with mild or subclinical levels of depression seek the reassurance from significant others that they are truly cared for in an effort to assuage their own feelings of insecurity and loneliness. However, when reassurance is provided, these individuals question its sincerity and seek further reassurances. Over time, the individual's excessive reassurance-seeking lead others to feel increasingly frustrated and hostile, which may result in withdrawal from or rejection of the target individual. This loss of social support precipitates the development of more serious depressive symptoms (Haeffel, Voelz, & Joiner, 2007). Empirical tests of Coyne's theory generally confirmed the proposition that depressed individuals provoke negative or ambivalent interactions in others, and are more likely to be rejected (Dryden, 1981; Hammen & Peters, 1978). In a recent review of the burgeoning stress generation literature, Joiner (2007) identified a number of additional processes through which depressed individuals actively generate their own interpersonal stress, and contribute to the chronicity and duration of their depression. These processes include engaging in negative feedback–seeking as a means of confirming negative self-views, avoidance of interpersonal conflict, and the elicitation of others' negative and biased representations of themselves (Hammen, 1991; Simons, Angell, Monroe, & Thase, 1993).

Another influential theory is the interpersonal theory of depression (Klerman, Weissman, Rounsaville, & Chevron, 1984), which views depression as a medical illness that is exacerbated by interpersonal problems in the individual's past or present in a stress-diathesis relationship. While the model recognizes the role of biological and psychological factors, they are viewed primarily from the perspective of how they influence the individual's present-day interactions with others. Similar to Coyne, Klerman et al. (1984) view depression as both a contributor to interpersonal difficulties and a product of those maladaptive interpersonal interactions. Interpersonal therapy for depression (IPT) thus emphasizes the resolution of interpersonal conflicts and mastery of current social roles.

INDIGENOUS ETIOLOGICAL MODELS

Given the hegemonic influence of Western psychiatry and psychology worldwide, many of the psychological models reviewed above have been widely accepted by Asian mental health professionals abroad. In contrast, few indigenous Asian models of depression have been described in the English-language literature, with most existing studies restricted to Chinese and Chinese American populations. Chinese laypeople, for example, tend to emphasize the somatic aspects of depressive experience, which overlaps phenomenologically with the concept of *shenjing shuairuo* (neurasthenia), translated as "weakness of the nerves" (Kleinman, 1982). Although the Chinese classification system outlines distinct diagnostic criteria for depressive neurosis and *shenjing shuairuo* respectively, the lay public tends to use the latter term to refer generically to a wide array of cognitive, psychological, and somatic symptoms, frequently attributed to psychosocial stress (D. F. Chang, Myers, et al., 2005; Kleinman, 1982). Psychosocial stress is seen as having direct psychological and physical health consequences (D. F. Chang, 2000), a view that may be traced back to traditional Chinese medical theories of psychological disorder. Use of the term *shenjing shuairuo*, however, has recently become much less popular, in part due to increasing exposure to Western models of illness (S. Lee, 1999). Similarly, a recent study of Chinese Americans found that those with traditional illness beliefs tended not to consider depression as a distinct disease entity (Yeung, Chang, et al., 2004). Rather, depression was frequently considered as part of the manifestations of a physical disorder or a bodily reaction to psychosocial stress.

Although space limitations prohibit a comprehensive comparative discussion of indigenous models of depression among all Asian ethnic groups, conceptual and empirical studies have described a similar tendency toward a holistic and relational conceptualization of mental health among other East Asian, South Asian, and Southeast Asian populations, with religion and spirituality figuring strongly among the latter two groups (Hussain & Cochrane, 2002; Malik, 2000; Westermeyer & Her, 2007).

CRITICAL APPLICATION OF KEY PSYCHOLOGICAL
MODELS TO ASIAN POPULATIONS

Despite the evidence supporting behavioral, cognitive-behavioral, and interpersonal theories of depression, studies have generally been limited to European or Euro-American samples. Nevertheless, there is growing interest in the cognitive processes underlying depressive risk in Asian populations, with some studies highlighting culture-specific aspects of cognitive vulnerability. In addition, the sociocentric emphasis in Asian cultural socialization is congruent with interpersonal theories of depression, suggesting their potential explanatory power among culturally identified Asian individuals.

Research suggests that cognitive and appraisal processes are central in the experience of depression among Asians (H. Chen, Guarnaccia, & Chung, 2003; Fry & Grover, 1982), as has been found in other groups. However, there appears to be some cultural variation in the specific cognitions associated with depression risk. Given the emphasis placed on interdependence over independence in Asian cultural contexts, self-perceptions tend to be grounded in an interpersonal framework, where the self is inextricably linked to one's social location and role relationships with others (Markus & Kitayama, 1991; Triandis, 1989). Within such a context, negative views of the self, as described in Beck's cognitive model, may have more adverse consequences when tied to the interpersonal context than when related to self-autonomy beliefs. Although direct tests of this cultural hypothesis are lacking, there are a few studies that lend some preliminary support. For example, two recent studies involving Chinese adolescents reported that low ratings of family and peer support and acceptance were among the strongest predictors of depressed mood (Greenberger, Chen, Tally, & Dong, 2000; Stewart et al., 1999). One study showed that such associations were significantly higher for Chinese compared to U.S. youth (Greenberger et al., 2000). Validation studies conducted in Singapore of two Asian-specific depression scales—the Asian Adolescent Depression Scale (Woo et al., 2004) and the Asian Children's Depression Scale (Koh et al., 2007)—found that negative socially oriented self-evaluation or *negative social self* (e.g., perceptions of social rejection or inadequacy compared to others) emerged as a culture-specific dimension of Asian depressive experience. In contrast, the relationship between self-efficacy (e.g., beliefs about one's ability to master challenges in the environment) and depression was somewhat weaker among Hong Kong Chinese compared to U.S samples (Stewart et al., 2005).

These findings, along with cultural theories suggesting that interpersonal and role functioning may play a stronger role than personal accomplishment in the development of self-esteem among more sociocentric individuals, lead us to the conclusion that interpersonal theories of depression may be particularly relevant in the etiology of depression in Asians. Although systematic research is needed, the emphasis on the interpersonal context and consequences of depression (Klerman et al., 1984) over biological and psychological factors provide a promising framework for understanding the interpersonally embedded nature of self-appraisal and depressive experience among Asian individuals.

With regard to specific maladaptive cognitions that may play a direct causal role in depression, E. C. Chang (1996) found that low optimism emerged as one of the strongest predictors of depressive symptoms for Asian Americans. For White Americans, pessimism was found to be one of the strongest predictors of depressive symptoms. While the finding for White Americans is consistent with Beck and colleagues' (1979) cognitive model of depression, which identified pessimism as a cognitive vulnerability, the findings for Asians suggest that pessimism does not produce the same negative outcomes for Asians. E. C. Chang (2001) hypothesized that given the Asian cultural emphasis on interpersonal harmony, pessimism may be an adaptive strategy used to anticipate potential negative consequences of one's behavior as a means of motivating oneself toward active problem-solving. Low optimism may be a more proximal risk factor, which would suggest that increasing optimistic thoughts may have more therapeutic benefit for depressed Asians than decreasing pessimistic thoughts.

With regard to the hopelessness theories of depression, a cross-cultural longitudinal study of adolescents found evidence that these theories appear to be valid in the Hong Kong cultural context. Stewart et al. (2005) reported that that cognitive errors (distortions) and hopelessness were strongly associated with depressed mood and suicidal ideation in both U.S. and Hong Kong samples. Furthermore, hopelessness was found to be a strong and unique predictor of suicidal ideation six months later, even after controlling for other cognitive variables, depressive symptoms, baseline suicidal ideation, and demographic characteristics.

Psychodynamic theories have been exported to China, Japan, and other Asian societies abroad (D. F. Chang, Tong, Shi, & Zeng, 2005; Ewing, 1991; Roland, 1996). However, few studies have tested the cultural validity of specific psychodynamic models of depression for Asians. Although not conceptualized in psychodynamic terms, a study of Asian American college students confirmed that maladaptive perfectionism was significantly associated with depressive symptoms (Yoon & Lau, 2008). This finding may be seen as consistent with Jacobson's (1954) view of depression as arising from an unstable and negative view of the self, which results in part from excessively high self-expectations. Yoon and Lau (2008), however, found that the relationship between maladaptive perfectionism and depression was moderated by interdependence concerns. Specifically, highly interdependent Asian American students appeared more vulnerable to depression when exhibiting perfectionistic tendencies. The crucial finding therefore, appears to confirm the significance of an interpersonal context for self-evaluation among Asian Americans, such that "the cultural orientation of interdependence may foster vulnerability to maladaptive perfectionism and may potentially amplify the distress associated with perfectionism through a process of cultural sensitization" (p. 97). This research highlights the potential importance of cultural orientation in moderating depression risk associated with hypothesized vulnerability factors, regardless of the etiological model applied.

Social Models of Depression

Whereas biological and psychological models of depression focus on the genetic and individual-difference side of the diathesis-stress relationship, social models tend to emphasize the sociocultural environment as a primary causal agent that renders certain groups more vulnerable to developing depression and other mood disorders.

Studies of both adults and children confirm the role of stressful environmental conditions in increasing risk for depression, particularly in the absence of social support or sufficient coping resources (Kessler, 1997). Specific stressors that have been linked to depression include suboptimal parenting environments, poor physical health, significant life events, disruptive life conditions, exposure to traumatic events, interpersonal problems, and poverty (Carr, 2008). In addition, epidemiological studies provide strong evidence that social status is a significant correlate of depression, with most studies demonstrating that women, unmarried persons, and those of lower education, income, or occupational prestige have higher rates of depression or depressive symptoms compared to men, married individuals, and those of higher socioeconomic status (SES) (Dohrenwend & Dohrenwend, 1981). The inverse relationship between SES and depression has been shown to be particularly stable for women, with research supporting a social-causation theory of depressive risk (Dohrenwend et al., 1992). Social causation theory views low SES as presenting barriers to the achievement of desired goals (e.g., wealth, respect, honor), which decrease opportunities for social mobility and increase exposure to stress and adversity. This increased exposure to aversive environmental conditions is thought to contribute to the overrepresentation of depression and other mental disorders within lower SES groups (Hollingshead & Redlich, 1958).

Although stress appears to play a causal role in depression as well as suicidal ideation and behavior (Rich & Bonner, 1987; Rudd, 1990), a number of personal and social factors have been shown to moderate the relationship between stress and depression. These include problem-solving skills, intelligence, an active coping style, self-esteem, the capacity for self-reflection, an internal locus of control, physical health, and the availability of a supportive social network.

Whereas stress has been found to be causally linked to depressive illness, the alternative causal path has also been explored, namely that depression or its correlates reciprocally contribute to the generation of stress, which in turn exacerbates the illness. As discussed previously (see "Interpersonal Models"), studies have confirmed that depressed individuals engage in a number of maladaptive social behaviors that contribute to interpersonal stress and subsequently prolong their depressive experience (Hammen, 1991; Simons et al., 1993).

CRITICAL APPLICATION OF KEY SOCIAL MODELS TO ASIAN POPULATIONS

Large-scale international studies conducted in such countries as Sri Lanka, Taiwan, China, Japan, and Korea generally confirm the higher prevalence of depression among women, the elderly, and lower-SES populations, providing cross-cultural evidence that social and environmental factors may play a critical role in the development of depression (Malhotra, Chan, & Ostbye, 2010; Jang et al., 2009; Hirokawa, 2005; Tsai, Chung, Wong, & Huang, 2005). Similarly, studies conducted in India and China in particular reveal that women have a much higher rate of suicidality and completed suicides compared to men (Phillips, Liu, & Zhang, 1999; Vijayakumar, 2005), a reversal of the typically observed gender disparity found in Western parts of the world.

In China, suicide among women accounts for more than half of the world's female suicides (Phillips, Liu, & Zhang, 1999). For the Chinese population under 60, female suicides outnumbered male suicides by an average of 26%; however, the prevalence among young *rural* women was 66% higher compared to the prevalence among young *rural* men (Phillips, Li, & Zhang, 2002). This last finding is consistent with the generally higher rates of suicide in rural compared to urban areas found across all age groups in China (Phillips et al., 2002). Ethnographic and sociological studies suggest that rural women's vulnerability to suicide may be linked to two key social and environmental factors (Phillips et al., 1999). The first is the extreme feelings of deprivation and hopelessness that many young rural women feel in response to their inability to access the material wealth, economic opportunities, and freedom from domesticity that they associate with life in China's urban areas. The second is the lack of geographically accessible emergency medical services, which combined with the easy availability of toxic pesticides results in more successful suicide attempts than in the West. A national case control psychological autopsy study involving family and friends of 519 completed suicides and 536 victims of other fatal injuries found that only 40% of the suicide group had a diagnosis of depression (Phillips et al., 1999); and 37% of the sample did not meet criteria for a diagnosable mental disorder. Multivariate analyses found that other risk factors for suicide besides the degree of depressive symptoms before death included a previous suicide attempt and the presence of a severe acute stress at the time of death (most often intense interpersonal conflicts such as a severe marital dispute or family conflict with other family members).

In Asian American samples, traditional sociodemographic and socioeconomic risk factors have not been consistently shown to be related to depression. This lack of consistency has been attributed in part to acculturation and immigration factors that may alter the meaning and significance of different social status markers. For example the Chinese American Psychiatric Epidemiological Study, which surveyed 1,747 Chinese American households in the greater Los Angeles area, found that sex, age, education, and income were not consistently associated with lifetime or current major depressive episode or dysthymia (Takeuchi et al., 1998). The authors suggested that traditional measures of socioeconomic status do not address the underemployment faced by immigrants who arrive with high levels of education but who cannot obtain high-paying jobs in the United States, due to employment bias or limited English proficiency. Subsequent analyses conducted to explore the surprising absence of a relationship between sex and depression/dysthymia found a significant interaction between sex and acculturation, with women in the high-acculturation group 3.1 times more likely than men to have dysthymia in their lifetime and 2.16 times more likely than men to have a lifetime depressive episode. However, in the low-acculturation group, women did not differ significantly from men in either lifetime depressive episodes or dysthymia (Takeuchi, et al., 1998).

The National Latino and Asian American Study (Alegria et al., 2004), a state-of-the-art epidemiological survey that included a nationally representative sample of Asian Americans, also failed to find solid evidence that women are more vulnerable to developing a depressive disorder than men. Rather, immigration and acculturation processes interacted to produce different risk profiles for Asian American women and men (Takeuchi et al., 2007). For example, foreign-born Asian American women were significantly less likely to have experienced a depressive disorder in their lifetime compared to U.S.-born women, although this was not found for current (12-month) depressive disorder. For Asian American men, the effects of immigration and acculturation were more circumscribed. Although nativity had no relationship to depression, Asian American men who immigrated less than 5 years prior to the interview exhibited a significantly lower rate of a depressive disorder than their U.S.-born counterparts, as did men who spoke excellent/good English compared to those had more limited language proficiency (Takeuchi et al., 2007).

Given that much of the research on depression in Asian populations has been generated in Western contexts where they are a minority group, a great deal of attention has been paid to understanding the impact of stressors related to immigration and minority status, as well as the moderating effects of ethnic and cultural identity on depressive risk.

The particular stressors involved in adjusting to a new cultural environment are collectively referred to as *acculturative stress* (Berry, 1998). Examples of such challenges include language difficulties, separation from loved ones, disruptions in family roles and dynamics, loss of social status, underemployment, and experiences of discrimination and oppression. A growing number of studies confirm the relationship between acculturative stress and depression or depressive symptomatology in Asians and Asian Americans (Beiser & Hou, 2006; Constantine, Okazaki, & Utsey, 2004; Grossman & Liang, 2008; Hwang & Ting, 2008; M. T. Kim et al., 2005; Noh, Kaspar, & Wickrama, 2007; Shen & Takeuchi, 2001; Shin, 1994; Takeuchi et al., 2007; Thomas & Choi, 2006). The impact of acculturation and acculturative stress has also been associated with adverse effects on Asian immigrant family functioning. For example, cultural distance results from differential rates of acculturation between parents and children and has been linked to adolescent depressive symptoms and decreased family cohesion (Tseng & Fuligni, 2000; Farver, Narang, & Bhadha, 2002).

Given the declines in social status experienced by many Asian immigrants—most of whom were majority group members in their countries of origin—particular attention has been paid to studying the effects of discrimination and other forms of minority stress on the mental health of Asian youth and adults (Beiser & Hou, 2006; Grossman & Liang, 2008). A recent study of Korean immigrants in Canada, for example, found that subtle forms of discrimination were associated with depressive symptoms more than overt forms (Noh et al., 2007). These findings suggest that although blatant forms of discrimination are painful and distressing, the uncertainties associated with subtle forms of discrimination, such as being ignored or treated rudely, require greater emotional and cognitive processing. Indeed, the relationship between subtle discrimination and depressive symptoms were almost entirely mediated by cognitive appraisal processes associated with helplessness, powerlessness, frustration, and intimidation. Although this was untested in their study, the authors hypothesized that the stresses associated with this appraisal process contribute to risk for depression among minority groups.

In an effort to devise strategies for inoculating Asian immigrants against the iatrogenic effects of chronic exposure to discrimination and other forms of stress, researchers have begun to examine possible protective factors that may be enhanced through individual, family, and community-based interventions. Given the importance of social relationships and the interdependent focus of self-identity for Asian individuals, investigating the effects of social support on depression risk appears to be a promising direction for research. Similar to what has been found in the mainstream literature, studies involving diverse Asian samples consistently find an inverse relationship between social support and depression across age groups (C. Cheng, 1998; Huang, Hwang, & Ko, 1983; Guerrero et al., 2006). However, the buffering hypothesis—namely that social support helps to mitigate stress-related depression— has received mixed support in studies involving Asians.

Although some studies of Asian adolescents found that social support buffered the effects of stress on depression (e.g., Brown, Meadows, & Elder, 2007; C. Cheng, 1997), others failed to replicate these results (e.g., Grossman & Liang, 2008). Some research involving elderly Chinese and Korean immigrants have found that emotional/companionship support did significantly predict lower levels of depression and higher positive affect. However, elderly immigrants who lived with their spouses and adult children had lower positive affect compared to those who lived alone (S. T. Wong, Yoo, & Stewart, 2007). An earlier study conducted by the same research team (S. T. Wong, Yoo, & Stewart, 2006) on changes in perceptions of family relationships among elderly Chinese and Korean immigrants offers some insights into this surprising finding. Specifically, participants reported feeling that they had lost status and authority within their families, becoming more peripheral members of the family. These findings may explain why the immediate presence of extended family members did not have a salutatory effect on mental health in the 2007 study.

Other investigators have also observed that Asian Americans are less likely than other ethnic groups to turn to their social support networks for assistance in coping with stress, due to interpersonal concerns such as saving face, avoiding criticism, or not burdening others (Taylor et al., 2004). Additional research is needed to further understand the role that social support plays in stress-related depression among diverse Asian groups and how the protective function of social support may covary with acculturation and changes in cultural orientation over time (Rhee, Chang, & Rhee, 2003).

Ethnic identity and cultural orientation have also been identified as possible protections against depression; however the mixed nature of the findings suggest the need for studies that clarify the conditions under which they are apt to be most influential. For example, a study of Southeast Asian refugees suggests that the moderating effect of ethnic identity on depression varied according to the specific nature of the stressor (Beiser & Hou, 2006). Specifically, when Southeast Asians were confronted with racial discrimination or unemployment, strong ethnic identification was associated with higher levels of depressed mood. However, when experiencing difficulties as a result of limited English skills, ethnic identity served a protective psychological function (Beiser & Hou, 2006).

With regard to cultural orientation, findings are similarly mixed, likely due in part to methodological and sampling variation across studies. Adherence to traditional cultural values was associated with psychological well-being for less acculturated Chinese immigrants (S. H. Lee, 2006), while a telephone survey of aging South Asians in Canada found that a stronger agreement with South Asian cultural values was significantly related to a higher probability of being depressed (Lai & Surood, 2008). On the other hand, Ryder, Alden, and Paulhus (2000) tested a bidimensional model of acculturation and found that the acquisition of mainstream culture (assimilation) is significantly associated with lower levels of depressive symptoms, whereas maintenance of traditional Chinese cultural values and practices had little effect on psychological well-being (Ryder et al., 2000).

Strengths, Weaknesses, and Alternatives in Applying Current Etiological Models of Mood Disorders to Asians

The current etiological models of mood disorders, including the biological, psychological and social models, were developed with the assumption that they are universal and are applicable across ethnic/racial groups. Thus far, studies on these etiological models have been predominantly conducted on Western populations, although a growing number of studies support the applicability of a diathesis-stress model of depression among Asians. Future studies are needed to examine whether genetic variations across races and ethnicities are modifiers of the biological models. In addition, the possible moderating and mediating effects of cultural factors on Asians' cognitive and social vulnerability to mood disorders will also need to be explored further.

TREATING MOOD DISORDERS IN ASIANS

Critical Appraisal of Major Treatment Approaches for Mood Disorders

Biological Approaches (Ethnopharmacology)

For both unipolar depression and bipolar disorder, psychotropics are the mainstay of biological treatment. Traditionally, tricyclic and tetracyclic antidepressants have been used for the treatment of unipolar depression. With the introduction of the selective serotonin reuptake inhibitors (SSRIs) (e.g., fluoxetine, paroxetine, luvoxamine, citalopram), dual-action serotonin-norepinephrine reuptake inhibitors (e.g., venafaxine, duloxetine), and other newer antidepressants (e.g., mirtazepine, nefazodone), the new generation of antidepressants are now increasingly being used as first-line medications for depression due to their more benign side effects. In addition to antidepressants, typical antipsychotic agents (e.g., chlorpromazine, haloperidol) are combined with antidepressants to treat patients with psychotic depression. Mood stabilizers (e.g., lithium, anticonvulsants such as valproic acid and lamotrigine) and some atypical antipsychotic drugs (e.g., olanzapine, quetiapine) are now used to treat mania as well as bipolar depression (Ukaegbu et al., 2008).

Genetic Polymorphism of Genes Encoding Drug-Metabolizing Enzymes

Studies have shown that there are interindividual and cross-ethnic variations in drug responses (Pi & Gray; 2000). Many medications, including practically all psychotropics, are dependent on one or more of the cytochrome P450 (CYP) enzymes for metabolism. Functionally, significant genetic variations exist in most of the CYPs, resulting in large differences in the activity of these enzymes in any given population. Individuals can be classified as extensive metabolizers (EMs), poor metabolizers (PMs), or slow metabolizers (SMs), depending on whether they carry genetic mutations that alter the amino acid structure and activity of the enzymes. Typically, the rate of genetic polymorphism varies substantially across ethnic groups, giving rise to unique profiles of genetic polymorphism for most ethnic groups. This may explain the dosing differences that have been reported among Asians compared to other populations in the treatment of mood disorders.

For example, CYP2D6 is involved in the metabolism of most antipsychotics, tricyclic antidepressants, SSRIs, and venlafaxine. About 33–50% of Asians appear to have forms of the enzyme that are significantly less active than the form typically found in Caucasians. This may partially explain the results in some studies showing that Asians have slower pharmacokinetic profiles and lower dose ranges compared to Caucasians of drugs metabolized by the CYP2D6.

Similarly, CYP2C19, which metabolizes diazepam and several antidepressants, is also found to have significant interethnic differences. Between 23% and 39% of Asians have a genetic variant with little or no activity of this enzyme, compared to only 2–10% of whites and 25% in African Americans. This may explain why more Asians compared to Caucasians can be categorized as slow metabolizers of the CYP2C19 (Pi & Gray, 2000).

TREATMENT OF ASIANS WITH MOOD DISORDERS USING ANTIDEPRESSANTS

Pi and Gray (1998) reviewed clinical data on treatment of depressed Asian Americans and reported that they required lower doses of antidepressants. Allen et al. (1977) studied 6 Asian males and 11 English male volunteers and found that Asians have significantly higher plasma levels of clomipramine after a single dose of 25 mg or 50 mg clomipramine. In another study, Pi et al. (1986) compared the pharmacokinetics of 50 mg desipramine in 20 Asian volunteers and 75 mg desipramine in 20 Caucasian volunteers and found that Asians achieved peak plasma concentrations in significantly less time (4.0 hours vs. 6.9 hours). Other pharmacokinetic studies, however, failed to demonstrate racial differences in antidepressant treatment. Rudorfer et al. (1984) gave a single 10-mg oral dose in 10 Chinese and 10 Caucasian volunteers, and found no difference in the metabolism between the two groups. Shimoda et al. (1995) treated 108 Japanese psychiatric patients with clomipramine, with doses titrated up to total doses ranging from 30 to 250 mg/day, and patients received the same dose for 14 days before blood sampling was collected. They found that none of the Asian subjects were PMs, and there was no difference in the blood clomipramine levels between Asians and patients from other races. The authors concluded that sampling differences and/or intraethnic variations of polymorphism may be the reason why no PMs were identified among the Asian subjects in this study. There are fewer studies are on the ethnopharmacological aspects of SSRIs. A related study by Hong et al. (2006) reported that Chinese depressed patients require lower dosages and lower plasma concentrations of sertraline compared to Caucasian patients to achieve clinical efficacy.

TREATMENT OF ASIANS WITH MOOD DISORDERS USING ANTIPSYCHOTICS

Similar to the use of antidepressants, some clinical surveys have shown that Asian patients may respond to lower doses of antipsychotics, although the data were not consistent. In a retrospective study involving 13 Asians and 13 white patients matched by age, sex, diagnosis, and chronicity, Lin and Finder (1983) found that Asians received about half the daily dose of antipsychotic that Caucasians received. Yet, such retrospective surveys may simply reflect prescribing patterns of clinicians who presumed Asians needed lower doses of psychotropics. In a more vigorously designed study, Potkin et al. (1984) gave 0.4 mg/kg haloperidol doses to 18 non–Asian American and 18 Chinese schizophrenic patients for 6 weeks and found the plasma haloperidol levels to be 52% higher in the Chinese patients than in the Americans. The findings of this and other similar studies provide evidence that a higher proportion of Asians have the CYP2D6 SM phenotype, which is involved with the metabolism of haloperidol.

TREATMENT OF ASIANS WITH MOOD DISORDERS USING BENZODIAZEPINES

In a pharmacokinetic study of alprazolam, Lin et al. (1988) examined the blood alprazolam concentrations in 14 American-born Asians, 14 foreign-born Asians, and 14 Caucasian healthy male volunteers. Both Asian groups had higher peak plasma concentrations and lower total plasma clearance than the white group, after both oral and intravenous administration of alprazolam. In another study, Ajir et al. (1997) found that Asians had higher serum concentrations and lower clearance of adinazolam than both their Caucasian and African American counterparts. Findings from this study suggest that Asians may require smaller doses of adinazolam than white patients to achieve similar blood levels.

TREATMENT OF ASIANS WITH MOOD DISORDERS USING LITHIUM

With mechanisms that remain unclear, studies have found that Asians may respond to lower doses and plasma levels of lithium. S. S. Chang et al. (1985) reported that optimal therapeutic lithium concentrations are 0.71 and 0.73 mEq/L for Chinese patients with bipolar depression living in Shanghai and Taipei respectively, compared with a mean level of 0.98 mEq/L for matched White American patients (Pi, & Gray, 2000).

Psychological Treatments

Research indicates that psychological treatments for depression, particularly behavioral, cognitive behavioral, and interpersonal therapies, are as effective as pharmacologic treatments in reducing symptoms of depression in the short term and provide longer-lasting protection against future relapse after treatment is withdrawn (Dobson et al., 2008; Gloaguen, Cottraux, Cucherat, & Blackburn, 1998). Additional benefits of psychological treatments include the reduction of psychosocial impairments associated with depression, absence of side effects, and lower treatment costs than pharmacologic treatment. We focus our brief discussion below to several of the most widely used and/or well-studied psychotherapies judged to be efficacious in treating depression. Typically, the treatments described below are delivered in one-on-one contexts, although some treatments have been adapted and tested in group formats as well.

BRIEF DYNAMIC THERAPIES

A number of brief dynamic therapies—lasting between 6 and 20 sessions, on average—have recently been shown to be efficacious in treating depression, although the empirical base remains somewhat more limited than that of behavioral treatments, cognitive and cognitive behavioral treatments, and interpersonal therapy for depression (Chambless & Ollendick, 2001). In general, brief dynamic therapies for depression focus on increasing clients' awareness and understanding of core conflicts that often originated from early relationships. These core conflicts contribute to ongoing dysfunctional patterns and processes that increase vulnerability to depression (Barkham, et al., 1996; Gallagher-Thompson & Steffen, 1994; Shapiro et al., 1994). Core aspects of these therapies include a focus on early childhood experiences as they affect current functioning, identification of core conflictual relationship themes, affective expression, the therapeutic relationship, and facilitation of insight.

In general, evidence suggests that these treatments are associated with greater symptom improvement compared to no-treatment controls, with some studies suggesting that they may be as efficacious as cognitive behavioral treatments under certain conditions. For example, in a recent study involving clinically depressed family caregivers of elderly relatives, Gallagher-Thompson and Steffen (1994) found that after 20 sessions of either cognitive behavioral or brief psychodynamic individual treatment, over 70% of the total sample reported significant symptom improvement posttreatment. No differences were found between the two treatment groups. However, clients who had been caregivers for less than 44 months showed greater improvement in the psychodynamic condition, whereas those who had been caregivers for at least 44 months showed greater improvement in the cognitive behavioral condition.

BEHAVIOR THERAPIES

Behavior therapies (BT) apply the tenets of learning theory to the modification of problem behaviors associated with mental disorders. In the case of depression, problem behaviors include behavioral withdrawal, poor social skills, and maladaptive coping skills, which are thought to decrease the rate of positive reinforcement and/or increase the rate of punishing experiences. As a result, BTs focus on correcting skill deficits, decreasing avoidance, and scheduling activities to increase the likelihood of reinforcement. Behavioral interventions for depression include social learning therapies (e.g., token economies), self-control therapy, and behavioral activation strategies. Although interest and research in purely behavioral approaches declined with the development of cognitive and cognitive behavioral approaches (CBT), recent research suggesting that specific behavioral techniques may produce comparable effects to CBT has led to renewed interest in behavioral approaches. For example, Jacobson and colleagues (1996) found that the behavioral activation component of CBT was just as effective as the full treatment, suggesting that it could be a more economical strategy for treating depression. Behavioral activation involves a package of behavioral interventions aimed at encouraging clients to become more actively engaged in their environments, thereby increasing contact with available sources of reinforcement (Hopko, Lejuez, & Hopko, 2004). Specific interventions include monitoring daily activities, assessing the pleasure and mastery associated with engagement in various activities, assigning increasingly more difficult tasks that have a higher probability to provide a sense of pleasure or mastery, cognitive rehearsal of scheduled activities, problem solving, and social skills training. A recent meta-analysis involving seventeen randomized controlled trials reported that behavioral activation was superior to controls and supportive therapy, and equal to CBT in reducing self-reports of depression symptoms (Ekers, Richards, & Gilbody, 2008).

COGNITIVE AND COGNITIVE BEHAVIORAL THERAPIES

One of the most well-established and well-studied cognitive behavioral therapies (CBT) is cognitive therapy (CT; Beck et al. 1979). CT stems from the notion that the way individuals interpret events affects the way they feel about those events and their subsequent coping behaviors (Hollon, Hammen, & Brown, 2002). The treatment thus focuses on helping patients identify and alter negative patterns of thinking, which in turn reduces negative affect and improves one's ability to cope. CT emphasizes a collaborative relationship between patient and therapist, such that treatment goals are collaboratively set, feedback is solicited and provided, and the patient is taught and practices with specific tools to increase independence in dealing with future stressors. The core of the treatment involves cognitive techniques aimed at replacing clients' maladaptive and schema-driven modes of information processing with more flexible and data-driven strategies. However, behavioral techniques, such as event scheduling and social skills training, are an important component of the treatment in the initial phase, particularly for more severely depressed patients.

Compared to psychodynamic treatments, CT is highly structured and problem-focused, which allows for symptom relief to be achieved in a relatively short period of time (16–20 sessions), although an additional phase of treatment may be added to address the underlying schemas that may maintain vulnerability to relapse (Young et al., 2001). Research has demonstrated that in addition to BT and interpersonal therapy, CT is one of most effective treatments for depression (Dobson, 1989; Elkin, Gibbons, Shea, & Shaw, 1996). Furthermore, CT/CBT compares favorably to that of pharmacotherapy in reducing depression among all but the most severely depressed individuals, and patients receiving CT are less likely to relapse following treatment termination than patients withdrawn from medication (Dobson et al., 2008; Hollon & Shelton, 2001).

INTERPERSONAL THERAPY

Interpersonal therapy (IPT) is a short-term individual outpatient treatment with strong empirical evidence supporting its efficacy in treating and preventing relapse in individuals with mild to moderate depression (Elkin et al., 1989; Weissman, Markowitz, & Klerman, 2000). Important theoretical influences include the interpersonal school of psychoanalysis (Sullivan, 1953) as well as empirical research demonstrating the effect of mood on life events and the stress-buffering role of social support. IPT adopts a biopsychosocial model of depression, with an emphasis on relationship issues that contribute to the patient's difficulties. Stemming from Klerman and colleagues' (1984) original interpersonal theory of depression, the goals of the treatment include improvement of current social functioning as well as the amelioration of depressive symptoms (Weissman et al., 2000). Standard IPT progresses in three phases involving a total of 16 sessions. The early phase (Sessions 1 through 4) consists of a comprehensive assessment of psychiatric symptoms and interpersonal functioning, psychoeducation regarding the medical model of depression, the patient's adoption of the sick role, and the specification of the interpersonal focus of treatment. The four potential foci defined by Klerman and colleagues are grief, interpersonal disputes, roles transitions, and interpersonal deficits. Unlike psychodynamic treatments, IPT stresses current rather than past conflicts. The middle phase (Sessions 4 through 12) consists of working through the chosen interpersonal focus area. The final phase (Sessions 13 through 16) emphasizes integration of the major interpersonal themes discussed previously and identifying and practicing new interpersonal coping strategies. This work is done while preparing the client for termination of the therapy. Strict adherence to the treatment model is an important component of its efficacy. Frank and colleagues (1991) found that patients who received more model-adherent IPT had a median survival time between episodes of 101.7 weeks compared to the 18.1 weeks reported for the patient group receiving less model-adherent IPT. The efficacy of IPT has been demonstrated in a number of randomized controlled trials, leading to its identification as an empirically supported, well-established treatment for depression.

CRITICAL APPLICATION OF PSYCHOLOGICAL TREATMENTS WITH ASIANS

Although BT, CT/CBT, and IPT are well-established treatments for reducing symptoms of depression in children, adolescents, and adults (Chambless & Ollendick, 2001), their efficacy for Asian Americans and other ethnic minorities has not been definitively established. In a comprehensive review, Miranda et al. (2005) reported that while six major studies found CBT to be as efficacious as pharmacotherapy in treating depression, none of the studies included sufficient subsamples of ethnic minorities. They also noted that in the landmark National Institute of Mental Health Treatment of Depression Collaborative Research Project (Elkin et al., 1989), which demonstrated the effectiveness of CBT and IPT compared to medications, only 11% of the sample were ethnic minorities, with insufficient power to conduct separate ethnic group analyses.

In our review of the empirical literature (restricted to studies published in English or Chinese, reflecting our limited language capacity), we identified only a handful of psychotherapy treatment studies that focused on Asian populations. The majority involved tests of CT or CBT with Chinese adult samples. We were unable to locate any randomized controlled trials of BT alone or IPT conducted with Asian Americans or Asians abroad. In the only study conducted with Asian Americans, Dai et al. (1999) treated elderly Chinese Americans with mild depression with eight sessions of CBT and compared them with a no-treatment control group. Those that received CBT reported a significant decrease in depressive and somatic symptoms, whereas there was no change in symptom distress for the controls. While this study provided preliminary evidence that CBT could be effective for Chinese American clients, it was hampered by the lack of random assignment to groups.

CBT was first introduced in mainland China with the publication of Ji and Xu's (1989) description of Beck's model of cognitive therapy in the influential *Chinese Journal of Mental Health*. A number of international training programs on cognitive therapy provide regular training and supervision by foreign CBT experts (Xu & Ji, 1996), with many of the supervisory activities occurring online via video conferencing. In many ways, the CBT practiced in China appears to be similar in content to the procedures described by Beck. Yet, the structure of services typically reflects the practice conventions and resource constraints in providing mental health care in China. For example, sessions rarely exceed 30 minutes, and patients are frequently seen on a walk-in basis rather than regular weekly sessions (D. F. Chang, Tong, et al., 2005). In the larger urban clinics, however, this appears to be changing gradually toward a more Western model. By 1996, 20 Chinese treatment studies had been published on CBT, leading Xu and Ji (1996) to conclude that CBT was generally effective for the treatment of a variety of disorders, including depression.

Although the studies discussed above involved tests of individual therapy, evidence is gathering to suggest that CBT groups may also be helpful for depressed Chinese populations. D. F. K. Wong (2008) conducted a randomized wait-list controlled trial of a CBT group for chronically depressed Chinese in Hong Kong. The treatment group received 10 sessions of group-administered manualized CBT. The intervention was based on preexisting manualized group treatments with a number of cultural adaptations. These adaptations included minor changes to improve treatment engagement, such as translating technical terms into colloquial language, as well as more substantive learning tools such as specially designed worksheets and exercises in Chinese to enhance skill development. In addition, the treatment had a strong interpersonal focus, in recognition of the complex role responsibilities and interpersonal dynamics that may be a particular source of stress for Chinese individuals. Results indicated that compared to the control group, individuals in the treatment group reported greater improvements in depressive symptoms and adaptive coping skills, and more substantial decreases in negative emotions and dysfunctional attitudes, with 40% achieving clinically significant improvements in depressive symptoms. Despite its promising findings and improved methodology, the study's use of a wait-list control does not rule out the possibility that treatment gains were due to the support received in the group setting and not to the active treatment itself.

In contrast to the research on CBT with Chinese patients, efficacy studies involving other Asian and Asian American groups have not been widely reported in the English language literature. However, it appears that these treatments are being widely practiced in countries across Asia (David, 2007), with international organizations convening to bring together researchers and practitioners. For example, the 2nd Asian Cognitive Therapy Conference was held in 2008 in Thailand with representatives from Korea, Japan, Malaysia, China, Taiwan, India, and other countries in Europe, South America, and the United States. We look forward to seeing more efficacy and effectiveness studies of CBTs on other Asian populations made available in the English language literature.

In the absence of randomized controlled trial data for BT or IPT for depression in Asians, we conclude that CBTs represent the current best practice for treating depression in Asian populations, though more data are needed. The highly structured, problem-focused, and directive nature of cognitive approaches has been viewed as compatible with traditional Chinese values of rationality, pragmatism, and respect for authority (B. S. K. Kim et al., 2002; Tung, 1984; E. C. Wong, Kim, Zane, Kim, & Huang, 2003). In addition, there is evidence that cognitive treatments are viewed as more credible than insight-oriented approaches, particularly among culturally identified Asian Americans (E. C. Wong et al., 2003). As a result, many clinicians feel that these techniques do not require much cultural adaptation to work with Asian patients, although client engagement and the acquisition of key concepts may be enhanced by using culturally congruent communication, adopting a didactic orientation, linking new concepts with more familiar indigenous belief systems, and being aware of how interpersonal norms and relational styles may inadvertently exacerbate problem behavior (e.g., via stigma or loss of face) (Hwang, Wood, Lin, & Cheung, 2006; D. F. K. Wong, 2008). However, randomized clinical trials are still needed to rigorously test the efficacy of CBT in Chinese American as well as other Asian American groups and determine what cultural adaptations, if any, are needed.

Additional evidence in support of cognitive approaches to depression is provided by a 2002 study that applied a school-based Chinese version of the Penn Optimism Program (POP) to a sample of Beijing schoolchildren (Yu & Seligman, 2002). The POP, developed at the University of Pennsylvania, has been shown to prevent future depressive symptoms in American children and young adolescents at risk by training them to challenge pessimistic causal explanations and apply alternative coping strategies when confronted with negative life events (Gillham et al., 1995;

Seligman, Reivich, Jaycox, & Gillham, 1995). Results found that when compared to the control group, Chinese schoolchildren receiving the culturally adapted POP had significantly reduced depressive symptoms and a greater improvement in optimistic explanatory style posttreatment, after controlling for pretest scores (Yu & Seligman, 2002). The POP was also shown to prevent depressive symptoms for up to 6 months posttreatment. Mediation analyses indicated that change in explanatory style mediated the treatment effect on depressive symptoms.

At present, there is a scarcity of studies examining the efficacy of psychodynamic and other insight-oriented therapies with Asians, although case reports indicate that it is being applied with Asian patients in the United States and abroad (D. F. Chang, Tong, et al., 2005; Roland, 1996). The majority of publications focus on psychodynamic case formulations or general guidelines for conducting insight-oriented treatments with Asian patients (e.g., Tung, 1991). As discussed, a frequently noted problem is the low credibility of dynamic therapies among more culturally identified Asians (e.g., E. C. Wong et al., 2003) given the preference for more problem-focused and directive approaches to treatment.

STRENGTH, WEAKNESSES, AND ALTERNATIVES TO APPLYING CURRENT TREATMENT APPROACHES FOR MOOD DISORDERS TO ASIANS

Clinicians who treat Asian patients with mood disorders generally administer the biological and psychosocial interventions that were developed in the West. They do it partly with the assumption that these treatments apply well across cultures and ethnicities, and partly because there is a lack of alternative treatments that have the same degree of empirical support. While there are few published RCTs on treatment of mood disorders among Asians, a large number of Asians are being treated everyday using conventional treatments developed in the West. Anecdotal experience suggests that Asians do respond to conventional treatments. Ethnopsychopharmacological studies and cross-cultural studies, however, have shown that some Asians may require different dosages of their psychotropic medications compared to Caucasians; and psychotherapy for traditional Asian patients may need to focus more on the interdependent nature of self-construction, and on the involvement of family members when possible. Further research is needed to understand how to tailor treatment to individuals' biology and culture, as well as to show how environmental factors, such as diet and concurrent use of herbal remedies, affect the outcomes of biological and psychosocial treatments for mood disorders in Asians.

Asian indigenous treatments such as the use of specific Chinese herbs and mind-body practices including meditation, yoga, *tai chi*, and *qi-gong* are also frequently used by Asian patients for symptom relief. Therefore, additional research is needed to examine their specific effects on depression, either as primary interventions or adjuncts to conventional psychiatric treatments for mood disorders. Cultural diversity, instead of being considered an obstacle for treatment, can serve as fertile ground for developing innovative treatment modalities that combine Eastern and Western healing traditions for the benefit of diverse patient populations. For example, mindfulness-based cognitive therapy integrates meditation and cognitive therapy and has been found to be effective in preventing relapse among those who have recurrent depression (Ma & Teasdale, 2004).

CONCLUSIONS

The current concept of mood disorder and its diagnostic criteria are rooted in Western cultures, and so are the etiological models and psychosocial treatment modalities of mood disorders. In addition, most of the rigorously designed biological and psychosocial interventions developed out of work with Western patient populations. In recent years, there appears to be increasing convergence in how clinicians in North America, Europe, and Asia diagnose, conceptualize, and treat depression. While there are very limited data available to assess how well conventional psychosocial models apply to Asians, the few published studies suggest that BT, CBT, and IPT may be efficacious. This is encouraging as it provides some support to claims that the behavioral, cognitive, and social mechanisms of depression are similar across diverse cultural groups. On the other hand, ethnopsychopharmacological studies have provided evidence of variations in drug metabolism profiles across ethnic groups, and cross-cultural studies have demonstrated that Asians with traditional beliefs have significantly different causal beliefs and help-seeking behaviors for depression. In working with Asian patients from diverse origins and cultural backgrounds, it is important to keep in mind the impact of possible biological variations and cultural differences in their vulnerability, expression, experience, and response to mood disorders. In addition, clinicians are advised to collaborate with patients to create shared narratives and understandings of the illness, and to discuss acceptable treatment options. Treatment for mood disorders among Asians may include medications, conventional psychotherapies, and indigenous forms of interventions that are supported by scientific evidence. Future research is needed to explore how to provide individualized treatment tailored to patients' genetic variations, illness explanatory models, and cultural values to achieve the best clinical outcomes.

REFERENCES

Alegria, M., Takeuchi, D., Canino, G., Duan, N., Shrout, P., Meng, X. L., et al. (2004). Considering context, place, and culture: The National Latino and Asian American Study. *International Journal of Methods in Psychiatric Research, 13*(4), 208–220.

Alegria, M., Chatterji, P., Wells, K., Cao, Z., Chen, C., Takeuchi, D., et al. (2008). Disparity in depression treatment among racial and ethnic minority populations in the United States. *Psychiatric Services, 59*,1264–1272.

Abramson, L. Y., Metalsky, G. I., & Alloy, L. B. (1989). Hopelessness depression: A theory-based subtype of depression. *Psychological Review, 96*(2), 358–372.

Ajir, K., Smith, M., Lin, K. M., et al. (1997). The pharmacokinetics and pharmacodynamics of adinazolam: Multi-ethnic comparisons. *Psychopharmacology 129,* 265–270.

Allen, J. J., Rack, P. H., &Vaddadi, K. S. (1977). Differences in the effects of climipramine on English and Asian volunteers: Preliminary report on a pilot study. *Postgraduate Medical Journal, 53*(Suppl 4), 79–86.

American Psychiatric Association. (1987). *Diagnostic and statistical manual of mental disorders* (3rd ed., rev.). Washington, DC: Author.

American Psychiatric Association. (1994). *Diagnostic and statistical manual of mental disorders* (4th ed., rev.). Washington, DC: Author.

Barkham, M., Rees, A., Stiles, W. B., Shapiro, D. A., Hardy, G. E., & Reynolds, S. (1996). Dose-effect relations in time-limited psychotherapy for depression. *Journal of Consulting and Clinical Psychology, 64*(5), 927–935.

Badner, J. A., & Gershon, E. S. (2002). Meta-analysis of whole-genome linkage scans of bipolar disorder and schizophrenia. *Molecular Psychiatry, 7*, 405–411.

Barreto, R. M., & Segal, S. P. (2005). Use of mental health services by Asian Americans. *Psychiatric Services, 56*(6), 746–748.

Beck, A. T., Rush, J., Shaw, B. F., & Emery, G. (1979). *Cognitive therapy of depression.* New York: Guilford.

Beiser, M. N., & Hou, F. (2006). Ethnic identity, resettlement stress, and depressive affect among Southeast Asian refugees in Canada. *Social Science and Medicine, 63*(1), 137–150.

Berry, J. W. (1998). Acculturative stress. In P. B. Organista, K. M. Chun, & G. Marín (Eds.), *Readings in ethnic psychology* (pp. 117–122). Florence, KY: Taylor & Frances/Routledge.

Brown, J. S., Meadows, S. O., & Elder, G. H., Jr. (2007). Race-ethnic inequality and psychological distress: Depressive symptoms from adolescence to young adulthood. *Developmental Psychology, 43*(6), 1295–1311

Busch, F. N., Ruden, M., & Shapiro, T. (2004) *Psychodynamic treatment of depression.* Washington, DC: American Psychiatric Press.

Carr, A. (2008). Depression in young people: Description, assessment, and evidence-based treatment. *Developmental Neurorehabilitation, 11*(1), 3–15.

Chambless, D. L., & Ollendick, T. H. (2001). Empirically supported psychological interventions: Controversies and evidence. *Annual Review of Psychology, 52,* 685–716.

Chang, D. F. (2000). The cultural validity of neurasthenia: Psychiatric diagnosis and illness beliefs in a Chinese primary care sample. Unpublished dissertation, University of California, Los Angeles.

Chang, D. F., Myers, H. F., Yeung, A., Zhang, Y., Zhao, J., & Yu, S. (2005). *Shenjing Shuairuo* and the DSM-IV: Diagnosis, distress, and disability in a Chinese primary care setting. *Transcultural Psychiatry, 42,* 204–218.

Chang, D. F., Tong, H., Shi, Q., & Zeng, Q. (2005). Letting a hundred flowers bloom: Counseling and psychotherapy in the People's Republic of China. *Journal of Mental Health Counseling, 27,* 104–116.

Chang, E. C. (1996). Cultural differences in optimism, pessimism, and coping: Predictors of subsequent adjustment in Asian American and Caucasian American college students. *Journal of Counseling Psychology, 43*(1), 113–123.

Chang, E. C. (2001). Cultural influences on optimism and pessimism: Differences in Western and Eastern construals of the self. In *Optimism and pessimism: Implications for theory, research, and practice* (pp. 257–280). Washington, DC: American Psychological Association.

Chang, S. S., Pandey, G. N., Yang, Y. Y., et al. (1985, May 19–24). Lithium pharmacokinetics: Inter-racial comparison. Paper presented at the annual meeting of the American Psychiatric Association, Dallas, TX.

Chen, C. N., Wong, J., Lee, N., Chan-Ho, M. W., Lau, J. T. F., & Fung, M. (1993). The Shatin Community Mental Health Survey in Hong Kong. *Archives of General Psychiatry, 50,* 125–133.

Chen, H., Guarnaccia, P. J., & Chung, H. (2003). Self-attention as a mediator of cultural influences on depression. *International Journal of Social Psychiatry, 49*(3), 192–203.

Cheng, C. (1998). Getting the right kind of support: Functional differences in the types of social support on depression for Chinese adolescents. *Journal of Clinical Psychology, 54*(6), 845–849.

Cheng, C. (1997). Role of perceived social support on depression in Chinese adolescents: A prospective study examining the buffering model. *Journal of Applied Social Psychology, 27*(9), 800–820.

Cheng, T. A. (1989). Symptomatology of minor psychiatric morbidity: A cross-cultural comparison. *Psychological Medicine, 19,* 697–708.

Chong, M. Y., Chen, C. C., Tsang, H. Y., Yeh, T. L., Chen, C. S., Lee, Y. H., et al. (2001). Community study of depression in old age in Taiwan: Prevalence, life events and socio-demographic correlates. *British Journal of Psychiatry, 178,* 29–35.

Clark, D. A., Beck, A. T., & Alford, B. A. (1999). *Scientific foundations of cognitive theory and therapy of depression.* Hoboken, NJ: Wiley.

Constantine, M. G., Okazaki, S., & Utsey, S. O. (2004). Self-concealment, social self-efficacy, acculturative stress, and depression in African, Asian, and Latin American international college students. *American Journal of Orthopsychiatry, 74*(3), 230–241.

Coyne, J. C. (1976). Depression and the response of others. *Journal of Abnormal Psychology, 85*(2), 186–193.

Dai, Y., Zhang, S., Yamamoto, J., Ao, M., Belin, T. R., Cheung, F., et al. (1999). Cognitive behavioral therapy of minor depressive symptoms in elderly Chinese Americans: A pilot study. *Community Mental Health Journal, 35*(6), 537–542.

David, D. (2007). Quo vadis CBT? Trans-cultural perspectives on the past, present, and future of cognitive-behavioral therapies: Interviews with the current leadership in cognitive-behavioral therapies. *Journal of Cognitive and Behavioral Psychotherapies, 7*(2), 171–217.

Dinh, T. Q., Yamada, A. M., Yee, B. W. (2009) A culturally relevant conceptualization of depression: An empirical examination of the factorial structure of the Vietnamese Depression Scale. *International Journal of Social Psychiatry, 55*(6), 496–505.

Dobson, K. S. (1989). A meta-analysis of the efficacy of cognitive therapy for depression. *Journal of Consulting and Clinical Psychology, 57,* 414–419.

Dobson, K. S., Hollon, S. D., Dimidjian, S., Schmaling, K. B., Kohlenberg, R. J., Gallop, R. J., et al. (2008). Randomized trial of behavioral activation, cognitive therapy, and antidepressant medication in the prevention of relapse and recurrence in major depression. *Journal of Consulting and Clinical Psychology, 76*(3), 468–477.

Dohrenwend, B. P., & Dohrenwend, B. S. (1981). Socioenvironmental factors, stress, and psychopathology. *American Journal of Community Psychology, 9*(2), 128–164.

Dohrenwend, B. P., Levav, I., Shrout, P. E., Schwartz, S., Naveh, G., Link, B. G., et al. (1992). Socioeconomic status and psychiatric disorders: The causation-selection issue. *Science, 255*(5047), 946–952.

Dryden, W. (1981). The relationship of depressed persons. In S. Duck & R. Gilmour (Eds.), *Personal relationships* (Vol. 3). London: Academic.

Dykman, B. M., Horowitz, L. M., Abramson, L. Y., & Usher, M. (1991). Schematic and situational determinants of depressed and nondepressed students' interpretation of feedback. *Journal of Abnormal Psychology, 100*(1), 45–55.

Ekers, D., Richards, D., & Gilbody, S. (2008). A meta-analysis of randomized trials of behavioural treatment of depression. *Psychological Medicine, 38*(5), 611–623.

Elkin, I., Gibbons, R. D., Shea, M. T., & Shaw, B. F. (1996). Science is not a trial (but it can sometimes be a tribulation). *Journal of Consulting and Clinical Psychology, 64*(1), 92–103.

Elkin, I., Shea, M. T., Watkins, J. T., Imber, S. D., Sotsky, S. M., & Collins, J. E. (1989). National Institute of Mental Health Treatment of Depression Collaborative Research Program: General effectiveness of treatments. *Archives of General of Psychiatry, 46,* 971–982.

Ewing, K. P. (1991). Can psychoanalytic theories explain the Pakistani woman? Intrapsychic autonomy and interpersonal engagement in the extended family. *Ethos, 19*(2), 131–160.

Farver, J. A. M., Narang, S. K., & Bhadha, B. R. (2002). East meets west: Ethnic identity, acculturation, and conflict in Asian Indian families. *Journal of Family Psychology, 16*(3), 338–350.

Frank, E., Kupfer, D. J., Wagner, E. F., & McEachran, A. B. (1991). Efficacy of interpersonal psychotherapy as a maintenance treatment of recurrent depression: Contributing factors. *Archives of General Psychiatry, 48*(12), 1053–1059.

Fry, P. S., & Grover, S. C. (1982). Cognitive appraisals of life stress and depression in the elderly: A cross-cultural comparison of Asians and Caucasians. *International Journal of Psychology, 17*(4), 437–454.

Gallagher-Thompson, D., & Steffen, A. M. (1994). Comparative effects of cognitive-behavioral and brief psychodynamic psychotherapies for depressed family caregivers. *Journal of Consulting and Clinical Psychology, 62*(3), 543–549.

Gloaguen, V., Cottraux, J., Cucherat, M., & Blackburn, I. (1998). A meta-analysis of the effects of cognitive therapy in depressed patients. *Journal of Affective Disorders, 49*(1), 59–72.

Greenberger, E., Chen, C., Tally, S. R., & Dong, Q. (2000). Family, peer, and individual correlates of depressive symptomatology among U.S. and Chinese adolescents. *Journal of Consulting and Clinical Psychology, 68*(2), 209–219.

Grossman, J. M., & Liang, B. (2008). Discrimination distress among Chinese American adolescents. *Journal of Youth and Adolescence, 37,* 1–11.

Guerrero, A. P. S., Hishinuma, E. S., Andrade, N. N., Nishimura, S. T., & Cunanan, V. L. (2006). Correlations among socioeconomic and family factors and academic, behavioral, and emotional difficulties in Filipino adolescents in Hawai'i. *International Journal of Social Psychiatry, 53,* 343–359.

Haeffel, G. J., Voelz, Z. R., & Joiner, T. E., Jr. (2007). Vulnerability to depressive symptoms: Clarifying the role of excessive reassurance seeking and perceived social support in an interpersonal model of depression. *Cognition and Emotion, 21*(3), 681–688.

Hammen, C. (1991). Generation of stress in the course of unipolar depression. *Journal of Abnormal Psychology,* 100(4), 555–561.

Hammen, C. L., & Peters, S. D. (1978). Interpersonal consequences of depression: Responses to men and women enacting a depressed role. *Journal of Abnormal Psychology,* 87(3), 322–332. *Psychiatry,* 52(4), 343–359.

Hirokawa, K. (2005). Perspectives of gender-role identity in mental health: A review focusing on Japanese cultural aspects. In J.W. Lee (Ed.), *Psychology of gender identity* (pp. 63–80). Hauppauge, NY: Nova Biomedical Books.

Hollingshead, A. B., & Redlich, F. C. (1958). *Social class and mental illness.* New York: Wiley.

Hollon, S. D., & Shelton, R. C. (2001). Treatment guidelines for major depressive disorder. *Behavior Therapy,* 32(2), 235–258.

Hollon, S. D., Hammen, K. L., & Brown, L. L. (2002). Cognitive-behavioral treatment of depression. In I. H. Gotlib & C. L. Hammen (Eds.), *Handbook of depression* (pp. 383–403). New York: Guilford.

Hong Ng, C., Norman, T. R., Naing, K. O., et al. (2006). A comparative study of sertaline dosages, plasma concentrations, efficacy, and adverse reactions in Chinese versus Caucasian patients. *International Clinical Psychopharmacology,* 21, 87–92.

Hopko, D. R., Lejuez, C. W., & Hopko, S. D. (2004). Behavioral activation as an intervention for coexistent depressive and anxiety symptoms. *Clinical Case Studies,* 3(1), 37–48.

Hsu, G. L. K., Wan, Y. M., Chang H., Summergrad P., Tsang, B. Y., & Chen, H. (2008). Stigma of depression is more severe in Chinese Americans than Caucasian Americans. *Psychiatry,* 71(3), 210–218.

Huang, H., Hwang, K., & Ko, Y. (1983). Life stress, attribution style, social support, and depression among university students. *Acta Psychologica Taiwanica,* 25(1), 31–47.

Hussain, F. A., & Cochrane, R. (2002). Depression in South Asian women's beliefs on causes and cures. *Mental Health, Religion, and Culture,* 5(3), 285–311.

Hwang, W.-C., & Ting, J. Y. (2008). Disaggregating the effects of acculturation and acculturative stress on the mental health of Asian Americans. *Cultural Diversity and Ethnic Minority Psychology,* 14(2), 147–154.

Hwang, W.-C., Wood, J. J., Lin, K., & Cheung, F. (2006). Cognitive-behavioral therapy with Chinese Americans: Research, theory, and clinical practice. *Cognitive and Behavioral Practice,* 13, 293–303.

Hwu, H. G., Yeh, E. K., & Chang, L. Y. (1989). Prevalence of psychiatric disorders in Taiwan defined by the Chinese Diagnostic Interview Schedule. *Acta Psychiatrica Scandinavica,* 79, 136–147.

Jacobson, E. (1954). Transference problems in the psychoanalytic treatment of severely depressive patients. *Journal of the American Psychoanalytic Association,* 2, 595–606.

Jacobson, N. S., & Anderson, E. A. (1982). Interpersonal skill and depression in college students: An analysis of timing of self disclosures. *Behavior Therapy,* 13, 271–282.

Jacobson, N. S., Dobson, K. S., Truax, P. A., Addis, M. E., Koerner, K., et al. (1996). A component analysis of cognitive-behavioral treatment for depression. *Journal of Consulting and Clinical Psychology,* 64, 295–304.

Jang, S. N., Kawachi, I., Chang, J., Boo, K., Shin, H. G., Lee, H., Cho, S. I., et al. (2009). Marital status, gender, and depression: Analysis of the baseline survey of the Korean Longitudinal Study of Aging (KLoSA). *Social Science & Medicine,* 69(11), 1608–1615.

Ji, J. L., & Xu, J. M. (1989). Cognitive-behavioral therapy. *Chinese Journal of Mental Health,* 3, 129–132.

Joiner, T. E. (2007). Depression's vicious scree: Self-propagating and erosive processes in depression chronicity. *Clinical Psychology: Science and Practice,* 7(2), 203–218.

Kaplan, H. I., & Sadock, B. J. (1995). *Comprehensive textbook of psychiatry* (6th ed., pp. 1559–1595). Baltimore: Williams and Wilkins.

Karasz, A., Dempsey, K., & Fallek, R. (2007). Cultural differences in the experience of everyday symptoms: A comparative study of South Asian and European American women. *Culture, Medicine, and Psychiatry,* 31(4), 473–497.

Katon, W., & Schulberg, H. (1992). Epidemiology of depression in primary care. *General Hospital Psychiatry,* 14, 237–247.

Kelsoe, J. R. (1995). Mood disorders: Genetics. In H. I. Kaplan & B. J. Sadock (Eds.), *Comprehensive textbook of psychiatry* (6th ed., pp. 1582–1595). Baltimore: Williams and Wilkins.

Kessler, R. C. (1997). The effects of stressful life events on depression. *Annual Review of Psychology,* 48, 191–224.

Kessler, R. C., McGonagle, K. A., Zhao, S., Nelson, C. B., Hughes, M., Eshleman, S., et al. (1994). Lifetime and 12-month prevalence of DSM-III-R psychiatric disorders in the United States: Results from the National Comorbidity Survey. *Archives of General Psychiatry, 51*, 8–19.

Kim, B. S. K., Li, L. C., & Liang, T. H. (2002). Effects of Asian American client adherence to Asian cultural values, session goal, and counselor emphasis of client expression on career counseling process. *Journal of Counseling Psychology, 49*(3), 342–354.

Kim, H., Lim, S. W., Kim, S., Kim, J. W., Chang, Y. H., Carroll, B. J., et al. (2006). Monoamine transporter gene polymorphisms and antidepressant response in Koreans with late-life depression. *Journal of the American Medical Association, 296*(13),1609–1618.

Kim, M. T., Han, H.-R., Shin, H. S., Kim, K. B., & Lee, H. B. (2005). Factors associated with depression experience of immigrant populations: A study of Korean immigrants. *Archives of Psychiatric Nursing, 19*(5), 217–225.

Kishi, T., Kitajima, T., Ikeda, M., Yamanouchi, Y., Kinoshita, Y., Kawashima, K., et al. (2009). CLOCK may predict the response to fluvoxamine treatment in Japanese major depressive disorder patients. *Neuromolecular Medicine, 11*(2), 53–57. Epub April 4, 2009.

Kleinman, A. (1982). Neurasthenia and depression: A study of somatization and culture in China. *Culture, Medicine, and Psychiatry, 6*(2), 117–190.

Klerman, G. L., Weissman, M. M., Rounsaville, B. J., & Chevron, E. S. (1984). *Interpersonal psychotherapy of depression.* Northvale, NJ: Aronson.

Koh, J. B. K., Chang, W. C., Fung, D. S. S., & Kee, C. H. Y. (2007). Conceptualization and manifestation of depression in an Asian context: Formal construction and validation of a children's depression scale in Singapore. *Culture, Medicine, and Psychiatry, 31*(2), 225–249.

Lai, D. W. L., & Surood, S. (2008). Predictors of depression in aging South Asian Canadians. *Journal of Cross-Cultural Gerontology, 23*(1), 57–75.

Lee, D. T. S., Kleinman J., & Kleinman, A. (2007). Rethinking depression: An ethnographic study of the experiences of depression among Chinese. *Harvard Review of Psychiatry, 15*(1),1–8.

Lee, D. T. S., Yip, A. S. K., Chiu, H. F. K., Leung, T. Y. S., & Chung, T. K. H. (2001). A psychiatric epidemiology study of postpartum Chinese women. *American Journal of Psychiatry, 158*, 220–226.

Lee, S. (1999). Diagnosis postponed: *Shenjing shuairuo* and the transformation of psychiatry in post-Mao China. *Culture, Medicine, and Psychiatry, 23*(3), 349–380.

Lee, S. H. (2006). Saliency of one's heritage culture: Asian cultural values and its interconnections with collective self-esteem and acculturation/enculturation as a predictor of psychological well-being of people of Chinese descent. Unpublished dissertation. Ohio State University.

Lewinsohn, P. M., Biglan, T., & Zeiss, A. (1976). Behavioral treatment of depression. In P. Davidson (Ed.), *Behavioral management of anxiety, depression, and pain* (pp. 91–146). New York: Brunner/Mazel.

Lewinsohn, P. M., & Graf, M. (1973). Pleasant activities and depression. *Journal of Consulting and Clinical Psychology, 41*(2), 261–268.

Lewinsohn, P. M., & Libet, J. (1972). Pleasant events, activity schedules, and depressions. *Journal of Abnormal Psychology, 79*(3), 291–295.

Lin, K.-M., & Finder, E. J. (1983). Neuroleptic dosage for Asians. *American Journal of Psychiatry, 140*, 490–491.

Lin, K-M, Lau, J., Smith, M., et al. (1988). Comparison of alprazolam plasma levels and behavioral effects in normal Asian and Caucasian male volunteers. *Psychopharmacology (Berl) 96*, 365–369.

Ma, S. H., & Teasdale, J. D. (2004). Mindfulness-based cognitive therapy for depression: Replication and exploration of differential relapse prevention effects. *Journal of Consulting and Clinical Psychology, 72*(1), 31–40.

Malhotra, R., Chan, A., & Østbye, T. (2010). Prevalence and correlates of clinically significant depressive symptoms among elderly people in Sri Lanka: Findings from a national survey. *International Psychogeriatrics, 22*(2), 227–236.

Malik, R. (2000). Culture and emotions: Depression among Pakistanis. In C. Squire (Ed.), *Culture in psychology* (pp. 147–162). New York: Routledge.

Markus, H. R., & Kitayama, S. (1991). Culture and self: Implications for emotion, cognition, and motivation. *Psychological Review, 98*, 224–253.

McWilliams, N. (1999). *Psychoanalytic case formulation.* New York: Guilford.

Miranda, J., Bernal, G., Lau, A., Kohn, L., Hwang, W., & LaFromboise, T. (2005). State of the science on psychosocial interventions for ethnic minorities. *Annual Review of Clinical Psychology, 1*(1), 113–142.

Noh, S., Kaspar, V., & Wickrama, K. A. S. (2007). Overt and subtle racial discrimination and mental health: Preliminary findings for Korean immigrants. *American Journal of Public Health, 97*(7), 1269–1274.

Nolen-Hoeksema, S. (1991). Responses to depression and their effects on the duration of depressive episodes. *Journal of Abnormal Psychology, 100*(4), 569–582.

Paykel, E. S. (Ed.). (1992). *Handbook of affective disorders* (2nd ed.). New York: Guilford.

Phillips, M. R., Liu, H., & Zhang, Y. (1999). Suicide and social change in China. *Culture, Medicine & Psychiatry, 23*, 25–50.

Phillips, M. R., Li, X., & Zhang, Y. (2002). Suicide rates in China, 1995–1999. *Lancet, 359*, 835–840.

Pi, E. H., & Gray, G. E. (1998). A cross-cultural perspective on psychopharmacology. *Essential Psychopharmacology, 2*, 233–262.

Pi, E. H., & Gray, G. E. (2000). Ethnopsychopharmacology for Asians. In J. O. Oldman & M. B. Riba (Series Eds.) & P. Ruiz (Vol. Ed.), *Review of Psychiatry Series: Vol. 19, No. 4: Ethnicity and psychopharmacology* (pp. 91–108). Washington DC, American Psychiatric Press.

Pi, E. H., Simpson, G. M., & Cooper, T. M. (1986). Pharmacokinetics of desipramine in Caucasian and Asian volunteers. *American Journal of Psychiatry, 143*, 1174–1176.

Potkin, S. G., Shen, Y., Pardes, H., et al. (1984). Haloperidol concentrations elevated in Chinese patients. *Psychiatry Research, 12*, 167–172.

Rhee, S., Chang, J., & Rhee, J. (2003). Acculturation, communication patterns, and self-esteem among Asian and Caucasian American adolescents. *Adolescence, 38*(152), 749–768.

Rich, A. R., & Bonner, R. L. (1987). Concurrent validity of a stress-vulnerability model of suicidal ideation and behavior: A follow-up study. *Suicide and Life-Threatening Behavior, 17*(4), 265–265.

Roland, A. (1996). *Cultural pluralism and psychoanalysis: The Asian and North American experience.* New York and London: Routledge.

Rudd, M. D. (1990). An integrative model of suicidal ideation. *Suicide and Life-Threatening Behavior, 20*(1), 16–30.

Rudorfer, M. V., Lane, E. A., Chang, W. H., et al. (1984). Desipramine pharmacokinetics in Chinese and Caucasian volunteers. *British Journal of Clinical Pharmacology, 17*, 433–440.

Ryder, A. G., Alden, L. E., & Paulhus, D. L. (2000). Is acculturation unidimensional or bidimensional? A head-to-head comparison in the prediction of personality, self-identity, and adjustment. *Journal of Personality and Social Psychology, 79*(1), 49–49.

Saint Arnault D., & Kim, O. (2008). Is there an Asian idiom of distress? Somatic symptoms in female Japanese and Korean students. *Archives of Psychiatric Nursing, 22*(1), 27–38.

Sartorius, N., Ustun, T. B., Costa e Silva, J. A., et al. (1993). An international study of psychological problems in primary care. *Archives of General Psychiatry, 50*, 819–824.

Seligman, M. E. P., Reivich, K., Jaycox, L., & Gillham, J. (1995). *The Optimistic Child.* New York: Houghton Mifflin.

Shapiro, D. A., Barkham, M., Rees, A., Hardy, G. E., Reynolds, S., & Startup, M. (1994). Effects of treatment duration and severity of depression on the effectiveness of cognitive-behavioral and psychodynamic-interpersonal psychotherapy. *Journal of Consulting and Clinical Psychology, 62*(3), 522–534.

Shen, B., & Takeuchi, D. T. (2001). A structural model of acculturation and mental health status among Chinese Americans. *American Journal of Community Psychology, 29*(3), 387–418.

Shimoda, K., Noguchi, T., Ozeki, Y., et al. (1995). Metabolism of clomipramine in a Japanese psychiatric population: Hydroxylation, desmethylation, and glucuronidation. *Neuropsychopharmacology, 12*, 323–333.

Shin, K. R. (1994). Psychosocial predictors of depressive symptoms in Korean-American women in New York City. *Women and Health, 21*(1), 73–82.

Simons, A. D., Angell, K. L., Monroe, S. M., & Thase, M. E. (1993). Cognition and life stress in depression: Cognitive factors and the definition, rating, and generation of negative life events. *Journal of Abnormal Psychology, 102*(4), 584–591.

Stewart, S. M., Betson, C., Lam, T. H., Chung, S. F., Ho, H. H., & Chung, T. F. C. (1999). The correlates of depressed mood in adolescents in Hong Kong. *Journal of Adolescent Health, 25*, 27–34.

Stewart, S. M., Kennard, B. D., Lee, P. W. H., Mayes, T., Hughes, C., & Emslie, G. (2005). Hopelessness and suicidal ideation among adolescents in two cultures. *Journal of Child Psychology and Psychiatry, 46*(4), 364–372.

Sullivan, H. S. (1953). *The interpersonal theory of psychiatry*. New York: Norton.

Takeuchi, D. T., Chung, R. C. Y., Lin, K. M., Shen, H., Kurasaki, K., Chun, C. A., et al. (1998). Lifetime and twelve-month prevalence rates of major depressive episodes and dysthmia among Chinese Americans in Los Angeles. *American Journal of Psychiatry, 155,* 1407–1414.

Takeuchi, D. T., Zane, N., Hong, S., Chae, D. H., Gong, F., Gee, G. C., et al. (2007). Immigration-related factors and mental disorders among Asian Americans. *American Journal of Public Health, 97*(1), 84–90.

Taylor, S., Sherman, D., Kim, H., Jarcho, J., Takagi, K. & Dunagan, M. (2004). Culture and social support: who seeks it and why? *Journal of Personality and Social Psychology, 87*(3), 354–362.

Thomas, M., & Choi, J. B. (2006). Acculturative stress and social support among Korean and Indian immigrant adolescents in the united states. *Journal of Sociology and Social Welfare, 33*(2), 123–143.

Triandis, H. C. (1989).Cross-cultural studies of individualism: Collectivism. In J. Berman (Ed.), *Nebraska symposium on motivation* (Vol. 37, pp. 41–133). Lincoln: University of Nebraska Press.

Tsai, Y. F., Chung, J. W. Y., Wong, T. K. S., & Huang, C. M. (2005). Preview comparison of the prevalence and risk factors for depressive symptoms among elderly nursing home residents in Taiwan and Hong Kong. *International Journal of Geriatric Psychiatry, 20*(4), 315–321.

Tseng, V., & Fuligni, A. J. (2000). Parent-adolescent language use and relationships among immigrant families with east Asian, Filipino, and Latin American backgrounds. *Journal of Marriage and the Family, 62*(2), 465–476.

Tung, M. (1991). Insight-oriented psychotherapy and the Chinese patient. *American Journal of Orthopsychiatry, 61,* 186–194.

Tung, M. (1984). Life values, psychotherapy, and east-west integration. *Psychiatry, 47*(3), 285–292.

Ukaegbu, C., Banks, J. B., Carter, N. J., & Goldman, L. S. (2008). Clinical inquiries: What drugs are best for bipolar depression? *Journal of Family Practice, 57*(9), 606–608.

Usturn, T. B., & Sartorius, N. (Eds.). (1995). *Mental illness in general health care: An international study*. West Sussex, UK: Wiley.

Vijayakumar, L. (2005). Suicide and mental disorders in Asia. *International Review of Psychiatry, 17*(2), 109–114.

Weiss, M. G., Doongaji, D. R., Siddhartha, S., Wypij, D., Pathare, S., Bhatawdekar, M., et al. (1992). The explanatory model interview catalogue (EMIC): contribution to cross-cultural research methods from a study of leprosy and mental health. *British Journal of Psychiatry, 160,* 819–830.

Weissman, M. M., Bland, R. C., Canino, G. J., Faravelli, C., Greenald, S., et al. (1996). Cross-national epidemiology of major depression and bipolar disorder. *Journal of the American Medical Association, 276,* 29–299.

Weissman, M. M., Markowitz, J. C., & Klerman, G. L. (2000). *Comprehensive guide to interpersonal psychotherapy*. New York: Basic Books.

Westermeyer, J., & Her, C. (2007). Western psychiatry and difficulty: Understanding and treating Hmong refugees. In J. P. Wilson, & C. S. Tang (Eds.), *Cross-cultural assessment of psychological trauma and PTSD* (pp. 371–393). New York: Springer Science + Business Media.

Wong, D. F. K. (2008). Cognitive behavioral treatment groups for people with chronic depression in Hong Kong: A randomized wait-list control design. *Depression and Anxiety, 25*(2), 142–148.

Wong, E. C., Kim, B. S. K., Zane, N. W. S., Kim, I. J., & Huang, J. S. (2003). Examining culturally based variables associated with ethnicity: Influences on credibility perceptions of empirically supported interventions. *Cultural Diversity and Ethnic Minority Psychology, 9*(1), 88–96.

Wong, F. K., Lam, Y. K., & Poon, A. (2010). Depression literacy among Australians of Chinese-speaking background in Melbourne, Australia. *BMC Psychiatry, 10,* 7.

Wong, S. T., Yoo, G. J., & Stewart, A. L. (2006). The changing meaning of family support among older Chinese and Korean immigrants. *Journals of Gerontology. Series B, Psychological Sciences and Social Sciences, 61B*(1), S4–S9.

Wong, S. T., Yoo, G. J., & Stewart, A. L. (2007). An empirical evaluation of social support and psychological well-being in older Chinese and Korean immigrants. *Ethnicity and Health, 12*(1), 43–67.

Woo, B. S. C., Chang, W. C., Fung, D. S. S., Koh, J. B. K., Leong, J. S. F., Kee, C. H.Y., et al. (2004). Development and validation of a depression scale for Asian adolescents. *Journal of Adolescence, 27*(6), 677–689.

World Health Organization (WHO). (1990). *Composite International Diagnostic Interview (CIDI): Version 1.0.* Geneva, Switzerland: Author.

World Health Organization. (1992). *The ICD-10 classification of mental and behavioral disorders: Clinical descriptions and diagnostic guidelines.* Geneva, Switzerland: Author.

Xu, J., & Ji, J. (1996). Cognitive therapy in China. In Y. X. Xu (Ed.), *Cognitive psychotherapy* (pp. 9–10). Guizhou, China: Guizhou Educational Press.

Yeung, A., Chan, R., Mischoulon, D., Sonawalla, S., Wong, E., Nierenberg, A. A., et al. (2004). Prevalence of major depressive disorder among Chinese-Americans in primary care. *General Hospital Psychiatry, 26*(1), 24–30.

Yeung, A., Chang, D., Gresham, R. L., Nierenberg, A. A., & Fava, M. (2004). Illness beliefs of depressed Chinese Americans in primary care. *Journal of Nervous and Mental Disease, 192*(4), 324–327.

Yeung, A., Kam, R. (2008). Ethical and cultural considerations in delivering psychiatric diagnosis: Reconciling the gap using MDD diagnosis delivery in less-acculturated Chinese patients. *Transcultural Psychiatry, 45*(4), 531–552.

Yeung, A., Yu, S. C., Fung, F., Vorono, S., & Fava, M. (2006). Recognizing and engaging depressed Chinese Americans in treatment in a primary care setting. *International Journal of Geriatric Psychiatry, 21*, 819–823.

Yoon, J., & Lau, A. S. (2008). Maladaptive perfectionism and depressive symptoms among Asian American college students: Contributions of interdependence and parental relations. *Cultural Diversity and Ethnic Minority Psychology, 14*(2), 92–101.

Young, J. E., Weinberger, A. D., & Beck, A. T. (2001). Cognitive therapy for depression. In D. H. Barlow (Ed.), *Clinical handbook of psychological disorders: A step-by-step treatment manual* (3rd ed., pp. 264–308). New York: Guilford.

Yu, D. L., & Seligman, M. E. P. (2002). Preventing depressive symptoms in Chinese children. *Prevention & Treatment, 5*, Article 9.

| 7 |

ANXIETY DISORDERS IN ASIANS

JANIE J. HONG

IDENTIFYING ANXIETY DISORDERS IN ASIANS

Current DSM Nosology and Criteria for Anxiety Disorders

The *DSM-IV-TR* lists and describes the following disorders as part of the anxiety disorders category: panic disorder (with or without agoraphobia), agoraphobia without a history of panic disorder, specific phobias, social phobia or social anxiety disorder (SAD), obsessive-compulsive disorder (OCD), post-traumatic stress disorder (PTSD) and acute stress disorder, and generalized anxiety disorder (GAD) (American Psychiatric Association [APA], 2000). At first glance, the large number of disorders represented appears to suggest a heterogeneous array of syndromes with little to tie them together, other than the vague marker of experiencing "anxiety." The disorders are, however, cohesively linked by a single, underlying feature: a tendency to overestimate the dangerousness of a particular trigger or situation. Individuals with anxiety disorders will characteristically adopt maladaptive coping behaviors to protect themselves from perceived danger. Whether it is isolating oneself socially, washing hands excessively to rid them of germs, avoiding all bridges out of a fear of heights, or refusing to watch television to avoid triggering of traumatic memories, the maladaptive coping strategies used negatively reinforce fears and can further exacerbate the interference and dysfunction caused by their anxieties. Determining which anxiety disorder a person has depends on what trigger or situation an individual perceives as threatening or dangerous. For example, individuals with panic disorder fear having another panic attack, whereas individuals with social phobia fear social situations in which they may be negatively evaluated or humiliated.

The following sections provide an overview of the phenomenology and epidemiology of each of the anxiety disorders. When possible, cross-cultural differences in the presentation and prevalence of the disorders are also discussed.

143

Specific Phobias

Specific phobias are the most common type of anxiety disorder (Grant et al., 2004). They are characterized by a persistent and excessive fear of clearly identifiable objects or situations; exposure to the phobic objects or situations invariably provokes an immediate, marked anxiety response. The *DSM-IV-TR* identifies the following subtypes that may be the focus of phobic fear: animal type (e.g., dogs, spiders, snakes), natural environment (e.g., storms, heights), blood-injection-injury, situational (e.g., driving, bridges, elevators), and other (e.g., fear of vomiting).

The *DSM-IV-TR* reports lifetime prevalence rates for specific phobias ranging between 7.2% and 11.3%; estimates tend to decline with age and vary by type of phobia (APA, 2000). Data from the National Epidemiologic Survey on Alcohol and Related Conditions (NESARC; Grant et al., 2004), which assessed a representative U.S. sample of 43,093 respondents for major *DSM-IV* anxiety, mood, and substance use disorders, indicate that the age of onset of most new cases is 5 years, with symptoms lasting an average of 20.1 years, and only 8% of those with the disorder seeking treatment specifically for it (Stinson et al., 2007). The likelihood of having a specific phobia appears to differ significantly among ethnic-race groups. While the overall lifetime and 12-month prevalence estimates were 9.4% and 7.1% respectively, Asian Americans showed the lowest rates among all ethnic-race groups identified, with a lifetime prevalence rate of 5.9% and a 12-month prevalence rate of 4.1%. Epidemiological studies of South Korean (Cho et al., 2007) and Japanese (Kawakami et al., 2005) adults show similarly low rates of the disorder (see Table 7.1).

Specific phobias offer a clear view of many of the processes that characterize the anxiety disorders. There is an overestimation of danger, a strong physiological anxiety response, and the use of maladaptive coping strategies to manage anxiety. The following case example helps illustrate these processes. John suffers from a severe phobic fear of spiders. While visiting a friend's home, he asks his friend to check all furniture and windows for possible spiders before he enters any room (i.e., overestimation of threat). At one point during the visit, after finally entering the living room, he sees cobwebs lining the top corner of the far room window. Immediately, he notices his heart begin to race, his breath become shallow, and his hands start to shake (i.e., physiological arousal). He then rushes out of the room and refuses to reenter for the remainder of the visit (i.e., maladaptive coping).

Panic Attacks, Panic Disorder, and Agoraphobia

Panic attacks are defined by the *DSM-IV-TR* as a discrete period of intense fear or discomfort that is accompanied by an abrupt onset of somatic or cognitive symptoms (e.g., heart palpitations, shortness of breath, fears of "going crazy") that reaches peak intensity within 10 minutes. A frequent misconception is that panic disorder is diagnosed and distinguished from other *DSM-IV-TR* anxiety disorders by the presence of panic attacks. Panic attacks can occur in the context of *all* of the anxiety disorders, not just panic disorder. The *DSM-IV-TR* identifies three types of panic attacks: (1) unexpected panic attacks; (2) situationally bound panic attacks; and (3) situationally predisposed panic attacks. Unexpected panic attacks are perceived as occurring without reason and without an identifiable internal or external situational trigger. By contrast, situationally bound and situationally predisposed panic attacks are both clearly cued by an identifiable trigger, and are

TABLE 7.1: Comparison of Adult Anxiety Disorder Prevalence Rates among Asians and Those Reported in the *DSM-IV-TR*

Disorder		Prevalence Rates among Asians	DSM-IV
Generalized Anxiety Disorder	1-yr:	Asian Americans: 1.1% (Grant, Hasin, Stinson, et al., 2005)	
		South Korea: 1% (Cho et al., 2007)	3%
		Japan: 1.2% (Kawakami et al., 2005)	
		China: 0.8% (Ma et al., 2009)	
	Lifetime:	Asian Americans: 1.9% (Grant, Hasin, Stinson, et al., 2005)	
		South Korea: 2.3% (Cho et al., 2007)	5%
		China: 1.2% (Ma et al., 2009)	
Panic Disorder	1-yr:	South Korea: 0.2% (Cho et al., 2007)	
		Taiwan: 0.2% (Weissman et al., 1997)	0.5%–1.5%
		Japan: 0.5% (Kawakami et al., 2005)	
	Lifetime:	South Korea: 0.4% (Cho et al., 2007)	
		Taiwan: 0.4% (Weissman et al., 1997)	1%–2%
Specific Phobias	1-yr:	Asian Americans: 4.1% (Stinson et al., 2007)	
		South Korea: 4.2% (Cho et al., 2007)	
		Japan: 2.7% (Kawakami et al., 2005)	
	Lifetime:	Asian Americans: 5.9% (Stinson et al., 2007)	7.2%–11.3%
		South Korea: 5.2% (Cho et al., 2007)	
Social Phobia	1-yr:	Asian Americans: 2.1% (Grant, Hasin, Blanco, et al., 2005)	
		South Korea: 0.2% (Cho et al., 2007)	
		Japan: 0.8% (Kawakami et al., 2005)	
	Lifetime:	Asian Americans: 3.3% (Grant, Hasin, Blanco, et al., 2005)	3%–13%
		South Korea: 0.2% (Cho et al., 2007)	
Obsessive-Compulsive Disorder	1-yr:	South Korea: 0.6% (Cho et al., 2007); 1.1% (Weissman et al., 1994)	0.5%–2.1%
		Taiwan: 0.4% (Weissman et al., 1994)	
	Lifetime:	South Korea: 0.8% (Cho et al., 2007)	2.5%
		Taiwan: 0.7% (Weissman et al., 1994)	
Post-traumatic Stress Disorder	1-yr:	South Korea: 0.7% (Cho et al., 2007)	
		Japan: 0.4% (Kawakami et al., 2005)	
	Lifetime:	South Korea: 1.7% (Cho et al., 2007)	8%

distinguished from one another by the probability of experiencing a panic attack when exposed to the feared trigger or situation (i.e., always has a panic attack vs. sometimes has a panic attack).

Panic disorder is diagnosed when an individual experiences recurrent, unexpected panic attacks, with at least one of the attacks being followed by a period of concerns about having more attacks, worry about the implications of the attack or its consequences (e.g., "What if I die?" "What if I go crazy?"), and/or significant changes in behavior related to the attacks (e.g., stops eating certain foods out of fear of having an attack). Agoraphobia is always assessed within the context of assessing panic disorder. Agoraphobia is defined by the fear of having a panic attack or panic-like sensations while being in places or situations in which escape may be difficult or help may not be readily available (e.g., being in crowds, at home alone, or on an elevator). As a result of their agoraphobic fears, individuals will avoid situations or endure them with marked distress or require the presence of a companion. Panic disorder and agoraphobia cannot be diagnosed without mention of the other, which leaves the following potential *DSM-IV* diagnoses: panic disorder without agoraphobia, panic disorder with agoraphobia, and agoraphobia without a history of panic disorder.

The age of onset for panic disorder with or without agoraphobia ranges from mid-to-late twenties to early thirties, with the peak likelihood of having the disorder being around age 25 years (Grant et al., 2006; Weissman et al., 1997). Similar ages of onset have been reported for individuals in Taiwan and South Korea (Weissman et al., 1997). Individuals with panic disorder with agoraphobia are more likely to seek treatment and do so sooner than those with panic disorder without agoraphobia (Grant et al., 2006; Kessler et al., 2006). Individuals with panic disorder, particularly those with agoraphobia, are most likely to first seek treatment from general medical settings (Kessler et al., 2006), which is consistent with the somatic focus of the disorder. The *DSM-IV-TR* reports prevalence rates as high as 60% in cardiology clinics.

Overall lifetime and 12-month prevalence rates for panic disorder with or without agoraphobia are reported by the *DSM-IV-TR* as ranging between 1–2% and 0.5–1.5%, respectively. These rates are lower than those found in the NESARC epidemiological study, which reports overall lifetime and 12-month rates for panic disorder with and without agoraphobia as being 5.1% and 2.1%, respectively (Grant et al., 2006). Asian Americans in the study showed a reduced risk for panic disorder with and without agoraphobia (lifetime = 2.1%; 12-month = 0.7%) and had the lowest estimates among all ethnic-racial groups identified. In a large epidemiological study in South Korea, investigators found even lower odds of the disorder, reporting lifetime and 12-month rates of 0.4% and 0.2%, respectively (Cho et al., 2007). Similarly low estimates have been reported in Japan (Kawakami et al., 2005) and Taiwan (Weissman et al., 1997). It is unclear, however, whether these East Asian estimates include individuals with a concomitant agoraphobia diagnosis.

Obsessive-Compulsive Disorder

Obsessive-compulsive disorder (OCD) is diagnosed when an individual suffers from recurrent obsessions and/or compulsions. Obsessions are unwanted, intrusive, inappropriate thoughts, images, or urges that cause marked anxiety or discomfort. Compulsions are defined as repetitive behaviors or mental acts that are completed with the goal of reducing or preventing distress. The drive to engage in compulsions may be to neutralize the distress caused by obsessions (e.g., handwashing in response to contamination fears) but can also be to rigidly apply specific rules (e.g., touching objects in a particular way) in the absence of an obsession.

Individuals with OCD are able to recognize (to varying degrees) that their obsessions and compulsions are excessive or unreasonable, but struggle to resist them, despite the distress and interference caused. From checking door locks to repeated showering to having recurrent disturbing sexual images, the profile of someone with OCD varies greatly. This has led researchers to consider ways to meaningfully distinguish the array of symptom presentations, which include the possibility of identifying OCD subtypes or its underlying mechanisms (see McKay et al., 2004 for review).

Common OCD symptom patterns include: (1) contamination or illness concerns with compulsive cleaning or washing; (2) pathological doubting of actions with checking rituals; (3) obsessions and/or compulsions related to symmetry, orderliness, and numbers; (4) hoarding rituals; and (5) obsessional slowness (Lochner & Stein, 2003). Individuals with OCD may also struggle with aggressive, religious, or sexual obsessions and engage in covert neutralizations or compulsions (e.g., thinking good thoughts or phrases to counter unwanted obsessions; Rachman, 1997, 1998). Among those seeking treatment, approximately 75% present with primarily cleaning or checking compulsions, while patients with exactness, hoarding, or slowness rituals tend to be underrepresented (Ball, Baer, & Otto, 1996).

Average age of onset for OCD is typically early to mid-twenties (Crino, Slade, & Andrews, 2005; Kessler, Berglund, et al., 2005). Peak age of onset for OCD appears to be bimodal, with peaks in childhood–early adolescence (childhood onset) and late adolescence–early adulthood (adult onset) (Fornaro et al., 2009). Age of onset has been reported to be earlier in men than in women (Castle, Deale, & Marks, 1995; Noshirvani, Kasvikis, Marks, Tsakiris, & Monteiro, 1991). Childhood-onset OCD is typically associated with greater symptom severity, higher rates of compulsions and comorbid tic disorders, and may have greater genetic loading than adult-onset OCD (Fornaro et al., 2009; Lochner & Stein, 2003). In a study of French OCD outpatients (n = 617), patients with an early age of onset (i.e., age 15 years or earlier) were more likely to show a gradual rise in symptoms than those with a later age of onset (i.e., age older than 15 years; Millet et al., 2004). A later age of onset was more associated with a sudden onset of symptoms, which may indicate the stronger role of precipitating environmental factors than for early-onset patients. Similar to past studies, the early-onset group showed a greater likelihood to have comorbid tic disorders.

Based on past community studies of adults, the *DSM-IV-TR* reports a lifetime prevalence of 2.5% and 12-month prevalence of 0.5–2.1% for OCD. As noted in the *DSM-IV-TR*, these rates may, however, be inflated and may not accurately reflect the true epidemiology of the disorder. More recent epidemiological studies support this notion and suggest that studies using *DSM-III* criteria are more likely to see higher rates (Crino, Slade, & Andrews, 2005). When using *DSM-IV-TR* criteria, which emphasize the presence of clinically significant distress and impairment, the rates are significantly lower (Crino et al., 2005; Kessler, Berglund, et al., 2005; Kessler, Chiu, et al., 2005). In the National Comorbidity Survey Replication (NCS-R), using a large nationally representative sample of U.S. adults (n = 9,282), participants underwent face-to-face diagnostic assessments of *DSM-IV* anxiety, mood, impulse-control, and substance use disorders (Kessler & Merikangas, 2004). Findings from the NCS-R indicated lifetime and 12-month prevalence estimates for OCD as 1.6% and 1%, respectively (Kessler, Berglund, et al., 2005; Kessler, Chiu, et al., 2005). Although similar rates have been noted (Weissman et al., 1994), prevalence rates in East Asian contexts appear to be lower than those reported by the *DSM* and those found in the United States and other Western contexts (see Table 7.1).

Despite the heterogeneity in clinical symptom profiles, the features and nature of the disorder (e.g., type of obsessions/compulsions, age of onset, gender differences) appear to be consistent across cultures (Juang & Liu, 2001; Matsunaga et al., 2000; Matsunaga & Seedat, 2007). For example, using a sample of Taiwanese OCD patients (n = 200), Juang and Liu (2001) found a mean age of onset of 23.4 years (with an earlier age of onset for men); the most common obsessions were those related to fears of contamination, pathological doubting, and need for symmetry, and the most common compulsions were checking, washing, and putting items in order. These findings parallel those found with OCD patient samples in the West.

Generalized Anxiety Disorder

The diagnostic marker of generalized anxiety disorder (GAD) is chronic, excessive, uncontrollable worry. Individuals are diagnosed with GAD if they (1) worry excessively for more days than not (over at least a 6-month period), (2) find it difficult to control their worry, and (3) experience a number of somatic or cognitive difficulties as a result of their worry and anxiety (e.g., easily fatigued, difficulties concentrating). The content of the individual's fears are less important than the degree to which the worries consume his life and the degree to which the person feels he has control over his worries. In other words, individuals with GAD tend to report worries common to most people (e.g., finances, personal health, list of to-do items, personal relationships) but, unlike their nonclinical counterparts, they report significant difficulty shifting their focus away from their worries and engaging in their lives.

The constellation of physiological symptoms characteristic of GAD differs from those typically associated with anxious arousal and those seen in the other anxiety disorders (Brown, Marten & Barlow, 1995). The most commonly reported symptoms are irritability, restlessness/feeling keyed up, muscle tension, easy fatigability, sleep difficulties, and concentration difficulties (Marten et al., 1993). These symptoms correlate more strongly with worry and GAD severity than do symptoms of anxious arousal (Brown et al., 1995), and are considered evidence supporting GAD as distinguishable from the other anxiety disorders.

In a telephone-based study of Hong Kong residents aged 15–60 years (n = 3,304), participants were asked a series of questions to assess for the presence of GAD and difficulties associated with the diagnosis (S. Lee, Tsang, Chui, Kwok, & Cheung, 2007). Similar to past U.S. studies, among the 4.1% of participants meeting criteria in the past 6 months, the three most commonly reported symptoms were "easily tired," "easily irritable," and "difficult to concentrate." Unlike past U.S. studies, however, a high percentage of the Hong Kong GAD sample (i.e., greater than 50%) also reported difficulties with heart palpitations and bowel movements. Reports of higher anxious arousal symptoms have also been found with Nepali GAD patients when compared to U.S. patients (Hoge et al., 2006).

The median age of onset for GAD is approximately 30 years (Grant, Hasin, Stinson, et al., 2005; Kessler, Berglund, et al., 2005). According to the *DSM-IV-TR*, the lifetime and 12-month prevalence rates for GAD are 5% and 3%, respectively. These rates are significantly higher than those reported by studies with Asian Americans and individuals living in East Asian contexts (see Table 7.1). For example, in the NESARC study, comparisons of GAD prevalence estimates among the identified white, black, Native American, Hispanic, and Asian American ethnic-race groups showed the Asian American sample having the lowest prevalence rates (lifetime = 1.9% and 12-month = 1.1%) among all ethnic-race groups and rates significantly lower than the white sample (lifetime = 4.6% and 12-month = 2.2%; Grant, Hasin, Stinson, et al., 2005).

In an epidemiological study conducted in China, 5,296 individuals aged 15 years or older were interviewed by psychiatrists and assessed for GAD (Ma et al., 2009). The results indicated an overall lifetime prevalence of 1.2%, with higher estimates for women than for men (1.7% vs. 0.7%). Among those who met criteria for lifetime GAD, 80% met criteria for another psychiatric disorder, with the most common comorbid disorder being major depressive disorder. The high rate of comorbidity is similar to that found in the NESARC study of U.S. adults, where nearly 90% of the individuals with GAD suffered from another psychiatric disorder (Grant, Hasin, Stinson, et al., 2005).

Post-traumatic Stress Disorder

Post-traumatic stress disorder (PTSD) is unique from other anxiety disorders in that the cause for the disorder is assumed to be known; that is, exposure to a traumatic event. The *DSM-IV-TR* specifies a traumatic event as being both (1) the direct personal experience of an event that involves actual or threatened death or serious injury, or a threat to the physical integrity of the self or others, and (2) a response to the event that involves intense fear, helplessness, or horror. Thus, for an event to be classified as traumatic, the person not only has to have a direct experience with a traumatic stressor but also must perceive the stressor as horrific or terrifying.

As a result of exposure to a traumatic event, individuals with PTSD suffer from (1) persistent reexperiencing of the traumatic event, (2) persistent avoidance of stimuli associated with the trauma and numbing of general responsiveness, and (3) persistent symptoms of increased arousal. The PTSD diagnosis is differentiated from acute stress disorder by the duration of symptoms only. For a PTSD diagnosis, symptoms must be present for at least 1 month, whereas for an acute stress disorder diagnosis symptoms must be present more than 2 days but less than 1 month.

Although the diagnosis first gained attention with men suffering from combat-related disorders, research indicates that combat exposure accounts for only a small proportion of those who develop the disorder (Prigerson et al., 2002). Traumatic events that are more commonly reported are physical attacks, witnessing a traumatic event happen to another person, childhood maltreatment (physical, sexual, and emotional), and serious accidents (Perkonigg, Kessler, Storz, & Wittchen, 2000). The prevalence of trauma exposure is relatively high (N. Breslau et al., 1998; Kessler, Sonnega, Bromet, Hughes, & Nelson, 1995; Norris, 1992; Prigerson, Maciejewski, & Rosenheck, 2002). For example, the National Comorbidity Survey, which conducted diagnostic surveys with a representative U.S. sample of 5,877 individuals aged 15–54 years, found 60.7% of men and 51.2% of women reported experiencing at least one traumatic event (Kessler et al., 1995). Despite the high prevalence of trauma exposure, the risk of developing PTSD is relatively low. Among those exposed to a traumatic event, 80–90% of individuals will not develop PTSD (Brunello et al., 2001). The *DSM-IV-TR* reports a lifetime prevalence rate of 8.0% in the adult U.S. population, which is similar to the NSC-R sample estimate of 6.8% (Kessler, Berglund, et al., 2005).

Gender differences exist in the likelihood of experiencing different traumas. Women are more likely to suffer molestation, rape, and sexual abuse traumas, whereas men are more likely to experience physical attacks, accidents, and threats involving a weapon (Perkonigg et al., 2000; Prigerson et al., 2002; Kessler et al., 1995). Even when exposed to the same type of trauma as men, women are twice as likely to develop PTSD and have a greater persistence of PTSD symptoms (Kessler et al., 1995, Kessler, 2000, Perkonigg et al., 2000). The reasons for the gender difference are not clear, though several hypotheses have been forwarded (for review see Nemeroff et al., 2006).

The prevalence rates for PTSD reported in South Korea and Japan are significantly lower than those reported in the United States (see Table 7.1). It is unclear whether the lower rates reported are due to reduced prevalence of trauma exposure or increased resilience to traumatic events. Although past epidemiological surveys of U.S. Vietnam War veterans found that being an ethnic minority increased the likelihood of exposure to combat-related traumas and risk of PTSD (Beals et al., 2002; Kulka et al., 1990), the surveys did not include Asian American/Pacific Islanders in their samples. The Hawaii Vietnam Veterans Project (HVVP) investigated whether Native Hawaiian and Japanese American Vietnam veterans would similarly support minority status as a predictor of higher combat trauma exposure and higher PTSD prevalence rates (Friedman, Schnurr, Sengupta, Holmes, & Ashcraft, 2004). The HVVP study interviewed and included 100 Native Hawaiian and 102 Japanese American veterans and compared findings from past epidemiological studies. The study found that the Native Hawaiian sample experienced war zone (trauma) exposure (i.e., combat exposure, exposure to atrocities and violence, deprivations, and being held as prisoners of war) at rates comparable to the white, black, and Hispanic samples from the National Vietnam Veterans Readjustment Study (NVVRS; Kulka et al., 1990). Although total war zone exposure for the Japanese American sample did not significantly differ from the Native Hawaiian or white samples, the group showed the lowest exposure rate in all categories assessed and had rates significantly lower than the black and Hispanic veterans.

PTSD prevalence rates in the HVVP study were lowest for the Japanese Americans (Friedman et al., 2004). Current PTSD prevalence rates for the white, black, Hispanic, and Native Hawaiian groups ranged between 11.8% and 27.0%, whereas the Japanese American group rate was only 1.9%. Similarly, the lifetime prevalence estimate for the Japanese Americans was 8.8%, while the lifetime estimates for the other groups ranged between 22.4% and 38.7%. Overall, findings from the HVVP study suggest that Japanese American Vietnam veterans, unlike the other ethnic minority groups sampled, were less likely to develop PTSD. Moreover, the lower prevalence rates could not be fully attributed to lower war zone trauma exposure.

Although disproportionately high rates of PTSD have been reported for Southeast Asian refugee populations (e.g., Kinzie et al., 1990), one published review of PTSD prevalence rates among refugee populations suggests the rates may be lower than previously contended (Fazel, Wheeler, & Danesh, 2005). In the review, the authors examined 20 interview-based studies of unselected refugee populations that have resettled in Western countries, and provided diagnoses of PTSD and other serious mental disorders. Cumulatively, the 20 studies provided data for nearly 7,000 adult refugees. When examining data from individuals with Southeast Asian origins, the PTSD prevalence rates ranged from 8% to 10%, which appear to be similar to that reported by the *DSM-IV-TR*. Similarly, a large epidemiological study (not included in the Fazel et al. review) found that Vietnamese refugees in Australia (n = 1,161) held a PTSD prevalence rate of 3.5%, which did not differ from that found among their Australian-born counterparts (n = 7,961; Silove, Steel, Bauman, Chey, & McFarlane, 2007). Despite these findings, the prevalence of trauma exposure is extremely high among refugee populations, with rates of 80% and higher, and the lowered prevalence rates may not apply to all Southeast Asian populations. For example, in a cross-sectional, interview-based study of a random sample of Cambodians living in California (n = 490), 100% of participants reported exposure to trauma before immigrating to the United States and had high rates of PTSD (62%, weighted; Marshall, Schell, Elliott, Berthold, & Chun, 2005). Further study is needed to examine the specific mental health needs of different Southeast Asian populations, particularly given the high degree of risk for developing PTSD.

Social Phobia

Individuals with social phobia—also known as social anxiety disorder—are highly fearful of social situations in which they are exposed to the possible scrutiny of others. They believe they are in danger of acting inappropriately and of being negatively evaluated and, consequently, being humiliated or embarrassed. Their fear of others' evaluations often leaves them predicting disastrous social consequences (e.g., "If I don't say something witty or clever, she will tell all her friends that I am undatable") and causes them to avoid feared situations or endure them with intense anxiety or distress. Exposure to their feared social or performance situations almost always causes high anxiety, which may take the form of a panic attack.

The *DSM-IV-TR* reports a relatively wide range in lifetime prevalence estimates for social phobia (i.e., 3% to 13%) and partially attributes the range to the varying thresholds used to determine distress and the number of social situations specifically assessed. Using data from the NESARC study, investigators found overall lifetime and 12-month prevalence estimates to be 5.0% and 2.8%, respectively, with higher rates among women than for men (Grant, Hasin, Blanco, et al., 2005). The mean age of onset was 15.1 years, with peak likelihood of onset at 5 years or younger and ages 13–15 years. Among those with the disorder, 97.1% reported at least one performance fear (e.g., speaking in public) and 82.2% reported at least one interaction fear (e.g., having a conversation with people they didn't know well, going to parties or other social gatherings). Asian Americans in the sample showed lower prevalence rates than the white race-ethnic group (12-month: 2.1% vs. 3.0%; lifetime: 3.3% vs. 5.5%). The reported rates for Asian Americans in the sample are, however, similar to the overall sample rates and are markedly higher than those reported in East Asian contexts (see Table 7.1).

Social anxiety arises when someone wants to attain a particular social goal (e.g., "be the life of the party") but worries she will not achieve that goal (Clark & Wells, 1995; Schlenker & Leary, 1982). In other words, to experience social anxiety, the situation must be personally meaningful and the person must doubt he will be socially successful in that situation. Individuals with SAD experience chronically high levels of social anxiety and tend to hold excessively high or unrealistic standards of social performance (e.g., "I must not stumble on my words"; "There must be no pauses in the conversation"; Clark & Wells, 1995). With these standards comes an overestimation of the meaningfulness of their actions ("I just laughed like an idiot, now everyone probably thinks I'm crazy") and the likelihood of negative social consequences ("Everyone is probably wondering how I even got invited to this party").

Perceptions of high social threat are thought to pressure the individual to prevent social failure, which then triggers increased self-focused attention or self-consciousness. Rather than helping the person avoid disapproval, increased self-focused attention can actually exacerbate anxieties and increase the likelihood of feared consequences. By focusing more on themselves, they are more likely to notice when they make minor social errors (e.g., stuttering, pause in conversation) and exaggerate how noticeable these errors are to others. Moreover, by being so focused on themselves, there is little room to notice others' actual reactions or ability to attend to social cues.

A disorder that closely resembles features of social phobia is Taijin-Kyofu-Sho (TKS). Although the *DSM-IV* has classified TKS as a culture-bound syndrome unique to Japan, the disorder has been identified in Korea (e.g., Choy et al., 2008; S. Lee & Oh, 1999), and symptoms of the disorder have been found in U.S. and other Western samples (e.g., Choy et al., 2008; J. Kim, Rapee, & Gaston, 2008; Kleinknecht, Dinnel, Kleinknecht, Hiruma, & Harada, 1997). TKS is characterized by an intense and excessive fear of embarrassing, offending, or even causing harm to others as a result of a person's perceived physical defects (e.g., blushing, trembling) or inappropriate social behavior. Social phobia and TKS are similar in that both feature fears of negative, interpersonal interactions that lead to avoidance of social situations and marked social impairment. Although fears of negative evaluation are prominent in both social phobia and TKS, the feared consequences of the negative evaluation are considered to be distinct (Kleinknecht et al., 1997; Dinnel, Kleinknecht, & Tanaka-Matsumi, 2002). Individuals with social phobia are primarily fearful of embarrassing *themselves*, whereas individuals with TKS are primarily fearful of embarrassing *others*.

Conceptually, the distinction fits with cultural differences in the importance of self vs. others in achieving social success and acceptance. In Western contexts, the individual is seen as the primary agent in determining social success, which likely explains the rise in self-focus seen among those with social phobia. Perceptions of high social threat by social phobia patients likely lead them to feel increased pressure to prevent social failure, which, in turn, triggers increased self-focused attention. In East Asian contexts, however, the role of others is just as important as (if not more than) the self in determining social success. This allocentric interpersonal focus may explain, in part, the development of fears reported by individuals suffering from TKS in East Asian contexts.

Despite the conceptual consistency with known cultural differences, research investigating the relationship between TKS and social phobia suggests a more complex picture. Choy and colleagues (2008) assessed the prevalence of characteristic TKS symptoms in samples of U.S. and South Korean social phobia patients. The results suggested a strong relationship between social phobia and TKS symptomatology for both U.S. and Korean samples. Symptoms considered unique to the offensive subtype of TKS were endorsed by 75% of both the U.S. and Korean social phobia patients and were associated with the severity of social anxiety symptoms. These findings are consistent with those found in nonclinical samples (Kleinknecht et al., 1997).

The study findings also challenged the proposed distinction between social phobia and TKS in their focus of fear (i.e., fear of embarrassing oneself vs. offending others) (Choy et al., 2008). For both the U.S. and Korean samples, fears of embarrassment to the self were stronger than fears of offending others. A subsample of the Korean patients included in the study met criteria for TKS. Patients with TKS appeared to have stronger fears of offending others *and* embarrassing themselves, than their nonoffensive social phobia counterparts. Overall, the findings indicate that TKS symptoms may not specific to East Asian cultures, may feature prominently among those with social phobia, and may be indicative of more severe difficulties with social anxiety.

Anxiety Disorders as a Whole

Data from the NESARC and NCS-R epidemiological studies have indicated 12-month prevalence estimates for having *any* anxiety disorder in the United States as 11.1% and 18.1%, respectively (Huang et al., 2006; Kessler, Chiu, et al., 2005). One-year prevalence estimates appear to be lower for Asians, with reported estimates of 6.9% for Asian Americans, 6.2% for Koreans, and 4.8% for Japanese (Cho et al., 2007; Huang et al., 2006; Kawakami et al., 2005). Table 7.1 lists the prevalence rates reported by the *DSM-IV-TR* for each of the anxiety disorders and compares these rates with those reported by epidemiological studies with different East Asian populations. Overall, the findings indicate prevalence rates among East Asian populations as being lower than those reported by the *DSM-IV-TR*.

Further investigation of epidemiological data suggests that the lower prevalence rates may be moderated by immigration status. Specifically, U.S. immigrants appear to be at a lower risk for developing or having a mood or anxiety disorder than those born in the United States of the same national origin (J. Breslau, Borges, Hagar, Tancredi, & Gilman, 2009; J. Breslau & Chang, 2006; Takeuchi et al., 2007). Using data from the NESARC study, J. Breslau and Chang (2006) compared lifetime prevalence rates of Asian Americans who reported being born in the United States (n = 282) with those who were foreign-born (n = 954). Lifetime prevalence for having any anxiety disorder was significantly higher among U.S.-born Asians than foreign-born Asians (17.8% vs. 9.1%). Parallel differences were found for social phobia (5.5% vs. 2.7%), panic disorder with agoraphobia (5.2% vs. 1.6%), specific phobia (8.6% vs. 5.0%), and GAD (3.4% vs. 2.0%). Despite the lower risk of having an anxiety disorder among the foreign-born Asians, the risk of developing an anxiety disorder rose with increasing length of time spent in the United States and reached a level similar to U.S.-born Asian Americans after the first 5 years postimmigration. These findings may help explain the significantly higher rates of social phobia seen in the NESARC Asian American sample (Grant, Hasin, Blanco, et al., 2005) than those reported by East Asian epidemiological studies (Cho et al., 2007; Kawakami et al., 2005).

Cultural Factors Relevant to the Assessment, Etiology, and Treatment of Anxiety Disorders in Asians

At present, the ways in which anxiety disorders are assessed, conceptualized, and treated have primarily been conceived within Western contexts with minimal consideration of cultural factors. Before discussing *how* our understanding of anxiety disorders may be culturally limited, it is important to identify *what* cultural differences may potentially influence the expression and severity of anxiety symptoms. Thus, the following section offers a brief description of psychological features that are considered important to well-being in Western contexts (e.g., being independent, self-confident, true to oneself) but may be less relevant in East Asian contexts. The cultural contrast in value placed on these features then serves as a foundation for discussing the strengths and weaknesses of Western approaches to assessing, understanding, and treating the anxiety disorders.

Self-Construal

An individual's self-view or self-construal helps shape beliefs about how to act, what to attend to (and potentially fear), and where to focus one's personal and social energies. Western, particularly North American, individuals tend to act and think in ways that are consistent with descriptions of an independent self-construal (Cousins, 1989; Singelis & Brown, 1995). An independent self-construal is characterized by the belief that each individual is defined by a unique cluster of traits, abilities, and preferences (Kanagawa, Cross, & Markus, 2001; Markus & Kitayama, 1991). Questions like What do I think? What do I value? and What am I feeling? help foster a sense of self-efficacy, self-awareness, and self-confidence, which are synonymous with social maturity and success.

East Asians tend to endorse the goals of group harmony or peaceful relations that are characteristic of an interdependent self-construal and collectivistic orientation (Hofstede, 1980, Markus & Kitayama, 1991). Embedded within a larger whole, interdependent individuals define the self by their relationships with significant others and predefined obligations and roles (Markus & Kitayama, 1991). Personal attributes and abilities are viewed as context specific, and behavior is shaped and regulated by expectations of an assumed role and the demands of others in a given situation (Cross & Madson, 1997; Cross, Morris, & Gore, 2002; Markus & Kitayama, 1991). In essence, questions like What is expected of me? How can I help the situation? and What does the other person need? help achieve the goal of group harmony, which, in turn, promotes personal social success and well-being (for review see Markus & Kitayama, 1991).

How individuals protect themselves from social alienation and distress is, in part, dependent on which social values are culturally promoted and how well they internalize the appropriate cultural norms. Relevant to the development of anxiety, East Asians tend to differ from Westerners in the degree to which they emphasize (or deemphasize) the importance of self-criticism, self-consistency, and saving face (Heine et al., 1999; Kitayama et al., 1997; Suh, 2002). Each of these differences are discussed in turn.

Self-Criticism

Having a positive self-image and high self-esteem are often considered critical to good mental health. Given the emphasis on autonomy, strategies to promote one's positive traits and unique abilities are likely effective in Western contexts. Consistent with this, numerous studies have shown that Western individuals hold cognitive biases and use self-enhancement strategies to help sustain a positive self-image (for review see Banaji & Prentice, 1994). Individuals are inclined to attribute personal successes to enduring personal traits (Gilbert & Malone, 1995), describe themselves as more unique (Taylor & Brown, 1988), and more likely to experience positive future life events than their peers (E. Chang, Asakawa, & Sanna, 2001; Heine & Lehman, 1995; Oishi, Wyer, & Colcombe, 2000). The wealth of evidence indicating such self-serving biases has established self-enhancement as a well-known Western phenomenon.

Within collectivistic contexts, however, self-enhancement strategies are likely less effective and having high self-esteem less important to well-being. Individuals are encouraged to preserve the group's integrity and place greater attention on the group's needs and esteem rather than their own. Emerging evidence suggests East Asians may use self-criticism, rather than self-enhancement, to facilitate psychological well-being and positive social feedback (Heine, 2003; Heine, Kitayama, & Lehman, 2001; Kitayama et al., 1997). Current interpretations of the data view self-criticism as part of a process that allows individuals to fit in socially with others and achieve the desired group harmony.

The following analogy helps illustrate the proposed functional role of self-criticism. Car owners routinely service their vehicles to check for potential problems and replace parts (e.g., oil change, tire rotations). It is to the owner's (and arguably the car's) advantage to pay for regular maintenance checks to prevent a more costly breakdown of the entire vehicle. In a similar way, East Asians may view personal traits and behaviors as contributing to the overall functioning of a group and find being aware of and changing potential negative self-characteristics is less costly than the loss of the entire group's integrity and esteem.

The suggested functionality of self-criticism in East Asian contexts starkly contradicts Western conceptions of self-criticism as a vulnerability factor for distress and the development of psychological disorders (Beck, 1983; Enns & Cox, 1997; Nietzel & Harris, 1990; Pyszczynski & Greenberg, 1986). Although self-criticism is typically associated with depression, studies suggest self-criticism may also be a pronounced feature among individuals suffering from anxiety (Cox et al., 2000; Cox, Fleet, & Stein, 2004). The relationship between anxiety and self-criticism appears to be particularly salient among those with social phobia.

Identity Consistency

Messages like "be yourself" and "do not change who you are" pervade Western contexts and suggest the importance of self-consistency to well-being. Several lines of research support the psychological benefit of promoting an integrated, stable set of personality traits and features (Allport, 1937; Deci & Ryan, 1991; Donahue et al., 1993; Seeman, 1983; Sheldon & Kasser, 1995) and the distressing effect of viewing oneself as inconsistent across social roles (Donahue et al., 1993; Roberts & Donahue, 1994; Hong & Woody, 2007). Moreover, individuals who view themselves as less autonomous are more likely to view themselves as inconsistent across different interpersonal situations (Koestner, Bernieri, & Zuckerman, 1992; Hong & Woody, 2007). Taken together, "being yourself" promotes a sense of personal integrity and the individualistic goal of following a coherent, internal set of beliefs, values, and goals.

East Asians tend to place value on the context-specific demands of a situation in determining behavior (Fiske, Kitayama, & Markus, 1998; Markus & Kitayama, 1991; Triandis, 1995). Unlike their Western counterparts, East Asians are more likely to attribute external causes to social events (Morris & Peng, 1994), place greater emphasis on situation-related factors in viewing others' behavior (Norenzayan, Choi, & Nisbett, 1999), and describe the self in more context-specific ways (Cousins, 1989; Kanagawa et al., 2001). To the extent that East Asians are more likely to explain or guide behavior based on situational demands, promoting a consistent self-view (i.e., "being yourself") would be less valued.

Using the Identity Consistency Index (ICI; Suh, 2002), data comparing Korean and Euro-(North) American samples indicate marked cultural differences in the endorsement of identity consistency (Hong & Woody, 2007; Suh, 2002) and in the relationship between identity consistency and well-being (Suh, 2002). The ICI asks respondents to rate the degree to which different personality traits (e.g., honest, cheerful, calculative, two-faced) describes them across a variety of interpersonal situations (e.g., with a close friend, with a parent, with a stranger). In both studies, Korean participants described themselves more inconsistently across situations than their Western counterparts. Moreover, Suh (2002) found that, for the U.S. sample, individuals who view themselves as more consistent across situations report more positive affect and less negative affect, whereas, for the Korean sample, consistency ratings are unrelated to positive or negative affect.

Face-Saving

The concept of "face" or "saving face" features prominently in East Asian cultures (H.-C. Chang & Holt, 1994; Ting-Toomey & Kurogi, 1998; Ting-Toomey et al., 1991). "Face" can be defined as an individual's perceived view of a favorable self-image within a relational context or network (Ting-Toomey, 1988). Within East Asian cultures, the goal of group harmony is promoted by active attempts to support the face of the group members and prevent the loss of personal face. Cross-cultural differences in the utilization of and preference for specific conversation and conflict resolution strategies appear to reflect the guiding principles of facework that are distinct to East Asian cultures (Gudykunst, 1987; Gudykunst et al., 1996; M.-S. Kim, 1994; M.-S. Kim & Kim, 1997; Oetzel, 1998; Leung, 1987; Peng & Nisbett, 1999). East Asians tend to adopt avoidant and cooperative conversational strategies, which include remaining silent to hide disagreement with others and conceding to the goals of the group over their own; such strategies have been described as prototypical of "face-honoring" moves (Oetzel, 1998a, 1998b; Ting-Toomey et al., 1991).

The benefits of face-honoring moves in East Asian contexts contradict their role in Western contexts, where social approval stems, in part, from showing self-confidence and disclosing personal strengths and traits to others. Consistent with an emphasis on one's individuality and unique identity, patients with social phobia tend to believe that the unmasking of negative self-characteristics will lead to social disapproval. Indeed, compared to their nonanxious counterparts, Western socially anxious individuals show reduced ability to self-disclose (Alden & Bieling, 1998; Walters & Hope, 1998); this lack of self-disclosure, presumably used to protect the self from disapproval, tends to elicit more negative interpersonal reactions and produce the very outcome socially anxious individuals are often trying to avoid (Alden & Bieling, 1998). Thus, the very strategies and behaviors that appear to be unfavorable to Westerners may be socially advantageous to East Asians.

In sum, East Asians, when compared to their Western counterparts, tend to view the self as more interdependent, and place greater value on noticing personal weaknesses in order to improve the self (i.e., self-criticism), adjust their identities and behaviors according to the demands of the situation (i.e., identity flexibility), and focus on communicating and acting in ways that preserve relationships with and face of all other persons involved (i.e., face-saving). Given these differences, the following section describes ways existing Western-based assessment strategies may be less appropriate for Asian populations.

Difficulties in Using Current Nosology and Assessment Measures for Identifying Anxiety Disorders in Asians

Although most epidemiological studies utilize interview-based or clinician-administered measures to assess the presence of different disorders, the majority of anxiety disorder assessment tools that are used in clinical settings are self-report measures that have been developed in the United States and other Western contexts. Self-report measures may be culturally limited in at least two ways: (1) Likert-type rating scales may be better suited for individuals holding a more independent self-view; and (2) the ways in which constructs are operationalized into measure items may be culturally biased.

Likert-Type Rating Scales

Many self-report questionnaires use Likert-type rating scales that ask respondents to rate the degree to which they agree with each provided statement or the extent to which each statement is true (of them). Inherent to this format is the assumption that individuals hold a core, stable set of beliefs or values that rises above situation-specific demands and expectations. The trait-like structure of self-report questionnaires conforms to the Western tendency to describe the self using inner psychological attributes and traits (Cousins, 1989; Kanagawa et al., 2001; Rhee, Uleman, Lee, & Roman, 1995) but may be ill-suited to reported East Asian preferences to describe themselves using situation-specific actions and behaviors (Cousins, 1989; Kanagawa et al., 2001). For example, in a study using the Twenty Statement Test, Japanese participants tended to respond to the question Who are you? by listing behaviors or actions (e.g., "I laugh a lot during conversations"), whereas American participants responded by listing context-free, internalized traits (e.g., "I am friendly") (Kanagawa, Cross, & Markus, 2001).

Concerns about the limitations of Likert-type self-report measures have been particularly pronounced in discussions of how best to assess Eastern beliefs about the contextual sensitivity and flexibility of one's identity, beliefs, and behaviors (Kanagawa et al., 2001; Markus & Kitayama, 1998). Consider, for example, measures of self-construal. These measures are designed to assess the degree to which an individual endorses either an independent or interdependent self-construal. At face value, the contextual sensitivity of an interdependent self-construal appears to be captured by asking how much an individual identifies with different interdependent values. The essence of all interdependent values is that one's identity and behaviors are highly situation-specific, which makes the imposition of trait-like statements on these measures difficult to answer. As an example, the Singelis (1994) Interdependent Self-construal scale item *I will stay in a group if it needs me, even when I am not happy with the group* theoretically presents as a difficult question for the interdependent individual. Endorsement of the item (i.e., strongly agree) would suggest the individual will behave in this manner irrespective of contextual concerns, whereas low endorsement would suggest the individual places little value on maintaining group harmony.

Findings from Levine et al.'s (2003) meta-analysis of self-construal measures further indicate that Likert-type self-report measures may appeal more to Western-based views of the self. To the extent that self-construal measures present both independent and interdependent items in a trait-like manner and Westerners view the self as a stable set of traits and attributes, the authors hypothesized that Westerners would endorse self-construal items in more consistent ways than East Asians. Across all studies reviewed by Levine et al., the Western samples' degree of identification with the two self-construal types differed in the expected directions; Westerners identified with an independent self-construal more than an interdependent self-construal (mean effect: $r = +.43$). By contrast, the difference between self-construal scores for East Asians varied across studies and was highly inconsistent (mean effect: $r = -.10$); six of nine effects were statistically significant in an unexpected direction and only two effects showed East Asians scoring significantly higher on interdependence than independence.

The difficulties associated with measuring self-construal likely generalize to clinical self-report measures of anxiety. Many of the questions listed on these measures are context-free and ask individuals to make judgments based on how much certain symptoms apply to them "on average." To the extent that East Asians are more context-dependent, it may be that existing self-report questionnaires are less accurate and fail to capture the actual degree to which certain symptoms endorsed are related to an individual's level of distress and impairment.

Operationalization of Constructs

Operationalizing psychological constructs like anxiety sensitivity or emotion suppression into self-report measure items is likely influenced by the cultural contexts in which the measures are developed. Given that current measures of anxiety and related constructs are primarily Western-based, it may be that they are influenced by Western values and interpretations so that they become less relevant to East Asian populations. As an example, the following section describes how development of the Revised Self-Monitoring Scale (RSMS; Wolfe, Lennox, & Cutler, 1986) may have been influenced by Western conceptions of the self-monitoring construct.

Conceptually, high self-monitoring is consistent with the interdependent social values of East Asian cultures. Individuals high in self-monitoring are highly responsive to social and interpersonal cues and regulate their self-presentations according to a desired public presentation or image (Snyder, 1987). Within collectivistic contexts, greater situational flexibility in self-presentation translates into a higher probability of social success. Self-monitoring scales are designed to differentiate individuals who alter their self-presentations according to perceived situational demands from those who do not (Gangestad & Snyder, 2000). Given that self-monitoring appeared to be closely tied to interdependent social goals, Hong (2005) hypothesized that the Koreans in her sample would score higher in self-monitoring than the Euro-Canadians. Contrary to expectation, however, the Euro-Canadian sample reported significantly higher levels of self-monitoring than the Korean sample.

What appear to be embedded within the RSMS are Western conceptions of social success. Consider the following RSMS item: *I have the ability to control the way I come across to people, depending on the impression I wish to give them.* Implicit to the item is that the individual is a sole agent to his social success and that the primary social goal is to achieve personal favor, rather than overall group harmony. While descriptions of high self-monitoring mirror East Asian values of self-flexibility and cross-situational sensitivity, actual measurement of self-monitoring appears to be colored by Western views of social success, which may make the construct less (rather than more) culturally syntonic for Asians.

Existing measures of anxiety also include assumptions of how best to assess anxiety, and these assumptions may be Western-specific. For example, research indicates that East Asians and Asian Americans score higher on Western measures of social anxiety (Okazaki, 1997, 2000, 2002; Okazaki & Kallivayalil, 2002; Okazaki, Liu, Longworth, & Minn, 2002), which directly contradicts epidemiological findings of lower rates of social phobia among Asians. When examining popular Western social anxiety measures, one finds that scores typically reflect the frequency to which individuals report experiencing social anxiety or the degree to which individuals endorse feelings of social anxiety as being characteristic of them in a variety of social situations. For example, the Social Phobia and Anxiety Inventory presents a series of social situations (e.g., "I feel anxious when entering social situations where there is a small group") and asks respondents to rate the frequency (e.g., Never, Infrequently, Sometimes, Frequently, Always) to which they experience anxiety in the presented situations (Turner, Beidel, Dancu, & Stanley, 1989). The measures, however, fail to assess perceptions of symptom severity or degree of functional impairment experienced by the respondent.

Implicit to the design of these questionnaires is the assumption that the frequency to which individuals experience anxiety in social situations invariably translates into their level of social distress or impairment. This assumption appears to be well founded among Westerners (Beidel et al., 1989; Heimberg et al., 1992; Herbert et al., 1991) but may not generalize to East Asian populations. Among Westerners, social anxiety measures serve well to identify individuals with a social phobia diagnosis, predict subjective levels of distress during social tasks (e.g., impromptu speech, role play), and predict avoidance of social situations (Beidel, Turner, Stanley, & Dancu, 1989; Heimberg, Mueller, Holt, Hope, & Liebowitz, 1992; Herbert, Bellack, & Hope, 1991).

It is unclear whether experiencing anxiety at a higher frequency across social situations is as functionally impairing or distressing to East Asians. Given the East Asian emphasis on the contextual demands of a situation, it may be that being characteristically "anxious" within social situations is not only perceived as less distressing but also as potentially advantageous to reading situation-specific social cues. To the extent that contextual sensitivity is important to achieving the East Asian social goal of group harmony, feelings of "anxiety" may be viewed as a level of arousal that is conducive to being alert to situation-specific cues and demands. Following this line of reasoning, among East Asians experiencing "anxiety" or arousal within a social situation may be interpreted less negatively than among Westerners, which may explain the cultural difference in social anxiety ratings.

The following section takes a closer look at how cultural differences in self-construal and social values may lead to different pathways to the development of an anxiety disorder, with particular focus on the role of cultural factors in social phobia.

PERSPECTIVES ON THE CAUSES OF ANXIETY DISORDERS IN ASIANS

Critical Appraisal of Major Etiological Models of Anxiety Disorders

Panic Disorder and Agoraphobia

One trait that has been closely tied to the development of panic disorder and agoraphobic fears is anxiety sensitivity (see Taylor, 1999, for review). Individuals with high anxiety sensitivity tend to interpret anxious bodily sensations (e.g., heart palpitations, dizziness, shortness of breath, depersonalization) as being physically, psychologically, and/or socially dangerous or harmful (Reiss & McNally, 1985). The original Anxiety Sensitivity Index (ASI; Reiss, Peterson, Gursky, & McNally, 1986) and the expanded Anxiety Sensitivity Index-Revised (ASI-R; Taylor & Cox, 1998) assess the degree to which an individual worries about the potential negative consequences of different anxiety sensations and are frequently used as measures of anxiety sensitivity. Using these measures, studies have shown that anxiety sensitivity prospectively predicts the future occurrence of panic attacks (Schmidt, Lerew, & Jackson, 1997, 1999; Schmidt, Zvolensky, & Maner, 2006), can predict the intensity and severity of future panic symptoms (Maller & Reiss, 1992), is associated with the development of panic symptoms independent of negative affect, and is significantly lowered after pharmacological and cognitive-behavioral interventions for panic disorder (Romano, van Beek, Cucchi, Biffi, & Perna, 2004; Simon et al., 2004; Smits, Powers, Cho, & Telch, 2004). Research has also shown that targeting high anxiety sensitivity directly can help reduce the likelihood of developing panic disorder or panic-related symptoms in the future (Gardenswartz & Craske, 2001; Schmidt et al., 2007).

The association between panic disorder and anxiety sensitivity may be less pronounced among Asians. In a factor analytic study of the ASI-R, results from a community sample of Koreans indicated a stronger correlation between anxiety sensitivity and depression than between anxiety sensitivity and anxiety (Lim, Yu, & Kim, 2007). These findings contradict assertions that anxiety sensitivity is more strongly associated with symptoms of anxious arousal than depression (Olatunji & Wolitzky-Taylor, 2009; Olatunji et al., 2009; Otto et al., 1995; S. Taylor, Koch, Woody, & McLean, 1996). In a 4-year longitudinal study of an ethnically diverse sample of U.S. adolescents (n = 2,356), investigators examined (1) whether overall ASI scores differed by ethnicity and (2) whether, for each ethnic group, ASI scores prospectively predicted the likelihood of having a panic attack (Weems, Hayward, Killen, & Taylor, 2002). When comparing overall ASI scores, both the Asian American and Hispanic samples reported significantly higher levels of anxiety sensitivity than the Euro-American sample. Despite the higher levels reported, scores on the ASI measure showed lower predictive utility for the Asian Americans than for the Euro-Americans. That is, Asian Americans scoring high in anxiety sensitivity did not significantly differ from low scorers in their likelihood to experience panic attacks. Moreover, the percentage of high-scoring Asian Americans who later experienced panic symptoms (both unexpected and cued) was significantly lower than that of their high-scoring Euro-American counterparts. Overall the data suggest that the strength and specificity of anxiety sensitivity as a risk factor for panic symptoms may be significantly lower for Asians than for Westerners.

Obsessive-Compulsive Disorder

Much as anxiety sensitivity has been implicated for panic disorder, inflated responsibility has been described as a core cognitive feature of OCD (Rachman, 1998, 2002; Salkovskis et al., 2000). Inflated responsibility (IR) is *the belief that one has power that is pivotal to bring about or prevent subjectively crucial negative outcomes. These outcomes are perceived as essential to prevent. They may be actual, that is, having consequences in the real world, and/or at a moral level* (Salkovskis, 1996). Studies indicate OCD patients report more beliefs related to responsibility than nonanxious and anxious controls (Freeston, Ladouceur, Gagnon, & Thibodeau, 1993; Salkovskis et al., 2000) and that OCD symptoms correlate with an increased sense of responsibility (Salkovskis et al., 2000). To illustrate the role of IR in OCD, imagine an individual has the intrusive thought "I may have left the stove on." Rather than dismissing the thought, he interprets the thought as a sign he has been somehow negligent and is responsible for preventing an impending house fire, so he proceeds to check his stove and sees that it is clearly off. As he walks away, he has the same intrusive thought "I may have left the stove on." He begins to doubt whether he actually turned the stove off, and doubts the memory of checking just a few moments earlier. He is unable to ignore or dismiss the urge to check because the potential consequences are too high and would be his fault. He returns to check the stove, walks away, and then repeats this same pattern another 30 times.

Rachman (2002) further specified the role of IR in OCD as a mechanism for checking compulsions. He also proposed that the act of repeated checking leads to increased doubting of one's memory and actions. Consistent with this, research indicates that increasing an individuals' sense of responsibility to prevent harm leads to increased frequency of checking compulsions among OCD patients (Arntz, Voncken, & Goosen, 2007) and that increased checking due to higher perceptions of responsibility leads to reduced memory vividness, detail, and confidence (Boschen & Vuksanovic, 2007).

Another cognitive factor that has been linked to OCD is perfectionism. Specifically, perfectionism is thought to increase perceptions of personal responsibility for negative events, which then increases checking behaviors as a way to prevent negative events from occurring (Bouchard, Rheaume, & Ladouceur, 1999). Consistent with this, perfectionism has been shown to predict checking behaviors and other OCD symptoms (Coles, Frost, Heimberg, & Rheume, 2003; Julien, O'Connor, Aardema, & Todorov, 2006; Moretz & McKay, 2009), and contribute to a larger overall factor of obsessive beliefs (Taylor, McKay, & Abramowitz, 2005). In addition to correlational data, research with postpartum parents has shown that obsessional beliefs, which include perfectionism and IR, prospectively predicted the severity of OCD symptoms but not general depression or anxiety symptoms (Abramowitz, Khander, Nelson, Deacon, & Rygwall, 2006). These findings suggest perfectionism and IR may play a causal role in the pathogenesis of OCD symptoms.

Studies in Japan also support a relationship between dysfunctional cognitive beliefs (i.e., IR and perfectionism) and OCD symptoms. Suzuki (2005) found, using a sample of Japanese college students, concerns for making mistakes predicted OCD symptom severity. The role of IR and perfectionism in checking behaviors has also been found with Japanese OCD patients (Matsunaga et al., 2001). Patients who were identified as having either primarily checking compulsions or both checking and washing compulsions reported significantly higher fears of making mistakes and doubting of their actions than individuals with primarily washing compulsions.

Cultural differences in levels of perfectionism and IR may exist. Using a sample of college students, R. Chang and Chang (2009) found that, compared to Euro-Americans, Asian Americans reported higher levels of negative perfectionism and lower levels of subjective well-being. Moreover, guilt and shame, which presumably are closely tied to feelings of responsibility, feature prominently in East Asian cultures and are thought to shape behavior in these cultural contexts (Bedford & Hwang, 2003). Despite evidence that Asians may be at higher risk for perfectionism and IR, it is unclear whether these cognitive factors play a similar role in OCD as has been found for Westerners. Indeed, the lower prevalence rates of OCD in East Asian countries suggest other factors may be contributing to the development of the disorder. Further cross-cultural work examining the role of these and other cognitive factors in the development of OCD is needed.

Generalized Anxiety Disorder

Several conceptual models have been forwarded to explain how GAD symptoms may develop and be maintained (for review see Behar, DiMarco, Hekler, Mohlman, & Staples, 2009). Despite the differences among the models, one common focus is on the function of worry as a way to avoid negative internal experiences and emotions. Worry is conceptualized as a maladaptive coping strategy for managing anxiety about the future and uncertain situations, and fosters suppression or avoidance of negative emotions that perpetuates the maintenance of GAD symptoms. In support of this, difficulties with emotion regulation and experiential avoidance have both been associated with GAD symptom severity (Roemer et al., 2009; Roemer, Salters, Raffia, & Orsillo, 2005). Moreover, research indicates that individuals with GAD (1) experience negative emotions (but not positive emotions) more intensely than healthy controls, individuals with social phobia, and individuals with depression; (2) have more difficulty describing and understanding their emotions than healthy undergraduates; and (3) engage in negative emotional coping strategies (e.g., excessive worry, emotional suppression) more frequently than healthy controls (Mennin, Heimberg, Turk, & Fresco, 2005; Mennin, Holaway, Fresco, Moore, & Heimberg, 2007).

It has been contended that East Asian cultures promote individual emotion suppression as a way to promote group harmony and preserve interdependent social goals (Butler, Lee, & Gross, 2007; Markus & Kitayama, 1991; Oyserman, Coon, & Kemmelmeier, 2002). Studies comparing Asian American and Euro-American nonclinical samples have suggested Asian Americans are more likely to suppress emotions on a daily basis and that suppressing negative emotions is *not* associated with feeling stronger negative emotions for Asian Americans, while it is for Euro-Americans (Butler et al., 2007; Gross & John, 2003). These data suggest that avoiding strong negative emotions may be less maladaptive for East Asians and Asian Americans than for their Western counterparts, and that the pathways by which GAD symptoms are maintained may culturally differ.

Post-traumatic Stress Disorder

Although exposure to a traumatic event is necessary for a PTSD diagnosis, only some individuals with a trauma history develop the disorder, while many others do not. One approach to understanding this discrepancy in the development of PTSD is a contemporary learning theory perspective (for review see Mineka & Zinbarg, 2006). According to this perspective, traumatic events that are perceived as uncontrollable and unpredictable are more likely to result in PTSD. This theory underscores the importance of the psychological mindset of the person experiencing the trauma; rather than the amount or severity of the actual trauma, it is the degree to which the person feels a sense of mental defeat during the trauma. Consistent with this, Dunmore and colleagues (2001) found that perceived mental defeat within 4 months of an assault predicted PTSD symptom severity at follow-up assessments 6 and 9 months after the assault. Individuals who have experienced prior traumas are more vulnerable to developing PTSD after a traumatic event (Ozer, Best, Lipsey, & Weiss, 2003), which, conceivably, may be due to a person being sensitized by past traumas to feel a lack of control and ability to resist the traumatic stressor.

There are data to suggest that Cambodian refugees experience two culturally specific types of panic attacks as part of a trauma-related disorder: orthostatically triggered panic attacks and neck-focused panic attacks (Hinton, Chhean, et al., 2005, Hinton, Pollack, et al., 2005). Neck-focused panic is characterized by worries that a neck vessel will rupture and is associated with autonomic arousal such as dizziness, blurry vision, and heart palpitations. Orthostatic panic attacks are associated with a sudden onset of dizziness and other somatic symptoms and fears of fainting, which leads the person to sit down. Hinton and colleagues have developed a culture-specific model of how these somatically focused panic symptoms are maintained; the model highlights both the role of trauma associations and increased anxiety sensitivity. Using this model, Hinton and colleagues have adapted existing cognitive behavioral therapy protocols to treat this unique constellation of symptoms, and have found the treatment to be highly effective (Hinton, Chhean, et al., 2005).

Role of Culture in the Etiology of Anxiety Disorders: An In-depth Look at Social Phobia

Prevalence rates for the anxiety disorders among Asians are markedly lower than those reported by the *DSM-IV-TR* and those found in Western samples (see Table 7.1). Although this appears to suggest Asians are less likely to struggle with anxiety, multiple cross-cultural studies comparing East Asian and Western populations have consistently shown *higher* levels of anxiety, particularly social anxiety, among East Asians (e.g., Norasakkunkit & Kalick, 2002; Okazaki, 1997, 2002; Zane & Yeh, 2002), as well as *higher* scores on factors implicated in the development or maintenance of different anxiety disorders (e.g., anxiety sensitivity, emotion suppression). Why is it that Asians are reporting greater difficulties with anxiety, and yet show lower rates of psychopathology? One explanation, in addition to the measurement difficulties previously discussed, may be that the pathways leading to the development of an anxiety disorder differs cross-culturally and that the factors considered maladaptive in one context may be less so in another.

One anxiety disorder that may be particularly susceptible to cultural influences is social phobia. Social anxiety arises partially as a function of an individual's level of doubt in his or her ability to act appropriately in social situations and to prevent negative social consequences (Schlenker & Leary, 1982). Given that perceptions of appropriate social behavior are shaped by cultural norms, what an individual fears might happen in a social situation and how others judge that person are likely influenced by culture.

Self-Construal and Social Anxiety

Several cross-cultural studies of social anxiety have assessed the relationship between self-construal patterns and social anxiety ratings (Dinnel, Kleinknecht, & Tanaka-Matsumi, 2002; Norasakkunkit & Kalick, 2002; Okazaki, 1997, 2000; Singelis et al., 1999). Overall, findings indicate interdependent self-construal ratings positively predict social anxiety whereas independent self-construal ratings negatively predict social anxiety. Moreover, self-construal appears to be a better predictor of social anxiety ratings than ethnicity alone (Okazaki, 1997, Dinnel et al., 2002).

In Okazaki's (1997) comparison of Asian and White American students, self-construal appeared to be a better predictor of social distress than ethnicity alone. When controlling for the variance associated with the other measures of distress, ethnicity failed to predict differences in depression and fears of negative evaluation. Self-construal, however, significantly predicted differences on both administered measures of social distress. Specifically, those who placed greater value on autonomy and the elaboration of personal characteristics (i.e., independent self-construal) and lower emphasis on maintaining peaceful relations with others (i.e., interdependent self-construal) were less likely to report social avoidance, distress in social situations, and fears of negative social evaluation.

Self-Criticism and Social Anxiety

Self-criticism appears to be uniquely associated with social phobia symptoms, above and beyond low mood difficulties. Cox and colleagues (2004) analyzed data from the National Comorbidity Survey (NCS; Kessler et al., 1994) and found that the relationship between self-criticism and social phobia remained significant after controlling for current emotional distress, neuroticism, and lifetime histories of mood, anxiety, and substance use disorders. Similarly, data comparing outpatients with social phobia, panic disorder, and major depressive disorder (MDD) indicated that self-criticism levels were similar between the MDD and social phobia groups and significantly higher than the panic disorder group, even when statistically controlling for symptoms of depression (Cox et al., 2000). An individual's likelihood of experiencing social distress has also been consistently linked with lower self-esteem ratings, memory biases for negative self-referent information, and self-critical beliefs (Alden & Wallace, 1995; Bouvard et al., 1999; Mansell & Clark, 1999).

Indirect Communication and Social Anxiety

Socially anxious individuals, however, often hold negative views of themselves and are fearful others will discover their perceived negative traits; these beliefs and fears reduce their willingness to disclose personally revealing information. Walters and Hope (1998) compared those diagnosed with social phobia to nonanxious subjects on a variety of social behaviors during an interaction task with a research confederate. The authors found that nonanxious participants faced the confederate more often and provided more information about themselves. In addition, social anxiety correlated positively with submissive behaviors; socially anxious participants were less likely to interrupt the confederate, brag, or give commands.

Lack of self-disclosure, presumably used to protect the self from disapproval, appears to elicit more negative interpersonal reactions and produce the very outcome socially anxious individuals are often trying to avoid. Within Western contexts, (positive) self-disclosure contributes to social success, and is likely related to an individual's level of self-confidence and use of self-enhancement strategies. By contrast, within East Asian contexts, indirect communication is typically promoted and viewed as an effective strategy to achieve face-work-related social goals.

Explaining Cross-Cultural Differences in Social Anxiety

Direct comparisons of social anxiety and cross-cultural research findings highlight a marked overlap between features that characterize socially anxious individuals and those that are promoted by East Asian cultures. Research indicates East Asians, when compared to their Western counterparts, tend to construe the self as less independent and more interdependent, be more self-critical, use more indirect communication strategies, and be more sensitive to (and subsequently shift behavior according to) the perceived wants of others. In parallel fashion, socially anxious Westerners endorse similar self-construal patterns, exhibit self-critical orientations, are less likely to self-disclose than their nonanxious counterparts, and are highly concerned about the opinions of others.

The apparent overlap may help explain why East Asians tend to report higher levels of social anxiety. Given that conceptualizations and descriptions of social anxiety draw primarily from Western cultural frames, (Western) social anxiety measures may not account for the markedly different social goals and strategies endorsed by East Asian cultures. The importance or emphasis placed on the constructs of self-consistency and self-criticism appears to markedly differ between East Asian and Western cultures. Self-flexible and self-critical views feature more prominently in East Asian contexts, which may suggest these constructs are more culturally normative than in Western contexts.

In line with past findings, Hong and Woody (2007) found that the Koreans in their study reported lower independent self-views and endorsed greater identity flexibility than their Euro-Canadian counterparts. Moreover, using data from the same samples, Hong (2005) found that the relationship between having an independent self-view and social anxiety ratings was mediated by East Asian social values (i.e., identity flexibility and self-criticism). To the extent that a less independent self-construal, more self-flexibility, and greater degrees of self-criticism are more culturally normative in East Asian cultures, elevated scores on social anxiety measures may also be more culturally normative. Meaning, East Asian reports of higher social anxiety may then be explained as a reflection of their affiliation with traits and behaviors that are advantageous and normative within East Asian cultures. This would also help explain the lower rates of actual impairment from social anxiety symptoms and social phobia diagnoses found in East Asian contexts.

Implications for Other Anxiety Disorders

The possible role of cultural factors in shaping the development and maintenance of a disorder likely extends beyond social phobia. As previously discussed, research has shown Asians scoring high on traits and behaviors that have been implicated for different anxiety disorders (e.g., anxiety sensitivity, perfectionism, emotion suppression), while having lower prevalence rates of the disorder. It may be that these traits and behaviors hold different meaning within East Asian contexts, and do not predict or contribute to the development of anxiety disorders in the same way they do for Western populations.

TREATING ANXIETY DISORDERS IN ASIANS

In this section, the effectiveness of pharmacotherapy and cognitive behavioral therapy (CBT) for the anxiety disorders is reviewed, and, when possible, the effectiveness of these treatments with Asians is discussed. The section concludes with potential strategies to address cultural factors in treatment (without reifying stereotypes) and a case example to highlight the strategies mentioned.

Pharmacotherapy

In general, the most commonly prescribed medications for the anxiety disorders are either benzodiazepines or antidepressants (for review see Dougherty, Rauch, & Jenike, 2002; Roy-Byrne & Cowley, 2002; Yehuda, Marshall, Penkower, & Wong, 2002). Due to risk of dependence and difficulties with withdrawal when discontinuing, benzodiazepines have been replaced by selective serotonergic reuptake inhibitors (SSRIs) and other similarly acting agents as first-line pharmacological treatments for the anxiety disorders. Long-term outcome studies indicate these medications are, overall, superior to placebo in relapse rates after treatment discontinuation (Thuile, Even, & Rouillon, 2008). Despite the improved efficacy over placebo, relapse rates tend to be high, particular for those disorders with a more chronic course (Thuile et al., 2008).

In a 3-year prospective study of benzodiazepine use in Taiwan, Fang and colleagues (2009) followed 187,413 individuals registered in the National Health Insurance Research Database. The investigators found that the prevalence of benzodiazepine use was approximately 2%, and that only 10–15% of those using benzodiazepines were longer-term users; the authors note that the rates reported are lower than those found in other studies. Results also indicated that, contrary to expectation, males were more likely to become long-term benzodiazepine users after receiving a prescription. Among those identified as long-term users, 62% had been diagnosed with a mental disorder, whereas only 20% of non-long-term users had a diagnosable mental disorder.

Kamijima and colleagues (2004) examined the efficacy of paroxetine, an SSRI agent, for OCD patients in Japan. Patients participated in a randomized, double-blind, placebo-controlled trial of the medication for a 12-week period. The results indicated that paroxetine was superior to placebo in reducing OCD symptoms. By the study's end, 50% of patients who received paroxetine were rated as "very much improved" or "much improved" versus 23% of those in the placebo condition.

Treatment response rates are similar to those reported by other studies on SSRIs for OCD (see Dougherty, Rauch, & Jenike, 2002).

Although the data suggest similar response rates to pharmacotherapy, Asians may differ in their willingness to seek such treatments. In a large, multisite U.S. study of primary care–setting patients, patients who endorsed having had a recent panic attack were asked how willing they would be to take medications for their panic symptoms (Hazlett-Stevens et al., 2002). When compared to their Euro-American counterparts, Asian American patients reported significantly lower willingness to consider medication for their symptoms.

Cognitive Behavioral Therapy

Over the years, cognitive behavioral therapy (CBT) has become one of the most studied and recommended therapies for the anxiety disorders (Butler, Chapman, Forman, & Beck, 2006; Hofmann & Smits, 2008). Although the details vary for the different disorders, the core strategies and principles presented to anxiety disorder patients are similar. Typically, anxiety disorder CBT protocols include a disorder-specific model of how symptoms are maintained, relaxation strategies to manage general anxious arousal, behavioral exposures (or experiments) targeting feared triggers and maladaptive coping strategies, and cognitive restructuring interventions targeting maladaptive beliefs. CBT sessions tend to be highly structured with a focus on teaching strategies to target presenting problems, and encourage collaboration between therapist and patient when developing a plan for how to practice skills learned in and outside of session.

In a review of meta-analyses examining the efficacy of CBT for different disorders, Butler and colleagues (2006) found that, for the anxiety disorders, CBT held strong effect sizes that were comparable to (if not superior to) pharmacotherapies. Follow-up data suggest that patients are more likely to maintain treatment gains after CBT ends than those who discontinue their medications. Hofmann and Smits (2008) conducted a meta-analysis of all randomized placebo-controlled trials examining the efficacy of CBT for anxiety disorders in adults, and found similarly encouraging results. CBT consistently was superior to placebo and had treatment outcome effect sizes in the medium to large range. Among all the anxiety disorders, CBT was shown to be most effective in reducing symptom severity for OCD. The meta-analysis did not indicate number of sessions or placebo modality (i.e., psychological vs. pill placebo) as significant moderators of the effects.

Although there are data supporting the efficacy of CBT for Asians (for review see Voss Horrell, 2008), the lack of consideration of cultural factors in CBT protocols may make them less optimal for individuals endorsing values and beliefs typically promoted by East Asian cultures. For example, in CBT, social phobia patients are typically encouraged to reduce the importance of others' evaluations and taught cognitive restructuring skills that suggest people typically pay little attention to others' behavior and that the predicted social consequences are exaggerated. Indeed, many of my past social phobia patients have told me that one of the most important lessons learned was "I'm not that important. People are not paying attention to me as much as I think they are." By learning that they are "not that important" my patients felt liberated from concerns of others' reactions and felt able to act according to their wants and values. While this lesson may be appropriate in Western cultural contexts, it may be less appropriate in East Asian ones. To the extent that interpersonal harmony is an important social goal and that individuals work to adapt their behavior to achieve that goal, others *do* notice individual behavior and individuals *are* that important. In East Asian contexts, rather than reduce the importance of others, it may be more helpful to focus on how being overly concerned with personal mistakes can actually prevent the achievement of group harmony.

Recommendations

Despite the potential limitations of Western-based assessment tools and CBT in addressing cultural factors, it is likely premature to abandon their use with Asian populations. Moreover, it is likely more unhelpful to immediately assume all Asians seeking treatment uphold East Asian beliefs and values, than it is to apply Western-based interventions with established treatment efficacy. Doing so may act to reify stereotypes and neglects the subtleties of each individual's presenting problems. Thus, the following strategies are recommended when approaching Asian patients in treatment. First, when using clinical assessment tools, review the scores with your patient and discuss whether the person agrees with the elevations and how impairing the elevations are to him/her. Note potential culturally based differences to help develop appropriate interventions. Second, when identifying problem behaviors or maladaptive coping strategies, work with the patient to understand the function of the behaviors and consider alternate, healthier coping strategies that are consistent with the person's cultural framework. Finally, develop treatment goals collaboratively with your patient and adapt interventions to meet the specified goals. The following case example highlights these recommendations.

CASE EXAMPLE

Joyce is a 23-year-old Korean American who is pursuing a master's degree in Fine Arts at a top Bay Area university. During her senior year in university, she began struggling with "really bad heart palpitations," which led her to be hospitalized and later diagnosed with panic disorder with agoraphobia.

Although Joyce initially sought treatment to help manage her panic symptoms, further assessment of her problems indicated that she also struggled with making decisions and reassurance-seeking/checking behaviors. For example, Joyce spoke to her parents or older sister by telephone "at least 4 or 5 times a day." During these calls, Joyce's family would check to make sure she had taken her medication, not experienced another panic attack, and/or completed all her school assignments. Joyce, in turn, would ask for help with decisions that ranged from which bus to take to the grocery store, to what time she should go to bed, to how to approach her professor about setting up a meeting. Joyce showed similar tendencies in her therapy sessions. She would rarely finish a sentence without saying "Do you think that makes sense?" or "Does that sound weird?" or "What do other people usually say?" Joyce also spent hours reviewing and rereviewing her homework, e-mails, and notes to make sure she "got it just right."

Diagnostically, Joyce's repeated seeking of reassurance and difficulties with indecisiveness could be viewed as symptoms of obsessive-compulsive disorder. These problems appeared to be exacerbated by her family's need to check in with her, which furthered her dependency on them. Moreover, the family's continual checking of Joyce's symptom status appeared to increase her sensitivity to and fear of somatic changes and, thus, increasing her vulnerability for future panic attacks. From a cognitive behavioral perspective, the goals of treatment were relatively clear: the patient needed to decrease sensitivity to somatic changes, learn how to assert personal boundaries (particularly with her family), reduce or eliminate reassurance-seeking behaviors, and increase tolerance of the uncertainty that comes with making decisions independently.

From an East Asian framework, however, such treatment goals could undermine the culturally valued goals of interdependence (particularly among family members) and group harmony. Moreover, Joyce was *not* seeking treatment for indecisiveness and likely would have viewed individuation from her family as irrelevant to her goal of reducing the frequency of her panic attacks. To promote such individuation would likely have reduced her willingness to stay (and her family's willingness to have her stay) in treatment.

Joyce's initial phase of treatment focused on explicitly targeting her panic disorder and agoraphobia symptoms. As treatment progressed and Joyce developed a stronger understanding of how certain behaviors (e.g., avoidance, checking for changes in bodily sensations) could exacerbate her fears, she began to question whether her interactions with her family were somehow contributing to her anxiety ("Do you think there's something wrong with always asking my family for advice?"). To help answer her questions, Joyce completed measures of OCD symptoms and beliefs. We reviewed the marked elevations on these measures and discussed the function of her compulsive reassurance-seeking and checking behaviors.

Through these discussions, Joyce identified two different reasons for her reassurance-seeking. The first reason fit with Western conceptualizations of OCD symptom maintenance: Joyce sought reassurance to reduce her discomfort and diffuse a sense of responsibility to prevent negative outcomes. This behavior, in turn, increased her sensitivity to triggering situations and her tendency to seek reassurance to relieve her discomfort. An example of this type of reassurance-seeking was asking her parents whether or not she should bring an umbrella with her to class.

The second reason had a more cultural explanation. Joyce valued the close ties she held with her family and felt that seeking their advice and opinions positioned her to make decisions that benefited not only her but also her family. For example, Joyce would frequently ask her parents how she should approach different social situations and did so because, to Joyce, being socially successful would show she had been raised well and would not cause a loss of face for her family. Joyce also insisted that seeking reassurance strengthened relations with her family; from asking her sister which makeup to buy, to asking her mother to stay on the phone with her and help her decide what to make for breakfast, to asking her father to check all her financial records to make sure she balanced her checkbook appropriately.

Using the distinction made in session, the second phase of treatment focused on increasing Joyce's ability to identify urges to seek reassurance because of anxiety and practice resisting these urges. For reassurance-seeking behaviors driven by the goals of interdependence and strengthening family ties, treatment focused on helping her elaborate on these values and developing ways to supplement existing behaviors to achieve these goals. For example, Joyce began calling her mother every Saturday morning and, rather than seeking advice or reassurance, she would spend the time talking about a television program that she and her mother both watch on Friday evenings.

At the end of treatment, Joyce no longer met criteria for panic disorder with agoraphobia, showed increased ability to make decisions without seeking reassurance, and reported stronger, deeper relationships with her parents and sister.

This case example highlights how following standard Western protocol may have reduced the effectiveness of treatment. Western therapy models carry the implicit assumption that all individuals hold values that are consistent with an individualistic cultural orientation and formulate a treatment plan based on this assumption. In the case of Joyce, these models recommend that treatment focus on explicating what Joyce wanted from her life, independent of what her family wanted from her, and working toward life goals that did not depend on her family to achieve them. What appeared to be effective for Joyce, however, was identifying and cultivating her collectivistic values and developing life goals that were necessarily interwoven with her family.

REFERENCES

Abramowitz, J. S., Khandker, M., Nelson, C. A., Deacon, B. J., & Rygwall, R. (2006). The role of cognitive factors in the pathogenesis of obsessive-compulsive symptoms: A prospective study. *Behaviour Research and Therapy, 44*, 1361–1374.

Alden, L. E., & Bieling, P. (1998). Interpersonal consequences of the pursuit of safety. *Behaviour Research and Therapy, 36*, 53–64.

Alden, L. E., & Wallace, S. T. (1995). Social phobia and social appraisal in successful and unsuccessful social interactions. *Behaviour Research and Therapy, 33*, 497–505.

Allport, F. (1937). *Personality: A psychological interpretation.* New York: Holt.

American Psychiatric Association. (2000). *Diagnostic and statistical manual of mental disorders* (Revised 4th ed.). Washington, DC: Author.

Arntz, A., Voncken, M., & Goosen, A. C. A. (2007). Responsibility and obsessive-compulsive disorder: An experimental test. *Behaviour Research and Therapy, 45*(3), 425–435.

Ball, S. G., Baer, L., & Otto M. W. (1996). Symptoms subtypes of obsessive-compulsive disorder in behavioral treatment studies: A quantitative review. *Behaviour Research and Therapy, 34*, 47–51.

Banaji, M. R., & Prentice, D. A. (1994). The self in social contexts. *Annual Review of Psychology, 45*, 297–332.

Beals, J., Manson, S. M., Shore, J. H., Friedman, M., Ashcraft, M., Fairbank, J. A., et al. (2002). The prevalence of posttraumatic stress disorder among American Indian Vietnam veterans: Disparities and context. *Journal of Traumatic Stress, 15*(2), 89–97.

Beck, A. T. (1983). Cognitive therapy of depression: New perspectives. In P. J. Clayton & J. E. Barnett (Eds.), *Treatment of depression: Old controversies and new approaches* (pp. 265–290). New York: Raven Press.

Bedford, O., & Hwang, K.-K. (2003). Guilt and shame in Chinese culture: A cross-cultural framework from the perspective of morality and identity. *Journal for the Theory of Social Behaviour, 33*, 127–144.

Behar, E., DiMarco, I. D., Hekler, E. B., Mohlman, J., & Staples, A. M. (2009). Current theoretical models of generalized anxiety disorder (GAD): Conceptual review and treatment implications. *Journal of Anxiety Disorders, 23*, 1011–1023.

Beidel, D. C., Turner, S. M., Stanley, M. A., & Dancu, C. V. (1989). The Social Phobia and Anxiety Inventory: Concurrent and external validity. *Behavior Therapy, 20*, 417–427.

Boschen, M. J., & Vuksanovic, D. (2007). Deteriorating memory confidence, responsibility perceptions, and repeated checking: Comparisons in OCD and control samples. *Behaviour Research and Therapy, 5*(9), 2098–2109.

Bouchard, C., Rheaume, J., & Ladouceur, R. (1999). Responsibility and perfectionism in OCD: An experimental study. *Behaviour Research and Therapy, 37*, 239–248.

Bouvard, M., Guerin, J., Rion, A. C., Bouchard, C., Ducottet, E., Sechaud, M., et al. (1999). Psychometric study of the social self-esteem inventory of Lawson et al. (1979). *European Review of Applied Psychology, 49*, 165–172.

Breslau, J., Borges, G., Hagar, Y., Tancredi, D., & Gilman, S. (2009). Immigration to the USA and risk for mood and anxiety disorders: Variation by origin and age at immigration. *Psychological Medicine, 39*, 1117–1127.

Breslau, J., & Chang, D. F. (2006). Psychiatric disorders among foreign-born and US-born Asian-Americans in a US national survey. *Social Psychiatry and Psychiatric Epidemiology, 41*, 943–950.

Breslau, N., Kessler R. C., Chilcoat, H. D., Schultz, L. R., Davis, G. C., & Andreski, P. (1998). Trauma and post-traumatic stress disorder in the community. *Archives of General Psychiatry, 55*, 626–632.

Brown, T. A., Marten, P. A., & Barlow, D. H. (1995). Discriminant validity of the symptoms constituting the DSM-III-R and DSM-IV associated symptom criterion of generalized anxiety disorder. *Journal of Anxiety Disorders, 9*, 317–328.

Brunello, N., Davidson, J. R. T., Deahl, M., Kessler, R. C., Mendlewicz, J., Racagni, G., et al. (2001). Posttraumatic stress disorder: diagnosis and epidemiology, comorbidity and social consequences, biology and treatment. *Neuropsychobiology, 43*, 150–162.

Butler, A. C., Chapman, J. E., Forman, E. M., & Beck, A. T. (2006). The empirical status of cognitive-behavioral therapy: A review of meta-analyses. *Clinical Psychology Review, 26*, 17–31.

Butler, E. A., Lee, T. L., & Gross, J. J. (2007). Emotion regulation and culture: Are the social consequences of emotion suppression culture-specific? *Emotion, 7*, 30–48.

Castle, D. J., Deale, A., & Marks, I. M. (1995). Gender differences in obsessive compulsive disorder. *Australian and New Zealand Journal of Psychiatry, 29*, 114–117.

Chang, E. C., Asakawa, K., & Sanna, L. J. (2001). Cultural variations in optimistic and pessimistic bias: Do Easterners really expect the worst and Westerners really expect the best when predicting future life events? *Journal of Personality and Social Psychology, 81*, 476–491.

Chang, H.-C., & Holt, G. R. (1994). A Chinese perspective on face as inter-relational concern. In S. Ting-Toomey (Ed.), *The challenge of facework*: Cross-cultural and interpersonal issues (pp. 95–132). Albany: State University of New York Press.

Chang, R., & Chang, E. C. (2009). Effects of socially prescribed expectations on emotions and cognitions in Asian and European Americans. *Cognitive Therapy and Research, 33*, 272–282.

Cho, M. J., Kim, J.-K., Jeon, H. J., Suh, T., Chung, I.-W., Hong, J. P., et al. (2007). Lifetime and 12-month prevalence of DSM-IV psychiatric disorders among Korean adults. *Journal of Nervous and Mental Disease, 195*, 203–210.

Choy, Y., Schneier, F. R., Heimberg, R. G., Oh, K., & Liebowitz, M. R. (2008). Features of the offensive subtype of Taijin-Kyofu-Sho in US and Korean patients with DSM-IV social anxiety disorder. *Depression and Anxiety, 25*, 230–240.

Clark, D. M., & Wells, A. (1995). A cognitive model of social phobia. In R. G. Heimberg, M. Liebowitz, D. A. Hope, & F. Schneier (Eds.), *Social phobia*: Diagnosis, assessment and treatment (pp. 69–93). New York: Guilford.

Coles, M. E., Frost, R. O., Heimberg, R. G., & Rheume, J. (2003). "Not just right experiences": Perfectionism, obsessive–compulsive features and general psychopathology. *Behaviour Research and Therapy, 41*, 681–700.

Cousins, S. D. (1989). Culture and self-perception in Japan and the United States. *Journal of Personality and Social Psychology, 56*, 124–131.

Cox, B. J., Fleet, C., & Stein, M. B. (2004). Self-criticism and social phobia in the US national comorbidity survey. *Journal of Affective Disorders, 82*, 227–234.

Cox, B. J., Rector, N. A., Bagby, R. M., Swinson, R. P., Levitt, A. J., & Joffe, R. T. (2000). Is self-criticism unique for depression? A comparison with social phobia. *Journal of Affective Disorders, 57*, 223–228.

Crino, R., Slade, T., & Andrews, G. (2005). The changing prevalence and severity of obsessive-compulsive disorder criteria from DSM-III to DSM-IV. *American Journal of Psychiatry, 162*, 876–882.

Cross, S. E., & Madson, L. (1997). Models of the self: Self-construals and gender. *Psychological Bulletin, 122*, 5–37.

Cross, S. E., Morris, M. L., & Gore, J. S. (2002). Thinking about oneself and others: The relational-interdependent self-construal and social cognition. *Journal of Personality and Social Psychology, 82*, 399–418.

Deci, E. L., & Ryan, R. M. (1991). A motivational approach to self: Integration in personality. In R. Dienstbier (Ed.), *Nebraska Symposium on Motivation*: Vol. 38. Perspectives in Motivation (pp. 237–288). Lincoln: University of Nebraska Press.

Dinnel, D. L., Kleinknecht, R. A., & Tanaka-Matsumi, J. (2002). A cross-cultural comparison of social phobia symptoms. *Journal of Psychopathology and Behavioral Assessment, 24,* 75–84.

Donahue, E. M., Robins, R. W., Roberts, B. W., & John, O. P. (1993). The divided self: Concurrent and longitudinal effects of psychological adjustment and social roles on self-concept differentiation. *Journal of Personality and Social Psychology, 64,* 834–846.

Dougherty, D. D., Rauch, S. L., & Jenike, M. A. (2002). Pharmacological treatments for obsessive compulsive disorder. In P. E. Nathan & J. M. Gorman (Eds.), *A guide to treatments that work* (2nd ed., pp. 387–410). New York: Oxford University Press.

Dunmore, E., Clark, D. M., & Ehlers, A. (2001). A prospective investigation of the role of cognitive factors in persistent posttraumatic stress disorder (PTSD) after physical or sexual assault. *Behaviour Research and Therapy, 39,* 1063–1084.

Enns, M. W., & Cox, B. J. (1997). Personality dimensions and depression: Review and commentary. *Canadian Journal of Psychiatry, 42,* 274–284.

Fang, S.-Y., Chen, C.-Y., Chang, I.-S., Wu, E. C.-H., Chang, C.-M., & Lin, K.-M. (2009). Predictors of the incidence and discontinuation of long-term use of benzodiazepines: A population-based study. *Drug and Alcohol Dependence, 104,* 140–146.

Fazel, M., Wheeler, J., & Danesh, J. (2005). Prevalence of serious mental disorder in 7000 refugees resettled in western countries: a systematic review. *Lancet, 365,* 1309–1314.

Fiske, A. P., Kitayama, S., & Markus, H. R. (1998). The cultural matrix of social psychology. In Gilbert, D. T., & Fiske, S. T. (Eds.), *Handbook of social psychology* (4th ed., Vol. 2, pp. 915–981). New York: McGraw-Hill.

Fornaro, M., Gabrielli, F., Albano, C., Fornaro, S., Rizzato, S., Mattei, et al. (2009). Obsessive-compulsive disorder and related disorders: A comprehensive survey. *Annals of General Psychiatry, 8,* 1–13.

Freeston, M. H., Ladouceur, R., Gagnon, F., & Thibodeau, N. (1993). Beliefs about obsessional thoughts. *Journal of Psychopathology and Behavioral Assessment, 15*(1), 1–21.

Friedman, M. J., Schnurr, P. P., Sengupta, A. S., Holmes, T., & Ashcraft, M. (2004). The Hawaii Vietnam Veterans Project: Is minority status a risk factor for posttraumatic stress disorder? *Journal of Nervous and Mental Disease, 192,* 42–50.

Gangestad, S. W., & Snyder, M. (2000). Self-monitoring: Appraisal and reappraisal. *Psychological Bulletin, 126,* 530–555.

Gardenswartz, C. A., & Craske, M. G. (2001). Prevention of panic disorder. *Behavior Therapy, 32,* 725–737.

Gilbert, D. T., & Malone, P. S. (1995). The correspondence bias. *Psychological Bulletin, 117,* 21–38.

Grant, B. F., Hasin, D. S., Blanco, C., Stinson, F. S., Chou, S. P., Goldstein, R. B., et al. (2005). The epidemiology of social anxiety disorder in the United States: Results from the National Epidemiologic Survey on alcohol and related conditions. *Journal of Clinical Psychiatry, 66,* 1351–1361.

Grant, B. F., Hasin, D. S., Stinson, F. S., Dawson, D. A., Goldstein, R. B., Smith, S., et al. (2006). The epidemiology of DSM-IV panic disorder and agoraphobia in the United States: Results from the National Epidemiologic Survey on alcohol and related conditions. *Journal of Clinical Psychiatry, 67,* 363–374.

Grant, B. F., Hasin, D. S., Stinson, F. S., Dawson, D. A., Ruan, W. J., Goldstein, R. B., et al. (2005). Prevalence, correlates, co-morbidity, and comparative disability of DSM-IV generalized anxiety disorder in the USA: results from the National Epidemiologic Survey on alcohol and related conditions. *Psychological Medicine, 35,* 1747–1759.

Grant, B. F., Stinson, F. S., Dawson, D. A., Chou, S. P., Dufour, M. C., Compton, W., et al. (2004). Prevalence and co-occurrence of substance use disorders and independent mood and anxiety disorders: Results from the National Epidemiologic Survey on Alcohol and Related Conditions. *Archives of General Psychiatry, 61,* 807–816.

Gross, J. J., & John, O. P. (2003). Individual differences in two emotion regulation processes: Implications for affect, relationships, and well-being. *Journal of Personality and Social Psychology, 85,* 348–362.

Gudykunst, W. B. (1987). Cross-cultural comparisons. In C. R. Berger & S. Chaffee (Eds.), *Handbook of communication science* (pp. 846–889). Thousand Oaks, CA: Sage.

Gudykunst, W. B., Matsumoto, Y., Ting-Toomey, S., Nishida, T., Kim, K., & Heyman, S. (1996). The influence of cultural individualism-collectivism on perceptions of communication in ingroup and outgroup relationships. *Communication Monographs, 54,* 295–306.

Hazlett-Stevens, H., Craske, M. G., Roy-Byrne, P. P., Sherbourne, C. D., Stein, M. B., & Bystritsky, A. (2002). Predictors of willingness to consider medication and psychosocial treatment for panic disorder in primary care patients. *General Hospital Psychiatry, 24,* 316–321.

Heimberg, R. G., Mueller, G. P., Holt, C. S., Hope, D. A., & Liebowitz, M. R. (1992). Assessment of anxiety in social interaction and being observed by others: The Social Interaction Anxiety Scale and the Social Phobia Scale. *Behavior Therapy, 23,* 53–73.

Heine, S. J. (2003). An exploration of cultural variation in self-enhancing and self-improving motivations. *Nebraska Symposium on Motivation, 49,* 101–129.

Heine, S. J., Kitayama, S., & Lehman, D. R. (2001). Cultural differences in self-evaluation: Japanese readily accept negative self-referent information. *Journal of Cross-Cultural Psychology, 32,* 434–443.

Heine, S. J., & Lehman, D. R. (1995). Cultural variation in unrealistic optimism: Does the West feel more invulnerable than the East? *Journal of Personality and Social Psychology, 68,* 595–607.

Heine, S. J., & Lehman, D. R. (1999). Culture, self-discrepancies, and self-satisfaction. *Personality and Social Psychology Bulletin, 25,* 915–925.

Heine, S. J., Lehman, D. R., Markus, H. R., & Kitayama, S. (1999). Is there a universal need for positive self-regard? *Psychological Review, 106,* 766–794.

Herbert, J. D., Bellack, A. S., & Hope, D. A. (1991). Concurrent validity of the Social Phobia and Anxiety Inventory. *Journal of Psychopathology and Behavioral Assessment, 13,* 357–368.

Hinton, D. E., Chhean, D., Pich, V., Safren, S. A., Hofmann, S. G., & Pollack, M. H. (2005). A randomized controlled trial of cognitive behavior therapy for Cambodian refugees with treatment resistant PTSD and panic attacks: A cross-over design. *Journal of Traumatic Stress, 18,* 617–629.

Hinton, D. E., Pollack, M. H., Pich, V., Fama, J. M., & Barlow, D.H. (2005). Orthostatically induced panic attacks among Cambodian refugees: Flashbacks, catastrophic cognitions, and associated psychopathology. *Cognitive and Behavioral Practice, 12,* 301–311.

Hofmann, S. G., & Smits, J. A. J. (2008). Cognitive-behavioral therapy for adult anxiety disorders: A meta-analysis of randomized placebo-controlled trials. *Journal of Clinical Psychiatry, 69,* 621–632.

Hofstede, G. (1980). *Culture's consequences.* Beverly Hills, CA: Sage.

Hoge, E. A., Tamrakar, S. M., Christian, K. M., Mahara, N., Nepal, M. K., Pollack, M. H., et al. (2006). Cross-cultural differences in somatic presentation in patients with generalized anxiety disorder. *Journal of Nervous and Mental Disease, 194,* 962–966.

Hong, J. J. (2005). *Social values and self-construal in the expression of social anxiety: A cross-cultural comparison.* Unpublished doctoral dissertation, University of British Columbia, Vancouver.

Hong, J. J., & Woody, S. R. (2007). Cultural mediators of self-reported social anxiety. *Behavior Research and Therapy, 45*(8), 1779–1789.

Huang, B., Grant, B. F., Dawson, D. A., Stinson, F. S., Chou, S. S., Saha, T. D., et al. (2006). Race-ethnicity and the prevalence and co-occurrence of Diagnostic and Statistical Manual of Mental Disorders, Fourth Edition, alcohol and drug use disorders and Axis I and II disorders: United States, 2001 to 2002. *Comprehensive Psychiatry, 47,* 252–257.

Juang, Y.-Y., & Liu, C.-Y. (2001). Phenomenology of obsessive-compulsive disorder in Taiwan. *Psychiatry and Clinical Neurosciences, 55,* 623–627.

Julien, D., O'Connor, K. P., Aardema, F., & Todorov, C. (2006). The specificity of belief domains in obsessive-compulsive symptom subtypes. *Personality and Individual Differences, 41,* 1205–1216.

Kamijima, K., Murasaki, M., Asai, M., Higuchi, T., Nakajima, T., Taga, C., et al. (2004). Paroxetine in the treatment of obsessive-compulsive disorder: Randomized, double-blind placebo-controlled study in Japanese patients. *Psychiatry and Clinical Neurosciences, 58*(4), 427–433.

Kanagawa, C., Cross, S. E., & Markus, H. R. (2001). "Who am I?" The cultural psychology of the conceptual self. *Personality and Social Psychology Bulletin, 27,* 90–103.

Kawakami, N., Takeshima, T., Ono, Y., Uda, H., Hata, Y., Nakane, Y., et al. (2005). Twelve-month prevalence, severity, and treatment of common mental disorders in communities in Japan: Preliminary finding from the World Mental Health Japan Survey 2002–2003. *Psychiatry and Clinical Neurosciences, 59,* 441–452.

Kessler, R. C. (2000). Posttraumatic stress disorder: The burden to the individual and to society. *Journal of Clinical Psychiatry, 61*(Suppl. 5), 13–14.

Kessler, R. C., Berglund, P., Demler, O., Jin, R., Merikangas, K. R., & Walters, E. E. (2005). Lifetime preva-lence and age-of-onset distributions of DSM-IV disorders in the national comorbidity survey replication. *Archives of General Psychiatry, 62*, 593–602.

Kessler, R. C., Chiu, W. T., Demler, O., & Walters, E. E. (2005). Prevalence, severity, and comorbidity of 12-month DSM-IV disorders in the national comorbidity survey replication. *Archives of General Psychiatry, 62*, 617–627.

Kessler, R. C., Chiu, W. T., Jin, R., Ruscio, A. M., Shear, K., & Walters, E. E. (2006). The epidemiology of panic attacks, panic disorder, and agoraphobia in the National Comorbidity Survey replication. *Archive of Psychiatry, 63*, 415–424.

Kessler, R. C., McGonagle, K. A., Zhao, S., Nelson, C. B., Hughes, M., Eshleman, S., et al. (1994). Lifetime and 12-month prevalence of DSM-III-R psychiatric disorders in the United States: Results from the national comorbidity survey. *Archives of General Psychiatry, 51*, 8–19.

Kessler, R. C., & Merikangas, K. R. (2004). The National Comorbidity Survey Replication (NCS-R): Background and aims. *International Journal of Methods in Psychiatric Research, 13*(2), 60–68.

Kessler, R. C., Sonnega, A., Bromet, E., Hughes, M., & Nelson, C. B. (1995). Posttraumatic stress disorder in the National Comorbidity Survey. *Archives of General Psychiatry, 52*(12), 1048–1060.

Kim, J., Rapee, R. M., & Gaston, J. E. (2008). Symptoms of offensive type Taijin-Kyofusho among Australian social phobics. *Depression and Anxiety, 25*, 601–608.

Kim, M.-S. (1994). Cross-cultural comparisons of the perceived importance of conversational constraints. *Human Communication Research, 21*, 128–151.

Kim, M.-S., & Kim, H.-J. (1997). Communication goals: Individual differences between Korean and American speakers. *Personality and Individual Differences, 23*, 509–517.

Kinzie, J. D., Boehnlein, J. K., Leung, P.K, Moore, L. J., Riley, C., & Smith, D. (1990). The prevalence of post-traumatic stress disorder and its clinical significance among Southeast Asian refugees. *American Journal of Psychiatry, 147*, 913–917.

Kitayama, S., Markus, H. R., Matsumoto, H., & Norasakkunkit, V. (1997). Individual and collective processes in construction of the self: Self-enhancement in the United States and self-criticism in Japan. *Journal of Personality and Social Psychology, 72*, 1245–1267.

Kleinknecht, R. A., Dinnel, D. L., Kleinknecht, E. E., Hiruma, N., & Harada (1997). Cultural factors in social anxiety: A comparison of social phobia symptoms and Taijin Kyofusho. *Journal of Anxiety Disorders, 11*, 157–177.

Koestner, R., Bernieri, F., & Zuckerman, M. (1992). Self-regulation and consistency between traits, attitudes and behaviors. *Personality and Social Psychology Bulletin, 18*, 52–59.

Kulka, R. A., Schlenger, W. E., Fairbank, J. A., Hough, R. L., Jordan, B. K., Marmar, C. R., et al. (1990). *Trauma and the Vietnam War generation: Report of findings from the National Vietnam Veterans Readjustment Study.* Philadelphia, PA: Brunner/Mazel.

Lee, S., Tsang, A., Chui, H., Kwok, K., & Cheung, E. (2007). A community epidemiological survey of general-ized anxiety disorder in Hong Kong. *Community Mental Health Journal, 43*, 305–319.

Lee, S.-H., & Oh, K. S. (1999). Offensive type of social phobia: Cross-cultural perspectives. *International Medical Journal, 6*(4), 271–279.

Leung, K. (1987). Some determinants of reactions to procedural models of conflict resolution: A cross-national study. *Journal of Personality and Social Psychology, 53*, 898–908.

Levine, T. R., Bresnahan, M. J., Park, H.-S., Lapinski, M. K., Wittenbaum, G. M., Shearman, S. M., et al. (2003). Self-construal scales lack validity. *Human Communication Research, 29*, 210–252.

Lim, Y.-J., Yu, B.-H., & Kim, J.-H. (2007). Korean Anxiety Sensitivity Index—Revised: Its factor structure, reliability, and validity in clinical and nonclinical samples. *Depression and Anxiety, 24*, 331–341.

Lochner, C., Stein, D. J. (2003). Heterogeneity of obsessive-compulsive disorder: A literature review. *Harvard Review of Psychiatry, 11*, 113–131.

Ma, X., Xiang, Y.-T., Cai, Z.-J., Lu, J.-Y., Li, S.-R., Xiang, Y.-Q., et al. (2009). Generalized anxiety disorder in China: Prevalence, sociodemographic correlates, comorbidity, and suicide attempts. *Perspectives in Psychiatric Care, 45*, 119–127.

Maller, R., & Reiss, S. (1992). Anxiety sensitivity in 1984 and panic attacks in 1987. *Journal of Anxiety Disorders, 6*, 241–247.

Mansell, W., & Clark, D. M. (1999). How do I appear to others? Social anxiety and processing of the observable self. *Behaviour Research and Therapy, 37,* 419–434.

Markus, H. R., & Kitayama, S. (1991). Culture and self: Implications for cognition, emotion, and motivation. *Psychological Review, 98,* 224–253.

Markus, H. R., & Kitayama, S. (1998). The cultural psychology of personality. *Journal of Cross-Cultural Psychology, 29*(1), 63–87.

Marshall, G. N., Schell, T. L., Elliott, M. N., Berthold, S. M., & Chun, C.-A. (2005). Mental health of Cambodian refugees 2 decades after resettlement in the United States. *Journal of the American Medical Association, 294,* 571.

Marten, P. A., Brown, T. A., Barlow, D. H., & Borkovec, T. D. (1993). Evaluation of the ratings comprising the associated symptom criterion of DSM-III-R generalized anxiety disorder. *Journal of Nervous and Mental Disease, 181*(11), 676–682.

Matsunaga, H., Kiriike, N., Matsui, T., Iwasaki, Koshimune, K., Ohya, K., et al. (2001). A comparative study of clinical features between pure checkers and pure washers categorized using a lifetime symptom rating method. *Psychiatry Research, 105,* 221–229.

Matsunaga, H., Kiriike, N., Matsui, T., Miyata, A., Iwasaki, Y., Fujimoto, K., et al. (2000). Gender differences in social and interpersonal features and personality disorders among Japanese patients with obsessive-compulsive disorder. *Comprehensive Psychiatry, 41,* 266–272.

Matsunaga, H., Seedat, S. (2007). Obsessive-compulsive spectrum disorders: Cross-national and ethnic issues. *CNS Spectrums, 12,* 392–400.

McKay, D., Abramowitz, J. S., Calamari, J. E., Kyrios, M., Radomsky, A., Sookman, D., et al. (2004). A critical evaluation of obsessive-compulsive disorder subtypes: Symptoms versus mechanisms. *Clinical Psychology Review, 24*(3), 283–313.

Mennin, D. S., Heimberg, R. G., Turk, C. L., & Fresco, D. M. (2005). Preliminary evidence for an emotion dysregulation model of generalized anxiety disorder. *Behavior Research and Therapy, 43,* 1281–1310.

Mennin, D. S., Holaway, R. M., Fresco, D. M., Moore, M. T., & Heimberg, R. G. (2007). Delineating components of emotion and its dysregulation in anxiety and mood psychopathology. *Behavior Therapy, 38,* 284–302.

Millet, B., Kochman, F., Gallarda, T., Krebs, M. O., Demonfaucon, F., Barrot, I., et al. (2004). Phenomenological and comorbid features associated in obsessive-compulsive disorder: Influence of age of onset. *Journal of Affective Disorders, 79,* 241–246.

Mineka, S., & Zinbarg, R. (2006). A contemporary learning theory perspective on the etiology of anxiety disorders: It's not what you thought it was. *American Psychologist, 61,* 10–26.

Moretz, M. W., & McKay, D. (2009). The role of perfectionism in obsessive-compulsive symptoms: "Not just right" experiences and checking compulsions. *Journal of Anxiety Disorders, 23,* 640–644.

Morris, M. W., & Peng, K. (1994). Culture and cause: American and Chinese attributions for social and physical events. *Journal of Personality and Social Psychology, 67,* 949–971.

Nemeroff, C. B., Bremner, J. D., Foa, E. B., Mayberg, H. S., North, C. S., & Stein, M. B. (2006). Posttraumatic stress disorder: A state-of-the-science review. *Journal of Psychiatric Research, 40*(1), 1–21.

Nietzel, M. T., & Harris, M. J. (1990). Relationship of dependency and achievement/autonomy to depression. *Clinical Psychology Review, 10,* 279–297.

Norasakkunkit, V., & Kalick, S. M. (2002). Culture, ethnicity, and emotional distress measures: The role of self-construal and self-enhancement. *Journal of Cross-Cultural Psychology, 33,* 56–70.

Norenzayan, A., Choi, I., & Nisbett, R. E. (1999). Eastern and Western perceptions of causality for social behavior: Lay theories about personalities and situations. In D. A. Prentice & D. T. Miller (Eds.), *Cultural divides: Understanding and overcoming group conflict* (pp. 239–272). New York: Russell Sage Foundation.

Norris, F. H. (1992). Epidemiology of trauma: Frequency and impact of different potentially traumatic events on different demographic groups. *Journal of Consulting and Clinical Psychology, 60,* 409–418.

Noshirvani, H. F., Kasvikis, Y., Marks, I. M., Tsakiris, F., & Monteiro, W. O. (1991). Gender-divergent aetiological factors in obsessive-compulsive disorder. *British Journal of Psychiatry, 158,* 260–263.

Oetzel, J. G. (1998a). The effects of self-construals and ethnicity on self-reported conflict styles. *Communication Reports, 11,* 133–144.

Oetzel, J. G. (1998b). Explaining individual communication processes in homogeneous and heterogeneous groups through individualism-collectivism and self-construal. *Human Communication Research, 25,* 202–224.

Oishi, S., Wyer, R. S., & Colcombe, S. J. (2000). Cultural variation in the use of current life satisfaction to predict the future. *Journal of Personality and Social Psychology, 78,* 434–445.

Okazaki, S. (1997). Sources of ethnic differences between Asian-American and white-American college students on measures of depression and social anxiety. *Journal of Abnormal Psychology, 106,* 52–60.

Okazaki, S. (2000). Asian American and white American differences on affective distress symptoms: Do symptom reports differ across reporting methods? *Journal of Cross-Cultural Psychology, 31,* 603–625.

Okazaki, S. (2002). Self-other agreement on affective distress scales in Asian Americans and white Americans. *Journal of Counseling Psychology, 49,* 428–437.

Okazaki, S., & Kallivayalil, D. (2002). Cultural norms and subjective disability as predictors of symptom reports among Asian Americans and white Americans. *Journal of Cross-Cultural Psychology, 33,* 482–491.

Okazaki, S., Liu, J. F., Longworth, S. L., & Minn, J. Y. (2002). Asian American–white American differences in expressions of social anxiety: A replication and extension. *Cultural Diversity and Ethnic Minority Psychology, 8,* 234–247.

Olatunji, B. O., & Wolitzky-Taylor, K (2009). Anxiety sensitivity and the anxiety disorders: A meta-analytic review and synthesis. *Psychological Bulletin, 135,* 974–999.

Olatunji, B. O., Wolitzky-Taylor, K., Elwood, L., Connolly, K., Gonzales, B., & Armstrong, T. (2009). Anxiety sensitivity and health anxiety in a nonclinical sample: Specificity and prospective relations with clinical stress. *Cognitive Therapy and Research, 33,* 416–424.

Otto, M. W., Pollack, M. H., Fava, M., Uccello, R., & Rosenbaum, J. F. (1995). Elevated Anxiety Sensitivity Index scores in patients with major depression: Correlates and changes with antidepressant treatment. *Journal of Anxiety Disorders, 9,* 117–123.

Oyserman, D., Coon, H. M., & Kemmelmeier, M. (2002). Rethinking individualism and collectivism: Evaluation of theoretical assumptions and meta-analyses. *Psychological Bulletin, 128,* 3–72.

Ozer, E., Best, S., Lipsey, T., & Weiss, D. (2003). Predictors of posttraumatic stress disorder and symptoms in adults: A meta-analysis. *Psychological Bulletin, 129,* 52–73.

Peng, K., & Nisbett, R. E. (1999). Culture, dialectics, and reasoning about contradiction. *American Psychologist, 54,* 741–754.

Perkonigg, A., Kessler, R. C., Storz, S., & Wittchen, H.-U. (2000). Traumatic events and post-traumatic stress disorder in the community: Prevalence, risk factors, and comorbidity. *Acta Psychiatrica Scandinavica, 101,* 46–59.

Prigerson, H. G., Maciejewski, P. K., & Rosenheck, R. A. (2002). Population attributable fractions of psychiatric disorders and behavioral outcomes associated with combat exposure among US men. *American Journal of Public Health, 92*(1), 59–63.

Pyszczynski, T., & Greenberg, J. (1986). Evidence for a depressive self-focusing style. *Journal of Research in Personality, 20,* 95–106.

Rachman, S. (1997). A cognitive theory of obsessions. *Behaviour Research and Therapy, 35,* 793–802.

Rachman, S. (1998). A cognitive theory of obsessions: Elaborations. *Behaviour Research and Therapy, 36,* 385–401.

Rachman, S. (2002). A cognitive theory of compulsive checking. *Behaviour Research and Therapy, 40,* 624–639.

Reiss, S., & McNally, R. J. (1985). The expectancy model of fear. In S. Reiss & R. R. Bootzin (Eds.), *Theoretical issues in behavior therapy* (pp. 107–121). London, England: Academic.

Reiss, S., Peterson, R. A., Gursky, D. M., & McNally, R. J. (1986). Anxiety sensitivity, anxiety frequency, and the predictions of fearfulness. *Behaviour Research and Therapy, 24,* 1–8.

Rhee, E., Uleman, J. S., Lee, H. K., & Roman, R. J. (1995). Spontaneous self-descriptions and ethnic identities in individualistic and collectivistic cultures. *Journal of Personality and Social Psychology, 69*(1), 142–152.

Roberts, B. W., & Donahue, E. M. (1994). One personality, multiple selves: Integrating personality and social roles. *Journal of Personality and Social Psychology, 62,* 199–218.

Roemer, L., Lee, J., Salters-Pedneault, K., Erisman, S., Mennin, D., & Orsillo, S. M. (2009). Mindfulness and emotion regulation difficulties in generalized anxiety disorder: Preliminary evidence for interdependent and overlapping contributions. *Behavior Therapy, 40,* 142–154.

Roemer, L., Salters, K., Raffa, S. D., & Orsillo, S. M. (2005). Fear and avoidance of internal experiences in GAD: Preliminary tests of conceptual model. *Cognitive Therapy and Research, 29*, 71–88.

Romano, P., van Beek, N., Cucchi, M., Biffi, S., & Perna G. (2004). Anxiety sensitivity and modulation of the serotonergic system in patients with PD. *Journal of Anxiety Disorders, 18*(3), 423–431.

Roy-Byrne, P. P., & Cowley, D. S. (2002). Pharmacological treatments for panic disorder, generalized anxiety disorder, specific phobia, and social anxiety disorder. In P. E. Nathan & J. M. Gorman (Eds.), *A guide to treatments that work* (2nd ed., pp. 337–365). New York: Oxford University Press.

Salkovskis, P. M. (1996). The cognitive approach to anxiety: Threat beliefs, safety-seeking behavior, and the special case of health anxiety and obsessions. In P. M. Salkovskis (Ed.), *Frontiers of cognitive therapy* (pp. 48–74). New York: Guilford.

Salkovskis, P. M., Wroe, A. L., Gledhill, A., Morrison, N., Forrester, E., Richards, C., et al. (2000). Responsibility attitudes and interpretations are characteristic of obsessive compulsive disorder. *Behaviour Research and Therapy, 38*, 347–372.

Schlenker, B. R., & Leary, M. R. (1982). Social anxiety and self-presentation: A conceptualization and model. *Psychological Bulletin, 92*, 641–669.

Schmidt, N. B., Eggleston, A. M., Woolaway-Bickel, K., Fitzpatrick, K. K., Vasey, M. W., & Richey, J. (2007). Anxiety Sensitivity Amelioration Training (ASAT): A longitudinal primary prevention program targeting cognitive vulnerability. *Journal of Anxiety Disorders, 21*, 302–319.

Schmidt, N. B., Lerew, D. R., & Jackson, R. J. (1997). The role of anxiety sensitivity in the pathogenesis of panic: Prospective evaluation of spontaneous panic attacks during acute stress. *Journal of Abnormal Psychology, 106*, 355–364.

Schmidt, N. B., Lerew, D. R., & Jackson, R. J. (1999). Prospective evaluation of anxiety sensitivity in the pathogenesis of panic: Replication and extension. *Journal of Abnormal Psychology, 108*, 532–537.

Schmidt, N. B., Zvolensky, M. J., & Maner, J. K. (2006). Anxiety sensitivity: Prospective prediction of panic attacks and Axis I pathology. *Journal of Psychiatric Research, 40*, 691–699.

Seeman, J. (1983). *Personality integration: Studies and reflections.* New York: Human Sciences Press.

Sheldon, K. M., & Kasser, T. (1995). Coherence and congruence: Two aspects of personality integration. *Journal of Personality and Social Psychology, 68*, 531–543.

Silove, D., Steel, Z., Bauman, A., Chey, T., & McFarlane, A. (2007). Trauma, PTSD, and the longer-term health burden amongst Vietnamese refugees: A comparison with the Australian-born population. *Social Psychiatry and Psychiatric Epidemiology, 42*, 467–476.

Simon, N., Otto, M. W., Smits, J. A. J., Nicolaou, D. C., Reese, H., & Pollack, M. H. (2004). Changes in anxiety sensitivity with pharmacotherapy for panic disorder. *Journal of Psychiatric Research, 38*, 491–495.

Singelis, T. M. (1994). The measurement of independent and interdependent self-construals. *Personality and Social Psychological Bulletin, 20*, 580–591.

Singelis, T. M., Bond, M. H., Sharkey, W. F., & Lai, C. S. Y. (1999). Unpackaging culture's influence on self-esteem and embarrassability: The role of self-construals. *Journal of Cross-Cultural Psychology, 30*, 315–341.

Singelis, T. M., & Brown, W. J. (1995). Culture, self, and collectivist communication: Linking culture to individual behavior. *Human Communication Research, 21*, 354–389.

Smits, J. A. J., Powers, M. B., Cho, Y. C., & Telch, M. J. (2004). Mechanism of change in cognitive–behavioral treatment of panic disorder: Evidence for the fear of fear mediational hypothesis. *Journal of Consulting and Clinical Psychology, 72*, 646–652.

Snyder, M. (1987). *Public appearances, private realities: The psychology of self-monitoring.* New York: Freeman/ Times Books/Henry Holt.

Stinson, F. S., Dawson, D. A., Chou, S. P., Smith, S., Goldstein, R. B., Ruan, W. J., et al. (2007). The epidemiology of DSM-IV specific phobia in the USA: Results from the National Epidemiologic Survey on alcohol and related conditions. *Psychology Medicine, 37*, 1047–1059.

Suh, E. M. (2002). Culture, identity consistency, and subjective well-being. *Journal of Personality and Social Psychology, 83*, 1378–1391.

Suzuki, T. (2005). Relationship between two aspects of perfectionism and obsessive-compulsive symptoms. *Psychological Reports, 96*, 299–305.

Takeuchi, D. T., Zane, N., Hong, S., Chae, D. H., Gong, F., Gee, G. C., et al. (2007). Immigration-related factors and mental disorders among Asian-Americans. *American Journal of Public Health, 97*(1), 84–90.

Taylor, S. (Ed.). (1999). *Anxiety sensitivity: Theory, research, and treatment of the fear of anxiety.* Mahwah, NJ: Erlbaum.

Taylor, S., & Cox, B. J. (1998). An expanded Anxiety Sensitivity Index: Evidence for a hierarchic structure in a clinical sample. *Journal of Anxiety Disorders, 12,* 463–483.

Taylor, S., Koch, W. J., Woody, S., & McLean, P. (1996). Anxiety sensitivity and depression: How are they related? *Journal of Abnormal Psychology, 105,* 474–479.

Taylor, S., McKay, D., & Abramowitz, J. S. (2005). Hierarchical structure of dysfunctional beliefs in obsessive-compulsive disorder. *Cognitive Behaviour Therapy, 34,* 216–228.

Taylor, S. E., & Brown, J. D. (1988). Illusion and well-being: A social psychological perspective on mental health. *Psychological Bulletin, 103,* 193–210.

Thuile, J., Even, C., & Rouillon, F. (2008). Long-term outcome of anxiety disorders: A review of double-blind studies. *Current Opinion in Psychiatry, 22,* 84–89.

Ting-Toomey, S. (1988). Intercultural conflict styles: A face-negotiation theory. In W. Gudykunst, L. Stewart, & S. Ting-Toomey (Eds.), *Communication, culture, and organizational processes.* Newbury Park, CA: Sage.

Ting-Toomey, S., Gao, G., Trubisky, P., Yang, Z., Kim, H. S., Lin, S. L., et al. (1991). Culture, face maintenance, and styles of handling interpersonal conflict: A study of five cultures. *International Journal of Conflict Management, 2,* 275–296.

Ting-Toomey, S., & Kurogi, A. (1998). Facework competence in intercultural conflict: An updated face-negotiation theory. *International Journal of Intercultural Relations, 22,* 187–255.

Triandis, H. C. (1995). *Individualism and collectivism.* Boulder, CO: Westview.

Turner, S. M., Beidel, D. C., Dancu, C. V., & Stanley, M. A. (1989). An empirically driven inventory to measure social fears and anxiety: The social phobia and anxiety inventory. *Psychological Assessment: A Journal of Consulting and Clinical Psychology, 1,* 35–40.

Voss Horrell, S. C. (2008). Effectiveness of cognitive-behavioral therapy with adult ethnic minority clients: A review. *Professional Psychology: Research and Practice, 39,* 160–168.

Walters, K. S., & Hope, D. A. (1998). Analysis of social behavior in individuals with social phobia and nonanxious participants using a psychobiological model. *Behavior Therapy, 29,* 387–407.

Weems, C. F., Hayward, C., Killen, J., & Taylor, C. B. (2002). A longitudinal investigation of anxiety sensitivity in adolescence. *Journal of Abnormal Psychology, 111,* 471–477.

Weissman, M. M., Bland, R. C., Canino, G. J., Faravelli, C., Greenwald, S., Hwu, H.-G., et al. (1997). The cross-national epidemiology of panic disorder. *Archive of Psychiatry, 54,* 305–309.

Weissman, M. M., Bland, R. C., Canino, G. J., Greenwald, S., Hwu, H. G., Lee, C. K., et al. (1994). The cross national epidemiology of obsessive compulsive disorder. The Cross National Collaborative Group. *Journal of Clinical Psychiatry, 55*(Suppl. 1), 5–10.

Wolfe, R. N., Lennox, R, D., & Cutler, B. L. (1986). Getting along and getting ahead: Empirical support for a theory of protective and acquisitive self-presentation. *Journal of Personality and Social Psychology, 50,* 356–361.

Yehuda, R., Marshall, R., Penkower, A., & Wong, C. M. (2002). Pharmacological treatments for posttraumatic stress disorder. In P. E. Nathan & J. M. Gorman (Eds.), *A guide to treatments that work* (2nd ed., pp. 411–445). New York: Oxford University Press.

Zane, N., & Yeh, M. (2002). The use of culturally-based variables in assessment: Studies on loss of face. In K. S. Kurosaki, S. Okazaki, & S. Sue (Eds.), *Asian American mental health: Assessment theories and methods* (pp. 123–137). New York: Kluwer Academic/Plenum.

| 8 |

SOMATOFORM DISORDERS IN ASIANS

Winnie W. S. Mak, Fanny M. Cheung, and Freedom Leung

IDENTIFYING SOMATOFORM DISORDERS IN ASIANS

Somatoform disorders are one of the most common mental disorders seen in primary health care settings (Ormel, Vonkorff, Ustün, Pini, Korten, & Oldehinkel, 1994). Individuals with somatoform disorders often enter health care systems with medically unexplained symptoms. Not only do they place a heavy toll on health care systems in terms of medical expenditures and human resources (Shaw & Creed, 1991), but they also experience frustration and dissatisfaction in the lengthy but often unproductive process. It is estimated that somatization posed an annual expenditure of US$256 billion on the health care system of the United States (Barsky, Orav, & Bates, 2005).

Somatoform disorders are often confused with the discussion of the somatization tendency among Asians. Part of the problem lies in the interchanged use of the terms by practitioners and researchers. Cheung (1998) noted that "somatization may be referred to as a psychiatric disorder, various patterns of illness behavior, forms of help-seeking related to bodily symptoms, or a combination of these concepts" (p. 42). In the present chapter, both somatoform disorders and the phenomenon of somatization are discussed in the context of how they are manifested among Asians.

Current DSM *Nosology and Criteria for Somatoform Disorders*

Somatoform disorders are a group of disorders in which people experience significant physical symptoms for which there is no apparent organic cause. These disorders cause clinically significant distress and/or psychosocial impairment. The physical symptoms are not under voluntary control, nor are they intentionally produced by the person. It is important to note that somatoform disorders are not the same as psychosomatic disorders, which are medical disorders in which people have an actual physical illness, such as an ulcer, that can be documented with medical tests and that is being worsened by psychological factors. A person with a somatoform disorder does not have a medical disease that can be documented by medical examinations or tests.

DSM-IV-TR (APA, 2000) includes seven disorders under the category of somatoform disorders: (1) somatization disorder, (2) undifferentiated somatoform disorder, (3) conversion disorder, (4) pain disorder, (5) hypochondriasis, and (6) body dysmorphic disorder, and (7) somatoform disorder not otherwise specified. In the following sections, we will briefly cover the major features of each of the somatoform disorders. Coverage of the disorders will vary depending on the body of evidence that we can find in the literature.

Somatization Disorder Among Asians

Somatization disorder is a polysymptomatic disorder that is characterized by a combination of pseudoneurological pain and gastrointestinal and sexual symptoms that have no apparent physical explanation. In the *DSM-IV-TR*, the diagnostic criteria for somatization disorder include: (1) a history of many physical complaints beginning before age 30 years that occur over several years; (2) at least four pain symptoms, two gastrointestinal symptoms, one sexual symptom, and one pseudoneurological symptom; (3) symptoms are not due to a medical condition or are excessive given a medical condition the person may be experiencing; and (4) symptoms are not intentionally produced or faked (APA, 2000).

The *DSM-IV-TR* states that the specific symptoms of somatization disorder may vary across cultures. For example, burning pains in the hands and the sensation of ants crawling under the skin are more frequent in Asia and Africa than in North America (APA, 2000). Some researchers have indicated that many individuals displaying subclinical somatization problem (below the clinical cutoff of eight required symptoms) also reported significant clinical distress and psychosocial impairment (Kroenke et al., 1997; Ledwig et al., 2001; Swartz, Landerman, George, Blazer, & Escobar, 1991), thus they questioned the validity of the arbitrary cutoff of eight required symptoms for diagnosing the disorder. In fact, a new diagnostic category of "multisomatoform disorder," which requires only three chronic physical symptoms, has been proposed and may be included in the *DSM-5* (Kroenke et al., 1997).

Prevalence studies indicated that while moderate degrees of somatization are common (Ledwig et al., 2001; Swartz et al., 1991), few people meet the diagnostic criteria for somatization disorder, ranging only from 0.2% to 2% among women and less than 0.2% in men (APA, 2000; Feder et al., 2001; Gureje et al., 1997; Katon, Sullivan, & Walker, 2001). Initial symptoms usually begin in adolescence, and diagnostic criteria are typically met before age 25 years (APA, 2000). Somatization disorder is considered to be a relatively chronic condition, and physical symptoms of patients with somatization disorder have been reported to covary with their emotional well-being. When individuals were anxious or depressed, they reported more physical complaints than when they were not anxious or depressed (Craig et al., 1993). Patients with somatization disorder often also report a host of psychosocial adjustment problems, such as truancy, poor work history, and marital difficulties (Katon, Sullivan, & Walker, 2001). Comorbidity is high with other psychiatric disorders, such as anxiety disorders, depression, substance abuse, personality disorders, and conversion disorder (Feder et al., 2001; Golding, Smith, & Kashner, 1991; Katon et al., 2001; Kirmayer, Robbins, & Paris, 1994; Noyes et al., 2001; Rief, Hiller, & Margraf, 1998).

In the United States, somatization is more common among lower socioeconomic status (SES) groups and people with less than a high school education. It is four times more common among African Americans than among European Americans, and considerably higher in Puerto Rico than on the U.S. mainland (Canino et al., 1987; Canino, Rubio-Stipec, & Bravo, 1988). Findings from a large-scale, cross-cultural study sponsored by the World Health Organization of somatization disorder and somatic symptoms in primary care patients among 14 countries (Gureje, Simon, Üstün, & Goldberg, 1997), however, revealed that the differences in the prevalence of somatization disorder across countries is a rather complex phenomenon and may involve many possible contributory factors such as stress level and condition of life in different countries. Gureje and colleagues (1997) found that the highest prevalence of somatization disorder was found in two Latin American cities: 17.7 % in Santiago, Chile, and 8.5% in Rio de Janeiro, Brazil. Another notable finding from the same study is the lack of differences in the prevalence of somatization disorder between industrialized and nonindustrialized countries. The lowest prevalence rate of somatization disorder was found in Verona, Italy, and Nagasaki, Japan (both at 0.1%), and Ibadan, Nigeria, and Manchester, U.K. (both at 0.4%). Many other countries, regardless of their cultural origins, reported comparable prevalence rate of somatization disorder: 1.5% in Shanghai, China; 1.8% in Bangalore, India; 1.7% in Seattle, U.S.A.; 1.3% in Berlin, Germany; 2.8% in Groningen, The Netherlands; 1.7% in Paris, France; and 1.3% in Athens, Greece (Gureje et al., 1997). Findings of this study suggest that cultural influences on somatoform disorders may be less prominent than previously thought.

In other epidemiological studies done among Asians and Asian Americans, the picture is more mixed. Elevated rates of somatization symptoms among Cambodian refugees (Hinton, Ba, Peou, & Um, 2000; Hinton, Um, & Ba, 2001) and Bhutanese refugees (van Ommeren et al., 2001) have been reported. Some researchers attributed this to the extreme stress and traumatic events that these groups of refugees were exposed to in their countries of origin. On the other hand, very low prevalence rates have been found among other Asians and Asian Americans. Based on data from the Epidemiologic Catchment Area (ECA) study, Asian Americans were found to have a lower prevalence of somatization disorder than European Americans (Zhang & Snowden, 1999). Chang (2002) also has summarized the prevalence of somatization across epidemiological studies done in different Asian regions/countries (Mainland China, Taiwan, Hong Kong, Korea). Across these studies, the lifetime prevalence rates of somatization were generally very low (0–0.2%) although they were comparable to that found among Asian Americans in the ECA.

Undifferentiated Somatoform Disorder Among Asians

Individuals are given this diagnosis when the physical complaints cannot be medically explained or the impairment exceeds what is expected based on the related medical condition and the complaints last for at least six months. The physical complaints can include fatigue, loss of appetite, gastrointestinal or urinary problems, and many others.

Conversion Disorder Among Asians

Individuals with conversion disorder lose motor or sensory functioning in a part of their bodies, mimicking neurological or other medical problems. The symptoms of conversion disorder resemble the pseudoneurological symptoms seen in somatization disorder, but with conversion disorder, the other kinds of symptoms of somatization disorder are not present. Some of the most common conversion symptoms are paralysis, blindness, aphonia, seizures, hearing loss, severe loss of coordination, and anesthesia in a limb. Conversion disorder typically involves one specific symptom, such as blindness or aphonia, but a person can have repeated episodes of conversion involving different parts of the body. Psychological stressor usually precedes the onset of the symptoms.

In the *DSM-IV-TR*, the diagnostic criteria for conversion disorder include: (1) one or more symptoms affecting motor or sensory functioning and suggesting a neurological or medical condition; (2) symptoms are related to psychological conflict or severe stress; (3) symptoms are not intentionally produced and cannot be explained by a medical condition; and (4) symptoms cause clinically significant subjective distress or psychosocial impairment or warrant medical evaluation (APA, 2000). The onset of conversion disorder is generally from late childhood to early adulthood, rarely before age 10 years or after age 35 years, but onset as late as the ninth decade of life has been reported (APA, 2000). The onset of conversion disorder is generally acute. Typically, individual conversion symptoms are of short duration. In most cases, symptoms will remit within two weeks. Recurrence is common, however, occurring in from one-fifth to one-quarter of individuals within 1 year, with a single recurrence predicting future episodes. Symptoms of paralysis, aphonia, and blindness are associated with a good prognosis, whereas tremor and seizures are not (APA, 2000).

Conversion symptoms were quite common during war time, when soldiers inexplicably became paralyzed or blind and therefore were unable to return to the front (Ironside & Batchelor, 1945; Marlowe, 2001; Ziegler, Imboden, & Meyer, 1960). Otherwise, conversion disorder is relatively rare. The prevalence of this disorder ranged from 11/100,000 to 500/100,000 in the general population (Akagi & House, 2001; APA, 2000). It has been reported in up to 3% of outpatients referrals to mental health clinics (Fink, Hansen, & Oxhøj, 2004). Studies of general medical/surgical inpatients have identified conversion symptom rates ranging between 1% and 14% (APA, 2000; Faravelli et al., 1997; Fink et al., 2004). The form of conversion symptoms often reflects local cultural ideas about acceptable and credible ways to express distress (APA, 2000).

Conversion disorder has been reported to be more common in rural populations, individuals of lower SES, and individuals less knowledgeable about medical and psychological concepts (Binzer & Kullgren, 1996). Higher rates of conversion symptoms are reported in developing regions, with the incidence generally declining with increasing development. The limited available evidence suggested that the diagnosis of conversion symptoms has declined in Western societies such as the United States and England (Hare, 1969), but has remained more prevalent in developing countries such as Libya (Pu, Mohamed, Imam, & El-Roey, 1986), China, and India (Tseng, 2001). The lower prevalence in the West may be a result of improved diagnostic practices, or perhaps of Western society's greater acceptance of the expression of emotional distress (Shorter, 1992). Another viewpoint is that conversion disorders are still prevalent today in the West but they take the form of conditions like Gulf War Syndrome, chronic fatigue syndrome, or other puzzling maladies (Showalter, 1997). In proposal for the *DSM-5*, conversion disorder is proposed to be reclassified under dissociative disorders (APA, 2010).

Pain Disorder Among Asians

The symptoms of pain disorder resemble the pain symptoms seen in somatization disorder, but with pain disorder, pain is the sole focus of complaint and the other kinds of symptoms of somatization disorder are not present. Although a medical condition may contribute to the pain, psychological factors are judged to play an important role in its onset, severity, exacerbation, or maintenance. In the *DSM-IV-TR* (APA, 2000), the diagnostic criteria for pain disorder include: (1) pain in one or more anatomical sites as primary focus of clinical presentation; (2) pain causes clinically significant subjective distress or psychosocial impairment; (3) psychological factors are thought to play an important role in the onset, severity, or maintenance of pain; and (4) symptom or deficit is not intentionally produced or faked. The *DSM-IV-TR* specifies two coded subtypes: (a) pain disorder associated with psychological factors, and (b) pain disorder associated with both psychological factors and a general medical condition. The first subtype applies where psychological factors are judged to play a major role in the onset or maintenance of the pain and any coexisting general medical condition is considered to be of minimal causal significance in the pain complaint. The second subtype applies where the experienced pain is considered to result from both psychological factors and some medical condition that could cause pain. In either case, the pain disorder may be acute (duration of less than 6 months) or chronic (duration of over 6 months).

Pain that causes significant distress or impairment in psychosocial functioning is widespread. It is estimated that, in any given year, 10–15% of adults in the United States have some form of work disability due to back pain (APA, 2000). The prevalence of pain disorder, however, is unknown. It is likely quite common among patients at pain clinics. It is diagnosed more frequently in women than in men and is very frequently comorbid with anxiety and mood disorders (APA, 2000). In most cases, the pain has persisted for years by the time the individual comes to the attention of the mental health profession. Important factors that appear to influence recovery from pain disorder are the individual's acknowledgment of pain; giving up unproductive efforts to control pain; participation in regularly scheduled activities (e.g., work) despite the pain; recognition and treatment of comorbid psychiatric problems; psychological adaptation to chronic illness; and not allowing the pain become the determining factor in his or her lifestyle. Individuals with greater numbers of painful body areas and higher numbers of general medical symptoms other than pain have a poorer prognosis (APA, 2000).

Hypochondriasis Among Asians

Hypochondriasis is characterized by the preoccupation with the anxiety of contracting a serious disease or with the idea that they actually have such a disease based on the person's misinterpretation of bodily symptoms or bodily functions. Individuals with hypochondriasis generally resist the idea that their problem is a psychological one that might best be treated by a mental health professional. In the *DSM-IV-TR* (APA, 2000), the diagnostic criteria for hypochondriasis include: (1) preoccupation with fears of contracting, or the idea that one has, a serious disease; (2) preoccupation continues despite medical reassurance; (3) the symptoms cause clinically significant distress or psychosocial impairment; and (4) symptoms last at least 6 months.

Hypochondriasis may be the most commonly seen somatoform disorder. The prevalence of hypochondriasis is estimated to be between 1–5% in the general population and 2–7% among primary care outpatients (APA, 2000). It occurs about equally often in men and women and can start at almost any age, although early adulthood is the most common age of onset. The course of the disorder is usually chronic, with waxing and waning symptoms over time. Individuals with hypochondriasis often also suffer from mood disorders, panic disorder, and somatization disorder (Creed & Barsky, 2004). Some researchers think hypochondriasis is closely related to anxiety trait and therefore prefer the term health anxiety to hypochondriasis (Taylor & Asmundson, 2004).

Body Dysmorphic Disorder Among Asians

Body dysmorphic disorder refers to the preoccupation of a slight or imagined defect in appearance. Relative to the physical anomaly, individuals' reactions are markedly excessive. This preoccupation causes significant distress and impairment in social, occupational, or other areas of functioning. The condition is found to be equally prevalent across males and females and may be particularly common among individuals seeking cosmetic surgery or dermatologic treatment, with reported rates of 6–15% (APA, 2000). In a sample of 566 adolescents, a prevalence of body dysmorphic disorder was found to be 2.2%, with African Americans reporting greater level of body dissatisfaction than their European American, Hispanic American, and Asian American (including Cambodian, Vietnamese, Filipino, and Asian nonspecific) counterparts (Mayville, Katz, Gipson, & Cabral, 1999). Much controversy has arisen on the nosology of body dysmorphic disorder, with some researchers arguing that it falls within the realm of obsessive-compulsive spectrum disorder (Phillips, McElroy, Hudson, & Pope, 1995). In the proposed revision of the *DSM-5*, the Somatic Symptoms Disorder Work Group recommends it be reclassified with anxiety and obsessive-compulsive spectrum disorders (APA, 2010). Others believed that as it involves body image distortion, it shares very little in common with other somatoform disorders that involve distress-induced physical symptoms (Mayou et al., 2005; Sharpe & Mayou, 2004).

Somatoform Disorder Not Otherwise Specified Among Asians

When individuals are presented with medically unexplained physical complaints that do not fit within specific disorders in the category, they are considered to have this diagnosis.

Proposed Classification in the DSM-5

Much discussion has been made in the reclassification of somatoform disorders for the upcoming edition of the *DSM*. As of May 2010, the Somatic Symptoms Disorder Work Group suggested that the overall diagnostic category of somatoform disorders to be changed to somatic symptoms disorders (APA, 2010). This proposed category will include not only somatoform disorders, it will also include psychological factors affecting medical condition and factitious disorders. With this change, somatoform disorder not otherwise specified will become somatic symptom disorder not otherwise specified. Moreover, a new encompassing disorder, complex somatic symptom disorder, is proposed, with somatization disorder, hypochondriasis, undifferentiated somatoform disorder, and pain disorder being reclassified to this new disorder. This new disorder is proposed in light of the somatic symptoms and preoccupation of these symptoms that are shared by the existing four disorders. As mentioned in the previous sections, body dysmorphic disorder is proposed to be reclassified under anxiety and obsessive-compulsive spectrum disorders; whereas conversion disorder is proposed to be reclassified under dissociative disorders. Finally, "medically unexplained symptoms" are proposed not to be considered as the core features of somatic symptoms disorders given the unreliability of their assessments and their implied and often problematic duality of the mind and the body. Nevertheless, given that the classification system for *DSM-5* has not been finalized, the above propositions are still subject to discussion and change.

Somatization Tendency Among Asians

In early studies of cultural psychiatry in the 1970s, the prevalence of somatic complaints presented by Chinese psychiatric patients was noted (Kleinman, 1977, 1982; Tseng, 1975). The tendency to present psychological distress in the form of somatic complaints and to delay psychiatric treatment was found particularly among patients with depression (Cheung, Lau, & Waldmann, 1980–1981). Although the tendency also prevails among individuals in non-Western cultures, including Asians living in the United States (Kleinman, 1980; Lee, Lei, & Sue, 2001; Lin, Inui, & Kleinman, 1982; Lin et al., 1992; Moore & Boehnlein, 1991), the discussion about its meaning and explanation among Chinese patients has been a subject of debate. In early studies of cultural psychiatry, post hoc cultural attributions, including the lack of psychological awareness, inadequate emotional vocabulary, and undifferentiated concrete level of thinking, were used to explain this tendency (Cheung, 1998).

Scholarly discourse and empirical research on somatization among Chinese psychiatric patients has illuminated the deficiencies of simplistic cultural explanations. Cheung (1995, 1998) illustrated the underlying contrast between the Western biomedical model of mental disorders and the holistic model of health adopted in Chinese medicine that contributed to the debate in somatization. Under the biomedical model, the somatization tendency is conceptualized as a masking of an underlying psychological disorder, such as depression, whereby psychological symptoms are suppressed. These biomedical approaches missed the complexity of the patterns of illness behavior through which somatization could inform the clinician about the subjective experience of the Chinese patients. In a holistic model of health, somatization could be understood in terms of the "phenomenology of discomfort and suffering, the process of communication, ways of coping and help-seeking, and the patient-doctor relationship" (Cheung, 1998, p. 42).

Recent research has indicated that the use of body-related verbal expressions in the Chinese language to describe a wide range of personal and social concerns, including feelings, thoughts, and images, is not equivalent to somatization (Tung, 1994). Studies also confirmed that presentation of somatic complaints does not preclude the presentation of affective and cognitive symptoms. For example, Y. P. Zheng, Xu, and Shen (1986) found that depressed patients described their suffering in both emotional and physical expressions. The somatic style of expressing emotions was not directly related to symptoms reported by patients if they were directly asked by the physician or when a symptom checklist was used (Cheung, Lau, & Waldmann, 1980–1981).

Cheung (1995) described somatization as an idiom of distress that is contextualized in a process of interpersonal communication between the patients and their social networks, as well as between the patients and the doctors. Chinese patients report different types of complaints, depending on their expectations about the nature of the consultation. The consultation experiences throughout their illness history would have shaped their interpretation and narratives of their suffering.

The reconceptualization of somatization as a culture-specific illness experience was a much more useful approach to understand patients' suffering and facilitate treatment planning (Cheung, 1985, 1995, 1998; Draguns, 1996). The somatization tendency and the situational orientation among Chinese patients may reflect common personality characteristics shaped by cultural factors. Understanding the patients' personality dynamics can help therapists to interpret the meaning of their illness behaviors and determine the appropriate course of intervention.

Strengths, Weaknesses, and Alternatives in Applying Current Nosology and Diagnostic Criteria for Identifying Somatoform Disorders in Asians

Just as many other diagnostic categories in the DSM, somatoform disorders lack distinct biological markers and are subject to sociocultural influences in the manifestation and experience of the illness. Thus, somatoform disorders, as they are presented in the DSM, are created under the dualistic conceptualization of health and medicine in the United States. According to Lee and Kleinman (2007), somatoform disorder was created as a residual category in the DSM. Individuals would only be diagnosed in this category of disorders when the possibility of all other Axis-I disorders are taken into account and excluded. Such a classification system gives primacy to psychological symptoms over somatic symptoms. On the other hand, Asians tend to conceptualize mind and body as a holistic whole. Rather than considering somatic and psychological symptoms as separate health experience, they consider them simultaneously under the nondualistic system (Lee & Kleinman, 2007). Thus, the conceptualization of somatoform disorders as distinctive from other psychological disorders is incompatible in traditional Asian, specifically Chinese, medicine. Since their introduction in the DSM-III, somatoform disorders are retained in the DSM-IV-TR although not without contention and criticisms (Mayou, Kirmayer, Simon, Kroenke, & Sharpe, 2005).

Slightly different from the classification of the DSM-IV-TR, the current version of the ICD (now in its 10th edition, ICD-10) set forth by the World Health Organization (1992) and the Chinese Classification of Medical Diseases used in Mainland China (now in its third edition,

CCMD-3; Chinese Psychiatric Society, 2001) share similar classification structure for somatoform disorders. Both ICD-10 and CCMD-3 categorize somatoform disorders with neurotic and stress-related disorders and divide somatoform disorders into the following specific categories: (1) somatization disorder, (2) undifferentiated somatoform disorder, (3) hypochondriacal disorder, (4) somatoform autonomic dysfunction, (5) persistent somatoform pain disorder, (6) other somatoform disorders, and (7) somatoform disorder, unspecified. In addition, both classification systems include neurasthenia as a separate, though related neurotic disorder. Although the overall prevalence of somatoform disorders according to ICD-10 (18.1%) and *DSM-IV* (20.2%) was similar, marked differences were found on specific disorders in a study done among internal medical inpatients in Denmark (Fink, Hansen, & Oxhøj, 2004). For example, according to the *DSM-IV* criteria, 1.5% and 10.1% of the 294 patients had somatization disorder and undifferentiated somatization disorder, respectively. On the other hand, based on the ICD-10 criteria, 5.2% and 0.7% had somatization disorder and undifferentiated somatization disorder.

Neurasthenia as a Distinct Category Among Asians

Neurasthenia was first identified by an American neurologist, George Beard, in 1869, to denote a cluster of physical symptoms related to a weakened nervous system (Beard, 1869; Yew Schwartz, 1999). It was characterized by physical symptoms including fatigue, physical or mental exhaustion, poor concentration, memory loss, headaches, and sleep disturbances, among a host of many other somatic complaints. It quickly gained popularity among physicians and the general public in the United States and Europe and was listed as "neurasthenia neurosis" in the *DSM-II* (APA, 1968). However, due to its nonspecific and ambiguous nature and indiscriminate use, its utility was called into question and it was dropped from *DSM-III* (APA, 1980; Yew Schwartz, 1999).

Neurasthenia was introduced to Japan and later to China in the early 1900s. It was translated as *shinkeisuijaku* in Japanese and *shenjing shuairuo* in Chinese, which actually are the same ideographically and mean "weakness of nerves" (Lee & Kleinman, 2007). Considered as a neurotic disorder, it encompassed somatic symptoms as well as affective and cognitive symptoms not unlike depression and anxiety disorders. Since its introduction, neurasthenia has become the most common psychiatric disorder up to the mid-1980s (P. Cheung, 1991). Eighty to ninety percent of the psychiatric outpatients in China were diagnosed with neurasthenia from the 1950s to 1980s (Kleinman, 1982). This popularity might be a result of the convergence of traditional Chinese health beliefs and the sociopolitical climate of the times. Given the holistic view of health in traditional Chinese medicine, psychological and physical symptoms are integrated and they are allowed to co-occur (Yew Schwartz, 1999). Being simultaneously somatic, cognitive, and emotional in nature, neurasthenia was congruent with the conception of this holistic system and was considered to be a socially acceptable way to express distress. Moreover, its introduction also coincided with the sociopolitical upheaval that was happening in communist China (Lin, 1992). People experienced tremendous tension with the government, with many suffering from physical and psychological hardships. To avoid being interpreted as showing discontent with the government (Kleinman, 1986), people reported having neurasthenia, which is regarded as a common medical condition.

However, several events since the 1980s led neurasthenia to lose its favor among Chinese psychiatrists (Lee, 1999). With the exclusion of neurasthenia in the *DSM-III* (APA, 1980) and the introduction of somatoform disorder, which gives dominance to somatic features at the exclusion of any affective symptoms, Chinese psychiatrists sensed the urgency to reconsider the diagnostic criteria of neurasthenia, especially with the introduction of the first edition of the Chinese Classification of Mental Disorders in 1981. In the following year, Kleinman (1982) published a study that examined the overlap between neurasthenia and *DSM-III* Axis I disorders. Out of the 100 outpatients with a diagnosis of neurasthenia at the Hunan Medical College, 87 could be rediagnosed with major depressive disorder, 69 with anxiety disorders, and 25 with somatoform disorders (Kleinman, 1982; D. F. Chang et al., 2005). More notably, those being rediagnosed as having depression responded favorably to tricyclic antidepressants (Lee & Kleinman, 2007). Similar results were found among Chinese studies with an overlap of 30% to 70% who were first diagnosed with neurasthenia having major depression (Zhang, 1989). Kleinman (1986) regarded this phenomenon as supporting the somatization tendency among Chinese and considered neurasthenia as a "biculturally patterned illness experience (a special form of somatization), related to either depression and other diseases, or to culturally sanctioned idioms of distress and psychosocial coping" (p. 115).

With the overlap between neurasthenia and depression found and the pressure to unify with ICD and *DSM*, Chinese psychiatrists relegated the diagnosis of neurasthenia as secondary to other psychological disorders in the Chinese Classification of Mental Disorders (CCMD). In the current version of the classification system (CCMD-3), a symptom hierarchy similar to that of the *DSM* was established for neurasthenia and the category of somatoform disorders to be consistent with ICD-10 and *DSM-IV-TR* (Lee & Kleinman, 2007). In the CCMD-3, neurasthenia was classified with a code of 43.5 within the category of hysteria, stress-related disorders, and neurosis (in ICD-10, it is coded F48 within F40–49 neurotic, stress-related, and somatoform disorders) and was listed behind all the somatoform disorders. Symptom criteria for neurasthenia in the CCMD-3 included predominance of weakness in cerebral and physical function, persistent mental fatigue, and physical fatigue and at least two of the following symptoms (1) affective symptoms (i.e., annoyance, tenseness, irritability, etc.); (2) excited symptoms (feelings of easy excitement); (3) muscular tensions, aches, pains, or dizziness; (4) sleep disturbance; and (5) other psychological and physiological disorder (i.e., palpitation, chest distress, impotence, menstrual disorder, etc.). The symptoms must last for at least three months and cause social impairment. Furthermore, any subtype of neurosis, depression, and schizophrenia must be excluded (Chinese Psychiatric Society, 2001).

Prevalence of Neurasthenia and Other Somatoform Disorders Among Asians

Despite the overlap found between neurasthenia and other psychological disorders, findings from more recent empirical studies indicated that neurasthenia is nosologically distinct from other disorders. In Chengdu, China, a prevalence of 5.5% to 6.3% was found Chinese patients in clinical settings (Liu & Song, 1986). In a nationwide epidemiological study, a lower prevalence of 1.3% was found in the general population in 12 areas of China (Epidemiological Study Group of Mental Disorders in 12 Areas in China, 1986). In a more recent clinical study of 139 patients at the Second Affiliated Xianga Hospital of Central South University in Hunan, China, 35.3% met the CCMD-2-R diagnosis of neurasthenia (D. F. Chang et al., 2005). Among the diagnosed, 19.4% were also diagnosed as having ICD-10 neurasthenia, 65.1% with *DSM-IV* diagnosis, including 30.6% with undifferentiated somatoform disorder, 22.4% with somatoform pain disorder, 4.1% with somatization disorder, and 2% with hypochondriasis. Thus, 44.9% of those with CCMD neurasthenia did not meet the criteria for any *DSM* diagnoses.

In the Chinese American Psychiatric Epidemiological Studies (CAPES), a prevalence of neurasthenia, as defined by the ICD-10, was found to be 6.4% among a random sample of 1,747 Chinese Americans in Los Angeles County (Y. P. Zheng et al., 1997). Among them, 43.7% met the diagnoses of *DSM* mood and anxiety disorders. In other words, the majority (56.3%) of individuals did not meet any current or lifetime *DSM* diagnoses. Based on the same epidemiological study (CAPES), 12.9% of the 1,747 Chinese Americans meet the Somatic Symptom Index (SSI) 5/5 criterion for somatization, as measured by the Symptom Checklist-90 Revised (SCL-90R) somatization score. Among them, 29.5% and 19.6% met the *DSM* criteria for depression and anxiety disorders, respectively (Mak & Zane, 2004). Findings from these studies indicated that neurasthenia is a distinct clinical condition experienced by Chinese that does not necessarily overlap with any Western diagnoses.

PERSPECTIVES ON THE CAUSES OF SOMATOFORM DISORDERS IN ASIANS

No research to date has examined the etiology of somatoform disorders specifically among Asians. The following sections will discuss some of the models that have been used in understanding the causes of somatoform disorders in general.

Critical Appraisal of Major Etiological Models of Somatoform Disorders

Psychobiological Models

Researchers have attempted to identify the psychobiological mechanisms underlying somatoform disorders (Sharpe & Bass, 1992). In response to common health complaints, individual differences exist in terms of the extent to which people can accept and tolerate them. For some, repeated stimulation of the nervous system may lead to habituation, for others, it may lead to sensitization. Neurobiological sensitization, or specifically limbic kindling, is proposed to be a basis for a spectrum of psychiatric disorders, including somatoform disorders (Teicher et al., 1993; Bell, 1994). Endogenous or exogenous stressors may cause an overstimulation of the limbic system. These stressors can be psychological, physical, or chemical. Such neurological hyperactivity may be manifested as overamplification of somatic and psychological responses. These subjective health complaints may activate the innate immune system, causing local inflammatory response that leads to enhanced symptoms (Dimsdale & Dantzer, 2007). Moreover, new stressors may cross-sensitize with the original stressor, causing sensitization by multiple sources of stress and at lower intensities (Bell, 1994). Thus, individuals may be comorbid with different psychiatric disorders (Eriksen & Ursin, 2002). In a sample of 264 patients presenting themselves at the outpatient clinic for multiple chemical sensitivity or idiopathic environmental intolerances, 35% of them were diagnosed with somatoform disorders, making it the most frequent *DSM-IV* diagnosis among the group (Bornschein, Hausteiner, Zilker, & Förstl, 2002).

In addition to the sensitization hypothesis, researchers have identified regional cerebral hypometabolism among 10 women with somatization disorder or undifferentiated somatoform disorder. Compared with controls, hypometabolism was found in the left and right precentral gyrus, left and right putamen, left and right nucleus caudatus, medial prefrontal lobes, postcentral gyrus, and thalamus on both sides (Hakala et al., 2002). These recent findings further point to the importance of exploring the neurobiological basis of somatization.

Psychological Models

In addition to sensitization happening at the neurological level, sensitization may also happen at the cognitive-emotional level (Brosschot, 2002). It was argued that individuals with somatoform disorders may have deficits in cognitive and interpersonal regulation of emotions (Waller & Scheidt, 2006). Thus, instead of managing their emotional arousal, they may selectively focus on their health complaints, leading to biased processing of this information. This attentional bias causes individuals to become more sensitive to physical sensations and more vulnerable to somatic illness (Brosschot, 2002). Somatic amplification, as measured by the Somatosensory Amplification Scale (SSAS), was found to explain 31% of the variance in hypochondriasis (Barsky & Wyshak, 1990). Thus, individuals with somatosensory amplification may have (1) increased vigilance to bodily sensations, (2) heightened tendency to focus on weak or infrequent sensations, and (3) greater tendency to appraise these sensations as abnormal or symptomatic of disease (Duddu, Isaac, & Chaturvedi, 2006).

The interaction between the neurobiological predispositions for experiencing strong physiological sensations when under stress with a maladaptive upbringing environment may create a psychological vulnerability for someone to develop different somatoform disorders. According to the cognitive activation theory of stress (CATS), individuals respond to health complaints based on the expectancies they have attached to the stimulus and the outcome. Pathology may develop over time as unspecific health complaints persist with the failure to cope with them through medical attention. This may result in sensitization in neural loops maintained by sustained attention and arousal (Eriksen & Ursin, 2004). Intense physiological sensations that habituate slowly will readily capture the attention focus of these individuals and lead to attention bias (sensation-driven attention bias). Research indicated that patients with somatoform disorders are more likely to experience sensation-driven attention bias in their cognitive processing (Lim & Kim, 2005;

Owens, Asmundson, Hadjistavropoulos, & Owens, 2004). Once people vulnerable for somatoform disorders notice physical symptoms, they are also more likely to overreact to them and make more negative attributions about them (sensation-driven cognitive appraisal bias). The exact form of the cognitive bias may vary, but most somatoform disorders seem to be characterized by worry about health and a tendency to catastrophize the symptoms (Kirmayer & Taillefer, 1997; Looper & Kirmayer, 2002).

In addition to this cognitive bias, people with somatoform disorders are also more likely to attribute their symptoms to organic causes and make vulnerability attributions (Rief, Nanke, Emmerich, Bender, & Zech, 2004). Based on their illness interpretations, they are more likely to seek medical examinations and have increased bodily scanning. Through past illness experiences, they are also more likely to develop cognitive distortions or schemas that prompt help-seeking and reassurance-seeking behaviors within the health system (Looper & Kirmayer, 2002). Frequent utilizers of the health care system were found to report less normalizing explanations for their common bodily sensations than low utilizers (Sensky, MacLeod, & Rigby, 1996). As a result, people with somatic symptoms may display abnormal illness behavior (Pilowsky 1969), which includes frequent health care utilization and doctor-switching to identify the medical causes of somatic symptoms, and frequent requests for medications and treatments (Duddu, Isaac, & Chaturvedi, 2006). Furthermore, avoidance of work, social tasks, and physical activity may develop due to functional limitations. They may complain of their symptoms to family members and their support network, who may reinforce these patterns through attention and taking away of social responsibilities (Kirmayer, 1999).

Social Models

Family history studies of somatoform disorders suggest that these disorders run in families, primarily among female relatives (Phillips, 2001). Anxiety and depression are common in the female relatives of people with somatization disorder (Garber, Walker, & Zeman, 1991). The male relatives of persons with somatization disorder also have higher than usual rates of alcoholism and personality disorders. Similarly, individuals with pain disorder tend to have family histories of psychological problems, most often pain disorder in the female relatives and alcoholism in the male relatives (Phillips, 2001). It is, however, not clear that the transmission of somatoform disorders in families has to do with genetics. A large study of over 3,400 twins could not determine whether genetics of shared environments were responsible for the aggregation within families of somatoform symptoms (Gillespie, Zhu, Heath, Hickie, & Martin, 2000). The children of parents with somatoform disorders may model their parents' tendencies to somatize distress (Craig, Boardman, Mills, Daly-Jones, & Drake, 1993). Parents who are somatizers also are more likely to neglect their children, and the children may learn that the only way to receive care and attention is to be ill. Some studies also indicated that individuals of somatoform disorders reported much childhood sickness and missing of school (Barsky, Wool, Barnett, & Cleary, 1994). They also tend to have an excessive amount of illness in their families while growing up, which may lead to memory bias of somatic problems (Pauli & Alpers, 2002). Chinese somatizers tended to report experiencing much more stress (daily hassles and financial strain) and less support from their family and friends than nonsomatizers (Mak & Zane, 2004).

Cultural Models

Somatization may be considered a cultural idiom of distress as the expression of physiological symptoms may be considered more acceptable than the expression of psychological symptoms among Asians and Asian Americans (Chen, 1995; Hong, Lee, & Lorenzo, 1995; Parker, Gladstone, & Chee, 2001; Tabora & Flaskerud, 1994). Cultural explanations along the lines of cultural values, language/semantic structure, and conception of health have been put forth to explain somatization among Asians and Asian Americans. Specifically, researchers have theorized that Chinese lack the vocabulary to express their emotions in psychological terms; therefore, they rely on physical metaphors to describe their affect (Kleinman, 1980; Kleinman & Kleinman, 1986). Some researchers claimed that Chinese somatize their affective states because they espouse the holistic conception of the mind and the body and do not differentiate the functions between these two systems (Chaplin, 1997; Kuo & Kavanagh, 1994). There are also some researchers who asserted that Chinese tend to suppress their negative emotions to preserve harmony in social interactions.

However, empirical evidence for the above explanations remains inconclusive. Studies have shown that when Chinese were directly asked about their distress, they can readily express it in psychological terms (Cheung, 1982; Cheung & Lau, 1982). Chinese psychiatric patients were able to acknowledge their affective states when they were directly asked (Cheung, Lau, & Waldmann, 1980–1981). They also were found to report different symptoms according to the settings in which they sought help (Cheung, 1982). Therefore, an alternative explanation may be that instead of replacing their psychological distress with somatic symptoms, Chinese are reporting different types of symptoms depending on the reporting situation and their routes of help-seeking.

In addition to the possible cultural influences on the somatizing tendencies among Asians and Americans, somatization may be comorbid with other psychiatric disorders. In the Chinese American Psychiatric Epidemiological Study (CAPES), using the SCL-90R somatization score, 12.9% of the 1,747 Chinese Americans meet the Somatic Symptom Index (SSI) 5/5 criterion for somatization. Among them, 29.5% and 19.6% of them met the *DSM* criteria for depression and anxiety disorders, respectively (Mak & Zane, 2004). A study on depressive symptom manifestation among 1,039 Taiwanese indicated that Chinese generally expressed more somatic complaints than cognitive-affective complaints; yet those who expressed depressive symptoms emphasized somatic symptoms less than did nondepressed respondents (H. Chang, 2007).

Furthermore, the somatization tendencies of Chinese may be in lieu of other psychiatric disorders. Rather than somatizing their depressive symptoms, recent clinical and epidemiological studies indicate that Chinese may be experiencing neurasthenia or *shenjing shuairuo*, independent from other Western diagnostic categories (D. F. Chang et al., 2005; Y. P. Zheng et al., 1997). Findings from these studies indicate that the reporting of somatic symptoms, as assessed by somatization, neurasthenia, or *shenjing shuairuo* by clinical and community samples might reflect their severe state of psychological distress that is comorbid with other psychiatric conditions. Moreover, these studies also showed that neurasthenia and *shenjing shuairuo* are distinct clinical conditions experienced by Chinese that do not necessarily overlap with any Western diagnoses.

Somatization tendencies were also related to help-seeking patterns, stress experiences, and the availability of social resources (Hoover, 1999). This issue is particularly salient among immigrant populations, whose experiences are often compounded by their lower access to health care, their level of stress and the social support they experienced and received in the host society. Research in help-seeking among Chinese showed that when the symptoms were perceived to be purely psychological in nature, Chinese prefer to rely on themselves or to seek the support of their friends or family. They would be more likely to seek medical or psychiatric attention if their symptoms were perceived to include a physical component (Cheung, 1987; Cheung, Lee, & Chan, 1983). Chinese Americans who met the Somatic Symptom Index 5/5 criterion were more likely to seek help from both Western and traditional Chinese doctors and to use both Western and traditional Chinese medicine than those who did not show signs of somatization. They were also more likely to seek help from psychiatrists, other medical doctors, and mental health specialists for their mental health problems than were nonsomatizers (Mak & Zane, 2004). Chinese Americans with somatoform disorders were also more likely to seek professional help than were those with depressive and anxiety disorders (Kung & Lu, 2008). All in all, the experience of somatization might be a result of severe psychological distress, excessive life strain, and a lack of social support in coping with stress among Asians and Asian Americans. Thus, the argument that Asians and Asian Americans translate their psychological distress into somatic symptoms appears to be oversimplifying the phenomenon of somatization as experienced by Asians and Asian Americans.

In addition to help-seeking behaviors, personality characteristics may provide the distal factors in explaining the individual differences in somatization tendency. Given that somatization is a common form of manifestation of psychopathology among the Chinese people, studying its relationship with culturally relevant personality features will inform the underlying dynamics of the illness experience. In particular, the interpersonal orientation emphasized in Chinese personality research would be relevant to the communicative nature of somatization. The development of the Chinese Personality Assessment Inventory (CPAI; Cheung, Leung, et al., 1996) using a combined emic-etic approach to include both universal and culturally relevant personality dimensions provided an opportunity for exploring this relationship.

The CPAI consists of a number of indigenously derived scales to assess culturally relevant personality and clinical features not readily available in Western personality measures. One personality factor, Interpersonal Relatedness, was found to be unique to the CPAI and contributed to the prediction of Chinese social behavior beyond the universal personality factors (Cheung, Leung, et al., 2001). The Interpersonal Relatedness factor includes scales that measures harmony, Renqing (reciprocal relationship orientation), and traditionalism. The Somatization scale of the CPAI focuses on the pattern of complaint presentation as part of the person's illness behavior (Cheung, 1995). Items on this scale cover the expression of personal and social distress in an idiom of physical symptomatology and the tendency to seek help for these distresses from medical practitioners instead of mental health professionals (Cheung, Leung, et al., 1996). The interpersonal dimension of illness behavior among Chinese patients suggests that the Interpersonal Relatedness factor of the CPAI is related to the somatization tendency.

Using the 1996 CPAI standardization sample, which consisted of 2,444 normal adults from different regions of Mainland China and Hong Kong, a multiple regression analysis was conducted. The four CPAI personality factors were entered to predict the Somatization scale. In particular, the additional contribution of the Interpersonal Relatedness factor beyond the other three universal personality factors was examined. The results showed that the Interpersonal Relatedness factor added another 16% to the variance explained by the other personality factors. The cumulative R^2 explained by all the CPAI personality factors was 50% (Cheung, Gan, & Lo, 2005). The contribution of individual CPAI personality scales to the prediction of Somatization further illustrated the specific personality features that were associated with the somatization tendency among normal Chinese people. Stepwise regression of the individual CPAI personality scales on the Somatization scale showed that Pessimism (vs. Optimism), Meanness (vs. Graciousness), Inferiority vs. Self-acceptance, and Emotionality scales that load on the Dependability factor are among the best predictors. In addition, high scores on the Face and Harmony scales, and low scores on the Flexibility and Modernization scales from the Interpersonal Relatedness factor were also strong predictors. In other words, individuals who tend to be more pessimistic, critical, emotional, and have a sense of inferiority while having a high concern for face and social harmony and are more traditional and less flexible are more likely to show a somatization tendency in their expression of distress.

Similar results were obtained with the revised version of the CPAI-2. Using the 2001 standardization sample data set, which consisted of a representative sample of 1,911 normal adults from different regions of Mainland China and Hong Kong (Cheung, Cheung, & Zhang, 2004), the regression results showed that the Interpersonal Relatedness factor added another 7% to the prediction of somatization beyond those contributed by the other three universal personality factors (i.e., Social Potency, Dependability, and Accommodation). The latter three personality factors from the CPAI-2 corresponded with the universal Big Five factors, whereas the Interpersonal Relatedness factor was unique to the CPAI-2 (Cheung, Cheung, Zhang, et al., 2008). Together, the four personality factors explained 47% of the total variance.

The contribution of the Interpersonal Relatedness factor to the prediction of somatization was even stronger in a large-scale clinical sample of Chinese psychiatric patients from Mainland China and Hong Kong (Cheung, Cheung, & Leung, 2008). A number of indigenously derived personality scales were particularly useful in predicting somatization among patients with depressive disorders. In particular, high scores in Traditionalism, Harmony and Ah Q Mentality (Defensiveness), and low scores in Family Orientation and Graciousness significantly predicted 46% of these patients' scores on Somatization. These personality correlates suggest when close family relationship is threatened, people who endorse more traditional values and social norms tend to avoid conflict and stigma associated with emotional distress and somatize their distress.

TREATING SOMATOFORM DISORDERS IN ASIANS

In recent years, more evidence on the efficacy of treatments for somatoform disorders has been published. This section will highlight some of the approaches that have been empirically supported in the treatment of somatoform disorders, as broadly defined by previous studies. Given very few clinical trials reported ethnic differences or focused on Asians or Asian Americans (Mak,

Law, Alvidrez, & Pérez-Stable, 2007), the evidence reviewed here is not specifically for Asians or Asian Americans.

Biological Approaches

Antidepressants in general were found to be efficacious in the treatment of different types of somatoform disorders. In a study of 67 patients with body dysmorphic disorder, fluoxetine (aka Prozac) was found to reduce obsessive-compulsive body dysmorphic disorder beliefs and behaviors compared with placebo (Phillips, Albertini, & Rasmussen, 2002). Another trial found venlafaxine (aka Effexor) to relieve reported pain of patients with multisomatoform disorder, but their somatic symptom scores showed no significant difference (Kroenke, Messina, Benattia, Graepel, & Musgnung, 2006). In a recent 12-week, randomized open-label trial of fluoxetine and sertraline (aka Zoloft) (Han et al., 2008), both fluoxetine and sertraline were found to reduce somatic symptoms (as measured by PHQ-15) and depressive symptoms (as measured by Beck Depression Inventory) among 45 patients with undifferentiated somatoform disorder at the end of treatment. No between-group differences were found. Three trials showed some effect of St. John's wort (Muller, Mannel, Murck, & Rahlfs, 2004; Volz, Murck, Kasper, & Moller, 2002) and opipramol (aka Insidon) (Volz, Moller, Reimann, & Stoll, 2000) for somatization-spectrum disorder (i.e., somatization disorder, abridged somatization disorder, undifferentiated somatoform disorder). However, Werneke (2005) commented that the exclusion of placebo responders after the placebo run-in phase in the Muller and colleagues' study (2004) may bias the results in favor of St. John's wort. Moreover, it must be noted that information on the optimum dosage, duration of treatment, or long-term outcome is still lacking. Thus, replication studies and more randomized controlled trials are necessary to clarify the effects of antidepressant medications on somatoform disorders (Sumathipala, 2007).

Few clinical trials on the treatment of somatoform disorders were found in the Chinese-language literature. Antidepressants were the most commonly used medications for treating somatoform disorders in Mainland China. Clinical trials on selective serotonin reuptake inhibitors (SSRIs) such as paroxetine (aka Paxil) (Jiang, Zhang, Sun, Zhang, & Shang-Guan, 2007; Xie & Deng, 2008; K. Zheng, Shi, & Liu, 2004), noradrenergic and selective serotonergic antidepressants (NaSSAs) such as mirtazapine (aka Remeron) (Zou, Wang, & Yang, 2006), and serotonin-norepinephrine reuptake inhibitors (SNRIs) such as venlafaxine (Xie & Deng, 2008) all demonstrated clinical significance in treating somatoform disorders. For paroxetine, it was found to reduce the number of self-reported depression and somatoform symptoms (Jiang et al., 2007; K. Zheng et al., 2004). Paroxetine was found to have similar effects as venlafaxine on 28 female patients with somatoform disorders on depression and anxiety symptoms, yet paroxetine showed fewer side effects (Xie & Deng, 2008). In another study, mirtazapine was found to reduce self-reported depression among 36 patients with somatoform disorders. Of the treated individuals, 85.6% had significant improvement in their somatoform symptoms (Zou, Wang, & Yang, 2006). It is noted that most of these studies have small sample sizes and are basic pre-post studies that lack a control group and a randomized design. Thus, more rigorously designed studies are necessary to further note the efficacy and effectiveness of antidepressants on Chinese with somatoform disorders.

Psychological Approaches

In recent systematic reviews of clinical trials (both nonrandomized and randomized) (Kroenke & Swindle, 2000; Kroenke, 2007; Nezu, Nezu, & Lombardo, 2001; Sumathipala, 2007), cognitive behavioral therapy (CBT) was found to be effective across a spectrum of somatoform disorders, including somatization disorder (Allen, Woolfolk, Escobar, Gara, & Hamer, 2006) and its lower threshold variants (i.e., abridged version of somatization disorder [McLeod, Budd, & McClelland, 1997; Sumathipala, Hewege, Hanwella, & Mann, 2000]), medically unexplained symptoms (Hellman, Budd, Borysenko, McClelland, & Benson, 1990; Lidbeck, 1997; Speckens et al., 1995), hypochondriasis (Barsky & Ahern, 2004; Clark et al., 1998; Visser & Bouman, 2001; Warwick, Clark, Cobb, & Salkovskis, 1996), and body dysmorphic disorder (Butters & Cash, 1987; Rosen, Reiter, & Orosan, 1995; Rosen, Saltzberg, & Srebnik, 1989; Veale, Gournay, Dryden, Boocock, Shah, Willson, & Walburn, 1996). The average effect size of CBT among the five published studies with this information was 1.78, which is considered a large effect. One nurse-administered intervention combined both antidepressants and cognitive behavioral therapy in the treatment of medically unexplained symptoms and was found to have a 16% difference compared to usual care (R. C. Smith et al., 2006). However, the format of CBT varies across studies, ranging from 30-minute individual session to 3-hour group session, and from 6 to 16 sessions. Moreover, content covers relaxation, stress management, exposure, and other components. Thus, the type of CBT administered was heterogeneous, and future studies need to replicate the findings and look into the components.

In addition to CBT, a psychiatric consultation letter written to the primary care physician on management strategies toward somatizing patients was found to improve physical functioning (Dickinson, Dickinson, deGruy, Main, Candib, & Rost, 2003) and reduce medical costs (Rost, Kashner, & Smith, 1994; G. R. Smith, Monson, & Ray, 1986; G. R. Smith, Rost, & Kashner, 1995), compared to usual care. However, such an approach did not reduce psychological distress, and none of the studies measured its effect in the reduction of somatic symptoms.

Attempts have also been done in assessing the effectiveness of training primary care physician in reattribution techniques compared with nonspecific psychosocial primary care in the treatment of patients with abridged somatization disorder. Reattribution basically involves three phases: (1) feeling understood, (2) changing the agenda, and (3) making the link (Goldberg, Gask, & O'Dowd, 1989; Sumathipala, 2007). Physical symptoms dropped in the reattribution group and the reduction was sustained at 6-month follow-up. However, improvement in physical functioning and reduction in depression and anxiety were no longer significant after controlling for baselines and covariates (Larisch, Schweickhardt, Wirsching, & Fritzsche, 2004). Thus, the effects of reattribution techniques were limited.

In all of the reviews, efficacy, and effectiveness studies on psychological approaches for somatoform disorders, effects were not analyzed separately by ethnic group, not to say on Asians and Asian Americans. All of the published studies found were conducted in Western countries, including the United States, United Kingdom, Netherlands, Australia, Sweden, and Germany. Thus, caution is necessary in evaluating the findings and applying the methods to patients who have different conceptions of the disorders, help-seeking patterns, and cultural values and beliefs.

CONCLUSION

The present chapter summarizes recent development in the understanding of the nosology, causes, and treatments of somatoform disorders and associated conditions. Based on our review of the literature, most of the studies conducted among Asians and Asian Americans focused on somatization rather than specific categories of somatoform disorders, and many studies are conducted either among Chinese samples or non-Asian samples. Thus, much more research needs to be done in examining the nosology, causes, and treatments of somatoform disorders for Asians and Asian Americans, particularly other non-Chinese Asian and Asian American groups. In this chapter, it is noted that there may be other forms of psychosomatic disorders (e.g., neurasthenia) that are distinct from somatoform disorders listed in the *DSM* yet are prevalent among Asians and Asian Americans. Researchers and clinicians need to pay attention to this possibility in studying and treating this population. Moreover, it may be worthwhile to consider the sociopolitical as well as the family context in which Asians and Asian Americans live so as to make better sense of their illness expression and reporting of somatic symptoms and somatization tendencies. Finally, although much clinical advance has been made in the treatment of somatoform disorders in the recent decade, very few studies included Asians and Asian Americans in their sampling, which limits the generalizability of the findings to this population. Given that Asians and Asian Americans constituted the majority of the world's population, it is imperative that empirical evidence be gathered in the development of a diagnostic system and treatment protocol that are sensitive and responsive to their needs.

REFERENCES

Akagi, H., & House, A. (2001). Epidemiology of conversion hysteria. In P. Halligan, C. Bass, & J. Marshall (Eds.), *Contemporary approaches to the study of hysteria* (pp. 73–86). Oxford: Oxford University Press.

Allen, L. A., & Woolfolk, R. L., Escobar, J. I, Gara, M. A., & Hamer, R. M. (2006). Cognitive-behavioral therapy for somatization disorder: A randomized controlled trial. *Archives of Internal Medicine, 166,* 1512–1518.

American Psychiatric Association (APA) (1968). *Diagnostic and statistical manual of mental disorders,* (2nd ed.). Washington DC: Author.

American Psychiatric Association . (1980). *Diagnostic and statistical manual of mental disorders* (3rd ed.). Washington, DC: Author.

American Psychiatric Association. (2000). *Diagnostic and Statistical Manual of Mental Disorders* (4th ed., text revision). Washington, DC: Author.

American Psychiatric Association. (2010). Somatoform disorders. Retrieved July 7, 2010 from http://www.dsm5.org/ProposedRevisions/Pages/SomatoformDisorders.aspx

Barsky, A. J., & Ahern, D. K. (2004). Cognitive behavior therapy for hypochondriasis: A randomized controlled trial. *Journal of the American Medical Association, 291,* 1464–1470.

Barsky, A. J., Orav, E. J., & Bates, D. W. (2005). Somatization increases medical utilization and costs independent of psychiatric and medical comorbidity. *Archives of General Psychiatry, 62,* 903–910.

Barsky, A. J., Wool, C., Barnett, M. C., & Cleary, P. D. (1994). Histories of childhood trauma in adult hypochondriacal patients. *American Journal of Psychiatry, 151,* 397–401.

Barsky, A. J., & Wyshak, G. (1990). Hypochondriasis and somatosensory amplification. *British Journal of Psychiatry, 157,* 404–409.

Beard, G. (1869). *American nervousness.* New York: Putnam.

Bell, I. R. (1994). Somatization disorder: Health care costs in the decade of the brain. *Biological Psychiatry, 35,* 81–83.

Binzer, M., & Kullgren, G. (1996). Conversion symptoms: What can we learn from previous studies? *Nordic Journal of Psychiatry, 50,* 143–152.

Bornschein, S., Hausteiner, C., Zilker, T., & Förstl, H. (2002). Psychiatric and somatic disorders and multiple chemical sensitivity (MCS) in 264 "environmental patients." *Psychological Medicine, 32,* 1387–1394.

Brosschot, J. F. (2002). Cognitive-emotional sensitization and somatic health complaints. *Scandinavian Journal of Psychology, 43,* 113–121.

Butters, J. W., & Cash, T. F. (1987). Cognitive-behavioral treatment of women's body-image dissatisfaction. *Journal of Consulting and Clinical Psychology, 55,* 889–897.

Canino, G. J., Bird, H. R., Shrout, P. E., Rubio-Stipec, M., Bravo, M., Martinez, R., et al. (1987). The prevalence of specific psychiatric disorders in Puerto Rico. *Archives of General Psychiatry, 44,* 727–735.

Canino, G. J., Rubio-Stipec, M., & Bravo, M. (1988). Psychiatric diagnostic classification in transcultural epidemiologic studies. *Acta psiquiátrica y psicológica de América Latina, 34,* 251–259.

Chang, D. F. (2002). Understanding the rates and distribution of mental disorders. In K. S. Kurasaki, S. Okazaki, S. Sue, *Asian American mental health: assessment theories and methods* (pp. 9–27). New York: Plenum Publishers.

Chang, D. F., Myers, H. F., Yeung, A., Zhang, Y., Zhao, J., & Yu, S. (2005). *Shenjing Shuairuo* and the DSM-IV diagnosis, distress, and disability in a Chinese primary care setting. *Transcultural Psychiatry, 42*(2), 204–218.

Chang, H. (2007). Depressive symptom manifestation and help-seeking among Chinese college students in Taiwan. *International Journal of Psychology, 42,* 200–206.

Chaplin, S. L. (1997). Somatization. In W. S. Tseng & J. Streltzer (Eds.), *Culture and psychopathology: A guide to clinical assessment,* (pp. 67–86). New York: Brunner/Mazel.

Chen, D. (1995). Cultural and psychological influences on mental health issues for Chinese Americans. In L. L. Adler & B. R. Mukherji (Eds.), *Spirit versus scalpel: Traditional healing and modern psychotherapy,* (pp. 185–196). Westport, CN: Bergin & Garvey.

Cheung, F.M. (1982). Somatization among Chinese: A critique. *Bulletin of the Hong Kong Psychological Society, 8,* 27–35.

Cheung, F. M. (1985) An overview of psychopathology in Hong Kong with special reference to somatic presentation. In W. S. Tseng & D. Y. H. Wu (Eds.), *Chinese culture and mental health* (pp. 287–304). Orlando, FL: Academic.

Cheung, F. M. (1987). Conceptualization of psychiatric illness and help-seeking behavior among Chinese. *Culture, Medicine, and Psychiatry, 11,* 97–106.

Cheung, F. M. (1995). Facts and myths about somatization among the Chinese. In T. Y. Lin, W. S. Tseng, & E. K. Yeh (Eds.), *Chinese society and mental health* (pp. 156–166). Hong Kong: Oxford University Press.

Cheung, F. M. (1998). Cross-cultural psychopathology. In C. D. Belar (Ed.), *Comprehensive psychiatry: Volume 10. Sociocultural and individual differences* (pp. 35–51). Oxford: Pergamon.

Cheung, F. M., Cheung, S. F., & Leung, F. (2008). Clinical utility of the Cross-Cultural (Chinese) Personality Assessment Inventory (CPAI-2) in the assessment of substance use disorders among Chinese men. *Psychological Assessment, 20,* 103–113.

Cheung, F. M., Cheung, S. F., & Zhang, J. X. (2004). What is "Chinese" personality? Subgroup differences in the Chinese Personality Assessment Inventory (CPAI-2). *Acta Psychologica Sinica, 36,* 491–499.

Cheung, F. M., Cheung, S. F., Zhang, J. X., Leung, K., Leong, F. T. L., & Yeh, K. H. (2008). Relevance of openness as a personality dimension in Chinese culture. *Journal of Cross-Cultural Psychology, 39,* 81–108.

Cheung, F. M., Gan, Y. Q., & Lo, P. M. (2005). Personality and psychopathology: Insight from Chinese studies. In W. S. Tseng, S. C. Chang, & M. Nishizono (Eds.), *Asian culture and psychotherapy: Implications for East and West* (pp. 21–39). Honolulu: University of Hawaii Press.

Cheung, F. M., & Lau, B. W. K. (1982). Situational variations of help-seeking behavior among Chinese patients. *Comprehensive Psychiatry, 23,* 252–262.

Cheung, F. M., Lau, B. W. K., & Waldmann, E. (1980–1981). Somatization among Chinese depressives in general practice. *International Journal of Psychiatry and Medicine, 10,* 361–374.

Cheung, F. M., Lee, S. Y., & Chan, Y. Y. (1983). Variations in problem conceptualization and intended solutions among Hong Kong students. *Culture, Medicine, and Psychiatry, 7,* 263–278.

Cheung, F. M., Leung, K., Fan, R. M., Song, W. Z., Zhang, J. X., & Zhang, J. P. (1996). Development of the Chinese Personality Assessment Inventory. *Journal of Cross-Cultural Psychology, 27,* 181–199.

Cheung, F. M., Leung, K., Zhang, J. X., Sun, H. F., Gan, Y., Song, W. Z., & Xie, D. (2001). Indigenous Chinese personality constructs: Is the Five-Factor Model complete? *Journal of Cross-Cultural Psychology, 32,* 407–433.

Cheung, P. (1991). Adult psychiatric epidemiology in China in the 80s. *Culture, Medicine, and Psychiatry, 15,* 479–496.

Chinese Psychiatric Society. (2001). *The Chinese classification of mental disorders* (3rd ed.). Shandong, China: Shandong Publishing House of Science and Technology. (CCMD-3)

Clark, D. M., Salkovskis, P. M., Hackmann, A., Wells, A., Fennell, M., Ludgate, J., et al. (1998). Two psychological treatments for hypochondriasis: A randomised controlled trial. *British Journal of Psychiatry, 173,* 218–225.

Craig, T. K. J., Boardman, A. P., Mills, K., Daly-Jones, O., & Drake, H. (1993). The South London somatisation study: I. Longitudinal course and the influence of early life experiences. *British Journal of Psychiatry, 163,* 579–588.

Creed, F., & Barsky, A. J. (2004). A systematic review of the epidemiology of somatisation disorder and hypochondriasis. *Journal of Psychosomatic Research, 56,* 391–408.

Dickinson, W. P., Dickinson, L. M., deGruy, F. V., Main, D. S., Candib, L. M., & Rost, K. (2003). A randomized clinical trial of a care recommendation letter intervention for somatization in primary care. *Annals of Family Medicine, 1,* 228–235.

Dimsdale, J. E., & Dantzer, R. (2007). A biological substrate for somatoform disorders: Importance of pathophysiology. *Psychosomatic Medicine, 69,* 850–854.

Draguns, J. G. (1996). Abnormal behaviour in Chinese societies: Clinical, epidemiological, and comparative studies. In M. H. Bond (Ed.), *The handbook of Chinese psychology* (pp. 412–428). Hong Kong: Oxford University Press.

Duddu, V., Isaac, M. K., & Chaturvedi, S. K. (2006). Somatization, somatosensory amplification, attribution styles, and illness behaviour: A review. *International Review of Psychiatry, 18,* 25–33.

Epidemiological Study Group of Mental Disorders in 12 Areas in China. (1986). 12 areas epidemiological survey of neuroses. *Chinese Journal of Neuropsychiatry, 19,* 87–91.

Eriksen, H. R., & Ursin, H. (2002). Sensitization and subjective health complaints. *Scandinavian Journal of Psychology, 43,* 189–196.

Eriksen, H. R., & Ursin, H. (2004). Subjective health complaints, sensitization, and sustained cognitive activation (stress). *Journal of Psychosomatic Research, 56,* 445–448.

Faravelli, C., Salvatori, S., Galassi, F., Aiazzi, L., Drei, C., & Cabras, P. (1997). Epidemiology of somatoform disorders: A community survey in Florence. *Social Psychiatry and Psychiatric Epidemiology, 32,* 24–29.

Feder, A., Olfson, M., Gameroff, M., Fuentes, M., Shea, S., Lantigua, R. A., et al. (2001). Medically unexplained symptoms in an urban general medicine practice. *Psychosomatics, 42,* 261–268.

Fink, P., Hansen, M. S., & Oxhøj, M.-L. (2004). The prevalence of somatoform disorders among internal medical inpatients. *Journal of Psychosomatic Research, 56,* 413–418.

Garber, J., Walker, L. S., & Zeman, J. (1991). Somatization symptoms in a community sample of children and adolescents: Further validation of the Children's Somatization Inventory. *Psychological Assessment, 3,* 588–595.

Gillespie, N. A., Zhu, G., Heath, A. C., Hickie, I. B., & Martin, N. G. (2000). The genetic aetiology of somatic distress. *Psychological Medicine, 30,* 1051–1061.

Goldberg, D., Gask, L., & O'Dowd, T. (1989). The treatment of somatization: Teaching techniques of reattribution. *Journal of Psychosomatic Research, 33,* 689–695.

Golding, J. M., Smith, R., & Kashner, T. M. (1991). Does somatization disorder occur in men? Clinical characteristics of women and men with multiple unexplained somatic symptoms. *Archives of General Psychiatry, 48,* 231–235.

Gureje, O., Simon, G. E., Üstün, T. B., & Goldberg, D. P. (1997). Somatization in cross-cultural perspective: A World Health Organization study in primary care. *American Journal of Psychiatry, 154,* 989–995.

Hakala, M., Karlsson, H., Ruotsalainen, U., Koponen, S., Bergman, J., Stenman, H., et al. (2002). Severe somatization in women is associated with altered cerebral glucose metabolism. *Psychological Medicine, 32,* 1379–1385.

Han, C., Pae, C.-U., Lee, B. H., Ko, Y.-H. Masand, P. S., Patkar, A. A., et al. (2008). Fluoxetine versus sertraline in the treatment of patients with undifferentiated somatoform disorder: A randomized, open-label, 12-week, parallel-group trial. *Progress in Neuropsychopharmacology and Biological Psychiatry, 32,* 437–444.

Hare, E. (1969). *Triennial statistical report of the Royal Maudsley and Bethlem Hospitals.* London: Bethlem and Maudsley Hospitals.

Hellman, C. J. C., Budd, M., Borysenko, J., McClelland, D. C., & Benson, H. (1990). A study of the effectiveness of two group behavioral medicine interventions for patients with psychosomatic complaints. *Behavioral Medicine, 16,* 165–173.

Hinton, D., Ba, P., Peou, S., & Um, K. (2000). Panic disorder among Cambodian refugees attending a psychiatric clinic: Prevalence and subtypes. *General Hospital Psychiatry, 22,* 437–444.

Hinton, D., Um, K., & Ba, P. (2001). Kyol goeu ("wind overload"): Part I. A cultural syndrome of orthostatic panic among Khmer refugees. *Transcultural Psychiatry, 38,* 403–432.

Hoover, C. R. (1999). Somatization disorders. In E. J. Kramer, S. L. Ivey, & Y. W. Ying (Eds.), *Immigrant women's health: Problems and solutions* (pp. 233–241). San Francisco, CA: Jossey-Bass.

Ironside, R., & Batchelor, I. R. C. (1945). The ocular manifestations of hysteria in relation to flying. *British Journal of Ophthalmology, 29,* 88–98.

Jiang, X., Zhang, J., Sun, Y., Zhang, Y., & Shang-Guan, S. (2007). Clinical studies of paroxetine hydrochloride in the treatment of somatoform disorder [in Chinese]. *Chinese Journal of Practical Medicine, 34,* 27–28.

Katon, W., Sullivan, M., & Walker, E. (2001). Medical symptoms without identified pathology: Relationship to psychiatric disorders, childhood and adult trauma, and personality traits. *Annals of Internal Medicine, 134,* 917–925.

Kirmayer, L. J. (1999). Rhetorics of the body: Medically unexplained symptoms in sociocultural perspective. In Y. Ono, A. Janca, M. Asai, & N. Sartorius (Eds.), *Somatoform disorders: A worldwide perspective* (pp. 271–286). Tokyo: Springer-Verlag.

Kirmayer, L. J., Robbins, J. M., & Paris, J. (1994). Somatoform disorders: Personality and the social matrix of somatic distress. *Journal of Abnormal Psychology, 103,* 125–136.

Kirmayer, L. J., & Taillefer, S. (1997). Somatoform disorders. In S. Turner & M. Hersen (Eds.), *Adult Psychopathology* (3rd ed., pp. 333–383). New York: Wiley.

Kleinman, A. (1977). Depression, somatization, and the "new cross-cultural psychiatry." *Social Science and Medicine, 11,* 3–10.

Kleinman, A. (1982). Neurasthenia and depression: A study of somatization and culture in China. *Culture, Medicine, and Psychiatry, 6,* 117–190.

Kleinman A. (1980). The cultural construction of illness experience and behavior: 2. A model of somatization of dysphoric affects and affective disorders. In A. Kleinman (Ed.), *Patients and healers in the context of culture: An exploration of the borderland between anthropology, medicine, and psychiatry,* (pp. 146–178). Berkeley: University of California Press.

Kleinman, A. (1986). *Social origins of distress and disease: Neurasthenia, depression, and pain in modern China.* New Haven, CT: Yale University Press.

Kleinman, A., & Kleinman, J. (1986). Somatization: The interconnections in Chinese society among culture, depressive experiences, and the meanings of pain. In A. Kleinman (Ed.), *Social origins of distress and disease: depression, neurasthenia, and pain in modern China* (pp. 449–490). New Haven, CT: Yale University Press.

Kroenke, K. (2007). Efficacy of treatment for somatoform disorders: A review of randomized controlled trials. *Psychosomatic Medicine, 69,* 881–888.

Kroenke, K. Messina, N., Benattia, I., Graepel, J., & Musgnung, J. (2006). Venlafaxine extended release in the short-term treatment of depressed and anxious primary care patients with multisomatoform disorder. *Journal of Clinical Psychiatry, 67,* 72–80.

Kroenke, K., Spitzer, R. L., deGruy, F. V., Hahn, S. R., Linzer, M. Williams, J. B., et al. (1997). Multisomatoform disorder: An alternative to undifferentiated somatoform disorder for the somatizing patient in primary care. *Archives of General Psychiatry, 54,* 352–358.

Kroenke, K., & Swindle, R. (2000). Cognitive behavioral therapy for somatization and symptom syndromes: A critical review of controlled clinical trials. *Psychotherapy and Psychosomatics, 69,* 205–215.

Kung, W. W., & Lu, P. C. (2008). How symptom manifestations affect help seeking for mental health problems among Chinese Americans. *Journal of Nervous and Mental Disease, 196,* 46–54.

Kuo, C. L., & Kavanagh, K. H. (1994). Chinese perspectives on culture and mental health. *Issues in Mental Health Nursing, 15,* 551–567.

Larisch, A., Schweickhardt, A., Wirsching, M., & Fritzsche, K. (2004). Psychosocial interventions for somatizing patients by the general practitioner: A randomized controlled trial. *Journal of Psychosomatic Research, 57,* 507–514.

Lee, J., Lei, A., & Sue, S. (2001). The current state of mental health research on Asian Americans. *Journal of Human Behavior in the Social Environment, 3,* 159–178.

Lee, S. (1999). Diagnosis postponed: *Shenjing shuairuo* and the transformation of psychiatry in post-Mao China. *Culture, Medicine, and Psychiatry, 23,* 349–380.

Lee, S., & Kleinman, A. (2007). Are somatoform disorders changing with time? The case of neurasthenia in China. *Psychosomatic Medicine, 69,* 846–849.

Lidbeck, J. (1997). Group therapy for somatization disorders in general practice: Effectiveness of a short cognitive-behavioural treatment model. *Acta Psychiatrica Scandinavica, 96,* 14–24.

Lim S., & Kim J. (2005). Cognitive processing of emotional information in depression, panic, and somatoform disorder. *Journal of Abnormal Psychology, 114,* 50–61.

Lin, K. M., Inui, T. & Kleinman, A. (1982). Sociocultural determinants of the help-seeking behavior of patients with mental illness, *Journal of Nervous and Mental Disease, 170*(2), 78–85.

Lin, K. M., Lau, J. K. C., Yamamoto, J., Zheng, Y. P., Kim, H. S., Cho, K. H., & Nagasaki, G. (1992). Hwa-Byung: A community study of Korean Americans. *Journal of Nerve Mental Disorders, 180*(6), 386–391.

Lin, T. Y. (1992). Neurasthenia revisited: Its place in modern psychiatry. *Psychiatric Annals, 22* (4), 173–187.

Liu, X. H., & Song, W. (1986). An epidemiological study of neuroses in Chengdu city. *Chinese Journal of Neuropsychiatry, 19,* 318–321.

Looper, K., & Kirmayer, L. J. (2002). Behavioral medicine approaches to somatoform disorders. *Journal of Consulting and Clinical Psychology, 70,* 810–827.

Mak, W. W. S., & Law, R.W., Alvidrez, J, & Pérez-Stable, E. J. (2007). Gender and ethnic diversity in NIMH-funded clinical trials: Review of a decade of published research. *Administration and Policy in Mental Health and Mental Health Services Research, 34,* 497–503.

Mak, W. W. S., & Zane, N. W. S. (2004). The phenomenon of somatization among community Chinese Americans. *Social Psychiatry and Psychiatric Epidemiology, 39*(12), 967–974.

Mayou, R., Kirmayer, L. J., Simon, G., Kroenke, K., & Sharpe, M. (2005). Somatoform disorders: time for a new approach in DSM-V. *American Journal of Psychiatry, 162*(5), 847–855.

Mayville, S., Katz, R., Gipson, M., & Cabral, K. (1999). Assessing the prevalence of body dysmorphic disorder in an ethnically diverse group of adolescents. *Journal of Child and Family Studies, 8,* 357–362.

McLeod, C. C., Budd, M. A., & McClelland, D. C. (1997). Treatment of somatization in primary care. *General Hospital Psychiatry, 19,* 251–258.

Moore, L. J. & Boehnlein (1991). Treating psychiatric disorders among Mien refugees from highland Laos. *Social Science and Medicine, 32*(9), 1029–1036.

Muller, T., Mannel, M., Murck, H., & Rahlfs, V. W. (2004). Treatment of somatoform disorders with St. John's wort: A randomized, double-blind and placebo-controlled trial. *Psychosomatic Medicine, 66,* 538–547.

Nezu, A. M., Nezu, C. M., & Lombardo, E. R. (2001). Cognitive behavioural therapy for medically unexplained symptoms: A critical review of the treatment. *Behavior Therapy, 32,* 537–583.

Noyes, R., Jr., Langbehn, D. R., Happel, R. L., Stout, L. R., Muller, B. A., & Longley, S. L. (2001). Personality dysfunction among somatizing patients. *Psychosomatics, 42,* 320–329.

Ormel, J. Vonkorff, M., Üstün, T. B., Pini, S., Korten, A., & Oldehinkel, T. (1994). Common mental disorders and disability across cultures: Results from the WHO Collaborative Primary Care study. *Journal of the American Medical Association, 272,* 1741–1748.

Owens, K. M. B., Asmundson, G. J. G., Hadjistavropoulos, T., & Owens, T. J. (2004). Attentional bias toward illness threat in individuals with elevated health anxiety. *Cognitive Therapy and Research, 28,* 57–66.

Pauli, P., & Alpers, G. W. (2002). Memory bias in patients with hypochondriasis and somatoform pain disorder. *Journal of Psychosomatic Research, 60,* 199–209.

Phillips, K. A. (2001). Body dysmorphic disorder. In K. A. Phillips, *Somatoform and factitious disorders* (pp. 67–94). Washington, DC: American Psychiatric Publishing.

Phillips, K. A., Albertini, R. S., & Rasmussen, S. A. (2002). A randomized placebo-controlled trial of fluoxetine in body dysmorphic disorder. *Archives of General Psychiatry, 59,* 381–388.

Phillips, K.A., McElroy, S.L., Hudson, J.I., & Pope, H.G., Jr. (1995). Body dysmorphic disorder: An obsessive-compulsive spectrum disorder, a form of affective spectrum disorder, or both? *Journal of Clinical Psychiatry, 56* (Suppl. 4), 41–51.

Pilowsky, I. (1969). Abnormal illness behaviour. *British Journal of Medicine and Psychology, 42,* 347–351.

Pu, T., Mohamed, E., Imam, K., & El-Roey, A. M. (1986). One hundred cases of hysteria in eastern Libya: A socio-demographic study. *British Journal of Psychiatry, 148,* 606–609.Rief, W., Nanke, A., Emmerich, J., Bender, A., & Zech, T. (2004). Causal illness attributions in somatoform disorders: Associations with comorbidity and illness behaviour. *Journal of Psychosomatic Research, 57,* 367–371.

Rief, W., Nanke, A., Emmerich, J., Bender, A., & Zech, T. (2004). Causal illness attributions in somatoform disorders: Associations with comorbidity and illness behaviour. *Journal of Psychosomatic Research, 57,* 367–371.

Rosen, J. C., Reiter, J., & Orosan, P. (1995). Cognitive-behavioral body image therapy for body dysmorphic disorder. *Journal of Consulting and Clinical Psychology, 63,* 263–269.

Rosen, J. C., Saltzberg, E., & Srebnik, D. (1989). Cognitive behavior therapy for negative body image. *Behavior Therapy, 20,* 293–404.

Rost, K., Kashner, T. M., & Smith, G. R. (1994). Effectiveness of psychiatric intervention with somatization disorder patients: Improved outcomes at reduced costs. *General Hospital Psychiatry, 16,* 381–387.

Sharpe, M., & Bass, C. (1992). Pathophysiological mechanisms in somatization. *International Review of Psychiatry, 4,* 81–97.

Sharpe, M. & Mayou, R. (2004) Somatoform disorders: a help or hindrance to good patient care? *British Journal of Psychiatry, 184,* 465–467.

Shaw, J., & Creed, F. (1991). The cost of somatization. *Journal of Psychosomatic Research, 35,* 307–312.

Sensky, T., MacLeod, A. K., & Rigby, M. F. (1996). Causal attributions about common somatic sensations among frequent general practice attenders. *Psychological Medicine, 26,* 641–646.

Shorter, E. (1992). *From paralysis to fatigue: A history of psychosomatic illness in the modern era.* New York: Free Press.

Showalter, E. (1997). *Hystories: Hysterical epidemics and modern media.* New York: Columbia University Press.

Smith, G. R., Monson, R. A., & Ray, D. C. (1986). Psychiatric consultation in somatization disorder: A randomized controlled study. *New England Journal of Medicine, 314,* 1407–1413.

Smith, G. R., Rost, K., & Kashner, T. M. (1995). A trial of the effect of a standardized psychiatric consultation on health outcomes and costs in somatizing patients. *Archives of General Psychiatry, 52,* 238–243.

Smith, R. C., Lyles, J. S., Gardiner, J. C., Sirbu, C., Hodges, A., Collins, C., et al. (2006). Primary care clinicians treat patients with medically unexplained symptoms: A randomized controlled trial. *Journal of General Internal Medicine, 21,* 671–677.

Speckens, A. E. M., van Hemert, A. M., Spinhoven, P., Hawton, K. E., Bolk, J. H., & Rooijmans, G. M. (1995). Cognitive behavioural therapy for medically unexplained physical symptoms: A randomized controlled trial. *British Medical Journal, 311,* 1328–1332.

Sumathipala, A. (2007). What is the evidence for the efficacy of treatments for somatoform disorders? A critical review of previous intervention studies. *Psychosomatic Medicine, 69,* 889–900.

Sumathipala, A. Hewege, S., Hanwella, R., & Mann, A. H. (2000). Randomized controlled trial of cognitive behaviour therapy for repeated consultations for medically unexplained complaints: A feasibility study in Sri Lanka. *Psychological Medicine, 30,* 747–757.

Swartz, M., Landerman, R., George, L., Blazer, D., & Escobar, J. I. (1991). Somatization disorder. In L. Robins & D. A. Regier (Eds.), *Psychiatric disorders in America* (pp. 220–257). New York: Free Press.

Tabora, B., & Flaskerud, J. H. (1994). Depression among Chinese Americans: A review of the literature. *Issues in Mental Health Nursing, 15,* 569–584.

Taylor, S., & Asmundson, G. J. G. (2004). *Treating health anxiety: A cognitive behavioral approach.* New York: Guilford.

Tseng, W. S. (1975). The nature of somatic complaints among psychiatric patients: The Chinese case. *Comprehensive Psychiatry, 16,* 237–245.

Tseng, W. S. (2001). *Handbook of cultural psychiatry.* San Diego, CA: Academic.

Tung, M. P. M. (1994). Symbolic meanings of the body in Chinese culture and somatization. *Culture, Medicine, and Psychiatry, 18,* 483–492.

van Ommeren, M., de Jong, J. T., Sharma, B., Komproe, I., Thapa, S. B., & Cardeña, E. (2001). Psychiatric disorders among tortured Bhutanese refugees in Nepal. *Archives of General Psychiatry, 58,* 475–482.

Veale, D., Gournay, K., Dryden, W., Boocock, A., Shah, F., Willson, R., et al. (1996). Body dysmorphic disorder: A cognitive behavioural model and pilot randomised controlled trial. *Behaviour Research and Therapy, 34,* 717–729.

Visser, S., & Bouman, T. K. (2001). The treatment of hypochondriasis: Exposure plus response prevention vs cognitive therapy. *Behaviour Research and Therapy, 39,* 423–442.

Volz, H. P., Moller, H. J., Reimann, I., & Stoll, K. D. (2000). Opipramol for the treatment of somatoform disorders results from a placebo-controlled trial. *European Neuropsychopharmacology, 10,* 211–217.

Volz, H. P., Murck, H., Kasper, S., & Moller, H. J. (2002). St John's wort extract (LI 160) in somatoform disorders: Results of a placebo-controlled trial. *Psychopharmacology (Berl), 164,* 294–300.

Waller, E., & Scheidt, C. E. (2006). Somatoform disorders as disorders of affect regulation: A development perspective. *International Review of Psychiatry, 18,* 13–24.

Warwick, H. M., Clark, D. M., Cobb, A. M., & Salkovskis, P. M. (1996). A controlled trial of cognitive-behavioural treatment of hypochondriasis. *British Journal of Psychiatry, 169,* 189–195.

Werneke, U. (2005). St. John's Wort improves somatoform disorders. *Evidence-Based Mental Health, 8,* 13.

World Health Organization. (1992). *The ICD-10 classification of mental and behavior disorders—Clinical descriptions and diagnostic guidelines.* Geneva, Switzerland: WHO.

Xie, X., & Deng, S. (2008). A comparative study of paroxetine in the treatment of woman somatization disorder [in Chinese]. *Acta Medicinae Sinica, 21,* 431–432.

Yew Schwartz, P. (1999). Neurasthenia. In E. J. Kramer, S. L. Ivey, & Y. W. Ying (Eds.), *Immigrant women's health: Problems and solutions* (pp. 242–248). San Francisco, CA: Jossey-Bass.

Zhang, A. Y., & Snowden, L. R. (1999). Ethnic characteristics of mental disorders in five U.S. communities. *Cultural Diversity and Ethnic Minority Psychology, 5,* 134–146.

Zhang, M. Y. (1989). The diagnosis and phenomenology of neurasthenia. A Shanghai study. *Culture, Medicine and Psychiatry, 13* (2), 147–161.Zheng, K., Shi, T., & Liu, X. (2004). Rehabilitation therapy for the elder inpatients with depressive symptom [in Chinese]. *Chinese Journal of Rehabilitation, 19,* 345–346.

Zheng, K., Shi, T., & Liu, X. (2004). Rehabilitation therapy for the elder inpatients with depressive symptom [in Chinese]. *Chinese Journal of Rehabilitation, 19,* 345–346.

Zheng, Y. P., Lin, K. M., Takeuchi, D., Kurasaki, K. S., Wang, Y., & Cheung, F. (1997). An epidemiological study of neurasthenia in Chinese-Americans in Los Angeles. *Comprehensive Psychiatry, 38,* 249–259.

Zheng, Y. P., Xu, L. Y., & Shen, Y. Q. (1986). Styles of verbal expression of emotional and physical experiences: A study of depressed patients and normal controls in China. *Culture, Medicine, and Psychiatry, 10,* 231–243.

Ziegler, F. J., Imboden, J. B., & Meyer, E. (1960). Contemporary conversion reactions: Clinical study. *American Journal of Psychiatry, 116,* 901–910.

Zou, H., Wang, Z., & Yang, R. (2006). Clinical studies of mirtazapine in the treatment of somatoform disorder [in Chinese]. *Journal of Clinical Psychosomatic Diseases, 12,* 28–29.

| 9 |

DISSOCIATION, CONVERSION, AND POSSESSION DISORDERS IN ASIANS

Wen-Shing Tseng and Cong Zhong

IDENTIFYING DISSOCIATION, CONVERSION, AND POSSESSION DISORDERS IN ASIANS

In this chapter, three disorders will be reviewed and discussed, namely: dissociation, conversion, and possession disorders in Asians. These three disorders are closely related, particularly concerning the core of their pathology and etiology, even though they are categorized as different disorders from a phenomenological point of view in the *Diagnostic and Statistical Manual of Mental Disorders* (*DSM*) classification system. The *DSM* system is basically descriptive in nature and based on clinical experiences with a mainly Western patient population, and some clinical disorders observed in Eastern patient populations are not adequately and suitably included. This is particularly true for the three disorders that are going to be reviewed in this chapter.

From a medical historical point of view, dissociation disorder and conversion disorder are considered merely subtypes of what was in the past called hysterical disorder. The term "hysteria" was invented in ancient times by Greek medical practitioners to refer to the acute onset of motor-sensory dysfunction and/or an alternate consciousness state of a transient nature, usually occurring in response to psychological stress. It was considered at the time to be a disorder of females, induced by an emotional cause (often sexual in nature), and believed to be due to the dislocation of the uterus; thus, it was named "hysteria" (literally meaning disorder of the uterus).

Current DSM Nosology and Criteria for Dissociation, Conversion, and Possession Disorders

Although hysteria was misnamed by interpreting it as a disorder caused by the dislocation of the uterus, the term "hysteria" is useful in referring to the acute mental and somatic conditions that usually occur in response to psychological stress. It is helpful clinically to manage a disorder of this nature by working on the cause of the disorder. Therefore, the term was used clinically in modern psychiatry throughout both the West and the East until 1980.

When the *DSM-II* was developed in the United States (APA, 1982), it undertook a radical change, using a descriptive approach and discarding the etiological base for classification. The etiological term "hysteria" was then abolished, and the original subtypes of hysteria, namely: dissociation and conversion, were split into different diagnostic categories, depending on their cardinal clinical symptomatologies.

However, in the International Statistical Classification of Diseases and Related Health Problems, Tenth Revision (ICD-10), revised in 1992 by the World Health Organization (WHO) for international use, even the ancient and misnamed term "hysteria" is no longer used, replaced by the compound diagnostic term "dissociative [conversion] disorders" for a diagnosis (F44) in ICD-10, referring to the hysteria disorder of the past. Regarding dissociative (conversion) disorders, ICD-10 reads: "The common themes that are shared by dissociative or conversion disorders are a partial or complete loss of the normal integration between memories of the past, awareness of identity and immediate sensations, and control of body movement." Under dissociative or conversion disorders are the subtypes of dissociative amnesia (F44.0), dissociative fugue (F44.1), dissociative stupor (F44.2), trance and possession disorders (F44.3), dissociative motor disorders (F44.4), dissociative convulsions (F44.5), dissociative amnesia, and sensory loss (F44.6), to include all the possible clinical manifestations that were referred to as hysteria in the past. Further, it is explained that: "All types of dissociated disorders tend to remit after a few weeks or months, if the onset is associated with a traumatic life event."

For the *DSM-IV-TM* (APA, 1994), published two years later in 1994, under the category of dissociative disorder, besides including the subtypes of dissociative amnesia (300.12), and dissociative fugue (300.13), similar to ICD-10, there are the additional subtypes of dissociative identity disorder (300.14) (formerly referred to as multiple personality disorder), and depersonalization disorder (300.6). As for conversion disorder, it is separately classified, under the group of somatoform disorders, and maintains its own category (300.11). The subtypes considered involve motor symptoms or deficit, sensory symptoms or deficit, and seizures or convulsions.

Thus, according to different classifications, different categories are used, and certain subtypes are included or neglected, reflecting the clinical situations that exist in various societies. An example is dissociative identity disorder (previously, multiple-personality disorder), a diagnostic term relatively commonly used in American society today, but not in Asian societies; whereas possession disorder is a clinical term used relatively frequently in Asia, while not in Western societies.

Spectrum from Normal to Pathological

In discussing the mental phenomena related to dissociation or possession, it is very important to entertain the concept of the spectrum from normal to pathological. It is the view taken in dynamic psychiatry (but not in descriptive psychiatry, which is adopted by the *DSM* classification system) that mental phenomena, including disorders, exist on a spectrum from normal to pathological rather than as clearly defined, static nosological disorders. This view is applicable particularly for phenomena relating to minor psychiatric disorders, such as anxiety, depression, or obsession, and more so regarding the phenomena of dissociation or possession.

Concerning the phenomena of dissociation, we know that many normal people go into a transient trance or dissociative state during their daily lives. To enter a trance or a dissociated mental condition during the practice of meditation is a well-known phenomenon, not to be confused with a pathological dissociative state. Between the normal and pathological conditions of dissociation, there is a unique phenomenon called *latah*, mainly observed among people in Malaysia. The person, after being startled, will suddenly fall into a trance state and behave like a different person—that is, an altered personality. In this condition the person will talk, act, and behave as if he/she is a different person, ignoring sociocultural restrictions and manifesting uninhibited and usually erotic behavior. Usually, the person will claim no recollection of what happened during the episode. Since neither the person nor others claim that he/she was possessed by "another" being, this is not categorized as a "possessed state." However, the audience's explanation is that the person is not him/herself during the attack, and, therefore, any behavior of an obscene but amusing nature during the episode is socially excused. Furthermore, on most such occasions, the *latah* episode occurs to a person who is not facing recognizable stress. The phenomenon tends to be provoked by others for the social function of amusement—with the person acting as a clown on social occasions. Thus, by nature, the majority of *latah* attacks are accepted as "ordinary" behavior by the local people. The only exception is when the person manifests harmful behavior toward him- or herself or others during the attack. Then the episode is labeled professionally as "malignant *latah*," implying that it is a morbid condition (Tseng, 2001, pp. 245–251). The phenomenon of *latah* is observed not only in Malaysia but also in other areas in Asia, for instance, as *imu* among the Ainu in Japan in the past, or *maili-mali* in the Philippines, *young-dah-het* in Burma, or *bah-tsche* in Thailand (Tseng, 2001, p. 250).

Possession, or the possessed state, is considered normal in two circumstances: when healers are possessed by guardian god(s) during a healing ceremony so that, in the name of the supernatural power, they can perform healing practices. This is observed in many folk healing practices of mediumship around the world, also known as shamanism; the other circumstance is when the client(s) becomes possessed during the healing ceremony. In this condition, the individual client will complain about his/her problems and request a way to remove or resolve them. More than one client can fall into a possessed state during the ceremony. This is known to occur in Zar cult ceremonies observed in Arabian societies, or Salvation cult ceremonies in Japan (Tseng, 2001, pp. 326–329).

The common features of these (normal) possessed states are that, under particular circumstances, with certain methods of induction, the person can enter into the possessed state by his/her own will, and can also at will reverse the state of being possessed and resume his/her ordinary condition. In other words, the state can be invoked for the needed period of time under the voluntary control of the person involved. Possessed states can also fulfill certain social functions, or healing practices. The normal phenomenon of a possessed state is different from pathological possession, which occurs as disturbing behavior.

Anthropological Studies of Phenomena

Concerning the trance and possession state, as observed in ordinary life in society, cultural anthropologist Erika Bourguignon (1973) carried out studies by drawing a worldwide sample of 488 societies (mostly traditional) from Murdock's Ethnographic Atlas. She reported that 437 (or 90%) of these societies have institutionalized some form of altered state of consciousness. Furthermore, she pointed out that there is a relationship between types of altered states manifested by the members of society and societal characteristics reflecting variations in complexity. Social complexity is defined sociologically by matters such as size of population or community, the complexity of jurisdictional hierarchy, stratification of the social structure, and so on. She pointed out that the less complex a society, the more likely it is to recognize a trance state, while a more complex society is more likely to recognize a possession trance.

Bourguignon (1976) interpreted trance as an intrapersonal psychic event. In contrast, possession involves the impersonation of another being on an occasion when there are witnesses. As such it is an interpersonal event because the witnesses and the audience have a crucial role to play in the event. In other words, a possession state, in contrast to a simple trance state, involves a much more complex psychic function.

Based on her studies of Sub-Saharan Africa, another anthropologist, Lenora Greenbaum (1973), speculated that mediumistic possession trance is more likely to exist in rigid societies than in more flexible ones. She interpreted the medium acting as the spirit, which may make it possible for the individual, the client, to be provided with solutions for some of his/her problems in ways that circumvent the rigid demands of the society. The client follows the social constraints in that he/she relies on an external authority, a spirit speaking through the medium, to get authorization for his actions.

In order to make a clear distinction between an institutionalized possessed state and a morbid possession disorder, anthropologist C. A. Ward (1980) suggested using the term "ritual possession" for the former and "pathological possession" for the latter. He elaborated further that ritual possession tends to occur to those who are respected by society, serve as religious persons or healers, and/or those who are "central" members of society; whereas, pathological possession often occurs to those who are "peripheral" members of society.

The distinction between central and peripheral members in terms of ritual and morbid possession is valid only in societies where folk healers are highly regarded. In some societies, they are not. For instance, it was found that in Japan and Taiwan there are several pathways a person may take to become a professional shaman: through formal selection and training of suitable candidates, or the self-conversion of a formal mentally ill person into a healer after self-training (Sasaki, 1969; Tseng, 1972). In Korea, it was called *shin-byung* (divine illness) when a person developed the mental disorder of possession first, and then converted into a shaman (Yongmi, 2000; Kim, 1973), which was interpreted dynamically as a mentally ill person projecting his distress into a shamanistic value, namely, an unconscious trial for reintegrating the disorganized ego to culturally approved norms. Therefore, a mentally sick person often converts into a folk healer after long, hard runs of coping with the distress.

In order to describe the situation in Asian societies and to utilize the data they reported based on the diagnostic criteria they used, the various forms of dissociation, conversion, and possession disorders will be reviewed and elaborated according to the groups of hysterical disorders, possession disorders, and the related clinical phenomena of epidemic hysteria, possession psychoses, and alternate-personality disorders.

Hysterical Disorders in Asians

CLINICAL MANIFESTATION OF HYSTERICAL DISORDERS

In this section, the clinical condition of hysteria will be reviewed as a diagnostic entity, as used clinically or in literature, which broadly includes the clinical phenomenon of an episode of emotional turmoil, a dissociative state, a conversion, or even a possession state, as used in the past or as currently used in Asian societies.

China

Gao (1996) reported clinical data on 675 cases of hysteria that had been treated in his general hospital in Shu County of Anhui Province in the northern part of China over a 10-year period, from 1983 to 1993. Most of the patients were farmers from the countryside. Gao reported that there were 102 male cases and 573 female cases, indicating a male/female ratio of 1:5.6, much greater prevalence among females. Of the cases, 102 were single, whereas 573 were married (16 cases divorced or lost spouses). Regarding their level of education, all were below junior high, and 385 cases (57.3%) were illiterate. The average age of first onset was about 32 years old, meaning the majority of them were married, young-adult women. Most of them had obvious psychological precipitating factors, which included family conflict (231 cases), family-plan-related problems (53 cases), problems relating to physical illness (120 cases), conflict in social life (96 cases), and, interestingly enough, emotional stress caused by unfavorable responses received from fortune-telling (44 cases). Many symptoms were noted for frequency of occurrence: emotional turmoil condition (372 cases), possessed state (250 cases), sleeping disturbance (279 cases), mannerisms (152 cases), headache (125 cases), convulsions (10 cases), and others. Gao pointed out that patients admitted to his general hospital with a diagnosis of hysteria occupied 5.4% of all admitted inpatients, a much higher admission rate than those reported from other countries (0.6–3%). He explained that hysteria is still a common disorder among uneducated, married, young-adult women in his serving area who develop acute, emotional reactions in response to mostly family-related conflict. It needs to be pointed out that, in Gaw's study, the diagnosis of hysteria was used broadly (as was done in the past) to include dissociation, conversion, and possession.

Concerning only conversion hysteria, Tang and his colleagues (1996) reported data from his psychiatric hospital in Nanchong City, Sichuang Province, in the central part of China. Among 48 cases diagnosed as conversion disorder and admitted to the hospital, in an urban setting, 12 cases were male, and 36 cases female, with a male/female ratio of 1:3. The average age was 31 years old, with most between the ages of 16 and 45. Manifested symptoms, by frequency of their occurrence, were mostly motor disturbances (54 times). These included convulsions (20 times), paralysis of extremities (14 times), aphasia (11 times), catatonic states (7 times), and stuttering (2 times). Sensory disturbances were noticed as well (34 times), which included: headache (18 times), numbness (8 times), foreign sensation in the throat (4 times), and pain over the body (4 times). There were also autonomic nervous system disturbances (14 times), including fainting (6 times), hyperventilation, nausea, and vomiting. As for the cause of the onset, it was revealed that there were psychological precipitating factors, such as emotional trauma (18 cases), family conflict (13 cases), physical fighting with others (8 cases), stress from physical illness (5 cases), and others.

FREQUENCY OF HYSTERICAL DISORDERS

Reports from China

Luo and Zhou (1984) investigated the diagnostic distribution of psychiatric patients who made visits to the emergency room at the Institute of Mental Health of Beijing Medical School, one of the major teaching institutes in Beijing. They reported that, during the 10-year period of 1972 to 1982, a total of 1,622 cases made emergency room visits. Among them, besides schizophrenia (15.5%), organic psychoses (7.1%), and other disorders, 820 cases (50.6%) were diagnosed as neuroses. Among these neurotic cases, almost all of them (781 cases, 95.2%) were diagnosed as hysteria. In these cases, the cardinal symptoms were convulsions (40.6%), emotional turmoil (31.1%), trance state (4.2%), and others. In other words, among the psychiatric patients who visited the emergency clinic, nearly half were diagnosed with hysteria, with major symptoms of convulsions or emotional turmoil.

A large-scale psychiatric epidemic study of minor psychiatric disorders was carried out in China in 1982, involving 12 geographic areas and nearly 7,000 people. From this study (Epidemic Survey Collaboration Team, 1986), it was reported that the overall prevalence rate for hysteria was 3.55 per 1,000 population of adults between the ages of 15 and 59. Among all neurotic disorders, hysteria was second only to neurasthenia, thus, it was a commonly observed minor psychiatric disorder. In rural areas, the rate was 5.00, while in urban areas, it was 2.09, indicating that the disorder was much more prevalent in rural areas. The disorder occurred much more frequently among females than males. For instance, in the area of Shangtong Province, the rate for women was 14.2, while that for men was merely 0.85.

Findings from India

A report was made by Dube (1970), based on an epidemiological study carried out by home visits in a census survey in the Agra region of Uttar Pradesh, northern India. Among 29,468 residents, he found 261 cases of conversion symptoms in the form of hysterical fits, with a prevalence rate of 8.9 per 1,000 population. He reported that females (mostly ages 15 to 24) constituted 96.1% of all cases. The role of caste, marital status, and educational level were found to be associated with the occurrence of hysteria.

Another report was made recently by Srinath and his associates (1993) concerning childhood hysteria observed in inpatient and outpatient psychiatric populations. They reviewed the case records for a one-year interval of inpatients admitted (n = 143) and outpatients visited (n = 640) at the Child and Adolescent Psychiatric Unit of the National Institute of Mental Health and Neuroscience, in Bangalore, South India. They found that, among these clinical cases, 30.8% (n = 44) of the inpatients and 14.8% (n = 95) of the outpatients were diagnosed with hysteria. The inpatient cases were mostly postpubertal, and, interestingly enough, their gender distribution was approximately even. Clinically, pseudoseizure was the most frequent presentation.

WANING OF THE DISORDER?

In addition to the prevalence of hysteria differing remarkably among various societies—being more prevalent in traditional and culturally restricted societies and less in culturally liberal and modernized societies—another trend that has been noticed by clinicians: That is, based on historical observation and clinical impression, the occurrence of hysteria is waning around the world in both traditional and modern societies. There was one follow-up epidemiological study carried out in rural areas of India supporting the declining trend of hysteria there.

Indian psychiatrist D. N. Nandi and associates (1992) reported the data that derived from their follow-up epidemiological studies carried out in two rural communities, Gambhirgachi and Paharpur, in West Bengal. The former was surveyed in 1972 and, 10 years later, in 1982; the latter was studied in 1972 and, 15 years later, in 1987. The total population of Gambhirgachi grew from 1,060 to 1,539 within 10 years. Over 90% of the villagers were Muslim, and the rest Hindu. The total population of Paharpur increased from 1,114 to 1,464 within 15 years. The villagers were divided almost equally between Hindu and Muslim. The results of the surveys indicated that the prevalence of hysteria declined considerably in these two villages, from 16.9 to 4.6 per 1,000 population and 32.3 to 2.05 per 1,000 population in Gambhirgachi and Paharpur, respectively. It is interesting that, associated with this remarkable decline in the prevalence of hysteria, there was a moderate increase in depression: from 37.7 to 53.3 per 1,000 population and 61.9 to 77.2 per 1,000 population in the two villages, respectively.

Nandi and his associates reported that, between these two surveys, besides the increase in population, there was clearly a visible change in the quality of life of the people. In 1972, most of the villagers had no work in the fields for a major part of the year. After the introduction of multiple crops and increased input in farming, people had work throughout the year and were paid higher wages. Along with this economic improvement, there was an increase in educational and health-care facilities. Nandi and his associates attribute the improvement in social status of women to the fall of the prevalence of hysteria.

Possession Disorders in Asians

Possession disorders are believed to occur in many parts of the world. Judging from the literature, it is still occurring in Asia, even in the present.

JAPAN

Besides the orthodox religion of *Sin-do*, traditionally Japanese are pantheists, believing animals (such as foxes, raccoons, dogs, snakes), trees, mountains, stones, and other subjects are all associated with spirits. According to Japanese folk legend, animal spirits, particularly the fox spirit, are commonly described. The spirit of the cunning fox can disguise itself into any human form, often a young lady, and play tricks on you. The Japanese commonly say *kitsune-ni-bakasareru*, literally meaning to be fooled by the spirit of a fox (*kitsune*). Perhaps related to this, when a person is possessed, people tend to interpret him or her as being possessed by an animal spirit, mostly a fox, and occasionally a dog or a cat (Daiguji, 1993; Eguchi, 1991). According to Kitanishi (1993),who studied possession phenomena in Japan, possession by the spirit of a fox is widespread geographically in Japan, whereas possession by the spirits of dogs and snakes only occurs in the southern part of Japan (such as Shikoku and Kushiu Islands), indicating that there are geographical differences. Furthermore, Kitanishi mentioned that the spirit of the animal that tends to possess people is believed to stay in certain households. The household with *tsukinomo-suji* (spirit lineage) tends to be looked down upon by others and is kept at a distance socially. It is speculated that such households may have originally been those of migrant families that wandered into the established village. Another explanation is that the possessing spirit was brought by a shaman to inhabit the designated household. It is generally believed that animal spirits will be transmitted through marriage and kept within a family. It is pointed out by Etusko (1991) that fox possession is becoming a rare phenomenon in contemporary Japan, but still a matter of concern in psychiatry is the metaphorical representation of possession by a fox.

KOREA

Perhaps because geographically Korea is close to Siberia, the practice of shamanism in Korea is believed by scholars to have existed from early history. Anthropological investigations of shamans and shamanism are well documented in recent publications (Harvey, 1979; Kendall, 1985). Possession by gods, deceased ancestors, or ghosts is still observed in the country.

Rhi (1993) reported his survey of 17 cases of patients who had been admitted to Seoul National University Hospital during the five-year period between 1983 and 1987. It needs to be pointed out that, clinically, the cases he reported were suffering from major psychiatric disorders (including mainly schizophrenia, and other psychoses) with secondary symptoms of possession, and only one case with a primary diagnosis of dissociative disorder. He described the subjects as possessed by the devil (*magui*), demon (*kuishin*), spirit (*shin*), soul of dead family members, and even the souls of living family members. He explained that the patients' complaints of various kinds of spirit possession and intrusion seemed to be largely related to the religious backgrounds of the patients and their families. He indicated that there were no cases among the samples he reviewed that were possessed by animals. However, he mentioned that there was one report in the literature according to which a patient, after killing a snake, acted as if he was possessed by the snake, sticking out his tongue as a snake does. The case was from the remote island of Cheju, where the snake is worshiped by the local people.

THAILAND

In Thailand, although most possessing beings are the spirits of animals or deceased persons, as elsewhere, there is a unique phenomenon by which a person can be possessed by the spirit of a living person. According to Suwanlert (1976), Thai people believe that *phii pob*, the soul of a living person, may come and go among people. When *phii pob* possesses you, you take the role of that living person. Possession by a living person's soul is observed mainly in northern Thailand.

Suwanlert described the following interesting case from among his reports. A 16-year-old girl was sent to live with her grandmother at age 2, when her father died. Many years later, when her mother remarried, she came back to live with her mother and her stepfather. One day, when she witnessed her drunken stepfather slap her mother during an argument, she suddenly acted differently, as if she was one of her stepfather's male friends who lived in the next village. It was clear to others that she was possessed by *phii pob*. In a male voice, she warned her stepfather that if he did not behave, the ancestor's spirit would punish him by breaking his neck. After the stepfather, in front relatives, promised that he would behave, the *phii pob*, the soul of the stepfather's friend, departed via the patient's mouth.

The case illustrates beautifully how a young girl, faced with a fearful situation, and without knowing how to deal with her drunken, abusive stepfather, turned herself (via a possession state) into a socially more powerful person and borrowed the authority of an ancestor to control her stepfather.

TAIWAN

In spite of governmental suppression during the Japanese occupation, shamanistic practices became popular again after World War II, when Taiwan was returned to China. Associated with this development, the phenomena of possession disorders became more visible than in the past. Wen (1996) conducted a community survey of a selected area in the south of Taiwan, and estimated that the people who had possession experiences (both ordinary and morbid conditions) were not less than 1 percent of the adult population. He pointed out that the traditional belief in pantheism and ancestor worship—belief in close relations and interaction with deceased ancestors—serves as the common ground for the frequent occurrence of possessed states. However, it is speculated that, in contrast to Japan, the belief in the possibility of interference from an ancestor spirit is more intense for people in Taiwan. This is reflected in concepts of fortune-telling, shamanism, and everyday language—such as, "If you disgrace your ancestors, their spirits will come to punish you," or "If you are in trouble, you may ask your ancestors' spirits to protect you."

During his investigation, Wen (1996) observed that, in both normal possession and possession disorders, a person can be possessed by spirits of at least 12 different ranks, according to the hierarchy of deities. This ranking goes from the lowest, wandering, wild spirit to a deceased infant's spirit, a deceased ancestor's spirit, the spirit of various historically recognized heroes or generals, then to Guanyin, Buddha, and finally, the Jade Emperor—the highest deity recognized in Chinese folklore. Thus, theoretically, a shaman needs to identify the kind of deity that possesses the client, and then try to be possessed by a higher ranking deity himself in order to overpower the client's spirit.

CHINA

According to the available literature, possession disorders are more frequently reported in the northeastern region of mainland China, including the areas previously called Manchuria and

Inner Mongolia. These areas are geographically close to Siberia, where anthropologists believe the practice of shamanism (in a narrow sense) originated.

In the Hebei Province of China (near Manchuria), Gaw and his colleagues (1998) studied clinical characteristics of 20 psychiatric patients admitted to 8 hospitals in the region, who believed they were possessed. All the patients were given the diagnosis of hysteria by local Chinese psychiatrists. The mean age of the patients was 37 years old. Most were women from rural areas with little education. Major events reported to precede possession included interpersonal conflicts. Possessing agents were thought to be spirits of deceased persons, deities, animals, and devils. The initial experiences of possession typically came on acutely, but often became chronic, relapsing illnesses.

According to Zhang (1992), a psychiatrist from the Mental Hospital of Liaoning Province (in Manchuria), there was a total of 4,714 forensic cases brought to the hospital for psychiatric evaluation. Of those cases, 52 (1.1%) had committed murder under possession disorders. Interestingly, among them, there were six groups of patients (with more than four people in each group) who carried out murder together. Most of them were family members or relatives who had developed a collective trance state or a "shared" possession state. In these conditions, they killed their victims with the conviction that the person was possessed by an evil that needed to be exorcized.

Following is a group murder case reported by Zhang (1992). Mr. and Mrs. Wang were a middle-age couple in their 50s. They had two sons. Mrs. Wang had a past history of possession episodes, claiming that she was often possessed by the spirit of her deceased mother-in-law. Their 24-year-old eldest son, after illegally cohabiting with his girlfriend, began to behave reclusively and strangely, claiming that he was a "headless evil" and intended to kill all of his family members. One night, hearing a noise on the roof, the mother suddenly fell into a possessed state, claiming that she was possessed by a shaman who had come to expel the headless evil from her son. She induced her husband, Mr. Wang, and her 18-year-old son, to fall into trance states. In these states, together they pounded 43 nails into the eldest son's body and stabbed him in the abdomen with a knife. As a result, the eldest son died. After the event, Mrs. Wang remained in a trance state for 10 days, claiming that she had expelled and killed the dangerous, headless evil. When she recovered from her trance state and learned that she had killed her son, she began to cry loudly.

Dynamically, a tempting interpretation is that the mother who psychologically lost her son to his girlfriend reacted with the belief that her son was evil. Her possessed state gave her an excuse to act out her wish to punish the unfilial (or emotionally betraying) son. Clinically, this is a case of associated or collective mental disorders, which takes place among the members of a family. The common belief in the person being possessed by evil and the need to conduct an exorcism were the bases for this family group of psychiatric disorders.

Possession Psychoses in Asians

Given the case described above, it becomes immediately clear that the distinction between possession disorder (of a hysterical nature) and possession psychoses is not merely a clinical matter, but also a forensic challenge, if the patient is involved in a crime.

The term "invocation psychosis" is still used by psychiatrists in some societies, including Japan. It refers to a psychotic condition characterized by the delusion of being possessed, in addition to other psychotic pictures, including hallucination, bizarre behavior, and thought disorder. This condition, even though manifested as a possession state, is different from possession disorder of a hysterical nature in that its onset is not necessarily sudden or in reaction to external stress, but may last a relatively long time, more than several weeks or months, and it does not respond favorably to any psychological treatment for underlying psychological stress. From a forensic point of view, the patient suffering from this condition is considered less responsible for criminal acts that he or she may commit.

Invocation psychosis should not be confused with "hysterical psychosis," which has been misused by some medical anthropologists to include all mental disorders in different cultures that are of a hysterical nature—namely, that have an acute onset and a brief, benign course. The culture-related specific disorders of *latah*, arctic hysteria, *amok*, and others have been included in this ill-defined term. In an entirely different way, some psychiatrists still use the term "hysterical psychosis" to refer to the clinical condition characterized by a brief and acute psychotic state, often occurring as a reaction to stress, associated with symptoms of a theatrical nature, and from which the patient tends to recover with a good prognosis, without mental sequels.

Altered Personality Disorder

Characteristically different from possession disorder is altered-personality disorder. In the latter there is no interpretation by either the patient or other people that the patient is possessed by "others." It is understood that the person alternates between (or among) different personalities, either in a trance state or without it. In other words, there is a psychological and not a supernatural interpretation of the phenomenon. Therefore, it is observed mainly in "modernized" societies, where folk beliefs of a supernatural nature have more or less diminished.

It is a common notion among psychiatrists that, in traditional societies, where trance and possession states are more frequent, the phenomena of altered-personality and multiple- personality disorders are seldom found. In contrast, in modern societies, possession disorders are rare or diminishing, and double- or multiple-personality disorders are becoming more prevalent.

According to Ross (1991), the frequency of diagnosed multiple-personality disorder in clinical populations increased exponentially during the 1980s. Reviewing the entire world literature, Greaves (1980) pointed out that not more than a couple of hundred cases (mainly in Western societies) have been reported since the beginning of this century. However, according to Ross, P. Coons, in 1986, estimated that 6,000 cases of multiple-personality disorders had been diagnosed in North America.

INDIA

In contrast, Adityanjee and his colleagues (1989) in India reported that only two cases of multiple-personality disorder had been reported in India in the past. They reportedly encountered three more cases over a period of three years at a psychiatric clinic in New Delhi. Based on their clinical experience, Adityanjee and his colleagues estimated that the frequency of this disorder was about 0.15 per 1,000 psychiatric outpatients per year at their clinic. They claimed there was a frequent diagnosis of possession disorder, but the diagnosis of multiple-personality disorder was rare.

JAPAN

A similar situation has been observed in Japan. In order to confirm the clinical impression of Japanese psychiatrists, Takahashi (1990) conducted a review of 489 psychiatric inpatients who were hospitalized during a 5-year period (1983–1988) in the psychiatric ward of the General Hospital of Yamahashi Medical College, where he worked. He reported that seven cases were diagnosed as dissociative disorders, but none were multiple-personality disorders. It may be criticized that he used psychiatric inpatients rather than outpatients for the study, but he claimed that his findings reflected the situation in Japan, namely, that multiple-personality disorders are rare and, instead, there are cases of dissociation and possession disorder.

Beyond the influence of diagnostic-practice patterns in different societies, there is good reason to speculate that, in association with the level of modernization—or the degree of belief in folk supernatural powers—there is a trend away from the possessed state to the altered-personality state.

If we think carefully, we will realize that the possession state and the altered-personality state are similar, except that the former is interpreted as the takeover of the self by an "external (supernatural) being," while the latter is the taking over of the self by an "internal (psychological) being," or another part of the self. Both offer mechanisms for avoiding taking responsibility for one's actions, but in different ways, based on the common beliefs shared by the people in the society.

Epidemic Hysteria in Asia

Epidemic mental disorders refer to mental disorders or pathological psychological reactions that occur among groups of people in a contagious way within a relatively short period of time in a particular social setting. The mental disorders may involve a small number of subjects or hundreds or even thousands collectively through the process of contagion in an endemic or epidemic fashion, and are therefore called "contagious" or "epidemic." Since mental disorders are transmitted or spread from one person to another, the nature of the transmission is understood to be psychological, closely related to the social atmosphere and community setting at the time, the common beliefs or attitudes shared by the group of people involved, and a part of the mechanism of group psychology.

During the past several decades, numerous cases of mental epidemics have been reported in scientific literature in both the East and West (Tseng, 2001, pp. 265–290). The psychiatric symptoms are usually manifested as hysterical conversion reactions (such as fainting, paralysis, or convulsions) or panic states (such as fear of disaster, danger, or death) and occasionally as delusional states or collective suicide. Here, the epidemic occurrences of hysteria in Asia will be briefly reviewed.

CHINA

Reviewing the literature published during the 10-year period from 1995 to 2005, Su and her colleagues (2007) found nearly 100 reports of mass hysteria describing a total of 80 events that occurred in China during this time. Analyzing the precipitating factors speculated to be the cause of these endemic occurrences, they reported that about 38% were related to public-health vaccinations (such as those for encephalitis), 20% to public-health medications (such as for parasites), 18% to environmental intoxication, and 24% to psychological factors (related to stress from examinations, or superstitious beliefs). It is interesting to note that biological factors were mainly considered to have provoked the endemic hysteria, while less attention was given to psychological factors.

In contrast, there was a report from Hong Kong by Wong and colleagues (1982) describing an epidemic of hysteria. A total of 413 school students were taken ill with symptoms from an alleged poisonous gas affecting two different geographic locations at the same time, but without influence on the residents in the neighboring areas. An epidemic survey was carried out. The results supported that there was no organic cause as initially speculated, and a cause of a psychological nature was confirmed.

MALAYSIA

Tan (1963) mentioned that epidemic hysteria was a rather common occurrence in the Malay area. According to him, in 1971 alone, a total of 17 episodes were noted by psychiatrists.

Teoh and his colleagues (1975) reported an episode of endemic hysteria that occurred among female dormitory students. This report described the psychological aspects of the epidemic in sufficient detail to allow us to elaborate on the cultural and group dynamics associated with the occurrence of epidemic hysteria. It is obvious that this outbreak centered around the headmaster's behavior, primarily his intrusion into the girls' private lives. However, since Malay culture provided no appropriate way to oppose his authority, mass hysteria became the only way to force him to recognize and change the source of the problem.

Psychiatric literature has shown that occasionally more than one member of a family may become mentally ill through a process of contagion—forming so-called "double insanity" or "family insanity" (*folie á deux* or *folie á famille* in French). The psychiatric condition may take the form of dissociation, conversion, delusion, or abnormal behavior. Although the phenomenon of folie á famille is considered rare, sporadic occurrences have been reported in the Philippines (Goduco-Angular & Wintrob, 1964), Malaysia (Woon, 1976), and Taiwan (Tseng, 1969).

The case reported by T. H. Woon (1976) concerned a Chinese-Malaysian family whose two young-adult brothers and one sister simultaneously developed dissociated conditions, creating sensational turmoil in a rural village in Malaysia. The situation occurred after their aged father, a village shaman, suffered a stroke, making it necessary to choose a successor from among his adult children. Affected by intense feelings of competition and the inability to handle these emotions, the siblings one after another developed dissociated conditions. Reviewing this contagious family mental disorder, it is apparent that, in addition to the existing premorbid personalities of the family members, a strong emotional bond among them facilitated the occurrence of the condition, particularly when they faced a stressful situation together. To share and to be involved by having a similar psychiatric condition appeared to be an alternative way for the siblings to deal with the common crisis they encountered. It is speculated that such an unusual, contagious reaction tends to be observed in societies where family ties are stressed.

Strengths, Weaknesses, and Alternatives in Applying Current Nosology and Diagnostic Criteria for Identifying Dissociation, Conversion, and Possession Disorders in Asians

The Acute and Transient Nature of Disorders—Making Community Surveys Difficult

Most clinical findings regarding dissociation, conversion, and possession disorders are available mainly from Asia, as reviewed here. In contrast, there is relatively little information available from America, particularly about Asian Americans, for comparison. It is speculated that there are fewer clinical conditions of these disorders and reports in literature are very scanty. Studies of these epidemic disorders by community surveys are relatively difficult, because the disorders tend to occur as acute disorders, with remittance within a short period of time; they are, therefore, less likely to be found in prevalence-focused community surveys. Furthermore, different sets of clinical diagnoses are applied in different societies, making meaningful comparison limited. However, this does not mean that these disorders have entirely disappeared in America, including among Asian Americans. There is still a clinical need to pay attention to these disorders and provide proper care for them.

Diagnostic Variations Needed for Clinical Work

The disorders described may show different clinical variations even in different Asian societies, so that diagnostic adjustment and special attention are needed in caring for them. A good example is that the clinical picture presented by most of the hysteria patients in India is different from that described in ICD-10 as well as *DSM-IV*. Psychiatrists from Manipal, India, Alexander and colleagues (1997), claimed that their proposed category of "brief dissociative stupor" is needed for their clinical work. Several studies from India (Das & Saxena, 1991; Saxena & Prasad, 1989) have revealed that up to 90% of the patients with dissociative disorders treated in the outpatient psychiatric clinic were classified as being in the "unspecified" or "atypical" categories of dissociative disorders of the *DSM-III* or *DSM-III-R*. Das and Saxena (1991) reported that 81% of their patients with dissociative disorders met the criteria for "simple" dissociative disorders, which are characterized simply by transient episodes of alternations in consciousness (manifested by a relative lack of responsiveness to the external environment) —namely, trance states. These states may be associated with some bizarre or convulsion-like motor movements, crying, shouting, or verbalizing thoughts. Alexander and associates (1997), based on their clinical experiences with psychiatric inpatients in a general hospital, reported that a significant number of the patients with dissociative disorders experienced recurrent episodes of unresponsiveness lasting for short periods (without convulsions, motor movements, or verbalization). Therefore, they suggested using the term "brief dissociative stupor" to describe their hysterical patients.

General Comments

It seems that, if we rely on worldwide clinical observation, it would be fair to say there is a great variety of clinical manifestations of hysteria-related disorders. The majority of cases exhibit the clinical syndrome of a simple trance-state disorder, which may be associated with a stupor, motor excitement, or emotional outburst. Beyond that, some cases manifest more specialized forms of disorders, including dissociated amnesia, depersonalization, or possession. Clearly there is a wide range of altered mental conditions relating to the function of consciousness, mental integration, and self-identity within normal life conditions, special conditions, and pathological conditions. Thus, within the spectrum of pathology, there is a need for more diagnostic subgroups to capture the whole perspective of this group of disorders. This is particularly true from a cross-cultural perspective.

PERSPECTIVES ON THE CAUSES OF DISSOCIATION, CONVERSION, AND POSSESSION DISORDERS IN ASIANS

Biological Models

There are fragmented clinical findings that suggest dissociative or possession conditions tend to occur within the same family. This is particularly true for dissociation or possession disorders that occur as double insanity or family insanity (Woon, 1976). Case reports made by Chinese forensic psychiatrists (Li, 2000; Zhang, 1996) support the findings that many dissociation or possession disorders have occurred among family members, including parents and siblings, who have committed crimes together during their dissociated or possessed states.

It is also commonly known that the family members of a shaman tend to evidence dissociation episodes, and they are considered potential candidates for future shamans (Kim, 1973; Tseng, 1972). Based on this information, biological factors as a predisposing cause cannot be entirely dismissed, and the biological bases for personality traits that tend to manifest dissociation should be considered for further investigation.

Psychological Models

Because most of the cases develop these disorders after being exposed to stress or conflicts in life, particularly relating to family, there is substantial reason to consider that such disorders are prominently related to psychological causes.

Many studies from the West have recently tried to demonstrate that certain early childhood traumas, including sexual abuse, tend to predispose certain personality traits (such as narcissistic, hysterical, or borderline-personality traits), which, in turn, make the person vulnerable to certain mental disorders. This type of study has not yet been done in Asia, and is awaiting further clinical investigation.

Clinical reports from the East tend to illustrate that the psychological stress the patient encountered and with which he or she had difficulty coping is usually caused by family-related problems such as conflict between mother-in-law and daughter-in-law; emotional problems between husband and wife; a wife suppressed by her husband or a daughter by her parents; affair problems between a man and a woman; and problems associated with forbidden sexual desire or behavior. In general, it can be said that a person is suppressed by others and, when there is no way socially or culturally to deal with it openly, he or she has to repress his or her feelings of resentment or hate, which tends to provoke the occurrence of conversion, dissociation, or an (hysterical) emotional turmoil reaction.

Social Models

Generally speaking, most clinicians and scholars tend to think that certain social and cultural environments favor the occurrence of hysteria-related disorders. The social environment is usually described as very traditional, rigid, and conservative, with many restrictions, making it difficult for people to express their feelings, to communicate their stresses, and to deal with their emotional conflicts openly. Dissociation, conversion, and possession become alternative choices for individuals, particularly those with vulnerable personalities facing severe emotional conflict or stress.

However, in some societies, people refuse to look at and examine the psychological perspective of such disorders, particularly in epidemic occurrences, and tend to look at biological factors as the cause for these collective mental disorders. There is a great need to improve the psychological understanding of such contagious, collective emotional disorders.

TREATING DISSOCIATION, CONVERSION, AND POSSESSION DISORDERS IN ASIANS

Biological Approaches

Most of the clinicians in Asia tend to prescribe medication for the management of dissociation, conversion, or possession disorders, simply because there is a need to "give some medication" to the patients as expected by them according to their illness behavior or help-seeking behavior. It is considered clinically that the clinical condition tends to improve not due to pharmacological effects, but through psychological effects. That is, the patient has the excuse of being recognized as ill by having medication, and, also, and most importantly, the excuse to recover from the ill condition after having the medication as long as the precipitating psychological stress has been resolved through psychological counseling of the patient and his or her family.

A caution is needed for severe cases, such as so-called possession psychosis, the malignant dissociation of *latah*, which have relatively unfavorable prognoses and do not respond to medication with suggestive natures. They need to be treated as psychotic patients with antipsychotic medications.

Psychological Approaches

Clearly, for psychologically induced mental disorders, there is little use for biological approaches to treatment except by utilizing placebo effects. A psychological approach is the best choice of treatment. To examine and reveal the underlying cause of the occurrence of these mental phenomena, and to work with the patient as well as the family on how to deal with and resolve the psychological problems is the correct treatment.

From a clinical point of view, it is very important not to explain to the family or even the patient that the patient is faking. This interpretation will invite resistance from the patient, and lead to his or her not recovering, and also may cause mistreatment by the family, based on the belief that the patient is pretending to be sick and calling for attention with secondary gain. Obviously, it would be counterproductive to give such an interpretation to the family.

Social Approaches

The most important characteristics of patients with hysteria-related disorders are their dramatic reactions to stress and the theatrical quality of their response to audiences—family members, friends, and other people surrounding the patient, including those who deliver care. The outcome of the disorder will vary depending on how these people conceive and understand the disorder, how they react toward the illness event, and how they deal with the patient during the hysterical attack.

Thus, there is a need for competent clinical skill, with dynamic knowledge and orientation, with which to approach patients, their family members, and surrounding people. Clearly there is room for improvement among clinicians on how to care for patients manifesting dissociation, conversion, or possession disorders. This is true not only for Asian clinicians but also for American mental health care providers as well.

Although these disorders may be treated directly by psychiatrists needing cultural knowledge to manage them (Tseng, 2003), most of the clinical conditions are treated by doctors in emergency settings or the inpatient setting of internal medicine (for adults cases) or the pediatric ward (for child or adolescent cases), with or without consulting with a psychiatrist. Only a few, usually severe cases may be treated at a psychiatric clinic or in an inpatient setting (Tseng & Streltzer, 2004). Therefore, doctors of other disciplines, including internal medicine, pediatrics, and neurology, need not only medical knowledge and skill to manage these patients, but also the ethnic and cultural knowledge and insight to care for them (Tseng & Streltzer, 2008).

CONCLUSION

Vicissitude of the Disorders

Although there is no strong statistical data to confirm this directly, based on clinical observations that have been made through time, it is the consensus among clinicians that there has been an obvious change in the frequency of hysteria from both historical and geographic perspectives. Generally, it has been noted that hysterical disorders, whether in simple, trance, possessed, or conversion forms, are gradually fading away in many societies in which they used to be prevalent. The reasons are unclear, but several possibilities can be offered. The nature of many societies is gradually changing and modernizing, with fewer traditional and conservative societies than there were in the past. People are becoming more educated and understanding better how to deal with emotional stress in more active, effective ways rather than in primitive ways. In today's society, when stress encountered in daily life is not tolerable, many people tend to indulge in substance abuse or drinking to deal with it. Thus, substance-induced trance and dissociation become substitutes for the primitive dissociative state that was frequently observed in the past.

Cultural Aspects of Hysteria-Related Disorders

There are basically five ways that culture impacts psychopathology—through psycho-pathogenic, -plastic, -selective, -facilitating, and -reactive effects (Tseng, 2001, pp. 177–193). We find this to be true when we examine the nature of hysteria-related disorders through the concept of how culture impacts psychopathology.

Based on contemporary psychiatric knowledge, hysteria is understood as a reaction to psychological stress. Yet, the nature of stress varies according to cultural background. In some societies, insoluble stress for a young person may be created by parental authority. Severe stress might also be experienced by a submissive wife who has no way of handling her husband's unfaithful behavior, or of dealing with a constantly overpowering and abusive mother-in-law. However, these stresses may not be important in societies where the rights of the individual are greatly valued and protected. Instead, breaking off a romantic relationship, the traumatic loss of a family member, or loneliness associated with aging may constitute major problems in life, which may or may not cause a hysterical reaction. Becoming depressed or indulging in excessive drinking or substance abuse may be other choices. Thus, culture has a *pathogenic* as well as a *patho-selective* effect with regard to hysteria.

Related to the core issue of altered consciousness, there are many ways to manifest hysteria-related disorders: as a simple emotional outburst, a simple trance, a specific dissociated condition, or a more complicated possessed state or altered personality. Thus, culture has a *patho-plastic* effect. Even with the possessed state, there are many "other beings" that can possess the person, depending on the kind of animal spirits or deities that are familiar to him and to others in the community. Thus, there are variations of Zar possession, fox spirit possession, and *phii pob* possession observed in different cultures.

A person claiming that he is possessed by the spirit of his deceased ancestor, for instance, needs to be believed by the people around him, or the morbid condition, if not responded to and reinforced by others, will not last long. Thus, culture contributes significantly to both the *patho-reactive* and the *patho-facilitating* effects. If family members, friends, and other people in the community regard the hysteria as a sign of weakness in the patient's personality, his inability to handle stress, and an unconscious calling for attention and help-seeking, then the severity of the disorder will be reduced and the morbid condition will not last long. Thus, hysteria is a psychological disorder very much bound by cultural settings. The vicissitude of the disorder is directly determined by the views, attitudes, and reactions shared by the culture toward the phenomenon.

Clinical Critics: Contemporary Ignorance (in the West)

It is obvious that, due to their current clinical situations and experiences, there is professional ignorance of hysteria-related mental conditions among psychiatrists in European and North American societies. The academic ignorance can be described in several areas (Tseng, 2001, pp. 332–333).

Due to the descriptive orientation in the present *DSM* system, the hysterical disorder is split into the different categories of dissociated and conversion disorder. This diverts attention from the basic element of the disorder, its reactive and defensive nature. The symbolic meaning and protective function of the disorder are disconnected from the sociocultural setting in which it takes place.

Associated with this is the neglect of possession disorder, which is still frequently observed in many non-Western societies. Instead, only the altered-personality disorder is included in the classification system. The epidemic occurrence of hysteria, or mass hysteria, which is still not infrequently observed in developing or developed societies, is not included in the classification system.

The ignorance about the disorders is primarily due to the rarity of trance, dissociation, and possession in modern Western societies. However, it needs to be recognized that, in non-Western societies, which comprise more than three-quarters of the world's population, these phenomena are still prevalent, and require continued clinical attention and consideration. Trance, dissociation, and possession are mental conditions experienced by human beings, whether ordinary, special, or morbid. They are predominantly psychologically related and attributed to cultural factors, and are unique, interesting, still mysterious, and deserving of greater attention.

REFERENCES

Adityanjee, Raju, G. S. P., & Khandelwal, S. K. (1989). Current status of multiple personality disorder in India. *American Journal of Psychiatry, 146*(12), 1607–1610.

Alexander, P. J., Joseph, S., & Das, A. (1997). Limited utility of ICD-10 and DSM-IV classification of dissociative and conversion disorders in India. *Acta Psychiatrica Scandinavica, 95,* 177–182.

American Psychiatric Association (APA). (1982). *Diagnostic and Statistical Manual of Mental Disorders* (2nd ed.). Washington, DC: Author. (*DSM-II*).

American Psychiatric Association (APA). (1994). *Diagnostic and Statistical Manual of Mental Disorders* (4th ed., text rev.). Washington, DC: Author. (*DSM-IV-TR*).

Bourguignon, E. (1973). World distribution and patterns of possession states. In R. Prince (Ed.), *Trance and possession states* (Proceedings of Second Annual Conference). Montreal: R. M. Bucke Memorial Society.

Bourguignon, E. (1976). Possession and trance in cross-cultural studies of mental health. In W. P. Lebra (Ed.), *Culture-bound syndromes, ethnopsychiatry, and alternate therapies.* Honolulu: University Press of Hawaii.

Daiguji, M. (1993). *Psychopathology of possession: Clinical examination of contemporary phenomenon* [in Japanese]. Tokyo: Seiwa Publisher.

Das, P. S., Saxena, S. (1991). Classification of dissociative states in DSM-III-R and ICD-10 (1989 draft). *British Journal of Psychiatry, 159,* 425–427.

Dube, K. C. (1970). A study of prevalence and biosocial variables in mental illness in a rural and an urban community in Uttar Pradesh, India. *Acta Psychiatrica Scandinavica, 46,* 327–359.

Eguchi, S. Y. (1991). Between folk concepts of illness and psychiatric diagnosis: Kitsune-tuski (fox possession) in a mountain village of western Japan. *Culture, Medicine, and Psychiatry, 15*(4), 421–452.

Etsuko, M. (1991). The interpretation of fox possession: Illness as metaphor. *Culture, Medicine, and Psychiatry, 15*(4), 453–477.

Epidemic Survey Collaboration Teams. (1986). Epidemic survey of neurotic disorders in 12 geographic areas [in Chinese]. *Chinese Neuropsychiatric Journal, 19,* 87–91.

Gao, Z. X. (1996). Clinical analysis of 657 cases of hysteria [in Chinese]. *Chinese Journal of Primary Medicine, 3*(4), 212.

Gaw, A. C., Ding, O., Levine, R. E., & Gaw, H. (1998). The clinical characteristics of possession disorder among 20 Chinese patients in the Hebei province of China. *Psychiatric Services, 49*(3), 360–365.

Goduco-Angular, C., & Wintrob, R. (1964). *Folie á famille* in the Philippines. *Psychiatric Quarterly, 38,* 278–291.

Greaves, G. B. (1980). Multiple personality disorder: 165 years after Mary Reynolds. *Journal of Nervous and Mental Disease, 168,* 577–596.

Greenbaum, L. (1973). Possession trance in Sub-Saharan Africa: A descriptive analysis of fourteen societies. In E. Bourguignon (Ed.), *Religion, altered states of consciousness, and social change.* Columbus: Ohio State University Press.

Harvey, Y. S. K. (1979). *Six Korean women: The socialization of shamans.* New York: West.

Kendall, L. (1985). *Shamans, housewives, and other restless spirits: Women in Korean ritual life.* Honolulu: University of Hawaii Press.

Kim, K.-I. (1973). Psychodynamic study of two cases of shaman in Korea [in Korean with English abstract]. *Korean Journal of Cultural Anthropology, 6,* 45–65.

Kim, Y.-Y. (2000). Shin-byung (divine illness) in a Korean woman. *Culture, Medicine, and Psychiatry 24*(4), 471–486.

Kitanishi, K. (1993). Possession phenomena in Japan. In *Possession Phenomena in East Asia.* Proceedings of the Fourth Cultural Psychiatry Symposium. Seoul: East Asian Academy of Cultural Psychiatry.

Lebra, T. S. (1976). Taking the role of supernatural "other": Spirit possession in a Japanese healing cult. In W. P. Lebra (Ed.), *Culture-bound syndromes, ethnopsychiatry, and alternate therapies.* Honolulu: University Press of Hawaii .

Li, C. P. (2000). *Practice and theory of forensic psychiatric assessment: Including analysis and discussion of 97 forensic cases* [in Chinese]. Beijing: Beijing Medical University Publisher.

Luo, H. C., & Zhou, C. S. (1984). Clinical analysis of 1,622 psychiatric emergency cases [in Chinese]. *Chinese Neuropsychiatric Journal, 17*(3), 137–138.

Nandi, D. N., Bznerjee, G., Nadi, S, & Nandi, P. (1992). Is hysteria on the wane? *British Journal of Psychiatry, 160,* 87–91.

Rhi, B. Y. (1993). Possession phenomena in Korea. In *Possession Phenomena in East Asia.* Proceedings of the Fourth Cultural Psychiatry Symposium. Seoul: East Asian Academy of Cultural Psychiatry.

Ross, C. A. (1991). Epidemiology of multiple personality disorder and dissociation. *Psychiatric Clinics of North America, 14*(3), 503–517.

Sasaki, Y. (1969). Psychiatric study of the shaman in Japan. In W. Caudill & T. Y. Lin (Eds.), *Mental health research in Asia and the Pacific.* Honolulu: East-West Center Press.

Saxena, S., & Prasad, K. V. S. R. (1989). DSM-III subclassification of dissociative disorder applied to psychiatric outpatients in India. *American Journal of Psychiatry, 14*(2), 261–262.

Srinath, S., Bharat, S., Girimaji, S., & Seshadri, S. (1993). Characteristics of a child inpatient population with hysteria in India. *Journal of American Academic Child and Adolescent Psychiatry, 32*(4), 822–825.

Su, P. Y., Tao, F. B., Sun, Q. H., & Zhou, X. R. (2007). Analysis of the epidemic characteristics of mass hysteria in schools from 1995 to 2004 in China [in Chinese]. *Chinese Journal of Epidemiology, 28*(3), 301–304.

Suwanlert, S. (1976). *Phii pob*: Spirit possession in rural Thailand. In W. P. Lebra (Ed.), *Culture-bound syndromes, ethnopsychiatry, and alternate therapies.* Honolulu: University Press of Hawaii.

Takahashi, Y. (1990). Is multiple personality really rare in Japan? *Dissociation, 3*(2), 57–59.

Tan, E. S. (1963). Epidemic hysteria. *Medical Journal of Malaya, 18,* 72–76.

Teoh, J. I., Soewondo, S., & Sidharta, M. (1975). Epidemic hysteria in Malaysian schools: An illustrative episode. *Psychiatry, 38,* 258–268.

Tang, D. L., Gen, Y. Y., & Xia, N. (1996). Clinical analysis of 48 cases of conversion hysteria [in Chinese]. *Sichuan Mental Health, 9*(4), 260.

Tseng, W. S. (1969). A paranoid family in Taiwan: A dynamic study of "folie famille." *Archives of General Psychiatry, 21,* 55–63.

Tseng, W. S. (1972). Psychiatric study of shamanism in Taiwan. *Archives of General Psychiatry, 26,* 561–565.

Tseng, W. S. (2001). *Handbook of cultural psychiatry.* San Diego: Academic.

Tseng, W. S. (2003). *Clinician's guide to cultural psychiatry.* San Diego: Academic.

Tseng, W. S., & Streltzer, J. (2004). *Cultural competence in clinical psychiatry.* Washington DC: American Psychiatry Publishing.

Tseng, W. S., & Streltzer, J. (2008). *Cultural competence in health care: A guide for professionals.* New York: Springer.

Ward, C. A. (1980). Spirit possession and mental health: A psycho-anthropological perspective. *Human Relations, 33*(3), 146–163.

Wen, J. K. (1996). Possession phenomena and psychotherapy [in Chinese]. In W. S. Tseng (Ed.), *Chinese mind and therapy.* Taipei: Laureate.

Wong, S. W., Kwong, B., Tam, Y. K., & Tsoi, M. M. (1982). Psychological epidemic in Hong Kong: I. Epidemiological study. *Acta Psychiatrica Scandinavica, 65*(6), 421–436.

Woon, T. H. (1976). Epidemic hysteria in a Malaysian Chinese extended family. *Medical Journal of Malaysia, 31,* 108–112.

World Health Organization (WHO). (1992). *International Statistical Classification of Diseases and Related Health Problems* (10th rev.). Geneva, Switzerland: Author. (ICD-10)

Zhang, X. F. (1992). A report of 32 cases with hysteria involved in homicide [in Chinese]. *Chinese Mental Health Journal, 6*(4), 175–176.

| 10 |

ANTISOCIAL BEHAVIOR AND EXTERNALIZING DISORDERS AMONG ASIANS, ASIAN AMERICANS, AND PACIFIC ISLANDER POPULATIONS

Sopagna Eap Braje, Jessica Murakami-Brundage, Gordon C. Nagayama Hall, Vivian Ota Wang, and Xiaojia Ge

INTRODUCTION

This chapter will focus on clinical issues related to the identification and treatment of externalizing symptoms among Asians, and Asian Americans and Pacific Islanders (AAPIs). Although the research on internalizing disorders among AAPIs is growing, externalizing problems among this population continues to be a neglected empirical topic. This oversight may be due to existing stereotypes of Asians and Asian Americans as docile and unassertive, traits inconsistent with externalizing disorders. Given the continued growth and heterogeneity of the population, as well as an accumulating body of research that contradicts the "model minority" stereotype, externalizing disorders and antisocial behavior among AAPI populations need to be better understood by mental health professionals.

Due to the broad categories of behavior that are included under antisocial behavior, only behaviors not addressed in other chapters, namely criminal behavior such as physical violence, domestic violence, and sexual aggression, will be discussed. This chapter will exclude substance and alcohol abuse, as well as antisocial personality disorder because these topics are discussed in separate chapters. Although this handbook is intended to focus on adult psychopathology, this chapter will include problem behaviors in children and adolescents to underscore the important developmental variables that contribute to adult antisocial behavior.

IDENTIFYING EXTERNALIZING DISORDERS AND ANTISOCIAL BEHAVIOR AMONG AAPIs

Mental health symptoms are dichotomized into two categories of symptom clusters: externalizing and internalizing disorders (Achenbach, 1982). Externalizing symptoms are also referred to as "undercontrolled" or "impulse control" behaviors, while internalizing symptoms are referred to as overcontrolled behaviors. Examples of externalizing disorders included in the *DSM-IV* are oppositional defiant disorder (ODD), conduct disorder (CD), attention deficit hyperactivity disorder (ADHD), antisocial personality disorder (see Chapter 9) and disorders of alcohol and drug dependence (see Chapter 4), while internalizing disorders include the majority of mood and anxiety disorders. Despite this distinction, it is important to note that externalizing and internalizing disorders often co-occur. Both categories are also associated with feelings of distress, either experienced by the individual or by others who are affected by the individual. This is particularly true for externalizing disorders, which often include antisocial behavior.

Antisocial behaviors describe acts that violate social rules and, more significantly, legal parameters. It includes rule violations that may be aggressive (e.g., destroying property, fighting, attacking others, threatening others) or nonaggressive (e.g., truancy, shoplifting, drug use). Antisocial behavior creates substantial financial and emotional costs to individuals and society in terms of victim and perpetrator treatment, and perpetrator incarceration. For example, antisocial behavior has serious health consequences for victims, including injury, death, disease, unwanted pregnancy, psychological harm, and interference with development (World Health Organization, 2002). Such health consequences may also occur for perpetrators who tend to associate with and become victimized by other perpetrators. The majority of persons who engage in antisocial behavior experience alcohol abuse or dependence, which exacerbates problems associated with antisocial behavior (Waldman & Slutske, 2000).

Examples of externalizing disorders characterized by antisocial behaviors include oppositional defiant disorder, conduct disorder, and antisocial personality disorder. According to the *DSM-IV*, oppositional defiant disorder describes individuals (usually children and adolescents) who exhibit negative, hostile, and defiant behavior toward adults and other figures of authority for a period of 6 months or more. Conduct disorder describes more serious symptoms that include behaviors that harm and encroach on the basic rights of others, such as aggression toward animals or/and people, destruction of property, theft, and serious rule violations that have persisted for 6 months or more. Meanwhile, antisocial personality disorder describes an individual that has a "pervasive pattern of disregard for the rights of others" (American Psychiatric Association, 2000, p.706). Personality disorders are thought of as "an enduring pattern of inner experience and behavior" (APA, 2000, p. 686) that deviates extensively from social and cultural norms. In the *DSM* multi-axial system, they are diagnosed on the second axis, suggesting that they are not as amendable to change as axis I psychiatric disorders. Individuals who engage in antisocial behavior may or may not meet criteria for one of these disorders. Indeed, most people have engaged in antisocial behavior. It is the severity and the repetition of such behavior that may warrant a diagnosis of ODD, CD, or ASPD.

In contrast, attention deficit hyperactivity disorder (ADHD) is diagnosed when individuals exhibit 6 or more symptoms of inattention (i.e., easily distracted, difficulty with organization, forgetful) and/or hyperactivity (i.e., excessive fidgetiness, excessive talking, difficulty remaining seated) with problems of impulsivity (i.e. difficulty with turn-taking, interrupts when others are talking) for a period of 6 months or more. Individuals diagnosed with ADHD do not necessarily engage in antisocial behavior, although rates of comorbidity with other externalizing (and internalizing) disorders are high (Beiderman, Newcorn, & Sprich, 1991). Additionally, ADHD in childhood may increase the risk of substance abuse later in life (Biederman et al., 1995, 1998).

Prevalence Rates of Externalizing Disorders and Antisocial Behavior Among Asians

There is a paucity of research on externalizing disorders and antisocial behavior among Asians and AAPI individuals. Findings from the available research are often contradictory. Therefore, although prevalence rates can be informative in describing the impact of externalizing disorders among a specific population, they do not completely explain the influence of culture on ethnic disparities in rates of mental health disorders.

Externalizing Disorders in Children and Adolescents

According to an epidemiological study of 541 Chinese adolescents from high schools in Hong Kong, externalizing disorders among Asian children and adolescents may be comparable to or slightly higher than rates for American children (Leung et al., 2008). Using the parent and youth version of the Chinese DISC-IV (Diagnostic Interview Schedule for Children Version 4), the authors found rates of 3.9 %, 6.8 %, and 1.7 % for ADHD, oppositional defiant disorder, and conduct disorder, respectively. Rates for ADHD and ODD are slightly higher and the rate for CD is slightly lower than rates reported in previous epidemiological studies conducted in the United States (Costello et al., 2004).

The research on externalizing disorders among Asian American children is inconclusive. Although Jang (2002) found lower rates of negative school behavior among Asian Americans compared to white, black, Hispanic, and Native Americans in a sample of 18,132 adolescents, other epidemiological studies suggest comparable levels of externalizing behavior problems among Asian American adolescents relative to other ethnic groups. Choi and Lahey (2006) found in a nationally representative sample of adolescents that Asian American youth showed similar rates of delinquent acts, and slightly higher rates of aggressive acts compared to European American youth. Relative to African Americans, they had higher rates of substance use and nonaggressive offenses. Still, other studies suggest higher rates for AAPI youth relative to other ethnic groups. Yao, Solanto, and Wender (1988) found hyperactivity prevalence rates of 8.8% among boys and 1.7% among girls in a sample of 250 Chinese American immigrants enrolled in first through sixth grade using the Conner's Teaching Rating Scale, which is higher than national averages for attention deficit hyperactivity disorder. Their study focused exclusively on hyperactivity, however, which in itself is not sufficient to receive a diagnosis of ADHD. The study also lacked a comparison group, making it difficult to conclude whether the higher rate of hyperactivity is due to cultural reasons or to classroom factors.

It is important to note that prevalence rates are affected by within-group variation. Loo and Rapport (1998) found greater behavioral problems among Hawaiian and European American male children relative to non–Hawaiian Asian American males in their study of 804 Hawaiian school children.

Criminal Behavior

The proportion of AAPI individuals arrested for rape, murder, and aggravated assault is lower than for any other ethnic group (Federal Bureau Investigation, 2004). The relatively few criminal offenses committed by individuals of AAPI descent often precludes them from being included in analyses examining rates of incarceration by race and ethnicity as noted by the lack of data on Asian Americans and Pacific Islanders in a report by the Bureau of Justice Statistics (2010). This glaring absence from criminal data perpetuates the conception of Asians as the "Model Minority" and suggests that violence and criminal activity is not a problem among Asian American populations. Because Asian Americans constitute a small percentage of the overall population in the United States, they are often excluded in large epidemiological estimates. For this reason, criminologists have shown little interest in the criminal behavior of Asian Americans.

Nevertheless, violence and illegal activity perpetrated by Asian Americans is a problem that warrants attention. The low estimates of Asian American criminality mask the existence of within-group variation with regard to criminal behavior and ignore pockets of violence in ethnic communities. For instance, Southeast Asian (Cambodian, Hmong, Laotian, and Vietnamese) youths have the highest rate of arrest among Asian Americans (Le, 2002) and are overrepresented in violence and crime statistics (National Council on Crime and Delinquency, 2003) relative to their proportion in the general population. Media reports also suggest that there is a strong presence of gang activity in ethnic enclaves in urban settings. For instance, the Jackson Street Boys originating in San Francisco's Chinatown; and the Color of Blood, and Sons of Death, originating in Richmond, California, have been implicated in a number of violent crimes occurring in the Bay Area over the last decade (Johnson, 2004; Zamora, 2003). The city of Oakland, California, estimates that there are 15 different Asian gangs within its Metropolitan area (City of Oakland Agenda Report, 2007).

The use of self-report data, however, may provide a more accurate reflection of criminal behavior among Asian Americans than criminal records (Hall, 2002). For instance, Hall and colleagues (2005) found that 30% of both Asian American and European American men endorsed engaging in sexually aggressive behavior in a study that included the largest sample of Asian American men studied to date.

Family Violence

Research on violence among Asian American families is limited, and results are often contradictory. Findings from the National Violence Against Women Survey (Tjaden & Thoennes, 2000) found no differences in physical assault against Asian American women compared with other ethnic groups. On the other hand, the 1993–1998 violence victimization rates reported by the Department of Justice Bureau of Justice Statistics indicate that AAPI males and females have the lowest rate of intimate partner violence of 1.9 and .3 per 1,000 persons over the age of 12, respectively (Rennison, 2002).

When domestic violence does occur, however, the circumstances surrounding the abuse are concerning. Bhuyan, Mell, Senturia, Sullivan, and Sharyne (2005) found that immigrant Cambodian woman reported self-blame related to their domestic abuse and attributed their victimization to fate (2005). A greater percentage of domestic disputes lead to homicide among Asian Americans and European Americans relative to other ethnic groups. Block and Christakos (1995) found in their study that intimate homicide accounted for 13% of all homicides among Asian Americans, which is higher than the proportion of intimate homicides for European Americans (11%) and Latinos (5%) and comparable of that to African Americans (14%).

Rates on child abuse for Asian Americans are also inconclusive. An examination of child welfare records for Los Angeles County found instances of physical abuse among 49 percent of immigrant Korean American families compared to 13 percent of all other families (J. Chang, Rhee, & Weaver, 2006) and 35 percent of all immigrant Chinese American families compared with 19 percent of all other families (Rhee, Weaver, Chang, & Wong, 2008). Lau et al. (2006), however, found in their self-report study that 33 % of Asian American parents reported use of minor assault (i.e. slapped, hit, spanked, pushed, grabbed) and 2.2 % reported major assault (kicked, bit, or hit with fist) toward their children. This is lower than rates of minor assault and major assault reported by European American (79.5 and 6 %), Hispanic (72 and 15.9 %), and black parents (73.2 and 11.5 %) in the National Comorbidity Survey from 1990–1992. When Asian American groups are broken further into sub-ethnic groups, Vietnamese Americans report even lower rates (13.8 and 1.5%) than Chinese Americans (38.1 and 1.8%) and Filipino Americans (38.8 and 2.5%). Parents with at least some college education were more likely and parents who immigrated to the United States later in life were less likely to report use of minor assault. Perceived discrimination and cultural conflict increased the likelihood of severe assault.

Current studies suggest inconsistent rates of externalizing symptoms and disorders for Asian and AAPI populations. In general, few studies indicate that externalizing symptoms are more of a problem among Asian and AAPI individuals relative to other ethnic groups. Although prevalence rates provide some insight into antisocial behavior among Asian and AAPI populations, there are several layers of complexity that clinicians should take into consideration when working with AAPIs with externalizing and antisocial disorders.

STRENGTHS, WEAKNESSES, AND ALTERNATIVES IN APPLYING CURRENT NOSOLOGY AND DIAGNOSTIC CRITERIA FOR IDENTIFYING EXTERNALIZING DISORDERS AND ANTISOCIAL BEHAVIOR

Among AAPIs

It is unknown whether the generally low rates of externalizing disorders constitute a real difference or whether AAPIs in the United States are misdiagnosed and underidentified with regard to externalizing disorders. Misdiagnosis can harm individuals, as it can lead to a mismatch in treatment goals and appropriate clinical interventions (e.g., medication).

On the other hand, the generally low rates of externalizing and antisocial behavior may constitute real differences in diagnoses. Asian culture traditionally emphasizes behavior consistent with social harmony and conformity (Kim & Markus, 1999). Thus, deviancy may be tolerated less in Asian culture than in Western cultures such as the United States, where uniqueness is more highly valued.

Underidentification may be less of a problem with regard to externalizing behavior problems among AAPI youth than internalizing behavior symptoms. Stereotypes of Asians may increase the likelihood that externalizing symptoms are recognized by professionals working with Asian American children. D. F. Chang and Sue (2003) found that stereotyping of Asian American children as passive, shy, and unassertive continues to persist and influence evaluations of what constitutes normal behavior. In their study, teachers were given vignettes describing undercontrolled, overcontrolled, or normal behaviors of a child who was identified as African American, Asian American, or European American. Teachers were more likely to perceive overcontrolled behaviors of an Asian American child as typical of their ethnic background, but normal and undercontrolled behaviors were more likely to be considered atypical of the child's ethnic background. These results suggest that Asian American children are less likely to be identified when exhibiting internalizing symptoms and more likely to be identified for externalizing symptoms, even for behaviors typically observed in children their own age.

Cultural differences may also differentially impact assessment tools of antisocial behavior. Fujii, Tokioka, Lichton, and Hishinuma (2005) examined the cultural validity of the HCR-20, a clinical rating scale for predicting violent behavior, among European Americans, Asian Americans, and Native Hawaiians. The HCR-20 had predictive validity for Asian Americans, Native Hawaiians, and European American psychiatric patients, but the predictive validity of individual items varied by ethnic group. For Asian Americans, impulsivity was the only significant predictor of violent behavior. For Native Hawaiians, age of violence initiation, relationship instability, and infeasibility of risk management plans predicted violence. Only age of violence initiation was predictive of violence behavior among European Americans. Because of the Asian American emphasis on saving face, Fujii et al. suggested that Asian Americans generally do not seek help unless symptoms are severe. As a result, only Asian Americans with severe psychiatric illness would be included in this psychiatric sample. Genetically determined factors (such as impulsivity) may be more predictive of violent behavior among patients with more severe psychiatric symptoms than situationally based factors (such as past history of antisocial behavior), which is more amendable to contextual changes. On the other hand, the items predicting violence among Native Hawaiians were related to context. The authors suggested that Native Hawaiians lack a construct for mental illness and instead refer to psychiatric symptoms as "pilikia," or "trouble occurs," underscoring the importance of context for shaping emotional and behavioral responses among Native Hawaiians. The study, however, lacked the necessary variables to support these explanations. Nevertheless, the study brings to light the cultural nuances associated with assessment and diagnostic tools.

In general, any ethnic differences should be interpreted with caution as such findings may inadvertently stigmatize specific cultural groups. Indeed, identification of externalizing disorders in children can be complex. Diagnoses are made based on clinical observation, as well as parent, teacher, and child report, which can vary widely based on the informant. Although some of these discrepancies may be due to contextual differences, others may be attributed to the informants and their awareness and sensitivity to psychological distress (Kazdin, Esveldt-Dawson, Unis, & Rancurello, 1998). Identification of externalizing disorders among different ethnic groups presents a particular challenge because behaviors are compared to what is considered culturally normal. As such, the threshold of when child and adolescent behavior is considered pathological is heavily influenced by culture. As noted above, Asian cultures tend to be high on collectivism and emphasize the maintenance of social harmony, suggesting that they have less tolerance for social deviance than a more individualistic culture. European American parents tend to socialize their children to be independent, and assertive behavior is encouraged. Asian children are expected to conform to social norms and parenting is more authoritarian than authoritative (Chao, 2001; Dornbusch, Ritter, Leiderman, Roberts, & Fraleigh, 1987).

Although Asian culture may be less tolerant of deviant behavior, AAPI parents may be less likely to perceive psychological and behavioral symptoms as problems that warrant intervention. Cross-cultural studies by Weisz and colleagues over the last two decades illustrate how cultural beliefs can influence the point at which the type of and intensity of a behavior is identified as a problem by parents. Weisz et al. (1988) compared the judgments of parents, teachers, and clinical psychologists on vignette descriptions of undercontrolled (i.e., disobedience) and overcontrolled (i.e., fear) behaviors of two children. Thais were less likely than Americans to perceive problems of undercontrolled and overcontrolled symptoms as serious and in need of attention compared to Americans and more likely to believe that behaviors will get better with time. Additionally, Lau et al. (2004) found in a study of 600 adolescents that ethnic minority parents, which included Asian American parents, reported significantly fewer externalizing symptoms on the Achenbach Behavior Rating Scale than their offspring when compared to European American parents. Lau et al. suggested that ethnic minority parents may be less sensitive to their children's symptoms due to their acculturative stress. Also having less familiarity with the concept of mental health likely causes them to be oblivious to specific symptoms. Both studies suggest that low rates of problems may be due to cultural differences in perceptions of problem behaviors.

When applying the diagnostic criteria for externalizing disorders to AAPI populations, clinicians should be familiar with issues related to socialization practices, clinical bias, cultural nuances in assessment tools, and perceptions of problem behaviors. These factors are likely to impact prevalence rates of externalizing disorders, as well as motivations to seek treatment.

PERSPECTIVES ON THE CAUSES
OF EXTERNALIZING DISORDERS AND
ANTISOCIAL BEHAVIOR AMONG ASIANS

Theories of antisocial behavior have commonly identified antisocial behavior that is serious and chronic, and typically aggressive (Moffitt, 1993). Another form of antisocial behavior is circumscribed, typically nonaggressive, and often begins and desists during adolescence. The former form of antisocial behavior, which often begins during childhood, is more likely to be genetically influenced, whereas the adolescence limited form is more prominently influenced by environmental processes (Moffitt, 1993). Although most researchers will agree that externalizing disorders are a product of psychological, social, and biological influences, understanding the separate etiological theories provides a strong foundation toward a more integrative and holistic explanatory model of externalizing disorders among Asians, Asian Americans and Pacific Islanders.

Biological/Genetic Models

Biological explanations of ethnic differences in antisocial behavior tend to evoke an uncomfortable, even contentious reaction from those in the mental health profession. As such, any discussion of biological factors that underlie disparities in antisocial behavior must be addressed carefully and thoroughly as to not inadvertently stigmatize ethnic groups. Nevertheless, a discussion of causal pathways toward antisocial and externalizing symptoms is incomplete without an understanding of genetic influences.

Recent work examining the role of genetics in explaining ethnic disparities in antisocial behavior and externalizing symptoms has focused on the identification of the role of candidate genes. In pursuit of this endeavor, both structural and functional genomics approaches have been used to identify candidate genes associated with antisocial behavior. Structural genomic approaches (e.g., mapping) provide information about the location, structure, and sequence of a candidate gene or genes. Functional approaches for candidate genes studies identify and define when and how gene products are associated with gene sequences (e.g., the neurotransmitters serotonin, dopamine, and monamine oxidase A in the case of antisocial behaviors). It should be noted that the following findings are preliminary and that most have not been replicated. However, they are mentioned here to spur additional research and to provide a basic understanding of biological influences on antisocial behavior.

There is evidence to suggest that certain types of genetic risk for antisocial behaviors and externalizing disorders may be consistent between individuals of Asian descent and those of European descent. For instance, diminished serotonergic activity may increase sensitivity to stimuli that elicit provocation and aggression and decrease sensitivity to stimuli associated with punishment (Spoont, 1992). Low serotonergic activity is associated with greater aggressive behavior in European American and Asian groups (Lee & Coccaro, 2001). Serotonergic transmitter dysfunction associated with aggression and conduct disorder has been identified on chromosome 17q12 region. In a sample of 153 European American male forensic patients, the 5-HTTLPR S allele at the 17q12 site (a polymorphism within the 5HT transporter promoter gene involved in serotonin function) was more commonly found among those with recurrent violent behavior (Retz et al., 2004). The 17q12 chromosomal region was also implicated in conduct disorder studies including 249 adolescents from consecutive admissions to treatment facilities for substance abuse and delinquency and their siblings and 4,493 community adolescents (Stallings et al., 2005). Liao, Hong, Shih, and Tsai (2004) also identified SLC64 as a possible candidate serotonin transporter gene at the 17q12 loci. In their study of 169 criminals and 111 community controls in Taiwan, violent criminals were identified as having a higher frequency of the 5-HTTLPR S allele than controls.

Because of the role of dopamine in brain reward and approach systems, some researchers have postulated associations between dopamine regulation, antisocial behaviors, and novelty-seeking. There is some evidence of DRD2 and DRD4 as candidate genes associated with conduct disorder in European American samples (Rowe et al., 2001) and DRD2 with conduct disorder in Han Chinese samples (Lu, Lee, Ko, & Lin, 2001). However, despite evidence of an association between DRD4 and novelty-seeking behavior, these results have been less convincing since they have not been replicated possibly due to substantial unknown moderators across studies (Schinka, Letsch, & Crawford, 2002).

Other findings on genetic risk have not been replicated with AAPI samples. For example, monoamine oxidase A (MAO-A) is crucial for the catabolic metabolism of monoamine neurotransmitters, and low activity associated with the MAO-A allele has been linked with antisocial behavior. Researchers have suggested that low MAO-A activity interacts with child maltreatment, an environmental variable, increasing risk for antisocial behavior. Caspi and colleagues (2002) studied the childhood maltreatment history (8% severe, 28% probable, 64% not maltreated) and MAO-A genotype (37% low activity allele, 63% high activity allele) of 442 white males in the longitudinal Dunedin Multidisciplinary Health and Development Study. Among boys having the combination of the low MAO-A activity allele and severe maltreatment, 85% developed some form of antisocial outcome (i.e., conduct disorder, violent behavior, disposition toward violence, antisocial personality disorder) by 26 years of age, whereas about 25% with low MAO-A activity who were not maltreated developed an antisocial outcome. Among those with the high activity MAO-A allele and severe maltreatment, approximately 42% developed an antisocial outcome, and 25% of those with the high activity allele and without maltreatment developed antisocial behavior. While the direct effects of the MAO-A allele were limited, child maltreatment was suggested as a potent risk factor for antisocial behavior, with child maltreatment in combination with low MAO activity creating the greatest risk for antisocial behavior.

Despite this seemingly robust finding, the association of low MAO-A activity and antisocial behavior was not replicated in an Asian sample. In a cohort of 631 males and females studied from childhood to adulthood, Widom and Brzustowicz (2006) found that the interaction of low MAO-A activity and childhood maltreatment (court-substantiated child abuse and neglect) was associated with violent and antisocial behavior (arrests, self-report, diagnoses) among European American participants, but not among non–European Americans (African Americans, Latino/a Americans, American Indians, and Pacific Islanders). It is difficult to draw conclusions specifically about the AAPI groups specifically in their study because separate analyses on the non–European American participants were not conducted.

Lu and colleagues (2003) found no direct effects of MAO-A on antisocial behavior among Chinese Han males. The uVNTR and EcoRV polymorphisms of the MAO-A gene, both individually and as a haplotype block (a number of genetic variants that are associated with one another), were studied among 41 men diagnosed with antisocial personality disorder and alcoholism, 50 diagnosed with antisocial personality disorder without alcoholism, 38 without either disorder as a jail control group, and 77 community controls. No significant association was observed between these two gene polymorphisms and antisocial personality disorder with alcoholism, either individually or for haplotype, or for antisocial personality disorder without alcoholism. Unfortunately, these researchers did not account for the confounding influence of child maltreatment, which has been shown to interact with low MAO-A activity producing antisocial behavior (Caspi et al., 2002; Foley et al., 2004). However, the Widom and Brzustowicz (2006) and Lu et al. (2003) study results underscore the need to study antisocial behavior across racial and ethnic populations.

It should be noted that researchers also have suggested that maltreatment is not the result of an exclusive environmental influence but how a child's genetic constitution contributes to behaviors that evoke maltreatment from their parents (Moffitt, 2005; Rutter et al., 2001). However, Jaffee et al. (2004) have suggested more severe forms of punishment may be more influenced by genes than less severe forms of punishment and found evidence that factors leading to maltreatment occur primarily in the environment rather than in the child.

Although obtaining gene location and function can be critical first steps toward understanding the genomics of antisocial behavior, what behavioral scientists have to offer is the understanding of the interrelationships and interactions between genes, environment, and behavior. Unfortunately, identifying and understanding specific genomic contributions associated with antisocial behavior has been limited by study participant samples that are not inclusive of broader racial, ethnic, and cultural populations.

Psychosocial Theories

Psychosocial models of ethnic differences in externalizing disorders and antisocial behavior generally have wider acceptance and greater empirical support than biological/genetic models. As discussed above, social theories are more applicable to antisocial behaviors that begin and desist in adolescence (Moffitt & Caspi, 2001).

A study by Jang (2002) integrated social learning theory (Akers, 1985) and social bonding theory (Hirschi, 1969) to explain antisocial behavior in 18,132 Asian Americans and non–Asian American adolescents. Social learning posits that association with deviant peers increases risk of deviancy. Social bonding theory suggests that while deviant motivation is universally experienced, deviant behavior is the result of broken bonds with conventional institutions. Jang hypothesized that Asian American adolescents are less deviant than their non-Asian counterparts because they are more attached, committed, associated, and involved in conventional institutions and their authority figures, activities, and peers and more likely to hold conventional beliefs. Therefore, Jang postulated that Asian American adolescents are more likely to value academic achievement, accept informal methods of social control, and less likely to associate with deviant peers. Asian American adolescents were significantly less likely to report engagement in school related deviant behaviors than non–Asian American adolescents (Jang, 2002). No significant difference was found on other types of deviant acts such as running away from home and criminal arrest.

Observed ethnic differences may be attributed to family characteristics (social economic status, family size, and family intactness), Asian Americans' commitment to education, and their association with nondeviant peers. Jang (2002) noted that, while school bonding variables were significant in explaining ethnic differences in deviant behavior, family bonding factors were not. Asian American adolescents did not report greater attachment to their parents than adolescents of other ethnic groups. However, family bonding was measured by affective ties and close communication with family members. Jang noted that cultural conflict may be an emerging problem during the adolescent time period in Asian American child-parent relationships, which may explain the low scores reported by Asian American adolescents. She further noted that lack of communication may be less of a problem in Asian culture where affective closeness is not traditionally emphasized. Instead, Asian parents rely on nonverbal means of exerting social control, which may have been cultivated at an early age and continue to have an effect despite the lack of close communication between Asian American parents and their adolescent children. Therefore, although Jang's study included a measure of family bonding, further research is necessary in order to understand the complex influence of family dynamics on Asian Americans' antisocial behavior.

Problems with Current Models

Existing models do not specifically address the role of culture in contributing to antisocial symptoms and externalizing disorders. One reason for this oversight is that the stigmatization attached to antisocial and externalizing disorders deters researchers from identifying specific aspects of culture that may contribute to or mitigate antisocial tendencies. Additionally, existing models are overly simplistic and do not integrate the role of culture and biology in explaining antisocial behavior among AAPI populations. In this section, we first identify specific aspects of Asian culture that may mitigate or increase antisocial behavior. Next we propose a more integrative model that incorporates cultural and genetic risk. What becomes clear is that the same cultural value may act as both a risk and a protective factor depending on the context and that any model of antisocial behavior is incomplete without considering the influence of genetic risk.

Risk and Protective Factors

Asian American parents tend to emphasize social harmony and discourage assertive behavior among their children (Ou & McAdoo, 1993), suggesting that Asian cultural values may be a salient protective factor against Asian American externalizing and antisocial behavior. Yet, the empirical literature on cultural factors has been contradictory and inconclusive. Wong (1999) found that adherence to Chinese culture was a protective factor against delinquency and acculturation to North American values was a risk factor among 315 Chinese Canadian youths aged 10–20. Conversely, ethnic identity was positively associated with delinquency among a sample of 54 adolescent Cambodian American males (Go & Le, 2005). In this study, Cambodian ethnic identity was associated with trauma and war experience. Meanwhile, Le and Stockdale (2008) found no relationship between ethnic identity and peer delinquency or serious violence among a sample of 329 Chinese, Cambodian, Laotian, and Vietnamese youth. Thus, ethnic identity in interdependent cultures is a broad construct and does not constitute a protective factor per se, especially given the amount of diversity within AAPI populations.

One reason for these conflicting findings is that the acculturative process and ethnic identity may be associated with either positive or negative experiences depending on the context and as such may not be as informative as other cultural variables. Social factors, unrelated to culture but associated with immigration or minority status, can increase risk of antisocial acts. In the Lau et al. study (2006), reported perceived discrimination and family conflict, and not nativity status or acculturation, were associated with parent report of severe assault against their children. Discrimination has also been found to increase risk of engaging in physical fighting and use of a weapon among Southeast Asian youth (Ho, 2008). This finding, however, may depend on ethnic identification. Deng, Kim, Vaughan, and Li (2010) found that ethnic identity moderated the relationship between perceived discrimination and adolescent delinquency. In their study of 311 Chinese American adolescents, they found that, among Chinese adolescents with a strong Chinese orientation, there was a positive association between perceived discrimination and delinquency while there was no relationship between perceived discrimination and delinquency among adolescents with a low Chinese orientation. This suggests that perceived discrimination can be risk factor for antisocial behavior but only among Chinese youth who are highly identified with their culture of origin.

The influence of cultural norms within the group may be more important than being a member of an interdependent group or identifying with it. Prosocial norms in an interdependent group create a proscription against antisocial behavior. Thus, engaging in antisocial behavior would result in "loss of face," an East Asian concept related to shaming of one's in-group (i.e., family). Although norms in many ethnic groups are prosocial, ethnic subgroups, such as gangs, may develop antisocial norms in which prosocial behavior is proscribed. In such subgroup contexts, failing to engage in antisocial behavior would result in loss of face (Hall, 2002).

However, AAPI youth may gravitate away from norms inherent to their culture of origin toward norms established by their peers. Rumbaut and Portes (2002) have observed that immigrant parents and their children tend to experience acculturative dissonance, which describes the differing rates of adaptation to the host culture exhibited by parents and their offspring. Acculturative dissonance may lead to increased family conflict, which in turn contributes to youth delinquency (Choi, He, & Hirachi, 2009).

Similar to youths from other ethnic groups, peer norms have been consistently shown to influence antisocial behavior among Asian American adolescents. Peer delinquency has been shown to be positively associated with delinquency for Cambodian, Korean, Japanese, Laotian, Mien, Vietnamese, and Chinese American adolescents (Go & Le, 2005; Kim & Goto, 2000; Le, Monfared, & Stockdale, 2005). Peer delinquency is also a stronger predictor of antisocial behavior in Asian American youths than parental influences, such as social support, attachment, and discipline (Kim & Goto, 2000; Le et al., 2005). Peers provide an important source of social support, particularly if acculturative dissonance is pronounced among families. Ethnically similar peers may have a better understanding of acculturative dissonance, which may result in their seeking each other out for emotional support. These same ethnic peer friendships may result in a group that is alienated from mainstream culture. The gravitation of second-generation youths to antisocial peer groups may reflect experiences of social marginalization as an identified member of a minority group.

Hall and Barongan (1997) posited that prosocial cultural norms in some self-identified ethnic groups having an interdependent orientation may attenuate risk factors for men's antisocial behavior. Supporting this hypothesis, Hall, Sue, and colleagues (2000) have demonstrated that loss of face is a protective factor against sexual aggression among Asian American men. Rates of self-reported sexually aggressive behavior were not significantly different between 377 European American and 91 Asian American men. However, Asian American men were significantly more concerned about loss of face than European American men. Concern about loss of face generally was a protective factor against sexual aggression among Asian Americans, but was not significantly associated with European American men's sexual aggression. European American men's sexual aggression was primarily determined by misogynous beliefs.

In a replication and extension of the Hall, Sue, et al. (2000) study, Hall and colleagues (2005) examined sexual aggression among 222 mainland Asian Americans, 127 Asian Americans in Hawaii, and 399 European Americans from the mainland and Hawaii. The study of ethnic minority (mainland) and ethnic majority (Hawaiian) Asian Americans was important to determine if loss of face is more pronounced in situations in which a group is a numerical minority versus a cultural variable. Results from that study mirrored those of Hall et al. (2000). Loss of face was a protective factor against sexual aggression among both the mainland and Hawaiian Asian American subsamples. Asian American men generally were more concerned than European American men about loss of face, and there was not a main effect for loss of face on sexual aggression among European Americans.

One might argue that Asian American men concerned about loss of face may have under-reported sexually aggressive acts. However, the study also found an association between loss of face and self-reported early physical and sexual abuse histories in Asian American men, but not European American men. Asian American males who are sexually or physically abused as children and learn the cultural value of loss of face may become aware that abusive relationships are nonnormative (Hall et al., 2005). They may not become perpetrators of abuse because they do not want to engage in behavior that is deviant and would result in loss of face. The attenuation of the effects of early physical/sexual abuse by loss of face is important, because early physical/sexual abuse has been found to be a risk factor for antisocial behavior (Caspi et al., 2002; Foley et al., 2004).

Hall and colleagues' (2005) ethnic-specific findings were not a function of actual or perceived minority status, as mainland Asian Americans and Asian Americans in Hawaii did not differ on a measure of loss of face. Additionally, perceived minority status was not significantly correlated with loss of face. The findings were also not a result of response bias, as loss of face was associated with both socially desirable and undesirable attitudes. Thus, loss of face may be a protective factor that is generally more relevant to Asian Americans, who have interdependent cultural origins, than to European Americans, whose culture is independent.

In a one-year follow-up of the Hall et al. (2005) study, Hall and colleagues (2006) identified four groups of men among 562 Asian Americans and 477 European Americans who: (1) were not sexually aggressive (N = 358; nonaggressors); (2) reported being sexual aggressive at the first assessment but not at the second (N = 120; desisters); (3) reported being sexually aggressive at the second assessment but not at the first (N = 39; initiators); and (4) reported sexual aggression at both assessments (N = 48, persisters). There were no ethnic differences in representation in these four sexual aggression trajectory groups. As in the previous studies (Hall et al., 2000; Hall et al., 2005), loss of face was a protective factor against sexual aggression for self-identified Asian Americans but not for European Americans.

These four sexual aggression trajectory groups are important to study because they correspond with chronic and transitory antisocial subtypes, which are assumed to differ in genetic vs. environmental influence (Moffitt, 1993). The one-year follow-up in the Hall et al. (2006) study did not allow a definitive determination of whether the participants' sexual aggression actually desisted or was chronic. Nevertheless, it is possible that some of the men in the sample had genetic risk for antisocial behavior that was attenuated by loss of face.

Toward an Integrated Model of Antisocial Behavior

The existence of ethnic differences is important because it implies differential genetic and environmental risk for antisocial behavior. It is important to consider how and to what degree the presumptions about racial, ethnic, and cultural differences are in biological, environmental, behavioral, and/or cultural underpinnings. Central to these issues is the question of whether cultural risk and protective factors exist and, if they do, how they enhance or attenuate genetic risk for antisocial behavior.

The study of race, ethnicity, culture, and antisocial behavior has been regarded as contentious in behavioral genomics research. This may be due to social and personal fears of the possible unwarranted group stigma and harms based on reinforcing genetic essentialism by identifying increased genetic risks for antisocial behavior that is greater for one group than for another. That said, what do cross-racial heritability studies tell us about antisocial behavior?

Although genetic risk for antisocial behavior across racial groups has not been adequately examined at this time, data suggest that an equal distribution of antisocial behavior exists (Zuckerman, 2003). Does this mean that there is an equal probability of genetic risk for antisocial behavior across population groups? How do ethnic and cultural contexts moderate antisocial behavior?

Race and ethnicity are often treated as categorical independent variables where most studies of purported racial and ethnic differences do not include adequate or consistent measures of race or ethnicity (Ota Wang & Sue, 2005). For example, self-identified racial and ethnic categories do not reveal the basis of ethnic differences or similarities, often ignore the great variability within racial and ethnic groups, and can be poor proxies for biological processes.

Race and ethnicity variables may be more useful in research designs if they are considered as moderators or mediators of behavior (Ota Wang & Sue, 2005). Thus, the basis of racial or ethnic differences should also be carefully conceptualized and measured. For example, acculturation and other cultural variables, such as interdependent cultural norms, may account for ethnic differences in a behavior.

Similar to child maltreatment interacting with genetic risk to produce antisocial behavior (Caspi et al., 2002; Foley et al., 2004), cultural norms may influence expression thresholds that may alter (e.g., trigger or prevent expression of) genetic diathesis. The *social push hypothesis* suggests that for those exposed to adverse early environments (e.g., child maltreatment), social influences (e.g., antisocial cultural norms) on antisocial behavior may camouflage genetic influences (Raine, 2002). Indeed, in a Swedish twin study, environmental influences on antisocial behavior (i.e., self-reported property offenses, drug-related offenses, violent offenses; $c^2 = 69\%$) were stronger than genetic influences ($a^2 = 1\%$) under conditions of neighborhood socioeconomic disadvantage, as determined by percentage of persons born outside Europe, North America, Australia, and New Zealand, educational level, unemployment level, net income, and crime rates (Tuvblad, Grann, & Lichtenstein, 2006). Under conditions of neighborhood socioeconomic advantage, genetic influences ($a^2 = 37\%$) were stronger than environmental influences ($c^2 = 13\%$).

Additionally, cultural norms may confer protection against genetic risk for antisocial behavior. Social order may be maintained in cultural contexts through informal social control, which involves social norms and structural constraints that are placed on people to limit their behavior and choices. According to the *social control hypothesis*, in settings of high social control, a large percentage of the people will exhibit the same phenotype (e.g., prosocial behavior) regardless of their genotypes, whereas in settings marked by low social control, people's choices and behaviors are more likely to reflect their genotype (Shanahan & Hofer, 2005). Given what we know about the interaction between genetic risk and cultural influences on antisocial behavior, a revised model is proposed below to explain the development of antisocial behavior.

A Genocultural Model of Antisocial Behavior

A proposed genocultural model of antisocial behavior is presented in Figure 10.1. Genetic factors create a risk for childhood antisocial behavior which, in turn, creates a risk for adolescent antisocial behavior. Although antisocial behavior that commences in adolescence may be directly influenced by genetic factors, it is more likely to be influenced by environmental processes (Moffitt, 1993). Other protective genetic factors may moderate genetic risk. Cultural moderators may also attenuate or exacerbate genetic risk. Our focus is on cultural moderators, although there are other environmental moderators of risk for antisocial behavior that are not necessarily culturally based, such as socioeconomic status, education, and child maltreatment.

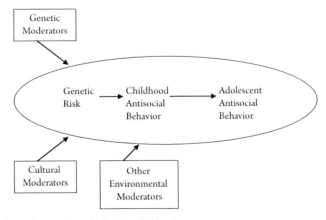

FIGURE 10.1: A Genocultural Model of Behavior.

We posit that group norms are stronger influences in groups that are interdependent and weaker in groups that are independent and have less identification with groups or group norms. Group influences are also likely to be stronger in ethnic groups that have norms of social control than in groups in which there is less social control. A cultural protective factor would be interdependent social norms. Such social control norms may be transmitted through families, peers, or both. Conversely, a cultural risk factor would be low social control norms in an independent context. Although low social control norms may be transmitted via families and peers, personal decisions concerning antisocial behavior may be as influential, if not more influential, in independent contexts. However, interdependency would increase risk for antisocial behavior in contexts where norms are antisocial.

In instances of increased genetic risk without an increased cultural risk, the presence of antisocial behavior would implicate genetic influences, whereas its absence would implicate cultural influences. An example of low or absent cultural risk would be a context in which there are social control norms. In instances of an increased cultural risk without genetic risk, the presence of antisocial behavior would implicate cultural influences, whereas its absence would implicate genetic influences. Low social control norms would be an example of environmental risk.

TREATING EXTERNALIZING AND ANTISOCIAL BEHAVIOR IN AAPIS

Before considering the treatment implications of the genocultural model, it is important to consider the application of current evidence-based treatments (EBTs) to externalizing disorders and antisocial behavior in AAPIs. The majority of EBTs for externalizing disorders and antisocial behavior utilize cognitive behavioral approaches, as well as a group format, and tend to focus on anger management. Meta-analyses of empirical studies over the past couple of decades indicate medium effect sizes for the treatment of anger in children and adolescents (Sukhodolsky, Kassinove, & Gorman, 2004) and medium-large effect sizes for the treatment of anger in adults (Del Vecchio & O'Leary, 2004) with less support available for the treatment of serious violent offenders (Howells et al., 2005). However, few EBTs have had a sufficient number of AAPIs to support the use of treatment protocols with Asian Americans (Hall & Eap, 2007), and the effectiveness of EBTs for externalizing disorders and antisocial behavior has not been evaluated in AAPI populations. This includes empirically supported treatments of externalizing behavior disorders among children, namely behavioral therapy and parent management training (Maughan, Christiansen, Jenson, Olympia, & Clark, 2005).

One exception is the Head Start Parent Training from the *Incredible Years*. Reid, Webster-Stratton, and Beauchaine (2001) found evidence of decreased behavioral problems at one-year follow-up for children of parents enrolled in the experimental condition compared with the control conditions among a sample of 637 families, which included 73 Asian American families. The study found no ethnic differences with regard to treatment response, suggesting that parent training may be an effective treatment for externalizing disorders among Asian American children. Although the investigators found support for the use of parent management training for preschool-age children, clinicians should be cognizant of how cultural norms regarding parenting practices (e.g. an emphasis on nonverbal communication) may affect outcomes.

In a meta-analytic review of 77 parent-training programs, Kaminiski, Valle, Filene, and Boyle (2008) identified several components of parent-training programs that were associated with higher effect sizes, including increasing positive parent-child interactions and emotional communication skills. However, it is not clear if such findings would be replicated with AAPI samples, since increasing emotional communication skills may go against cultural norms. Additionally, increasing positive parent-child interactions may be a reasonable goal of treatment. However, the characteristics of positive parent-child interactions are culturally derived, and clinicians should be cognizant of both their clients' communication styles and preferences. Interestingly, there is some evidence that Asians and Asian Americans are more likely than European Americans to use *and* benefit from social support that does not involve explicit disclosure of distress (Kim, Sherman, & Taylor, 2008). Since acculturative dissonance has emerged as a prominent risk factor in antisocial behavior among AAPI youth, parent training and family treatment may also need to address such conflict. It is possible that acculturative dissonance and other risk factors for antisocial behavior in AAPIs (e.g., perceived discrimination) may moderate treatment outcome.

Clinicians should also consider the marginalized status of AAPIs in society, particularly when implementing cognitive behavioral approaches for anger management. According to Huesmann's script theory (1988), individuals who perceive the world as a dangerous place are more prone to violence than those who see the world as a safe place. While it is reasonable to assume that this theory is applicable to AAPIs, clinicians should be careful not to assume that their clients' hostile perceptions of others are largely inaccurate, especially with clients who have experienced repeated instances of racism and colonialism, as is the case with Native Hawaiians (McMullin, 2005). Unfortunately, existing violence prevention and treatment programs often fail to recognize the oppressive sociopolitical contexts in which they operate, instead focusing on the perceived faults of the individual (Ginwight & Cammarota, 2002). Rather than trying to refute "dysfunctional" beliefs (e.g., "People are discriminating against me."), it is advised that clinicians focus instead on reducing overgeneralization and dichotomous thinking (e.g., "Everyone is out to get me."), while acknowledging the validity of their clients' experiences.

Despite the lack of EBTs for Asian Americans, Guerrero, Goebert, Alicata, and Bell (2009) suggest that mental health professionals working with Asian Americans should have knowledge and familiarity of cultural concepts such as *ethnic identity, collective self concept, acculturation, culture congruency,* and *bicultural self-efficacy.* In addition to the cultural concepts suggested by Guerrero et al., current studies by Hall and colleagues underscore the role of specific cultural values (e.g., loss of face) in shaping behavior and preventing deviancy. For example, rather than avoiding loss of face in therapy for the purpose of reducing a client's distress, clinicians may choose to explore the importance of saving face as a motivator for change. Similarly, when the norms of an individual's reference group are prosocial, clinicians should emphasize such norms; when reference group norms are antisocial, it is important for individuals to distance themselves from such groups and find prosocial groups to identify with (Hall, 2002). Group therapists are in a unique position of facilitating the development of a prosocial group that individuals can identify with, particularly when prosocial leaders emerge within the group.

THE GENOCULTURAL MODEL AND TREATMENT

Researchers have advocated for the development of interventions for antisocial behavior that are based on contemporary aggression theories (Gilbert & Daffern, 2010). Treatment grounded in the genocultural model addresses the complex interactions between genetic risk, cultural variables, and an individual's larger societal context. Individuals engaging in antisocial behavior in environments under low prosocial control may benefit from environments with high prosocial control. Similarly, individuals engaging in antisocial behavior in environments under high antisocial control (e.g., gangs) may benefit from environments with high prosocial control. Individuals who engage in antisocial behavior in environments with high prosocial control may require more intensive interventions.

A genocultural treatment approach should also address specific aspects of culture that may be contributing or protecting an individual from antisocial behaviors. In this chapter, a number of cultural variables have been identified as potential risk/protective factors for antisocial behavior in AAPIs, including ethnic identity, interdependence, and loss of face. Level of acculturation and experiences of discrimination are also important clinical considerations. Once a case conceptualization is formulated based on an understanding of an individual's risk and protective factors, clinicians are then able to tailor their treatments to reduce risk factors and increase protective factors to the extent possible. For example, the importance of saving face through prosocial behavior (or through the remittance of antisocial behavior) may be explored through motivational interviewing. The *good lives model* (Ward, 2002) suggests that targeting an offender's personal goals and values is motivating and may lead to change. Understanding an individual's culturally derived value system (e.g., interdependence) is an important and potentially powerful treatment consideration.

More broadly speaking, the genocultural model suggests that treatment should also address the larger context in which an individual is located. Programs that incorporate critical pedagogies recognize the larger context in which antisocial behavior occurs. Trinidad (2009) presented a compelling case study of a "contextually grounded" intervention, "Towards *Kuleana* (responsibility)," for Native Hawaiian youth in Hawai'i. The program, which consisted of a student-run organic farm, included critical pedagogy (i.e., questioning dominant paradigms by raising "critical consciousness"), community youth development, and Hawaiian epistemology to promote wellness and the prevention of violence. According to Trinidad:

> Many programs for minority youth superimpose values and ways of being that are contrary to the youths' native culture. A focus on community epistemology is essential in understanding the specific needs of a cultural group, and challenges colonial assumptions about learning that contradict indigenous values. (p. 490)

Such programs, although not well established or empirically validated, offer culturally derived alternatives to programs that are well established but have not been validated with AAPIs.

CONCLUSION

Antisocial behavior and externalizing disorders are problems that have serious and noxious societal consequences. Externalizing disorders cover a diverse range of antisocial behaviors. The research on these classes of disorders is poorly understood with regard to the Asian and AAPI population, perhaps as a result of existing "model minority" stereotypes that characterize this population. Generally, prevalence rates suggest that externalizing symptoms among Asian and AAPI individuals are lower or comparable to that of other ethnic groups. Among Southeast Asian Americans, the problem of antisocial behavior is even more frequent and pervasive relative to their population in the United States. Their neglect in the empirical literature suggests that the research is lagging behind the needs of the community.

The factors that affect the diagnosis of externalizing disorders may be one contributing factor to the low prevalence rates. Although, Asian Americans are more likely to be diagnosed with an internalizing than an externalizing disorders relative to other ethnic groups (Nguyen et al., 2004), it is unclear whether this trend is due to clinician bias or a product of true ethnic differences. Among Asian American children, teachers are more likely to consider internalizing problems as less alarming than externalizing problems (D. F. Chang & Sue, 2003), suggesting that bias may actually increase the likelihood that externalizing symptoms are identified. Studies also suggest that the beliefs that emotional distress and behavioral problems are time limited (Weisz et al., 1988) and driven by context may influence the types of individuals that are seen in a clinical context (Fujii et al. 2005), perhaps limiting prevalence rates to only those individuals experiencing severe symptoms. For Asian American families, the experience of acculturative dissonance within families may provide some validity to the contribution of context to mental health symptoms.

Current models explaining antisocial behavior and externalizing disorders do not take into consideration cultural and social risk factors that are specific to Asian and AAPI populations. Additionally, biological/genetic models are not well integrated with social models.

Future studies need to examine the interaction of biological factors (such as low serotonergic activity, the effect of DRD2 and DRD4 as candidate genes, and low MAO-A activity) with cultural and social variables (such as acculturative dissonance, loss of face, and discrimination experiences) in order to understand fully the etiology of antisocial behavior and externalizing disorders among Asian, Asian American, and Pacific Islander populations. If cultural norms of social control attenuate genetic risk for antisocial behavior, an intervention based on the genocultural model could preserve or enhance such cultural norms. However, preserving and enhancing interdependent cultural norms associated with social control is antithetical to pressures to acculturate to independent norms in the United States. Moreover, most interventions for antisocial behavior focus on individuals and not on group norms that may be prosocial or antisocial (Hall et al., 2005). Such an individual focus may be appropriate among interdependent individuals. Nevertheless, the identification of culture-specific patterns of risk and protection for antisocial behavior would imply the need for more culture-specific intervention and prevention.

In this chapter, we proposed a genocultural model of aggression that emphasizes an individual's cultural context, risk, and protective factors. Given the lack of evidence-based treatments for AAPIs, specifically for the treatment of antisocial behavior and externalizing disorders, it is important that treatments be developed based on culturally sensitive models of aggression, such as the genocultural model. Research in the area of treatment for AAPIs demonstrating antisocial behavior is especially limited, though we anticipate such research to grow as the needs of the population become more prominent.

AUTHOR NOTES

Work on this article was supported by National Institute of Mental Health grants R01 MH58726 and R25 MH62575. We thank Deborah Capaldi and Temi Moffitt for their comments on an earlier version of this article.

Correspondence concerning this article should be addressed to Sopagna Eap Braje, California School of Professional Psychology-San Diego, Alliant International University, 10455 Pomerado Road, San Diego, CA 92131–1799. E-mail: sbraje@alliant.edu

REFERENCES

Achenbach, T. M. (1982). *Developmental psychopathology* (2nd ed.). New York: Wiley.

Akers, R. (1985). *Deviant behavior: A social-learning approach.* Belmont, CA: Wadsworth.

American Psychiatric Association. (2000). *Diagnostic and statistical manual of mental disorders* (4th ed., text rev.). Washington, DC: Author.

Biederman, J., Newcorn, T., & Sprich, S. (1991). Comorbidity of attention deficit hyperactivity disorder with conduct, depressive, anxiety, and other disorders. *American Journal of Psychiatry, 148,* 564–577.

Biederman, J., Wilens, T., Mick, E. Faraone, S., & Spencer, T. (1998). Does attention deficit hyperactivity disorder impact the developmental course of drug and alcohol abuse and dependence? *Biological Psychiatry, 44,* 269–273.

Biederman, J., Wilens, T., Mick, E., Milberger, S. Spencer, T., & Faraone, S. (1995). Psychoactive substance use disorder in adults with attention deficit hyperactivity disorder: effects of ADHD and psychiatric comorbidity. *American Journal of Psychiatry, 152,* 1652–1658.

Bhuyan, R., Mell, M., Senturia, K., Sullivan, M., & Sharyne, S. (2005). Women must endure according to their karma. *Journal of Interpersonal Violence, 20,* 902–921.

Block, C. R., & Christakos, A. (1995). Intimate partner homicide in Chicago over 29 years. *Crime and Delinquency, 41,* 496–526.

Bureau of Justice Statistics. (2010). *Number of State Prisoners Declined by Almost 3,000 During 2009; Federal Prison Population Increased by 6,800.* Retrieved on September 7, 2010, from http://bjs.ojp.usdoj.gov/content/pub/press/pim09stpy09acpr.cfm.

Caspi, A., McClay, J., Moffitt, T. E., Mill, J., Martin, J., Craig, I., et al. (2002, August 2). Role of genotype in the cycle of violence in maltreated children. *Science, 297,* 851–854.

Chang, J., Rhee, S., & Weaver, D. (2006). Characteristics of child abuse in immigrant Korean families and correlates of placement decisions. *Child Abuse and Neglect, 30,* 881–891.

Chang, D. F., & Sue, S. (2003). The effects of race and problem type on teachers' assessments of student behavior. *Journal of Clinical and Consulting Psychology, 71,* 235–242.

City of Oakland Agenda Report. (2007). Retrieved on August 1, 2010, from http://clerkwebsvr1.oaklandnet.com/attachments/17261.pdf.

Chao, R. (2001). Extending research on the consequences of parenting style for Chinese Americans and European Americans. *Child Development, 72,* 1832–1843.

Choi, Y., He, M., & Harachi, T. W. (2009). Intergenerational cultural dissonance, parent-child conflict and bonding, and youth problem behaviors among Vietnamese and Cambodian immigrant families. *Journal of Youth Adolescence, 37,* 85–96.

Choi, Y., & Lahey, B. B. (2006). Testing the model minority stereotype: Youth behaviors across racial and ethnic groups. *Social Science Review, 84,* 419–452.

Costello, E. J., Mustillo, S., Keeler, G., & Angold, A. (2004). Prevalence of psychiatric disorders in childhood and adolescents. In B. L. Levin, J. Petrilla, K. D. Hennessy (Eds.), *Mental health services: A public health perspective* (pp. 111–128). New York: Oxford University Press.

Del Vecchio, T., & O'Leary, K. D. (2004). Effectiveness of anger treatments for specific anger problems: A meta-analytic review. *Clinical Psychology Review, 24,* 15–34.

Deng, S., Kim, S. Y., Vaughan, P. W., & Li, J. (2010). Cultural orientation as a moderator of the relationship between Chinese American adolescents' discrimination experiences and delinquent behaviors. *Journal of Youth and Adolescence, 39,* 1027–1040.

Dornbusch, S., Ritter, P., Leiderman, P., Roberts, D., & Fraleigh, M. (1987). The relation of parenting style to adolescent school performance. *Child Development, 58,* 1244–1257.

Federal Bureau of Investigation. (2004). *Crime in the United States: Uniform crime reports.* Washington, DC: Federal Bureau of Investigation, U.S. Department of Justice.

Foley, D. L., Eaves, L., J., Wormley, B., Silberg, J. L., Maes, H., H., Kuhn, J., et al. (2004). Childhood adversity, MAO-A genotype, and risk for conduct disorder. *Archives of General Psychiatry, 61,* 738–744.

Fujii, D. E. M., Tokioka, A. B., Lichton, A. I., & Hishinuma, E. (2005). Ethnic differences in prediction of violence risk with the HCR-20 among psychiatric patients. *Psychiatric Services, 56,* 711–716.

Gilbert, F., & Daffern, M. (2010). Integrating contemporary aggression theory with violent offender treatment: How thoroughly do interventions target violent behavior? *Aggression and Violent Behavior, 15,* 167–180.

Ginwright, S., & Cammarota, J. (2002). New terrain in youth development: The promise of a social justice approach. *Social Justice, 29,* 82–95.

Go, C. G., & Le, T. N. (2005). Gender differences in Cambodian delinquency: The role of ethnic identity, parental discipline, and peer delinquency. *Crime and Delinquency, 51,* 220–237.

Guerrero, A. P. S., Goebert, D. A., Alicata, D., & Bell, C. K. (2009). Striving for a culturally responsive process in training health professionals on Asian American and Pacific Islander youth violence prevention. *Aggression and Violent Behavior, 14,* 499–505.

Hall, G. C. N. (2002). Culture-specific ecological models of Asian American violence. In G. C. N. Hall & S. Okazaki (Eds.), *Asian American psychology: The science of lives in context* (pp. 153–170). Washington, DC: American Psychological Association.

Hall, G. C. N., & Barongan, C. (1997). Prevention of sexual aggression: Sociocultural risk and protective factors. *American Psychologist, 52,* 5–14.

Hall, G. C. N., DeGarmo, D. S., Eap, S., Teten, A. L., & Sue, S. (2006). Initiation, desistance, and persistence of men's sexual coercion. *Journal of Consulting and Clinical Psychology, 74,* 732–742.

Hall, G. C. N., & Eap, S. (2007). Empirically-supported therapies for Asian Americans. In F. T. L. Leong, A. Inman, A. Ebreo, L. Yang, L. Kinoshita, & M. Fu (Eds.), *Handbook of Asian American psychology* (2nd ed., pp. 449–467). Thousand Oaks, CA: Sage.

Hall, G. C. N., Sue, S., Narang, D. S., & Lilly, R. S. (2000). Culture-specific models of men's sexual aggression: Intra- and interpersonal determinants. *Cultural Diversity and Ethnic Minority Psychology, 6,* 252–267.

Hall, G. C. N., Teten, A. L., DeGarmo, D. S., Sue, S., & Stephens, K. A. (2005). Ethnicity, culture, and sexual aggression: Risk and protective factors. *Journal of Consulting and Clinical Psychology, 73,* 830–840.

Hirschi, T. (1969). *Causes of delinquency.* Berkeley: University of California Press.

Ho, J. (2008). Community violence exposure of Southeast Asian American adolescents. *Journal of Interpersonal Violence, 23,* 136–146.

Howells, K., Day, A., Williamson, P., Bubner, S., Jauncey, S., Parker, A., et al. (2005). Brief anger management programs with offenders: Outcomes and predictors of change. *Journal of Forensic Psychiatry and Psychology, 16,* 296–311.

Huesmann, L. R. (1988). An information processing model for the development of aggression. *Aggressive Behavior, 14,* 13–24.

Jaffee, S. R., Caspi, A., Moffitt, T. E., & Taylor, Alan. (2004). Physical maltreatment victim to antisocial child: Evidence of an environmentally mediated process. *Journal of Abnormal Psychology, 113,* 44–55.

Jang, J. J. (2002). Race, ethnicity, and deviance: A study of Asian American and non-Asian American adolescents in American. *Sociological Forum, 17*, 647–679.

Johnson, J. B. (2004, June 13). From Southeast Asia to a violent East Bay: Gang rivalries turn immigrants' hopes into urban misery. *SF Gate.* Retrieved on October 10, 2011, from http://articles.sfgate.com/2004-06-13/news/17431665_1_first-gang-asian-ethnic-group.

Kaminiski, J. W., Valle, L. A., Filene, J., & Boyle, C. L. (2008). A meta-analytic review of components associated with parent training program effectiveness. *Journal of Abnormal Child Psychology, 36*, 567–589.

Kazdin, A. E., Esveldt-Dawson, K., Unis, A. S., & Rancurrello, M. D. (1983). Child and parent evaluation of depression and aggression in psychiatric inpatient children. *Journal of Abnormal Child Psychology, 11*, 401–413.

Kim, H., & Markus, H. R. (1999). Deviance or uniqueness, harmony or conformity? A cultural analysis. *Journal of Personality and Social Psychology, 77*, 785–800.

Kim, T. E., & Goto, S. G. (2000). Peer delinquency and parental social support as predictors of Asian American adolescent delinquency. *Deviant Behavior, 21*, 331–347.

Kim, H. S., Sherman, D. K., & Taylor, S. E. (2008). Culture and social support. *American Psychologist, 63*, 518–526.

Lau, A. S., Garland, A. F., Yeh, M., McCabe, K. M., Wood, P. A., & Hough, R. L. (2004). Race/ethnicity and inter-informant agreement in assessing adolescent psychopathology. *Journal of Emotional and Behavioral Disorders, 12*, 145–156.

Lau, A. S., Takeuchi, D. T., & Alegria, M. (2006). Parent-to-child aggression among Asian American parents: Culture, context, and vulnerability. *Journal of Marriage and Family, 68*, 1261–1275.

Le, T. (2002). Asian Pacific Islander and delinquency: A review of literature and research. *The Justice Professional, 15*, 57–70.

Le, T. N., Monfared, G., & Stockdale, G. D. (2005). The relationship of school, parent, and peer contextual factors with self-reported delinquency for Chinese, Cambodian, Laotian or Mien, and Vietnamese Youth. *Crime and Delinquency, 51*, 192–219.

Le, T. N., & Stockdale, G. (2008). Acculturative dissonance, ethnic identity, and youth violence. *Cultural Diversity and Ethnic Minority Psychology, 14*, 1–9.

Lee, R., & Coccaro, E. (2001). The neuropsychopharmacology of criminality and aggression. *Canadian Journal of Psychiatry, 46*, 35–44.

Leung, P. W. L., Hung, S., Ho, T. P., Lee, C., Liu, W., Tang, C., & Kwong, S. (2008). Prevalence of DSM-IV disorders in Chinese adolescents and the effects of an impairment criterion. *European Child and Adolescent Psychiatry, 17*, 452–461.

Liao, D., Hong, C., Shih, H., & Tsai, S. (2004). Possible association between serotonin transporter promoter region polymorphism and extremely violent crime in Chinese males. *Neuropsychobiology, 50*, 284–287.

Loo, S. K., & Rapport, M. D. (1998). Ethnic variations in children's problem behaviors: A cross-sectional, developmental study of Hawaii school children. *Journal of Child Psychology and Psychiatry, 39*, 567–575.

Lu, R., Lee, J., Ko, H., & Lin, W. (2001). Dopamine D2 receptor gene (DRD2) is associated with alcoholism with conduct disorder. *Alcoholism: Clinical & Experimental Research, 25*, 177–184.

Lu, R., Lin, W., Lee, J., Ko, H., & Shih, J.C. (2003). Neither antisocial personality disorder nor antisocial alcoholism is associated with the MAO-A gene in Han Chinese males. *Alcoholism: Clinical and Experimental Research, 27*, 889–893.

Maughan, D. R., Christiansen, E., Jenson, W. R., Olympia, D., & Clark, E. (2005). Behavioral family training as a treatment for externalizing behaviors and disruptive behavior disorders: A meta-analysis. *School Psychology Review, 34*, 267–286.

McMullin, J. (2005). The call to life: revitalizing a healthy Hawaiian identity. *Social Science and Medicine, 61*, 809–820.

Moffitt, T. E. (1993). Adolescence-limited and life-course-persistent antisocial behavior: A developmental taxonomy. *Psychological Review, 100*, 674–701.

Moffitt, T. E. (2005). The new look of behavioral genetics in developmental psychopathology: Gene-environment interplay in antisocial behaviors. *Psychological Bulletin, 131*, 533–554.

Moffitt, T. E., & Caspi, A. (2001). Childhood predictors differentiate life-course persistent and adolescence-limited antisocial pathways, among males and females. *Development and Psychopathology, 13*, 355–375.

National Council on Crime and Delinquency (2003). *Under the microscope: Asian and Pacific Islander Youth in Oakland.* Oakland, CA: Asian Pacific Islander Youth Violence Prevention Center.

Nguyen, L., Arganza, G. F., Huang, L. N., Laio, Q., Nguyen, H. T., & Santaigo, R. (2004). Psychiatric diagnoses and clinical characteristics of Asian American youth in children's servies. *Journal of Child and Family Studies, 13,* 483–495.

Ota Wang, V., & Sue, S. (2005). In the eye of the storm: Race and genomics in research and practice. *American Psychologist, 60,* 37–45.

Ou, Y., & McAdoo, H. P. (1993). Socialization of Chinese American children. In H.P MsAdoo (Ed), *Ethnicity: Strength in Diversity* (pp. 245–270). Newberry Park, CA: Sage.

Raine, A. (2002). Biosocial studies of antisocial and violent behavior in children and adults: A review. *Journal of Abnormal Child Psychology, 30,* 311–326.

Reid, M. J., Webster-Stratton, C., & Beauchaine, T. P. (2001). Parent training in Head Start: A comparison of program response among African American, Caucasian, and Hispanic mothers. *Prevention Science, 2,* 209–227.

Rennison, C. (2002). *Criminal victimization 2001: Changes 2000–01 with trends 1993–2001.* Washington, DC: U.S. Department of Justice, Bureau of Justice Statistics.

Retz, W., Retz-Junginger, P., Supprian, T., Thome, J., & Rosier, M. (2004). Association of serotonin transporter promoter gene polymorphism with violence: Relation with personality disorders, impulsivity, and childhood ADHD psychopathology. *Behavioral Sciences and the Law, 22,* 415–425.

Rhee, S., Weaver, D., Chang, J., & Wong, D. (2008). Child maltreatment among immigrant Chinese families: Characteristics and patterns of placement. *Child Maltreatment, 13*(3), 269–279.

Rowe, D. C., Stever, C., Chase, D., Sherman, S., Abromowitz, A., & Waldman, I. D. (2001). Two dopamine genes related to reports of childhood restrospective inattention and conduct disorder symptoms. *Molecular Psychiatry, 6,* 429–433.

Rumbaut, R. G., & Portes, A. (2002). *Ethnicities: Coming of age in immigrant America.* Berkeley: University of California Press.

Rutter, M., Pickles, A., Murray, R., & Eaves, L. (2001). Testing hypotheses on specific environmental causal effects on behavior. *Psychological Bulletin, 127,* 291–324.

Schinka, J. A., Letsch, E. A., & Crawford, F. C. (2002). DRD4 and novelty seeking: Results of meta-analyses. *American Journal of Medical Genetics, 114,* 643–648.

Shanahan, M. J., & Hofer, S. M. (2005). Social context in gene-environment interactions: retrospect and prospect. *Journals of Gerontology. Series B, Psychological Sciences and Social Sciences, 60B,* 65–76.

Spoont, M. R. (1992). Modulatory role of serotonin in neural information processing: Implications for human psychopathology. *Psychological Bulletin, 112,* 330–350.

Stallings, M. C., Corley, R. P., Dennehey, B., Hewitt, J. K., Krauter, K. S., Lessem, J. M., et al. (2005). A genome-wide search for quantitative trait loci that influence antisocial drug dependence in adolescence. *Archives of General Psychiatry, 62,* 1042–1051.

Sukhodolsky, D. G., Kassinove, H., & Gorman, B. S. (2004). Cognitive-behavioral therapy for anger in children and adolescents: A meta-analysis. *Aggression and Violent Behavior, 9,* 247–269.

Tjaden, P. & Thoennes, N. (2000). *Full report of the prevalence, incidence, and consequences of violence against women: Findings from the National Violence Against Women Survey* (Publication 183781). Washington, D. C.: National Center Justice.

Trinidad, A. M. O. (2009). Toward kuleana (responsibility): A case study of a contextually grounded intervention for Native Hawaiian youth and young adults. *Aggression and Violent Behavior, 14,* 488–498.

Tuvblad, C., Grann, M., & Lichtenstein, P. (2006). Heritability for adolescent antisocial behavior differs with socioeconomic status: Gene-environment interaction. *Journal of Child Psychology and Psychiatry, 47,* 734–743.

Waldman, I. D., & Slutske, W. S. (2000). Antisocial behavior and alcoholism: A behavioral genetic perspective on comorbidity. *Clinical Psychology Review, 20,* 255–287.

Ward, T. (2002). Good lives and the rehabilitation of offenders: Promises and problems. *Aggression and Violent Behavior, 7,* 513–528.

Weisz, J. R., Suwanlert, S., Chaiyasit, W., Weiss, B., Walter, B. R., & Anderson, W. W. (1988). Thai and American perspectives on over- and undercontrolled child behavior problems: Exploring the threshold model among parents, teachers, and psychologists. *Journal of Consulting and Clinical Psychology, 56,* 601–609.

Widom, C. S., & Brzustowicz, L. M. (2006). MAO-A and the "cycle of violence": Childhood abuse and neglect, MAO-A genotype, and risk for violent and antisocial behavior. *Biological* Psychiatry, *60*, 684–689.

Wong, S. K. (1999). Acculturation, peer relations, and delinquent behavior of Chinese-Canadian youth. *Adolescence, 34*, 108–119.

World Health Organization (2002). *World report on violence and health.* Geneva, Switzerland: Author.

Yao, K., Solanto, M. V., & Wender, E. H. (1988). Prevalence of hyperactivity among newly immigrant Chinese-American children. *Journal of Developmental and Behavioral Pediatrics, 9*, 367–373.

Zamora, J. H. (October 2003). Asian gang violence escalates in the East Bay: No one even recalls origins of the rivalries. Retrieved on October 10, 2011, from http://articles.sfgate.com/2003–10-19/bay-area/17514421_1_girl-s-slaying-gang-shootings.

Zuckerman, M. (2003). Are there racial and ethnic differences in psychopathic personality? A critique of Lynn's (2002) racial and ethnic differences in psychopathic personality. *Personality and Individual Differences, 35*, 1463–1469.

| 11 |

EATING DISORDERS IN ASIANS

LILLIAN HUANG CUMMINS, JANICE DELGADO LEHMAN,
AND REBECCA CHUN LIU

While in the past eating disorders (EDs) have been most commonly associated with white, upper-middle class, adolescent females in Westernized countries, their numbers are steadily increasing among men and women of diverse racial/ethnic, cultural, socioeconomic, and geographic backgrounds (Davis & Yager, 1992; Dolan, 1991; Pate, Pumariega, Hester, & Garner, 1992; Pike & Walsh, 1996; Ritenbaugh, Shisslak, Teufel, & Leonard-Green, 1996; Root, 1990b; Smith, 1995; Smolak & Striegel-Moore, 2001). Such reports have stimulated increased interest in the presentation of EDs in non-Western and nonwhite populations and have led to the suggestion that the study of EDs in diverse groups is essential to improving our understanding of how sociocultural influences may be related to their development (Dolan, 1991; Smith, 1995; Smolak & Striegel-Moore, 2001).

EDs are among the most lethal of psychiatric illnesses, with estimated mortality rates ranging from 0.3% to as high as 20% (Keel & Herzog, 2004; Keel & Mitchell, 1997; Nielsen, 2001). Their global prevalence appears to be on the rise (Crago, Shisslak, & Estes, 1996; Pate et al., 1992; Striegel-Moore & Bulik, 2007), yet EDs often go unrecognized and untreated in ethnic minorities or are only acknowledged after they have already progressed to a more severe stage (Cachelin, Rebeck, Veisel, & Striegel-Moore, 2001; K. H. Gordon, Perez, & Joiner, 2002; King, 1993; Pike & Walsh, 1996; Root, 1990b). For example, despite having a similar frequency of ED behaviors as non-Asian participants, Asian patients were found to have significantly lower rates of referral for more thorough evaluation (Franko, Becker, Thomas, & Herzog, 2007). Interventions occurring earlier in the course of certain EDs have been related to improved outcomes (Eisler et al., 1997). The importance of early recognition combined with the likelihood that EDs may often go unidentified in ethnic minorities make the study of EDs in nonwhite populations an even more critical endeavor.

The traditional misconception that EDs do not occur in nonwhite or non-Western populations extends to Asians and Asian Americans. In the past, researchers have suggested, perhaps mistakenly, that Asian populations may be less prone to EDs due to stereotypically smaller body frames in general as well as traditional Asian cultural values that associate larger body sizes with success and happiness (Cachelin, Veisel, Barzegarnazari, Striegel-Moore, 2000; S. Lee, 1993a; World Health Organization [WHO], 2004). Recent studies have demonstrated that Asian and Asian American populations are experiencing EDs and their symptoms (see Cummins, Simmons, & Zane, 2005 for a review), and in some areas and populations these prevalence rates may be on the rise (R. A. Gordon, 2001; Hsu & Lee, 1993). However, while the research on EDs in Asian populations has increased significantly in the last decade, much is still unknown with regard to how the specific sociocultural experiences of Asians and Asian Americans may impact the identification, assessment, etiology, and treatment of EDs.

The term "Asian" has been applied to an enormous diversity of populations in terms of ethnicity, nationality, history, and geography. The focus of this textbook, and therefore this chapter, will be on research that has been conducted with East Asian populations, both individuals living in their countries of origin and those of East Asian descent that are living in North America. There is a significant amount of research on EDs in general that has been conducted in the United Kingdom and some in particular that has focused on Asian populations; however, due to historical migration patterns, these British Asian populations have tended to be more heavily of South Asian descent (Cummins & Lehman, 2007). As a result, while some of these investigations may be mentioned here, they will not be the focus of this chapter. Some researchers have begun to study EDs in Asian populations in other European countries, Australia, and South Africa, yet this literature is still quite limited; thus, when referring to Asian populations living in more Westernized countries, this chapter will concentrate on research that has been conducted in the United States and Canada. Finally, while the study of EDs and their symptoms in male populations is an important and growing field, the majority of the literature is still focused on females. Therefore, this review is presented with the caveat that what we currently know about EDs, their prevalence, etiology, and treatment is mostly applicable for female populations, and where we discuss those few studies that have included men, we have made an effort to state so clearly.

IDENTIFYING EDS IN ASIANS

Current DSM-IV-TR Nosology and Criteria

Currently, the most commonly used criteria for the diagnosis of EDs are outlined in the *Diagnostic and Statistical Manual of Mental Disorders, Fourth Edition, Text Revision* (*DSM-IV-TR*; American Psychiatric Association [APA], 2000). Three categories of EDs are described there: anorexia nervosa (AN), bulimia nervosa (BN), and eating disorder not otherwise specified (EDNOS). The key clinical feature of AN is the refusal to maintain a minimally accepted standard of weight. Individuals with AN typically lose weight either by restricting their caloric intake or by binge eating and purging their food. In BN, low weight is not the focus so much as recurrent episodes of binge eating followed by inappropriate compensatory behaviors used to prevent weight gain. Compensatory behaviors in BN can be either purging (i.e., vomiting, laxative abuse, etc.) or nonpurging (i.e., fasting, excessive exercise, etc.). Finally, a third diagnostic category, known as EDNOS, is intended to capture those individuals who have disorders of eating that do not meet the criteria for either

AN or BN. Interestingly, while the "not otherwise specified" diagnoses in the *DSM* are typically reserved for a residual group, the majority of individuals with EDs likely fall into this category (Striegel-Moore & Bulik, 2007; Wonderlich, Joiner, Keel, Williamson, & Crosby, 2007). A large proportion of those with EDNOS are represented by individuals who meet the research criteria for binge eating disorder (BED), a possible third type of ED that has been proposed (APA, 2000). This syndrome features recurrent episodes of binge eating without compensatory behaviors. In BED, binge episodes are characterized by feelings of loss of control, extremely rapid eating, eating when not hungry, eating alone, and having feelings of disgust or depression regarding eating episodes (APA, 2000).

Anorexia Nervosa

In 2003, Hoek and van Hoeken reviewed the literature on the prevalence and incidence of diagnosable EDs and found that most large epidemiological studies of AN had been conducted in the US and Western Europe. Across this literature, they found an average prevalence rate of 0.3% among young females. A recent national study conducted in the United States found a lifetime prevalence of 0.6% (0.3% for men and 0.9% for women) for AN (Hudson, Hiripi, Pope, & Kessler, 2007).

AN in Asian Populations

Among Asian countries, Japan has been most typically identified as having rates of AN that may be more comparable to more Westernized countries (APA, 2000; R. A. Gordon, 2001). Nevertheless, many epidemiological studies there have found a relatively low prevalence rate of diagnosable AN (Nakamura et al., 2000; Tsai, 2000). While case reports of AN were published in Japan prior to 1970, most large epidemiological studies were not conducted until the 1980s. These generally indicated a rise in the prevalence of AN during this time; however, while these patterns of increasing incidence may have been similar to those found in the United States and Western Europe, overall rates still tended to be lower (R. A. Gordon, 2001; Nogami, 1997; Tsai, 2000). For example, Kuboki, Nomura, Ide, Suematsu, and Araki (1996) reported on two epidemiological surveys that asked physicians throughout Japan to report any cases of AN according to *DSM-III-R* (APA, 1987) criteria over a year's time. The first survey in 1985 found a prevalence of 2.9–3.7 per 100,000 in the general population, and the second survey conducted in 1992 found a prevalence of 3.6–4.5 per 100,000. More recently, a study of medical inpatients and outpatients in Niigata Prefecture found a point prevalence of 2.65 per 100,000 for AN using *DSM-IV* (APA, 1994) criteria (Nakamura et al., 2000). While it is difficult to compare these findings with the prevalence rates described above for more Westernized countries due to methodological differences in the approaches of these investigations, it appears that rates of AN in Japan are lower than those found in more Westernized countries whether clinical or nonclinical samples are examined (Tsai, 2000).

In Hong Kong, rates of AN have also been found to be relatively low compared to more Westernized countries. For example, one early study found no cases of AN among male and female college students using *DSM-III-R* (APA, 1987) criteria (S. Lee, 1993b), and a community-based study using *DSM-III* (APA, 1980) criteria found a lifetime prevalence rate of only .03% among 7,229 men and women (C. Chen et al., 1993). However, researchers have contended that these low rates for AN may have been influenced by symptom patterns that appeared to differ from the traditional, Western-based diagnostic criteria; namely, as investigators began to report on the first cases of AN in Hong Kong, they found that patients did not express a fear of fatness or body image concerns (R. A. Gordon, 2001; S. Lee, 2001). More recently however, weight concern appears to have become more normative in Hong Kong, and accordingly the incidence of diagnosable AN may be increasing as well (R. A. Gordon, 2001; Hsu & Lee, 1993; S. Lee, 2001).

Reports from other Asian countries such as mainland China (Chun et al., 1992), Korea (R. A. Gordon, 2001), and Singapore (Kok & Tian, 1994) describe low rates of AN. Researchers suspect that these may be on the rise; however, few reliable epidemiological surveys exist to confirm these assumptions (R. A. Gordon, 2001; S. Lee, 2001).

AN in Asian American Populations

Two initial studies with multiethnic samples (i.e., white, black, Asian, and Hispanic) found no differences in rates of AN across ethnic groups (Cachelin et al., 2000; le Grange, Stone, & Brownell, 1998). However, these findings may be questionable given problems with small sample sizes and a lack of clinical interviews to confirm diagnoses (Cummins et al., 2005). Only one other study that overcame these shortcomings was found in the literature. In 1999, the Epidemiological Catchment Area (ECA) study collected data from several ethnic groups living in five community catchment areas across the United States: New Haven, Connecticut; Baltimore, Maryland; St. Louis, Missouri; Durham, North Carolina; and Los Angeles, California. Using *DSM-III* (APA, 1980) criteria, this study again found no significant differences in rates of AN between the Asian and white samples, reporting a lifetime prevalence of 0.6% for the Asian group as compared to 0.9% for whites (Zhang & Snowden, 1999).

Bulimia Nervosa

Since criteria for BN was established in 1980, researchers in the United States and Western Europe have found a fairly consistent prevalence rate of 1.0% for BN among young women (Fairburn & Beglin 1990; Hoek & van Hoeken, 2003). In the United States, the lifetime prevalence of BN has been reported as 1.0% (0.5% for men and 1.5% for women; Hudson et al., 2007).

BN in Asian Populations

In their review, Pike and Mizushima (2005) suggested that there has been at least a 6-fold increase in EDs in Japan over the last 25 years. Interestingly, a self-report survey of female college and nursing students in Japan categorized 2.9% as having BN (Kiriike et al., 1988); however, it is important to consider that this study employed a self-report instrument to diagnose BN and did not confirm these diagnoses with a clinical interview, a method which may result in a high rate of false positives (Hsu, 1996). Kuboki et al. (1996) found a prevalence of 1.3–2.5 per 100,000 among all treated cases in Japan for the year 1992, and more recently Nakamura et al. (2000) estimated a point prevalence of .52 per 100,000 for BN among medical patients. Once again, however, whether studies utilized clinical or nonclinical samples, it appears that these rates of BN in Japan are lower than those typically found in more Westernized countries (Tsai, 2000).

Investigations in Hong Kong and China have reported very low rates of BN among male and female college students (Chun et al., 1992; S. Lee, 1993b). In Seoul, Korea a more recent study categorized 4.6% of a sample of college students and 1.5% of a sample of high school students as having BN; however, again this investigation only used cutoff scores from the BULIT-R (Thelen, Farmer, Wonderlich, & Smith, 1991) to define BN and did not confirm these prevalence rates with diagnostic interviews (Ryu, Lyle, & McCabe, 2003). Similar to rates of AN, while BN is presenting in individuals living in Asian countries and may be on the rise in Japan (Nogami, 1997), overall rates are lower when compared to those from more Westernized countries.

BN in Asian American populations

In the United States, two studies on the correlates of BN among high school students reported no differences in prevalence rates between ethnic groups when comparing white, black, Asian, Hispanic, American Indian, and "other" students (Gross & Rosen, 1988; Johnson, Lewis, Love, Lewis, & Stuckey, 1984). Similarly, two studies with adult women found no differences in rates of probable BN across samples of Hispanic, white, black, and Asian women (Cachelin et al., 2000; le Grange et al., 1998). In contrast, two investigations with mostly college-age samples reported lower rates of possible BN among Asian American women when compared to European American or Caucasian women (Nevo, 1985; Tsai & Gray, 2000). However, as mentioned previously, most of these studies either lacked a large enough sample size to detect differences among ethnic groups or did not utilize clinical interviews to confirm diagnoses. As a result, it is difficult to know whether findings of no differences between Asian Americans and other ethnic groups were compromised by a lack of power, and given the current research it is impossible to establish the true prevalence of BN among Asian Americans.

EDNOS and BED

In their review on the prevalence and incidence of EDs, Hoek and van Hoeken (2003) did not even address rates of EDNOS, citing the extreme heterogeneity of syndromes that fall within this category as a reason for the difficulty in summarizing the research. Nevertheless, approximately 60% of individuals with an ED diagnosis meet criteria for EDNOS rather than other ED diagnoses (Fairburn & Walsh, 2002; Wonderlich et al., 2007). Estimates suggest that between 4% to 6% of men and women in the general population have an EDNOS (Herzog & Delinsky, 2001), and one study found that more than 40% of women who sought treatment at an ED clinic would have received a diagnosis of EDNOS (Herzog, Hopkins, & Burns, 1993). Interestingly, research has suggested that sociocultural variables likely play a greater role in influencing the development of subclinical EDs as compared to AN and BN (Wildes, Emery, & Simons, 2001). Thus, while those individuals who meet criteria for EDNOS are a large and important part of the picture, especially in terms of the growing rates of EDs globally, the literature is significantly lacking in this area.

Similarly, because the criteria for BED is still considered "in need of further research," very few large epidemiological studies have been conducted to establish the prevalence of this diagnosis as of yet. In a preliminary review, Hoek and van Hoeken (2003) concluded tentatively that the prevalence of BED is at least 1%. Hudson et al.'s (2007) national U.S. study found a lifetime prevalence of 2.8% (2.0% for men and 3.5% for women) for BED.

In Asian countries, Nakamura et al. (2000) found in their study of the 5-day prevalence of EDs that across all medical facilities in Japan's Niigata Prefecture 80 patients were reported with *DSM-IV* (APA, 1994) EDs; of these, 51.3% were diagnosed with AN, 8.8% were diagnosed with BN, and 40.0% with EDNOS. A recent study of 1,245 schoolgirls in mainland China found no cases of AN or BN that met full diagnostic criteria but did identify seven cases of BED (Huon, Mingyi, & Oliver, 2002). Beyond these two studies, our review of the literature found no investigations that looked specifically at rates of EDNOS or BED in Asian or Asian American populations.

Strengths, Weaknesses, and Alternatives in Applying Current Nosology and Diagnostic Criteria

A Common Language

Certainly there are important advantages to having a common language by which researchers and clinicians can communicate about EDs: it allows researchers a means by which they can operationalize eating pathology and build a body of research around specific issues, it enables the exchange of information between the research and practice worlds, and it provides an efficient way by which past and future clinicians and/or multidisciplinary teams may communicate about a particular case. In their review, Franko, Wonderlich, Little, & Herzog (2004) recognized the importance of ED classification for influencing research agendas, policy issues, funding efforts, third-party reimbursement, and treatment strategies. Specific to the *DSM-IV-TR* categorization of EDs, Wonderlich et al. (2007) also noted in their recent review that there are many advantages to the current system. These include the ability to diagnose EDs reliably utilizing clinical interviews and the evidence of diagnostic validity for AN, BN, and BED in that they differ in their longitudinal patterns, evidence-based treatment findings, and, interestingly, cross-cultural presentations. By example, AN presents across cultures and in the absence of the influence of Westernization, whereas BN appears to be culture-bound (Keel & Klump, 2003). As the study of EDs "goes global," the ability for investigators to have a common means by which they can communicate and build on previous literature is even more vital.

This need is apparent when examining the literature on EDs among Asian populations. Because the criteria for AN and BN were initially established in the *DSM* in 1980, much of the research with Asian populations has been conducted during the time when the diagnostic criteria for these disorders were themselves evolving. As a result, the various classification systems (i.e., *DSM-III*,

DSM-III-R, DSM-IV) utilized throughout the research have caused some difficulty in comparing findings across studies (Cummins et al., 2005; Tsai, 2000). While researchers have criticized specific diagnostic criteria for both AN and BN (see Franko et al., 2004 for a review), the current classification system provides investigators the opportunity to build a body of research by studying essentially the same constructs over time.

Limitations of Current Approaches

Despite these advantages, it is clear that the current classification system for EDs has many limitations. Researchers have questioned the validity of the AN, BN, and EDNOS diagnoses, the validity of the AN and BN subtypes, and the utility of specific criteria (Franko et al., 2004). A review of the research on diagnosable EDs among Asian populations reveals even more ways in which our reliance on the current DSM system limits our ability to know more about how problematic eating behaviors are presenting in diverse groups.

For instance, while AN and BN can be diagnosed reliably, accurate diagnosis requires rigorous assessment. As noted in the review above, some studies have estimated diagnostic prevalence by evaluating whether individuals meet criteria according to self-report questionnaires, yet research suggests that a face-to-face interview is necessary to accurately assess for diagnosis (Hsu, 1996). As a result, for studies attempting to diagnose EDs, researchers have recommended a two-stage design wherein individuals are first screened with a self-report symptom measure and then high scorers are examined using a semistructured interview (Fairburn & Beglin, 1990). However, this process is both time-consuming and costly, and large epidemiological studies of diagnosable EDs in Asian or Asian American populations are already few and far between. Even when such studies have been conducted, their findings may not be available outside of that country; for example, it has been reported that two two-stage design studies of EDs in Thailand have been published in the Thai language (Jennings, Forbes, McDermott, Juniper, & Hulse, 2006), yet most Western researchers have no way to access these findings. While we have noted above where investigations have not utilized the two-stage design, dismissing these studies outright because diagnoses may have been unreliable would make the literature on the prevalence of AN and BN in Asian populations virtually nonexistent.

The occurrence of diagnosable EDs is also extremely low in the general population. As described previously, rates of AN and BN range from about 0.3% to only as high as 1% in more Westernized countries. Given the expectation that prevalence rates would be lower in Asian countries, very large samples are necessary to detect even a few cases of diagnosable EDs. Similarly, in countries such as the United States, where Asian Americans are estimated to be about 3.6% of the total population (U.S. Census Bureau, 2001), very large samples are necessary to detect diagnosable EDs and, if desired, to have enough power to detect between-group differences in prevalence rates among ethnic groups.

Finally, in their recent review of the classification of EDs, Wonderlich et al. (2007) recognized that most research investigating the specific criteria for ED diagnoses has been conducted with young, Caucasian women from more Westernized countries. This calls into question the validity of these criteria for Asian populations (Cummins et al., 2005). Current methods of diagnosing

EDs require the endorsement of a specific symptom set, yet different patterns of symptom presentation may exist cross-culturally. Because various permutations are possible in terms of meeting *DSM* criteria, even individuals who have the same ED diagnosis may differ in the types of symptoms they express. Researchers have suggested that this misuse of Western criteria sets has contributed to misleading findings when prevalence rates of EDs are studied in non-Western and nonwhite populations (King, 1993; Wildes et al., 2001).

One notable example where this may have been the case is the weight phobia criterion that is required for a diagnosis of AN. While the inclusion of this criterion has been questioned across cultures, as mentioned previously, much of the initial argument was based on those cases reported by Lee and colleagues in Hong Kong in which a fear of fatness was absent (Franko et al., 2004). In fact, a historical and cross-cultural review of the literature on AN suggests that while the syndrome itself exists cross-culturally, the particular symptom of weight concern may be culture-bound (Keel & Klump, 2003). In fact, this questioning of the weight phobia criterion has even motivated the proposal of a "culture-independent diagnostic criteria" set for AN in which culturally appropriate alternatives for explaining food avoidance (e.g., adherence to spiritual beliefs, somatic complaints such as abdominal pain or bloating) are delineated (Woodside & Twose, 2004).

Other variations in symptom presentation may be culturally based as well. For example, studies with Chinese populations have noted that individuals with AN tend to engage in restricting rather than purging (Lai, 2000), and individuals with BN tend to engage in laxative abuse rather than vomiting (S. Lee, Hsu, & Wing, 1992). While it is certainly possible that there may be other ways in which EDs present differently for Asian populations, the manifestation of AN without weight phobia, which may cause Asian women to be diagnosed with EDNOS instead, is currently the most well established.

Expanding Our Cultural Understanding of EDs

While the *DSM* is currently the most commonly utilized, other diagnostic standards, such as Feighner's criteria for AN (Feighner et al., 1972) and the *International Statistical Classification of Diseases and Related Health Problems, 10th revision* (ICD-10; WHO, 1992) criteria have also been employed in this research. While these diagnostic methods may provide broader categories by which cultural variations in the presentation of EDs might be studied, it remains to be seen whether utilizing these alternatives would solve any of the issues raised by the *DSM* since none have been employed as consistently. In contrast to these already-established criteria, new models for the classification of EDs have recently been proposed that may provide an interesting framework for the study of cultural similarities and differences. For example, Williamson, Gleaves, and Stewart (2005) have proposed a three-dimensional model in which EDs are conceptualized based on three symptom dimensions: binge eating, fear of fatness-compensatory behaviors, and extreme drive for thinness. Such a symptom-focused approach would allow for wider exploration of possible variations in eating pathology that may be culturally influenced.

Even more inclusive is the transdiagnostic approach proposed by Fairburn and colleagues (Fairburn, Cooper, & Shafran, 2003), which suggests a single diagnostic category, "eating disorder."

This model is based on the idea that there is more in common among AN, BN, and EDNOS than there is to separate them. The authors argue that these disorders share the same core psychopathology (i.e., the overvaluation of control over shape, weight, and eating) and the same distinctive clinical features (e.g., restricting, purging, overexercise, body checking, and binge eating) that are maintained by similar psychopathological processes (i.e., perfectionism, low self-esteem, mood intolerance, and interpersonal difficulties). They also point to the fluctuating longitudinal course of the disorders (i.e., patients often move from one diagnostic category to another over time).

This trend toward inclusivity in how EDs are defined may be quite beneficial to the study of eating pathology in diverse populations such as Asians and Asian Americans. Certainly, as our ways of defining EDs have broadened over time—from the *DSM-III* in 1980, which only listed AN and BN, to our current *DSM-IV-TR* (APA, 2004), which provides criteria for four possible EDs—there has also simultaneously been diversification in the types of populations where EDs appear to be presenting. Interestingly, while increases in the incidence of AN are still up for debate, researchers have noted a rise in the more relatively "recent" disorders of BN and BED (Hoek & van Hoeken, 2003; Hudson et al., 2006). At the same time, more and more studies have noted that men and women of varying ethnicities and countries of origin are experiencing EDs. While these trends may be unrelated or may merely be artifacts of greater attention to these issues, it is likely that as we become more inclusive in our ways of defining EDs, we may also open our minds to more possibilities in terms of cultural variations in their presentation.

Given the difficulties enumerated above in studying diagnosable EDs, many researchers have turned their focus to the study of the relative prevalence of ED symptoms such as body image disturbance, binge eating, purging, and restricting. These symptoms, which tend to present more frequently in general populations, can be assessed more easily than multisymptom syndromes. Some of these symptoms (i.e., body dissatisfaction, dieting) have also been identified as risk factors for developing diagnosable EDs (Stice, 1999). In addition, by looking at specific ED symptoms, researchers can study how ethnic and cultural variation may be related to different types of problematic eating attitudes and behaviors without being confined to Western-based symptom patterns alone. We now turn to a review of the major etiological models of EDs, an area which, as it applies to Asians and Asian Americans, has been informed greatly by the study of specific ED symptoms.

PERSPECTIVES ON THE CAUSES OF EDS IN ASIANS

Critical Appraisal of Major Etiological Models of EDs

The etiology of EDs has been theorized from a number of biological, psychological, and social perspectives. However, it is widely known that EDs are multifactorial in terms of etiology and maintenance, and almost all theorists today will agree that no single model can fully account for ED development and expression in a given individual. The major models within each view will be reviewed briefly in the following section as a starting point for better understanding the causal perspectives of these complex disorders.

Biological Models

Genetic studies

While previously sociocultural and family models dominated the landscape in terms of the research on the etiology of EDs, the last decade has produced a plethora of genetic and biological research that has clearly established the importance of these factors in the development of EDs (Bulik, 2004). Family studies have found a higher lifetime prevalence of EDs among the relatives of individuals with EDs, and this trend occurs across the diagnoses of AN, BN, and EDNOS such that family members of individuals with one diagnosis are at risk for the other ED types as well (Bulik, 2004; Striegel-Moore & Bulik, 2007). In addition, twin studies have established that AN and BN are familial with more than half (58–83%) of the variation in risk possibly accounted for by genes (Bulik, 2004; Klump & Culbert, 2007), and initial studies have also found substantial heritability for binge eating in the absence of purging behaviors (Striegel-Moore & Bulik, 2007).

These findings have guided researchers to pursue molecular genetic studies to more specifically identify possible relevant genes. Association studies, which compare the genes of individuals who exhibit the trait of interest with the genes of those who do not, have targeted systems implicated in feeding, appetite, weight regulation, and mood. These include genes associated with serotonergic or dopaminergic function and other genes related to fasting metabolism and control of energy expenditure (Bulik, 2004). Linkage studies focus on the genome with the goal of identifying areas of the chromosome that may contain genes that influence the trait of interest. Utilizing these methods, researchers have begun to refine the genes of focus, showing promise with those involved in the serotonin, brain-derived neurotrophic factor, and ovarian hormone systems (Klump & Culbert, 2007). However, the field is still in its infancy and thus far no single gene or set of genes has consistently appeared to be tied to either AN or BN (Bulik, 2004).

Neuroimaging and Neurotransmitter Studies

Both neuroimaging techniques, which evaluate abnormalities in both brain structure and function, and studies of brain neurotransmitter levels have also contributed to our understanding of the biological etiology of EDs. Structural neuroimaging (i.e., computerized tomography and magnetic resonance imaging) studies suggest a relationship between EDs and changes in brain structures; however, while a few cases have demonstrated these changes after recovery and weight restoration, it is still unclear whether these brain alterations indicate an underlying vulnerability to EDs or are a consequence of starvation (Barbarich-Marsteller & Marx, 2007; de Zwaan, 2003). Similarly, functional neuroimaging techniques (i.e., positron emission tomography, single photon emission tomography, magnetic resonance spectroscopy, and functional magnetic resonance imaging) have found differences in blood flow and metabolic rate for certain areas of the brain in individuals with EDs, and neurotransmitter studies suggest alterations in the brain serotonin and dopamine activity of individuals with EDs. However, once again this area of study is quite recent, and more research is necessary to elucidate whether these changes are related to underlying dysfunction or are secondary to starvation (Barbarich-Marsteller & Marx, 2007; de Zwaan, 2003).

The majority of studies investigating biological and genetic contributions to the etiology of EDs have been conducted in the United States or Western Europe and none that were reviewed for this chapter described the ethnicity of their participants. Nevertheless, Nogami (1997) indicated that some endocrine studies have been conducted in Japan and that most of these have resulted in similar findings to those investigations from more Westernized countries.

Psychological Models

Psychodynamic Theory

Psychodynamic psychology, which views symptoms as symbolically meaningful phenomena that stem from earlier life experiences, is perhaps the longest-standing psychological model by which EDs have been conceptualized. AN and BN have both been theorized from a variety of psychoanalytic perspectives, including drive theory, object relations, ego, and self psychology (see Dare & Crowther, 1995, for a fuller discussion). Across them all, the etiological underpinning is that ED symptoms are the unconscious symbolic expression of internalized conflicts that originated in earlier developmental stages.

In psychodynamic thinking, the focus is on the meaning of the symptoms and the psychological function of the individual's experience with and need for the ED. The earliest psychoanalytic models viewed the somatic state as a symbolic picture of psychological trauma. For example, vomiting could be understood as an attempt to eliminate the unwanted symbol of sexual trauma, and the bodily wasting of AN could reflect an unconscious identification with a relative who died in an emaciated state (Dare & Crowther, 1995). Contemporary theories tend to focus more on object relations, conceptualizing EDs as symptomatic of disturbances in interpersonal relationships and self-concept. In particular, seminal theorists such as Bruch (1973) and Selvini-Palazzoli (1974) saw the eating disordered individual's relationship to food as an expression of separation difficulties with the maternal object, or mother figure.

Although psychodynamic theories have been widely cited in the ED literature, research has mainly been in the form of exploratory case studies. There has been some empirical support connecting object relations disturbances with bulimic symptomatology in larger samples of both clinical and nonclinical undergraduate women in the United States (Becker, Bell, & Billington, 1987; Patton, 1992). However, it is unclear whether such findings are applicable for Asian American women, as these studies have typically not specified the ethnic breakdown of their participants. At the current time, there have yet to be psychodynamic theory-oriented studies in East Asian or Asian American populations that are cross-cultural or culturally informed.

Attachment Theory

During the past thirty years, attachment theory has become one of the most important conceptual frameworks for understanding affect regulation and human relationships (Tasca, Balfour, Ritchie, & Bissada, 2007). According to the theory, a person's earliest attachment experience with a primary caregiver determines his or her later attachment style, or the template for how he or she perceives and responds to others (Bowlby, 1988). Insecure attachment has been linked to negative outcomes such as low self-esteem and lower academic achievement, as well as psychopathology such as EDs (Eggert & Klump, 2007).

Psychodynamic and family systems–oriented models have long advocated the central role of attachment disruption in the development of EDs (i.e., Humphrey & Stern, 1988; Masterson, 1977; Selvini-Palazzoli, 1978). Attachment theorists propose that the problems with separation and individuation that are often seen in individuals with EDs stem from insecure or anxious attachment to the primary caregiver. It has been asserted that the attachment-related disturbances of women with EDs include parents who may have been emotionally unavailable, overly intrusive, or inconsistent in their responses, selectively encouraging and ignoring behaviors based on their own needs rather than their child's (Krueger, 1990). Thus, a reversal of the healthy attachment relationship occurs, and the child may come to refuse food in order to establish a boundary, or to binge in order to gain nurturance. (Bruch, 1978).

Overall, research suggests that secure attachment is inversely associated with ED symptomatology (Heesacker & Neimeyer, 1990; Kenny & Hart, 1992). Correspondingly, studies using adult attachment measures have shown that women with clinical and subclinical levels of EDs are more likely to be insecurely attached than those without eating pathology (Eggert & Klump, 2007). In particular, the insecure-resistant attachment style has been most consistently associated with disordered eating (Salzman, 1997; Suldo & Sandberg, 2000; Troisi, Di Lorenzo, Alcini, & Nanni, 2006).

Women with EDs have been found to display insecure attachment that is characterized by separation anxiety (Heesacker & Neimeyer, 1990). To date, there has been one study with an Asian population examining separation anxiety. Edman and Yates (2004) found an association between separation anxiety and disordered eating attitudes among Chinese and Malaysian college students in Malaysia. Four types of separation anxiety were measured, including general separation anxiety, school phobia, distress when away, and harm to family. It is unclear which of these types were elevated in the sample, but the authors concluded that separation anxiety does also seem to manifest itself in terms of ED symptoms among Chinese and Malaysian females.

Cognitive Behavioral Theory (CBT)

Cognitive behavioral models combine behavioral concepts derived from learning theory with the central tenet of the cognitive model: that one's thoughts influence one's emotions and behavior. In the field of EDs, both behavioral and cognitive behavioral (CBT) models have been postulated. While there have been limitations in their ability to account for the origins of disordered eating, the major strength of these models has been their amenability to generating empirically supported, effective treatment strategies (Fairburn, 1997; Garner et al., 1993).

According to CBT models of AN, the main disturbance stems from distorted ideas about weight and food intake. The AN patient's belief that she is overweight, when in fact she is not, has been viewed as an essentially cognitive phenomenon (De Silva, 1995). Cognitive distortions specific to EDs have been identified (i.e., "If I put on one pound, I'll keep gaining weight"), with the idea that such thoughts are never critically examined and thus contribute to the persistence of problematic behaviors. The patient's starvation therefore stays justified by her own faulty logic. Additionally, weight control is positively reinforced from many sources, including the social pressure to diet and responses of concern and attention from others (Garner & Bemis, 1985).

CBT models of BN attempt to explain the basic psychopathology and special features of the disorder. One of the most comprehensive models is the "cognitive-social learning model" proposed by Wilson (1989). In it, sequential elements of BN include the cognitions, fear, dieting, binge eating, purging, and postpurge psychological effects. A key aspect is the violation of the diet, which presumably happens because of the effects of prolonged starvation or negative affect. The cognitive distortions (i.e., "I have failed, so might as well keep eating") and negative affect (i.e., initial anxiety reduction gives way to guilt, depression, lower self-esteem, and worry) that ensue serve to maintain the binge-purge cycle of BN (Wilson, 1989).

Research with Caucasian samples suggests that half of patients who complete CBT-based treatment will have a total cessation of binge and purge behaviors and improved attitudes toward weight and shape (Agras & Apple, 2002). Some studies have found as much as an 80% reduction in binge eating frequency, with follow-up studies demonstrating continued improvement for up to six years posttreatment (Agras, Rossiter, & Arnow, 1994; Fairburn et al., 1993; Fairburn & Brownell, 2002). A fuller discussion of CBT treatment models and their effectiveness in the general population will be presented in the treatment section. At the present time there do not appear to be any large-scale studies on the use of CBT, or any other specific psychotherapy interventions for EDs, with Asian and Asian American populations.

Social Models

Family Systems Theory

Family systems theories regard the family as an organized whole in which each individual serves as a contributing member of that whole (S. Minuchin, 1974; P. Minuchin, 1985). EDs are seen as having functional significance in stabilizing and maintaining the status quo of the family system. There have been numerous studies conducted on Caucasian females residing in Westernized countries that have linked eating pathology to dysfunctional patterns of family functioning (Bruch, 1973; Garfinkel, 1983; S. Minuchin, 1975; Selvini-Palazzoli, 1974; Strober & Humphrey, 1987; Yager, 1982). The main theoretical concepts that frequently appear in this literature are family cohesiveness, expression of feelings, conflict resolution, and parental control (Bailey, 1991; Root, 1990).

The earliest studies to look at familial factors in ED etiology within an Asian population were conducted in Japan. Ishikawa, Iwata, and Hirano (1960) and Shimosaka (1961) observed common parental characteristics in AN patients' family backgrounds, such as overprotective, overly involved mothers and fathers who lacked firmness and leadership and/or were too attached to their daughters (Ishikawa, 1984). More recently, Koide and Hasegawa (1992) found patients with EDs to feel a sense of helplessness due to their mothers' inability to perceive their needs appropriately, and their fathers' inability to use their influence. Similarly, Tsukahara and Shimosaka (1994) observed the attitudes of fathers of patients with EDs in family sessions and multiple interview formats and found that they tended to adopt an indifferent, nonconfrontational stance within the family.

The most studied dimension of familial patterns with Asian populations has been disturbance within the mother-daughter relationship. Haudek, Rorty, and Henker (1999) found that Asian American women with higher levels of eating problems perceived their mothers as less caring than those without eating pathology. While maternal caring and control seem to be implicated, characteristics like maternal jealousy and competition do not seem to be as salient for Asian Americans with EDs as has been observed in Caucasian samples (Rorty & Yager, 2000).

Feminist Theory

Broadly speaking, feminist psychological theories explore how being female in nonegalitarian, male-dominated cultures shape and impact the mental health of the girls and women living in such societies. In the realm of body image, feminist theorists have viewed appearance standards as vehicles for the oppression of women and have long noted the negative impact of Western society's objectification of the female body (Bartky, 1990; Bordo, 1993; Brownmiller, 1984). Objectification theory (Fredrickson & Roberts, 1997) focuses on the ways in which sexual objectification of women's bodies may account for mental health risks that disproportionately affect females, such as EDs. As women's bodies have been socially sanctioned as objects for the use, consumption, and pleasure of others, EDs are seen as passive strategies that reflect the lack of power females have to control the objectification of their bodies by all members of society, including themselves.

There has been some empirical support for feminist theory–based predictions of body dissatisfaction and disordered eating in East Asian populations. Comparing the feminist model-derived "social change" hypothesis with the sociocultural model-based "media influence" hypothesis with Chinese, Korean, and American college women, Jung and Forbes (2007) found the former to be more accurate in predicting ED symptoms. Researchers found the highest body dissatisfaction with the group that underwent the greatest recent social changes (the Korean sample). Results supported the feminist social change theory, which says that any rapid social shifts toward gender equality will be countered by increasingly unrealistic appearance standards for women and greater pressure to achieve them. In turn, these pressures are expected to result in increased body dissatisfaction and ED symptoms.

Western women's anxiety about their physical appearance and body dissatisfaction has been well documented, with consistent evidence that even those who are not overweight generally express a desire to be thinner (Cash, Winstead, & Janda, 1986; Jackson, Sullivan, & Rostker, 1988; Mintz & Betz, 1986). Research on body dissatisfaction in Caucasian females has demonstrated that many women show a discrepancy between their real and ideal weight, engaging in both safe and dangerous food-restriction strategies (Ogden, 2002). While research analyzing body dissatisfaction in minority groups is not as plentiful, the literature on Asian groups suggests that there is cause for concern. In the United States, Franko and Striegel-Moore (2002) reviewed body image research with adolescents and found that within each Asian ethnic group, high body dissatisfaction was associated with disordered eating behaviors and low self-esteem. Likewise, Mintz and Kashubeck (1999) found that compared with their Caucasian counterparts, Asian American college women reported lower levels of self-esteem and more body dissatisfaction. In China and

Japan, negative body image and the prevalence of ED tendencies have also been reported as relatively higher when compared to rates in Western society (Davis & Katzman, 1998; A. M. Lee & Lee, 1996; S. Lee, 1993; Pike & Borovoy, 2004).

Culture-Specific Theories: Thin Ideal Internalization

Much has been written about the shrinking female body image ideal in the latter half of the 20th century and the media's increased focus on dieting, propagation of the thin ideal, and active promotion of eating disordered behaviors (Garner, Garfinkel, Schwartz, & Thompson, 1980; Snow & Harris, 1986). Given the 20th-century rise in EDs and related societal shifts in beauty standards, it is generally accepted that such sociocultural factors play a major role in ED etiology and maintenance. According to sociocultural models, exposure to thinness ideals, internalization of them, and the experience of discrepancy between actual and ideal self lead to the body dissatisfaction and dietary restriction associated with EDs. Evidence suggests that media exposure to the thin ideal, or social pressure about thin-ideal internalization, increases females' more immediate body image concerns (see Striegel-Moore & Bulik, 2007, for a fuller review).

What underlies much of the current literature on the development of EDs in Asians and Asian Americans is the sociocultural model, which attributes increased eating pathology in non-Western populations to exposure to Western thinness ideals and beauty standards (Stice, 2001; Stice & Shaw, 2002). The model posits that pressure to be thin promotes internalization of the thin ideal and body dissatisfaction, which then places individuals at risk for dieting, negative affect, and eating pathology (Stice, 1994). Contrary to earlier hypotheses predicting that ethnic minorities would be at lower risk for eating disordered behaviors due to less cultural pressure to be thin (i.e., Stice, 1994; Striegel-Moore, Silberstein, & Rodin, 1986), evidence has demonstrated significant differences among minority groups in terms of thinness ideal internalization. For example, Shaw, Ramirez, and Trost (2004) found that Asians and Caucasians evidenced significantly more internalization of the thin ideal than did blacks and Hispanics, and posited that ethnic groups may have reached parity in terms of eating disturbances because sociocultural pressures for thinness have become so widespread. Preliminary empirical evidence suggests that Asian American women experience similar pressure for thinness levels as Caucasian females (Phan & Tylka, 2006; Tylka & Subich, 2004).

Authors have increasingly commented on how thinness ideals have been a part of East Asian cultures for centuries, and have noted that there is actually a narrower range of acceptable body weights that may only increase susceptibility to EDs (Kennedy, Templeton, Gandhi, & Gorzalka, 2004; Mukai, Crago, & Shisslak, 1994). Stark-Wroblewski, Yanico, and Lupe (2005) found that a higher level of thin ideal internalization in Japanese and Chinese international students in the United States was not associated with general acculturation level. In addition to lending support for the sociocultural model of EDs in an East Asian population, researchers concluded that a thin ideal may already be well embedded within the female gender role of some East Asian cultures, a notion which has been supported by research with Japanese and Chinese samples (i.e., S. Lee, 1991; Mukai et al., 1994). Thus, more recent authors actively encourage clinicians to look beyond acculturation level indicators and instead consider specifically the extent to which clients are aware of and have internalized the thin ideal, as it applies to their specific individual and cultural context.

Culture-Specific Theories: Westernization/Industrialization

Sociocultural theorists contend that Western cultural values occupy a principal role in the etiology of disordered eating (Warren et al., 2005); so much so, in fact, that EDs have even been deemed "the price paid for Western civilization" (Bemporad, 1996). However, while many theorists have viewed the thinness ideal as the central cultural value that influences non-Western populations in the development of eating pathology, there are other aspects of modernization and industrialization that may help to account for the presence of EDs around the world. The emergence of EDs in the United States and Europe coincided with a number of sweeping societal changes in the second half of the 20th century, including the rise of a consumer economy, increasing conflicts in family and intergenerational relationships, and upheavals in traditional sex roles (R. A. Gordon, 2001). Some theorists have linked the rise of EDs in the West to female identity crises following the cultural upheavals of the 1960s (R. A. Gordon, 2000).

In the 1980s, researchers predicted that as Western cultural norms became more influential around the world, EDs would become more common in countries that had not seen or recognized the disorders before (Prince, 1985). The only non-Western countries reporting EDs before 1990 were Japan and Chile (R. A. Gordon, 2001). After 1990, EDs were reported for the first time in countries such as China, South Korea, Singapore, South Africa, Nigeria, Mexico, Argentina, Brazil, and India. Indeed, one landmark study conducted in Fiji, which evaluated eating disorder symptoms just one month after the introduction of television in 1995 and again three years later, found a significant increase in the presence of disordered eating among schoolgirls (Becker, Burwell, Herzog, Hamburg, & Gilman, 2002). These apparently newly emerged incidences of EDs shared the commonality of occurring in either highly urbanized, developed economies, or areas that were witnessing rapid market changes with an associated impact on the status of women in that society (R. A. Gordon, 2001). Accordingly, it has been argued that disordered eating is now bound less to "Westernization" than to the global culture of "modernity" (C. Lee, 1998; Littlewood, 1995).

Researchers in the United States have paid particular attention to Japan because of its early reports of EDs and economic rise during the 20th century. In the 1960s, Japanese clinicians attributed increasing rates of AN to post–World War II changes in traditional family structure (Pike & Borovoy, 2004). Likewise, researchers have since given as a possible reason the fact that many of the same tensions that arose in Western industrial societies (i.e., increased emphasis on individualism, altered societal expectations of female roles, the expanding impact of consumerism and media) have been in evidence in Japan as well (White, 1993). However, some warn that while certain aspects of cultural transition in the United States and Japan appear similar on the surface, the meaning and response to changes in gender role and culture differ in important ways that cannot be overlooked (see Pike & Borovoy, 2004, for a fuller discussion).

In much of the literature that seems to support the association between Westernization and increased rates of EDs, exactly which aspects of Westernization lead to increased susceptibility to eating pathology still remain unclear. In a study of first-year medical students in China, nearly 80% admitted to a fear of gaining weight or becoming fat (Chun et al., 1992). This was consistent with later findings of widespread dieting among Chinese adolescents (Huon, Walton, & Lim, 1999). Focusing on the role of modernization in Chinese society, some have noted that this departure from traditional values and practices may be partly attributable to a growing problem of obesity among Chinese youth (R. A. Gordon, 2001).

Other reports have demonstrated that Western influence, which is stronger in urbanized settings, may lead to the development of more ED symptoms (S. Lee & Lee, 2000). Comparing females in cities with varying degrees of modernization, authors found the highest eating disordered attitudes among those living in more urban areas, such as Hong Kong. Theorists have also cited recent rapid industrialization, increased media exposure to Western ideals, and the rise in consumerism as contributing factors to the rise of EDs in native Korean females when compared with Korean Americans (Ko & Cohen, 1998). Authors posit that Westernization itself, for those born in a Western culture, does not lead to increased eating pathology, whereas the unfamiliarity and newness of Western ideals within another culture may create more disordered eating attitudes (Ko & Cohen, 1998). As is needed throughout this body of literature, authors have called for further studies aimed at elucidating the relationship of Westernization and EDs.

Strengths, Weaknesses, and Alternatives in Applying Current Etiological Models of EDs to Asians

Biological Models

The results of current genetic research provide support for the theory that some significant part of the etiological picture with EDs is biological in nature. However, it is still unclear how these genetic factors interact with the psychosocial forces that also appear to be quite relevant to our understanding of how EDs develop. Striegel-Moore & Bulik (2007) have proposed a "mixed model," in which genetics account for the core symptoms (e.g., restricting, binge eating, self-induced vomiting) which have persisted both historically over time and across cultures. At the same time, the culture of a particular time or place might provide an explanatory context for the expression of certain symptoms. By example, they cite the culturally mediated presentation of AN in Asian populations, noting that the core symptom of low body weight has been observed for centuries and likely has genetic underpinnings, while contextual factors which support that symptom (e.g., refusal to eat due to somatic complaints of bloating versus weight phobia) may vary by culture and environment. Similarly, researchers have noted that while genetic research provides important evidence of biological contributions to etiology, most of this work has been conducted with samples from more Westernized countries in which the thin ideal is ubiquitous and therefore it is impossible to extract the impact of these environmental factors (Keel & Klump, 2003). One notable exception to this is the genetic research that has been conducted in Japan (Nogami, 1997); still, future research utilizing families or twin studies in non-Western countries could help elucidate this complex relationship (Keel & Klump, 2003).

Psychological Models

While psychodynamic conceptualizations of ED etiology were certainly the earliest theories hypothesized, they have largely been based on clinical and anecdotal observations of those who have historically presented in treatment settings: young, middle- to upper-class, Caucasian females in more Westernized countries. This may restrict the relevance and applicability of core theoretical constructs, such as the separation-individuation process, that may differ for Asian populations. By example, with family interdependence being a salient cultural value, it has been widely cited that Asian American adolescents often experience delayed autonomy from their parents compared to other ethnic groups (Kwak, 2003).

Similarly, it is important to note that although Bowlby (1973) emphasized the universality of attachment theory, research to support this has been somewhat mixed. There seems to be significant cross-cultural variance in the infant-caregiver attachment bond (McCarthy, 1998). For example, it was found that Japanese infants display more distress upon separation from the caregiver than infants in the United States, and less avoidant behavior upon return (Takahashi, 1990). One must consider the cultural variation in the degree to which caregivers encourage either exaggerated dependence or independence in their children, as well as the differing types and levels of parental demands and expectations for children across various cultures (Grossman & Grossman, 1990). For instance, research has suggested that both Chinese and Chinese American mothers feel it is not only acceptable but desirable for parents to actively intrude in their children's lives (Chiu, 1987). Such cultural variations must be considered and incorporated into the conceptualization and application of attachment and family-related theoretical models and research literature.

While interventions based on cognitive-behavioral models are often suggested as appropriate treatment approaches for Asian American populations due to their solution-focused, concrete, and specific nature, it is unclear whether cognitive-behavioral frameworks are applicable when considering the etiology of EDs for these groups. To date, no studies have investigated the presentation of cognitive distortions or negative affect related to body image and disordered eating among Asian or Asian American populations. In addition, the relevance of these theories for Asian populations may be difficult to evaluate with empirical investigations as researchers have noted that Asian cultures value the avoidance of negative thinking (Uba, 1994). Similarly, cognitive behavioral etiological theories may seem less pertinent for Asians or Asian Americans, who tend to view their actions through the lens of community and familial expectations more so than individual motivations (Sue & Sue, 2003). For a fuller discussion of how culturally based variables may impact the utilization of CBT for eating disorders with Asian populations, please refer to the section on treatment below.

Social Models

Certainly the social etiological theories for EDs are based in more of a collectivistic mindset in terms of the contributions of family and environment. Asian families, which have been described as having high parental expectations, more rigid hierarchies, and fewer demonstrations of affection and praise (Yee, DeBaryshe, Yuen, Kim, & McCubbin, 2007), might seem to be ideal environments in which to evaluate family systems theories that suggest the importance of family dynamics such as overcontrol, emotional inhibition, and conflict avoidance to the etiology of EDs. However, most of the current literature is limited by correlational designs, which can only report the coexistence of certain family dynamics and ED symptoms but cannot prove any causality between the two. It has been noted that parenting styles (i.e., authoritarian) that have been associated with negative outcomes in Caucasian families do not have similar relationships in Asian families (Yee et al., 2007). Thus, those family factors that may have previously been identified as contributing to EDs must be evaluated with caution and sensitivity toward the varying cultural meanings of dynamics in Asian families.

For decades, etiological research on EDs has focused mainly on sociocultural and familial influences, yet very few specific replicated factors have emerged consistently (Striegel-Moore & Bulik, 2007). Because most research on EDs has been conducted with Caucasian females in more Westernized countries, investigations with Asian populations are uniquely positioned to explore hypotheses regarding feminist and culture-specific theories of ED etiology. While there is much variation in women's roles and experiences, thin ideal exposure and internalization, and Westernization and industrialization among Caucasian women in Western countries, extending this research to Asians and Asian Americans expands more broadly that diversity, providing even more variation to aid us in better understanding these complex relationships (Cummins et al., 2005). For example, a recent study examined the relationship between the concepts of enmeshment, the cultural values of independence and interdependence, and their influence on ED etiology (Tomiyama & Mann, 2008). A positive correlation was found between the value of independence and ED symptomology. This study makes a case for the possibility of strong identification with more of an interdependent ethnic identity as being a possible protective factor for the development of EDs. However, other studies (e.g., Phan & Tylka, 2006) examining ethnic identity as a factor in EDs have found conflicting evidence.

As Katzman and Lee (1997) pointed out, further examination into the presentations and permutations of EDs in different societies may highlight the pressures placed on women globally, and "provide an alternative laboratory in which to examine the impact of societal changes and stresses on women's sense of their self and body" (p. 386). Researchers are just beginning to move beyond overinclusive concepts such as Westernization and acculturation to develop a fuller understanding of the specific cultural meanings of ED symptoms such as self-starvation, bingeing, and purging. For example, psychiatrist and anthropologist Littlewood (1995) asserted that Asian women, in the absence of a fear of fatness, engage in food refusal to instrumentally achieve self-determination when confronted with ambivalent cultural demands. Similarly, S. Lee (1995) described one Chinese AN patient's behavior as "symbolizing a loss of voice in a social world perceived to be solely oppressive" (p. 31). By broadening constructs with multicultural populations, feminist authors have suggested alternative ways of organizing thinking about EDs (i.e., as a problem of disconnection, transition, and oppression rather than dieting, weight, and fat phobia), which in turn may lead to an expanded vocabulary for conceptualization, treatment, and recovery.

Because more effective treatments can be developed when we know the causes of a disorder, efforts to identify the complex biopsychosocial forces that cause EDs are an important endeavor. As this work continues, it is still necessary to create effective interventions for those currently suffering with EDs; thus, the next section of this chapter turns to a review of what is currently known about the treatment of EDs.

TREATING EDS IN ASIANS

Given that EDs have the highest morbidity of any other psychiatric diagnosis, adequate treatment should be of the utmost concern. In most inpatient settings, treatment generally follows a multi-disciplinary team approach, (i.e., nutritionists, medical doctors, psychiatrists, and mental health clinicians). Due to the complexity and severity of these illnesses, maintaining a team approach when working on an outpatient basis is also useful, however, this is rarely seen outside of a hospital setting. While all of the treatments presented in this section were originally normed on a white population, the applicability of the various modalities to working with Asian populations will be discussed. Though inpatient hospitalization might be necessary in cases where there is increased medical or suicidal risk, the bulk of ED treatment will likely be conducted through an outpatient model (Wilson, Grilo, & Vitousek, 2007) and thus will be the focus of this section.

Critical Appraisal of Major Treatment Approaches for EDs

Biological Treatment Approaches

ANOREXIA NERVOSA

Pharmacotherapy used to treat EDs continues to be a controversial area of study. Over the past few decades, antidepressants, opiate antagonists, antipsychotics, and mood stabilizers have been used to treat AN in both inpatient and outpatient clinical settings (Attia & Schroeder, 2005). Medication may be more effective at improving the psychological symptoms (e.g., obsessions with food, distorted body image concerns) rather than having a direct impact on weight gain (Attia et al., 1998, Bulik et al., 2007). Attempts have been made, with little success, to examine the efficacy of medication in restoring weight for AN patients in critical and acute phases of their disorder as well as how much of an impact its use can have on preventing relapse (Attia et al., 1998; Barbarich et al., 2004; Halmi et al., 1986).

Hormonal treatments have also been attempted with both female and male patients with AN (e.g., Hill et al., 2000; Klibanski et al., 1995; Miller et al., 2005). Miller, Grieco, and Klibanski (2005) found that administering testosterone to female patients with AN significantly improved depressive mood symptoms. Klibanski et al. (1995) administered estrogen/progesterone to a group of 48 women with AN and found that after 6 months, they did not differ significantly from the control group with regard to bone loss. Hill et al. (2000) placed a sample of patients on growth hormone and found that this reduced the time to regain stable heart rates in patients that had previously been orthostatic.

Nutritional counseling is another method of treatment often recommended for AN. Through the introduction of meal planning as well as psychoeducation on the biological impact of starvation, patients/families can obtain necessary information regarding the gravity of the condition. Ideally, this would motivate behavioral change. A few studies, however, cite the ineffectiveness of this method alone without psychological treatment (Halmi et al., 2005; Pike et al., 2003; Serfaty et al., 1999). Used in conjunction with medication and psychotherapy, this can prove to be more effective (Wilson et al., 2007). Researchers have also attempted to use nutritional supplements (e.g., zinc) to increase weight gain with some success (Birmingham et al., 2004). Further research is necessary to study the efficacy of such interventions.

BULIMIA NERVOSA

Pharmacological treatments of BN appear to have more success than those for AN. According to Chavez and Insel (2007), antidepressants, antiemetics, and anticonvulsants have all been used to treat BN, with the selective serotonin reuptake inhibitor (SSRI) fluoxetine (Prozac) being the most studied medication. This is also the only drug that has been approved by the U.S. Food and Drug Administration to treat EDs. It not only appears to have a positive impact on disordered eating and body image perceptions but has also been found to decrease bingeing and vomiting behaviors (Chavez & Insel, 2007; Beumont et al., 1997; Goldstein et al., 1995; Romano et al., 2002). It may also have the added benefit of improving symptoms of depression and anxiety in patients with BN as well; however, findings appear to be inconsistent across studies in this regard (Chavez & Insel, 2007; Beumont et al., 1997; Goldstein et al., 1995; Romano et al., 2002). Wilson, Grilo, and Vitousek (2007) concur with this finding but also highlight that antidepressants combined with CBT appear to be no more effective at treating BN than CBT alone.

EDNOS AND BED

In searching for literature examining the use of medication to treat EDNOS, no studies were discovered. It seems intuitive, however, to assume that using medication to target particular symptoms of subclinical EDs (e.g., purging, restricting behavior, depressive/anxious symptoms) would have similar outcomes as when they are used with clinically diagnosed EDs. Still, more studies are needed to further investigate the usefulness of medications in treating EDNOS.

Like BN, antidepressants and anticonvulsants have been used to treat BED and have been found to assist in reduction of bingeing episodes as well as depressive symptoms and body image concerns (Arnold et al., 2002; Chavez & Insel, 2007; Hudson et al., 1998). Additionally, studies have examined the use of the SSRIs sertraline (McElroy et al., 2000) and citalopram (McElroy et al., 2003) in decreasing binge behavior as well as body weight. It was unclear, however, what impact these two medications had on reducing depressive symptoms in these participants. The latter study also found that topiramate, an anticonvulsant, had a similar impact on binge behavior and body weight but no impact on mood symptoms. Appetite suppressants, such as sibutramine, have also been found to reduce bingeing episodes as well as decrease depressive symptoms in patients with BED (Appolinario et al., 2003; Chavez & Insel, 2007).

Psychological Treatment Approaches

PSYCHODYNAMIC PSYCHOTHERAPY

Psychodynamic psychotherapy has been used to treat both AN and BN. Theories underlying psychodynamic treatment posit that ED symptoms are a manifestation of a "struggling inner self," that serves a specific function for patients (Costin, 1999, p. 109). Symptoms are not immediately targeted. Instead, the work revolves around encouraging the expression of unconscious concerns as a means to alleviate the need to engage in eating disordered behaviors (Costin, 1999). Some psychodynamic therapies focus on the use of transferences between the therapist and patient in order to understand how interpersonal dynamics contribute to the patient's need for the ED symptoms (Costin, 1999). However, there is little empirical research on the efficacy of psychodynamic treatments. Bachar et al. (1999) suggested that the use of self-psychological interventions proved to be more effective at creating lasting change in symptoms of AN, whereas CBT created short-term change but had a greater incidence of relapse. Critics of this type of approach argue that attempting to conduct explorative and insight-oriented therapy with a patient who has a malnourished brain would prove to be ineffective as he or she would not likely be able to engage in the work at an optimal cognitive level (Costin, 1999). Additionally, this type of work can take several years, and the lack of focus on targeting symptoms could put patients at risk for serious medical complications that may not be as well addressed in therapy.

COGNITIVE-BEHAVIORAL TREATMENTS

While a vast number of psychological modalities are used to treat AN and BN, the most empirically supported psychological treatments involve a cognitive behavioral component. These have been found to reduce binge/purge behaviors, disordered eating attitudes, and restrictive eating (Agras et al., 2000; Bailer et al., 2004; Carter et al., 2003). Bulik et al. (2007) reviewed numerous evidence-based treatment studies published between 1980 and 2005 for AN. The treatment modalities evaluated in these studies included medication alone, medication plus CBT, CBT alone, as well as other adaptations of behavior therapy. The two studies rated as "good" for AN, were both family-oriented treatments with adolescents that will be discussed in the next section (Bulik et al., 2007). Nine other studies were rated as "fair," six of which involved treating adults through individual CBT, interpersonal psychotherapy (IPT), cognitive analytic therapy (CAT), or family therapy. Cognitive behavioral approaches have been found to have greater efficacy in treating BN, and the National Institute for Clinical Excellence (NICE) committee's comprehensive study on the efficacy of various treatments for EDs gave the grade of "A" to manualized CBT for treating BN, indicating that they deem it to be at the highest level of effectiveness when compared to other types of treatment (NICE, 2004; Wilson et al., 2007).

Christopher Fairburn's manualized Oxford approach is the most widely known empirically supported treatment program used to understand and treat those with BN (Fairburn, Marcus, & Wilson, 1993). Emphasizing the critical roles of both cognitive and behavioral factors in the maintenance of the disease, the model posits that sociocultural pressures to be thin lead some women to overvalue the importance of body weight and shape (Fairburn, 1997). The BN patient's restrict-binge-purge cycle disrupts learned satiety that regulates food intake while, psychologically, increased distress and lower self-esteem reinforce the conditions that lead to perpetuating this cycle. As this self-sustaining process develops, binge eating provides negative reinforcement of BN maintenance and becomes a means of regulating negative affect by distracting from sources of distress (Wilson & Pike, 2001). Treatment focuses on breaking these dysfunctional coping strategies and creating a healthy, flexible pattern of eating, as well as decreasing overconcern with body image. This type of treatment typically consists of up to 20 individual sessions over a 5-month period but could also be conducted in group therapy format (E. Chen et al., 2003; Nevonen & Broberg, 2006; Wilson et al., 2007).

Similar to BN, treatments for BED include CBT using both individual and/or group treatment models (Chavez & Insel, 2007). These types of treatment can reduce binge episodes, restricting that leads to compensatory bingeing and negative body image as well as thought distortions around food (Hilbert & Tuschen-Caffier, 2004; Wilfley et al., 2002). They have also been found to be effective at temporarily reducing depressive symptoms. A manualized CBT treatment for BED was adapted from a model created to treat BN (Fairburn, Marcus, & Wilson, 1993). This was considered the best treatment available at the time of the NICE study and received the grade of an "A" for the treatment of BED (NICE, 2004; Wilson et al., 2007). The model follows a three-stage process through which the patient receives psychoeducation around eating and nutrition and develops alternative strategies to binge behavior. The patient is then taught to challenge negative thoughts and self-talk, as well as to reintroduce triggering foods in a healthy way. The final phase focuses on planning for the future, creating realistic food and body expectations for oneself, and avoiding relapse (Fairburn, 1995).

INTERPERSONAL PSYCHOTHERAPY (IPT)

IPT has also been cited as an effective method of treating both BN and BED (Fairburn et al., 1993; Wilson et al., 2007). It utilizes a nondirective format and focuses on recognizing how interpersonal issues in the patient's life might be perpetuating his or her ED. The focus is more on how interpersonal patterns can serve to maintain an eating disordered lifestyle and less on behavioral symptom management. In Fairburn et al.'s (1993) study, those patients administered either IPT or CBT had a 95% symptom reduction rate after a period of 12 months. IPT was also given a grade of "B" by the NICE committee's 2004 treatment guidelines, endorsing it as a useful alternative to manualized CBT for the treatment of BN (NICE, 2004; Wilson et al., 2007). Similar to the studies conducted on BN, Wilfley et al. (1993; 2002) found IPT to be just as effective for individuals with BED, finding symptom remission rates of greater than 70% for those patients administered CBT and IPT (Wilfley et al., 2002).

DIALECTICAL BEHAVIOR THERAPY (DBT)

Newer research has examined the efficacy of DBT for treating BN (Safer, Telch, & Agras, 2001). Researchers randomly assigned 31 mostly Caucasian women to either 20 weekly, 50-minute sessions of DBT, most of which were adapted from Linehan's (1993) skills training manual, or to a waiting-list control group. In the adapted model for treating BN, eating disordered behaviors are seen as the patient's attempts to control painful emotional states. The focus of treatment is on teaching patients skills to better cope with affect dysregulation as a means to diminish eating disordered behavior. At the end of the study, 28.6% of participants were abstinent from binge/purge behaviors, 35% of the patients reduced their binge eating behavior by 88% and purging behavior by 89%, and 35% remained symptomatic and continued to meet criteria for BN. None of the participants in the individual DBT therapy group dropped out of treatment. DBT also teaches patients valuable skills with regard to acceptance of particular body attributes that may be contributing to the eating disordered behavior (Delinsky & Wilson, 2006; Hayes, 2004; Wilson et al., 2007).

DBT has also been found to decrease binge behavior, depressive symptoms, and body image distortions, but does not appear to have significant impact on weight for individuals with BED (Chavez & Insel, 2007; Telch, Agras, & Linehan, 2001). In Telch, Agras, and Linehan's (2001) study, 44 women with BED were assigned to two treatment groups, receiving DBT and a control. After 20 sessions of DBT following an adapted model similar to that offered for BN, 82% reported no bingeing. Of these women 56% maintained abstinence for 6 months after treatment ceased. The NICE (2004) study deemed DBT as an effective alternate treatment for BED, giving it a grade of "B" (Wilson et al., 2007).

SELF-HELP

Other methods of treatment for BN include guided self-help (i.e., Banasiak, Paxton, & Hay, 2005; Palmer, et al., 2002; Wilson et al., 2007) as well as CBT self-administered through a CD-ROM (Murray, Pombo-Carril, & Bara-Carril, 2003). A number of studies have been conducted on the efficacy of self-help treatments for BED, including self-guided CBT as well as psychoeducational approaches to understanding ED behaviors (Grilo, 2007; Peterson et al., 1998). According to the NICE (2004) review, these approaches received a grade of "B," indicating a high level of efficacy (Wilson et al., 2007). Of the self-help approaches, the self-guided CBT approaches seem to be most efficacious (Grilo & Masheb, 2005). In a study comparing self-guided CBT with behavioral weight loss and a control, the self-guided CBT group achieved a 50% remission rate, while the other groups had less than half that amount (Grilo & Masheb, 2005).

Social Treatment Approaches

FAMILY THERAPY

While a variety of social treatments exist for AN, probably the most researched treatments to date incorporate behavioral intervention with family therapy in adolescents. Age is likely to be a factor in the efficacy of these treatments, as the longer one has been ill, the less potential the patient has for recovery, particularly patients who have had the illness for more than 10 years (Strober, Freeman, & Morrell, 1997). The "Maudsley Method" (Lock et al., 2001; Dare & Eisler, 1997) of therapy for adolescents with AN is a three-phase model that focuses first on refeeding (for medical stability), then shifts toward building family support and cohesion; increasing autonomy, awareness, and patient self-monitoring; and improving the family's ability to cope with environmental and emotional stressors. A recent 5-year follow up study on Maudsley-type family therapy found that 75% of patients reported no ED symptoms and only 8% reported turning to using purge behaviors instead of restricting to lose weight (Eisler et al., 2007).

The debate regarding the efficacy of family-based therapy versus individual treatment continues to be mixed. Robin et al. (1994) discovered that a Maudsley-like family treatment was more effective than ego-oriented individual therapy with adolescents. Ball and Mitchell (2004) found individual CBT treatment to be just as effective as the Maudsley-type family therapy. Other researchers have recommended a purely CBT treatment model aimed at motivating behavioral change (Garner, Vitousek, & Pike, 1997; Vitousek, Watson, & Wilson, 1998). In their recent review, Chavez and Insel (2007) note that the literature on treating adults with AN offers a less clear picture of what psychological treatments are most efficacious, and it has been suggested that family-based treatments may not be as effective in adult populations with AN (Bulik et al., 2007).

Le Grange, Lock, and Dymek (2003) examined the efficacy of family-based therapy for working with adolescents with BN by adapting the manualized, Maudsley method of treatment created for AN (Lock et al., 2001; Dare & Eisler, 1997). The personality and temperamental differences between AN and BN patients were cited as important considerations when adapting this to work with BN. Women with BN reported more troubled childhood experiences, had more difficulty identifying and articulating emotions, were more impulsive and self-rejecting, and sought the approval of others more often than patients with AN. In the original Maudsley model, families are responsible for "refeeding" their child; this adaptation also placed responsibility on the parents for preventing binge/purge behavior. The family goal is to foster more autonomy and create clearer, more appropriate roles. Researchers believe this program will be highly effective in treating BN as it accounts for many of the differences between it and AN. However, controlled treatment studies are necessary to support its efficacy.

Other forms of family therapy have been used as a type of sociocultural treatment for EDs. Dallos (2004) discussed the efficacy of integrating attachment and narrative theories into family therapy with ED patients. Using narratives with patients with EDs externalizes the problem by focusing on the sociocultural influences that may have precipitated it, rather than blaming particular family influences. Dallos (2004) created a four-stage intervention, which combined narrative and attachment theory for working with families to treat AN (see Dallos, 2004, for more details).

Another modality of family therapy examined by Scholz and Asen (2001) utilizes a multiple family treatment model for AN. The researchers followed 37 families who participated together in a variety of treatments ranging from intensive 5 days per week to 1-day treatments repeated every three weeks. Results of the 18-month program showed a reported increase in closeness between family members and increased autonomy and independence on the part of the parents, no longer relying on the doctors and staff for their needs. Patients also displayed symptomatic improvement, a reduction in relapses, a reduction in length of stay, and more intensive and effective work with family issues and conflicts. The lack of a control group in the sample does not support the generalizability of the study. However, future research using a controlled experimental design, particularly with families from diverse backgrounds, would prove to be extremely valuable to the treatment literature.

FEMINIST THERAPY

Various treatment approaches based on feminist theories of etiology have also been reviewed in the literature (Cummins & Lehman, 2007). Frank (1999) offered the idea of "culture-wise" parenting as a desirable way of preventing negative body image in adolescent females. She argued that parents who can view the sociocultural environment critically can serve as a buffer for their daughters and help them to resist negative cultural messages about body image. This method would require parents to make changes in their own attitudes (i.e., mothers not complaining about their own weight, and fathers not objectifying women). It would also be important for parents to explain cultural differences to their daughters with respect to body image and size, as the cultural body image ideal is often the thin, white woman (Frank, 1999). Feminist therapies have also been suggested for use in the treatment of EDs (Garner & Needleman, 1997). Principles that have been described as key to feminist therapy for EDs include: a recognition of the role that social oppressions play in the development of disordered eating, the minimization of hierarchy between client and therapist, an emphasis on women's strengths and relationships, and a commitment to empowering women to engage in personal and social change (Piran, Jasper, & Pinhas, 2004; Sands, 1998; Sesan & Katzman, 1998). Additionally, feminist therapy urges more of a focus on body acceptance versus food intake and dieting behaviors that can cause more self-criticism (Bergner et al., 1985). While these approaches may be quite useful to consider when treating EDs in Asian populations, no empirical evidence currently supports their efficacy.

Strengths, Weaknesses, and Alternatives in Applying Current Treatment Approaches for EDs to Asians

It is clear, given the high mortality rate associated with EDs and the dramatic and long-standing impact that these disorders can have on individuals and their families, that the identification of effective treatments for EDs is of urgent necessity. Nevertheless, our current understanding of efficacious treatments for AN is extremely limited, with family therapy the only currently recommended treatment for adolescents and no single approach clearly identified as the treatment of choice for AN in adults (Chavez & Insel, 2007). The picture is somewhat more promising for BN and BED. CBT and IPT have clearly demonstrated effectiveness in treatment studies, and other newer approaches such as DBT may also be quite efficacious. Pharmacotherapy may also be a useful strategy, especially in conjunction with psychotherapy and in cases where there is other comorbid psychopathology. Nevertheless, even the "best" treatments that research has presently been able to identify for EDs are only 30–50% effective, meaning many of those patients who are able to receive such treatments are still showing only limited to no improvement or are dropping out of therapy (Wilson et al., 2007).

This does not include the outcomes for individuals with EDs who are either not identified as needing treatment or who do not seek treatment. Recent studies in the United States demonstrate that clinicians are less likely to assess ethnic minority women for an ED, that minority women are disproportionately less likely to seek care for an ED when compared to their Caucasian counterparts, and that even when they seek care, they are less likely to actually receive treatment for an ED (Becker et al., 2003; Striegel-Moore & Bulik, 2007). While the literature examining the etiology and prevalence of EDs in Asian populations is on the rise, the same cannot be said for research on the treatment of EDs in these populations. Upon analyzing the studies discussed above examining treatment for AN, BN, and EDNOS/BED, it was found that the vast majority of them focused primarily on Caucasian populations or made no mention of the ethnicity of participants. The majority of studies considering ED treatment in non-Caucasian populations tend to take either a nonspecific or all-inclusive stance, examining a variety of cultural groups at the same time (i.e., Gilbert, 2003; Harris & Kuba, 1997; Kempa & Thomas, 2000). Very few studies exist that examine ED treatment in a specifically Asian or Asian American population. As a result of this, the following discussion will attempt to incorporate all of the inclusive as well as exclusive studies but will focus on applying treatments normed primarily on Euro-American populations to Asian and Asian American patients.

PHARMACOTHERAPY AND MEDICAL INTERVENTION

Cultural values significantly impact the patient's willingness to seek treatment as well as his/her ongoing adherence. According to Sue and Sue (1987), it is considered shameful in many Asian cultures to seek help outside of the family for emotional support related to mental illness. Thus, concern for loss of face and the stigma against help-seeking outside of the family could be significant barriers impeding access to the treatment of EDs. Keeping this value in mind, Asian patients might be more willing to consult with their general medical doctor regarding symptoms and may be more open to trying pharmacotherapy if prescribed by a primary care provider as opposed to a psychiatrist. Sodowsky et al. (1995) suggest that Asian American patients are more likely to present with somatic concerns (see Chapter 8 of this text for a fuller discussion of somatization in Asians), and providers should be aware of how to carefully link these to an understanding of the psychological implications of ED behaviors. Taking a psychoeducational standpoint might be one way in which this information can be conveyed without disrespecting the patient's cultural values regarding psychotherapy.

PSYCHOLOGICAL AND SOCIAL TREATMENTS

According to Wilson, Grilo, and Vitousek's (2007) review, it appears that ED treatments with the highest level of efficacy involve a cognitive behavioral component whether administered through family therapy, individual, or self-directed approaches. Tong et al. (2005) reported on five case studies of males in China with EDs and described CBT and family therapy as being successful with three of the five cases, dramatically improving the symptoms of one in particular. However, they did not go into detail as to how the treatment modalities were adapted to work with the Chinese patients. Some have recognized the individualistic nature of CBT interventions and recommended modification keeping a more collectivistic approach in mind with Asian populations (Sue & Sue, 2003). To investigate this, Wong et al. (2003) examined how culturally based variables (ethnic identity, white identity, values, self construal, and mental health beliefs) impacted 136 Asian American college students' perceptions of therapy credibility for both cognitive therapy (CT) and time-limited psychodynamic therapy (TLDP) for depression. Two of the factors, ethnic identity and self-construal (independence vs. interdependence), were found to have significant interactions with the treatment variables. While participants with low levels of white identity found the CT approach more credible than TLDP, those with high levels of white identity did not rate the approaches differently. Additionally, those who endorsed a greater self-construal as independent found CT more credible than TLDP; there was no difference for less-independent participants. This study highlights the importance of taking cultural considerations to a deeper level of understanding by examining what Asian or Asian American culturally based factors might contribute to treatment compliance, success, or failure. It also alludes to how a cognitive therapy like CBT might be more easily accepted by Asian and Asian American patients who view themselves as more independent but less white-identified. However, it is important to note that this study evaluated the credibility of a CBT treatment for depression; future research might better elucidate how cultural factors could impact the use of CBT for the treatment of eating disorders in Asian populations.

The Maudsley model (Lock et al., 2001; Dare & Eisler, 1997) is one of the best researched treatments for AN as well as BN. This structured, family-focused model is likely to be well adapted to working with patients from collectivistic cultures. The method could prove to be quite useful in working with young adult patients in college situations, or even married individuals, by employing the support of partners, friends, and children to help the patient in the same role as the parents would take from the initial model. Collective societal values brought to the treatment by Asian families might also work to improve the efficacy of such therapy, though little to no research has been conducted to assess this. Because the Maudsley model implements a structured format, there is less of a focus on deep-seated family dynamics that might be shameful or difficult to talk about, though these are addressed at a surface level later in the treatment. Narrative and attachment oriented therapies (e.g., Dallos, 2004) are likely to be difficult for Asian patients, as families might be less willing to explore maladaptive family narratives outside of the family home. A multiple family therapy model (e.g., Scholz & Asen, 2001) may prove useful for Asian families in that it allows them to receive support from one another and other families. However, conflict with the value of saving face may prevent many Asian families from participating in this type of treatment.

GENERAL TREATMENT CONSIDERATIONS

A few studies (i.e., Leong, 1986, Wong et al., 2003) have examined factors to consider regarding general psychotherapeutic treatment with Asians and Asian Americans. First, consider the patient, his or her family's understanding of psychotherapy, and what specific cultural values might be inherently contradicted through the process (e.g., saving face). Additionally, treatment clinics can be better equipped to be more sensitive to language and specific cultural differences by including clinicians from a variety of Asian cultures on their treatment teams. Clinicians from a non-Asian ethnic background as well as those from dissimilar Asian backgrounds than their patients can work to become more aware of biases and stereotypes that they hold which may interfere with the process of therapy (Leong, 1986). Also, having a better understanding of Asian ethnic identity development could improve one's awareness of cultural conflicts in treatment. Atkinson, Morten, and Sue (1979) offer a comprehensive stage model for understanding ethnic identity development in Asian Americans and internal and external conflicts that might arise as a result of transition through developmental stages.

Cummins and Lehman (2007) discuss a conceptual framework through which a clinician can conceptualize working with Asian patients with EDs. This Cultural and Social Environmental (CASE) model (Hong & Ham, 2001) suggests two dimensions that may be useful when strategizing how to treat Asian Americans with EDs in a culturally responsive manner. The first factor, cultural context, emphasizes the need to consider the worldview and value orientation of the client. This consists of the client's cultural identification and its manifestations; for instance, collectivism versus individualism is often highlighted as an important aspect for clinicians to assess. This value orientation can be manifested in many ways with regard to disordered eating symptoms in Asian Americans. For example, for some, the balancing act between the collectivistic beliefs of their family of origin and the individualistic ideals they are expected to uphold in their social environ-ments can prove difficult to manage, and these conflicts may be manifested in the eating and body image attitudes that the individual expresses. Taking special care to attend to possible cultural and familial influences on the developmental aspect of negative body image may also include consider-ing locus of control issues within the family dynamic, another value orientation that can be cultur-ally based. Kempa and Thomas (2000) suggest that "the model minority" label might also be an element of Asian worldview that would be important to consider in treatment. Acknowledging perfectionistic tendencies and normalizing "good enough" success-oriented strategies could also be useful interventions.

The second dimension in the CASE model is the social environmental context. Many researchers have written about the possible impact of gender roles and gender discrimination in the development of EDs (e.g., Smolak & Murnen, 2001). Racial/ethnic differences and discrimi-nation may also be important factors for ethnic minority women in the etiology of problematic eating behaviors and attitudes (Smolak & Striegel-Moore, 2001). Just as women are particularly subject to physical objectification and a thin body ideal, ethnic minority women must addition-ally contend with that ideal most often being presented in the form of more typically Caucasian facial features and body types (Hall, 1995; Root, 1990). It is important for clinicians to keep in mind that exposure to these ideals, and the external and internal racism that can result, are woven throughout the social environmental context for Asian American women with eating concerns. Gilbert (2003) suggests that certain CBT restructuring and challenging interventions might be useful at treating negative self-schemas and irrational belief systems created by cultural standards of beauty stereotypes.

In addition, as racial differences are most clearly identified through physical appearance, racialized features and an individual's perceptions of these could be important factors to con-sider when treating EDs. In their comprehensive review, C. Lee and Zhan (1998) cite several studies that found young Asian Americans to score significantly lower than Caucasian or African American youths on measures of physical self-esteem. Phinney (1989) discovered that across other minority ethnic groups (including Hispanic and African American), Asian American youths were found to be most dissatisfied with their physical appearance and were more likely to desire Caucasian physical features if allowed the opportunity. Thus, the question of level of internalized racism is an important area of exploration related to Asian American women's per-ceptions of their physical appearances. These factors, along with other environmental stressors that may be particular to Asian Americans, should be addressed when modifying therapeutic interventions to be more culturally appropriate for this population. Positive coping strategies for dealing with internalized racism and external oppression would also be useful treatment inter-ventions (Kempa & Thomas, 2000).

Harris and Kuba (1997) offer an intriguing blend of feminist, psychodynamic, and behav-ioral therapies for EDs and suggest four necessary components to successful treatment of EDs in women of color: medical management of symptoms, integration of life span influences for identity development (e.g., adolescent pressures), recognition of ethnic identity conflicts, and respect for the patient's community and culture. They also give helpful suggestions for using one's under-standing of ethnic identity developmental stages to inform symptom presentation and targeting in treatment. For example, someone at the encounter or dissonance stage of identity development might present with purging symptoms as an expression of the conflict she experiences between the two cultures. The researchers suggest implementing some grief work around the loss of one or both of her ethnic identities (i.e., Asian vs. American) as a means to alleviate symptoms.

PREVENTION

Unfortunately, most individuals with eating disorders never receive treatment and, even for those that do, relapse is quite common. In particular, Asians who display disordered eating behaviors are often not referred for further evaluation (Franko et al., 2007). As a result, researchers have turned to the development of prevention programs with the hopes of intervening earlier in the development of the risk factors (e.g., body dissatisfaction, dieting) that often lead to diagnosable eating disorders (Stice & Hoffman, 2004). In general, research suggests that prevention programs can be successful not only at reducing risk factors for eating pathology but also at lowering current rates and preventing future increases in rates of disordered eating symptoms (Stice & Hoffman, 2004). Unfortunately, the research is significantly lacking regarding prevention programs specifically focused toward Asian and Asian American populations. A few researchers have suggested that focusing on ethnic identity as a strength (Warren et al., 2005) and particularly, the value of interdependence, as being a possible protective factor against the development of EDs (Tomiyama & Mann, 2008). One study examined a prevention program focusing on the use of cognitive dissonance to combat thin ideal internalization, body image disturbance, and ED symptoms across three different ethnic groups (Rodriguez et al., 2008). Findings indicated improvement across all targeted areas of focus for all ethnic groups with no significant differences between groups. This demonstrates a hopeful area for future study with regard to prevention and treatment of EDs in diverse ethnic populations.

FUTURE RESEARCH

Culturally sensitive assessment and treatment are integral to success in combating EDs. Given the substantial lack of research focusing on treatment in non-Caucasian populations, a number of research areas could prove useful at informing the literature. It would be useful to see how specific psychotherapy interventions fare among the different Asian populations. The examination of cultural context in treatment is also a necessary area of study. Wong et al. (2003) suggested that specific cultural factors be broken down by how they impact patients' feelings about treatment modalities and style. Additionally, a number of researchers (i.e., Gilbert, 2003; Harris & Kuba, 1997; Kempa & Thomas, 2000) have suggested the need to examine how acculturation, ethnic identity development, internalized oppression, and perfectionism impact ED behaviors in Asians and Asian Americans. Gilbert (2003) also emphasizes the importance of specifying ethnic identity labels (e.g., Asian vs. Asian American vs. Japanese American) and what they mean to participants in creating sample populations so that an accurate representation of different people's experiences can be achieved. Given our current lack of knowledge about the treatment of EDs in general and the growing incidence of EDs worldwide, such explorations of the cultural aspects of ED treatment with more diverse populations are of vital importance.

REFERENCES

Agras, W. S., & Apple, R. F. (2002). Understanding and treating eating disorders. In F. W. Kaslow & T. Patterson (Eds.), *Comprehensive handbook of psychotherapy: Cognitive-behavioral approaches* (pp. 189–212). Hoboken, NJ: Wiley.

Agras, W. S., Rossiter, E. M., & Arnow, B. (1994). One-year follow-up of psychosocial and pharmacologic treatments for bulimia nervosa. *Journal of Clinical Psychiatry, 55,* 5, 179–183.

Agras, W. S., Walsh, B. T., Fairburn, C. G., Wilson, G. T., & Kraemer, H. C. (2000). A multicenter comparison of cognitive behavioral therapy and interpersonal therapy for bulimia nervosa. *Archives of General Psychiatry, 57,* 459–466.

American Psychiatric Association (APA). (1980). *Diagnostic and statistical manual of mental disorders* (3rd ed.). Washington, DC: Author.

American Psychiatric Association. (1987). *Diagnostic and statistical manual of mental disorders* (3rd rev. ed.). Washington, DC: Author.

American Psychiatric Association. (1994). *Diagnostic and statistical manual of mental disorders* (4th ed.). Washington, DC: Author.

American Psychiatric Association. (2000). *Diagnostic and statistical manual of mental disorders* (4th ed., text rev.). Washington, DC: Author.

Appolinario, J. C., Bacaltchuk, J., Sichieri, R., Claudino, A. M., Gody-Matos, A., Morgan, C., et al. (2003). A randomized, double-blind, placebo-controlled study of sibutramine in the treatment of binge eating disorder. *Archives of General Psychiatry, 60,* 1109–1116.

Arnold, L., McElroy, S., Hudson, J., Welge, J., Bennett, A., & Keck, P. (2002). A placebo controlled, randomized trial of fluoxetine in the treatment of binge eating disorder. *Journal of Clinical Psychiatry, 63*(11), 1028–1033.

Atkinson, D. R., Morten, G., & Sue, D. W. (1979). *Counseling American minorities: A cross-cultural perspective.* Dubuque, IA: Brown.

Attia, E., Haiman, C., Walsh, B., & Flater, S. (1998). Does fluoxetine augment the inpatient treatment of anorexia nervosa? *American Journal of Psychiatry, 155*(4), 548–551.

Attia, E., & Schroeder, L. (2005). Pharmacologic treatment of anorexia nervosa: Where do we go from here? *International Journal of Eating Disorders, 37,* S60–S63.

Bachar, E., Latzer, Y., Kreitler, S., & Berry, E. M. (1999). The contributions of self psychology to the treatment of anorexia and bulimia. *Journal of Psychotherapy Practice and Research, 8,*115–128.

Bailer, U., de Zwaan, M., Leisch, F., Strnad, A., Lennkh-Wolfsberg, C., El-Giamal, N., et al. (2004). Guided self-help versus cognitive-behavioral group therapy in the treatment of bulimia nervosa. *International Journal of Eating Disorders, 35*(4), 522–537.

Bailey, C. A. (1991). Family structure and eating disorders: The Family Environment Scale and bulimic-like symptoms. *Youth and Society, 23,* 2, 251–272.

Ball, J., & Mitchell, P. (2004). A randomized controlled study of cognitive behavior therapy and behavioral family therapy for anorexia nervosa patients. *Eating Disorders, 12*(4), 303–314.

Banasiak, S., Paxton, S., & Hay, P. (2007). Perceptions of cognitive behavioural guided self-help treatment for bulimia nervosa in primary care. *Eating Disorders, 15*(1), 23–40.

Bartky, S. L. (1990). *Femininity and domination: Studies in the phenomenology of oppression.* New York: Routledge.

Barbarich, N. C., McConaha, C. W., Halmi, K. A., Gendall, K. A., Sunday, S. R., & Gaskill, J. (2004). Use of nutritional supplements to increase the efficacy of fluoxetine in the treatment of anorexia nervosa. *International Journal of Eating Disorders, 35*(1), 10–15.

Barbarich-Marsteller, N. C., & Marx, R. (2007). What is neuroimaging and how can it be used to improve the treatment of eating disorders? *Eating Disorders, 15,* 273–275.

Becker, A. E., Burwell, R. A., Herzog, D. B., Hamburg, P., & Gilman, S. E. (2002). Eating behaviours and attitudes following prolonged exposure to television among ethnic Fijian adolescent girls. *British Journal of Psychiatry, 180,* 509–514.

Becker, A. E., Franko, D. L., Speck, A, & Herzog, D. B. (2003). Ethnicity and differential access to care for eating disorder symptoms. *International Journal of Eating Disorders, 33,* 205–212.

Becker, B., Bell, M., & Billington, R. (1987). Object relations ego deficits in bulimic women. *Journal of Clinical Psychology, 43, 1,* 92–95.

Bemporad, J. R. (1996). Self-starvation through the ages: Reflections on the pre-history of anorexia nervosa. *International Journal of Eating Disorders, 19, 3,* 217–237.

Bergner, M., Remer, P., & Whetsell, C. (1985). Transforming women's body image: A feminist counseling approach. *Women and Therapy, 4,* 25–38.

Beumont, P. J., Russel, J. D., Touyz, S. W., Buckley, C., Lowinger, K., Talbot, P. et al. (1997). Intensive nutritional counseling in bulimia nervosa: A role for supplementation with fluoxetine. *Australian and New Zealand Journal of Psychiatry, 31,* 514–524.

Birmingham, C., Goldner, E., & Bakan, R. (2004). Controlled trial of zinc supplementation in anorexia nervosa. *International Journal of Eating Disorders, 15,* 251–255.

Bordo, S. (1993). Unbearable weight: Feminism, western culture, and the body. Berkeley: University of California Press.

Bowlby, J. (1973). *Attachment and loss: Volume 1. Separation: Anxiety and anger.* New York: Basic Books.

Bowlby, J. (1988). *A secure base: Parent-child attachment and healthy human development.* New York: Basic Books.

Brownmiller, S. (1984). *Femininity.* New York: Linden.

Bruch, H. (1973). Eating disorders: Obesity, anorexia nervosa, and the person within. New York: Basic Books.

Bruch, H. (1978). *The golden cage: The enigma of anorexia nervosa.* Cambridge, MA: Harvard University Press.

Bulik, C. M. (2004). Genetic and biological risk factors. In J. K. Thompson (Ed.), *Handbook of eating disorders and obesity* (pp. 3–16). Hoboken, NJ: Wiley.

Bulik, C. M., Berkman, N. D., Brownley, K. A., Sedway, J. A., & Lohr, K. N. (2007). Anorexia nervosa treatment: A systematic review of randomized controlled trials. *International Journal of Eating Disorders, 40*(4), 310–320.

Cachelin, F. M, Rebeck, R. Veisel, C., & Striegel-Moore, R. H. (2001). Barriers to treatment for eating disorders among ethnically diverse women. *Eating Disorders, 30,* 269–278.

Cachelin, F. M., Veisel, C., Barzegarnazari, E., & Striegel-Moore, R. H. (2000). Disordered eating, acculturation, and treatment-seeking in a community sample of Hispanic, Asian, black, and white women. *Psychology of Women Quarterly, 24,* 244–253.

Carter, F., McIntosh, V., Joyce, P., Sullivan, P., & Bulik, C. (2003). Role of exposure with response prevention in cognitive-behavioral therapy for bulimia nervosa: Three-year follow-up results. *International Journal of Eating Disorders, 33*(2), 127–135.

Cash, T. F., Winstead, B. A., & Janda, L. H. (1986). The great American shape-up. *Psychology Today, 20, 4,* 30–37.

Chavez, M., & Insel, T. R. (2007). Eating disorders: National Institute of Mental Health perspective. *American Psychologist, 62* (3), 159–166.

Chen, C., Wong, J., Lee, N., Chan-Ho, M., Lau, J. T., & Fung, M. (1993). The Shatin community mental health survey in Hong Kong. *Archives of General Psychiatry, 50,* 125–133.

Chen, E., Touyz, S., Beumont, P., Fairburn, C., Griffiths, R., Butow, P., et al. (2003). Comparison of group and individual cognitive-behavioral therapy for patients with bulimia nervosa. *International Journal of Eating Disorders, 33*(3), 241–254.

Chiu, L. H. (1987). Child-rearing attitudes of Chinese, Chinese-American, and Anglo-American mothers. *International Journal of Psychology, 22,* 409–419.

Chun, Z. F., Mitchell, J. E., Li, K., Yu, W. M., Lan, Y. D., Jun, Z., et al. (1992). The prevalence of anorexia nervosa and bulimia nervosa among freshman medical college students in China. *International Journal of Eating Disorders, 12,* 209–214.

Costin, C. (1999). *The eating disorder sourcebook: A comprehensive guide to the causes, treatments, and prevention of eating disorders.* Los Angeles: Lowell House.

Crago, M., Shisslak, C. M., & Estes, L. S. (1996). Eating disturbances among American minority groups: A review. *International Journal of Eating Disorders, 19,* 239–248.

Cummins, L. H., & Lehman, J. D. (2007). Eating disorders and body image concerns in Asian American women: Assessment and treatment from a multicultural and feminist perspective. *Eating Disorders, 15,* 217–230.

Cummins, L. H., Simmons, A. M., & Zane, N. W. S. (2005). Eating disorders in Asian populations: A critique of current approaches to the study of culture, ethnicity, and eating disorders. *American Journal of Orthopsychiatry, 75*, 553–574.

Dallos, R. (2004). Attachment narrative therapy: Integrating ideas from narrative and attachment theory in systemic family therapy with eating disorders. *Journal of Family Therapy, 26*, 40–65.

Dare, C., & Crowther, C. (1995). Psychodynamic model of eating disorders. In G. I. Szmukler, C. Dare, & J. Treasure (Eds.), *Handbook of eating disorders: theory, treatment and research* (pp. 125–139). New York: Wiley.

Dare, C., & Eisler, I. (1997). Family therapy for anorexia nervosa. In D. Garner & P. D. Garfinkel (Eds.), *Handbook of treatment for eating disorders* (2nd ed., pp. 333–349). Chichester, England: Wiley.

Davis, C., & Katzman, M. A. (1998). Chinese men and women in the United States and Hong Kong: Body and self-esteem ratings as a prelude to dieting and exercise. *International Journal of Eating Disorders, 23*, 99–102.

Davis, C., & Yager, J. (1992). Transcultural aspects of eating disorders: A critical literature review. *Culture, Medicine, and Psychiatry, 16*, 377–394.

De Silva, P. (1995). Cognitive-behavioural models of eating disorders. In G. I. Szmukler, C. Dare, & J. Treasure (Eds.), *Handbook of eating disorders: theory, treatment and research* (pp. 141–153), New York: Wiley.

De Zwaan, M. (2003). Basic neuroscience and scanning. In J. Treasure, U. Schmidt, & E. van Furth (Eds.), *Handbook of eating disorders* (2nd ed., pp. 89–102). West Sussex, England: Wiley.

Delinsky, S., & Wilson, G. (2006). Mirror exposure for the treatment of body image disturbance. *International Journal of Eating Disorders, 39*(2), 108–116.

Dolan, B. (1991). Cross-cultural aspects of anorexia nervosa and bulimia: A review. *International Journal of Eating Disorders, 10*, 67–78.

Edman, J., & Yates, A. (2004). Eating attitudes among college students in Malaysia: An ethnic and gender comparison. *European Eating Disorders Review, 12*, 190–196.

Eggert, J., Levendosky, A., & Klump, K. (2007). Relationships among attachment styles, personality characteristics, and disordered eating. *International Journal of Eating Disorders, 40*, 149–155.

Eisler, I., Dare, C., Russell, G. F. M., Szmukler, G., le Grange, D., & Dodge, E. (1997). Family and individual therapy in anorexia nervosa: A 5-year follow-up. *Archives of General Psychiatry, 54*, 1025–1030.

Eisler, I., Simic, M., Russell, G., & Dare, C. (2007). A randomised controlled treatment trial of two forms of family therapy in adolescent anorexia nervosa: A five-year follow-up. *Journal of Child Psychology and Psychiatry, and Allied Disciplines, 48*(6), 552–560.

Fairburn, C. G. (1995). *Overcoming binge eating.* New York: Guilford.

Fairburn, C. G. (1997). Eating disorders. In D. M. Clark and C. G. Fairburn (Eds.), *Science and practice of cognitive behaviour therapy* (pp. 209–241). Oxford: Oxford University Press.

Fairburn, C. G., & Beglin, S. J. (1990). Studies of the epidemiology of bulimia nervosa. *American Journal of Psychiatry, 147*, 401–408.

Fairburn, C. G., & Brownell, K. D. (2002). *Eating disorders and obesity: A comprehensive handbook.* New York: Guilford.

Fairburn, C., Cooper, Z., & Shafran, R. (2003). Cognitive behaviour therapy for eating disorders: a "transdiagnostic" theory and treatment. *Behaviour Research and Therapy, 41*(5), 509.

Fairburn, C., Jones, R., Peveler, R., & Hope, R. (1993). Psychotherapy and bulimia nervosa: Longer-term effects of interpersonal psychotherapy, behavior therapy, and cognitive behavior therapy. *Archives of General Psychiatry, 50*(6), 419–428.

Fairburn, C. G., Marcus, M. D., & Wilson, G. T. (1993). Cognitive-behavioral therapy for binge eating and bulimia nervosa: A comprehensive treatment manual. In C. G. Fairburn, & G. T. Wilson (Eds.), *Binge eating: Nature, assessment and treatment* (pp. 361–404). New York: Guilford.

Fairburn, C., & Walsh, B. T. (2002). Atypical eating disorders (eating disorder not otherwise specified). In C. G. Fairburn & K. D. Brownell (Eds.), *Eating disorders and obesity: A comprehensive handbook* (2nd ed., pp. 171–177). New York: Guilford.

Feighner, J. P., Robins, E., Guze, S. B., Woodruff, R. A., Jr., Winokur, G., & Munoz, R. (1972). Diagnostic criteria for use in psychiatric research. *Archives of General Psychiatry, 26*, 57–63.

Frank, M. (1999). Raising daughters to resist negative cultural messages about body image. *Women and Therapy, 22*, 88.

Franko, D. L., Becker, A. E., Thomas, J. J., & Herzog, D. B. (2007). Cross-ethnic differences in eating disorder symptoms and related distress. *International Journal of Eating Disorders, 40*, 156–164.

Franko, D. L., & Striegel-Moore, R. H. (2002). The role of body dissatisfaction as a risk factor for depression in adolescent girls: Are the differences black and white? *Journal of Psychosomatic Research, 53, 5*, 975–983.

Franko, D. L., Wonderlich, S. A., Little, D., & Herzog, D. B. (2004). Diagnosis and classification of eating disorders. In J. K. Thompson (Ed.), *Handbook of eating disorders and obesity* (pp. 58–80). Hoboken, NJ: Wiley.

Fredrickson, B. L., & Roberts, T. (1997). Objectification theory: Toward understanding women's lived experiences and mental health risks. *Psychology of Women Quarterly, 21*, 173–206.

Garfinkel, P. E. (1983). A comparison of characteristics in the families of patients with anorexia nervosa and normal controls. *Psychological Medicine, 13, 4*, 821–828.

Garner, D. M., & Bemis, K. M. (1985). Cognitive therapy for anorexia nervosa. In D. M. Garner and P. E. Garfinkel (Eds.), *Handbook of psychotherapy for anorexia nervosa and bulimia* (pp. 123–150). New York: Guilford.

Garner, D. M., Garfinkel, P. E., Schwartz, D. T., & Thompson, M. (1980). Cultural expectations of thinness in women. *Psychological Reports, 47*(2), 483–491.

Garner, D. M., & Needleman, L. D. (1997). Sequencing and integration of treatments. In D. M. Garner & D. E. Garfinkel (Eds.), *Handbook of treatment for eating disorders* (2nd ed., pp. 50–63). New York: Guilford.

Garner, D. M., Rockert, W., Davis, R., Garner, M. V., Olmsted, M., & Eagle, M. (1993). Comparison of cognitive-behavioral and supportive-expressive therapy for bulimia nervosa. *American Journal of Psychiatry, 150*, 37–46.

Garner, D., Vitousek, K., & Pike, K. (1997). Cognitive-behavioral therapy for anorexia nervosa. In D. M. Garner & P. E. Garfinkel (Eds.), *Handbook of treatment for eating disorders* (2nd ed., pp. 94–144). New York: Guilford.

Gilbert, S. C. (2003). Eating disorders in women of color. *Clinical Psychology Scientific Practice, 10*, 444–455.

Goldstein, D., Wilson, M., Thompson, V., & Potvin, J. (1995). Long-term fluoxetine treatment of bulimia nervosa. *British Journal of Psychiatry, 166*(5), 660–666.

Gordon, R. A. (2000). Eating disorders: Anatomy of a social epidemic. New York: Blackwell.

Gordon, R. A. (2001). Eating disorders east and west: A culture-bound syndrome unbound. In M. Nasser, M. Katzman, & R. A. Gordon (Eds.), *Eating disorders and cultures in transition* (pp. 2–16). New York: Taylor & Francis.

Gordon, K. H., Perez, M., & Joiner Jr., T. E. (2002). The impact of racial stereotypes on eating disorder recognition. *International Journal of Eating Disorders, 32*, 219–224.

Grilo, C. M. (2007). Guided self-help for binge eating disorder. In J. Latner & G. T. Wilson (Eds.), *Self-help for obesity and binge eating.* New York: Guilford.

Grilo, C., & Masheb, R. (2005). A randomized controlled comparison of guided self-help cognitive behavioral therapy and behavioral weight loss for binge eating disorder. *Behaviour Research and Therapy, 43*(11), 1509–1525.

Gross, J., & Rosen, J. C. (1988). Bulimia in adolescents: Prevalence and psychosocial correlates. *International Journal of Eating Disorders, 7*, 51–61.

Grossmann, K. E., & Grossman, K. (1990). The wider concept of attachment in cross-cultural research. *Human Development, 33, 2*, 31–47.

Hall, C. C. I. (1995). Asian eyes: Body image and eating disorders of Asian and Asian American women. *Eating Disorders, 3*, 8–19.

Halmi, K., Agras, W., Crow, S., Mitchell, J., Wilson, G., Bryson, S., et al. (2005). Predictors of treatment acceptance and completion in anorexia nervosa: Implications for future study designs. *Archives of General Psychiatry, 62*(7), 776–781.

Halmi, K. A., Eckert, E. D., LaDu, T. J., & Cohen, J. (1986). Anorexia nervosa: Treatment efficacy of cyproheptadine and amitriptyline. *Archives of General Psychiatry, 49*, 177–181.

Harris, D. J., & Kuba, S. A. (1997). Ethnocultural identity and eating disorders in women of color. *Professional Psychology: Research and Practice, 28* (4), 341–347.

Haudek, C., Rorty, M., & Henker, B. (1999). The role of ethnicity and parental bonding in the eating and weight concerns of Asian-American and Caucasian college women. *International Journal of Eating Disorders, 25, 4,* 425–433.

Hayes, S. C. (2004). Acceptance and commitment therapy and the new behavior therapies: Mindfulness, acceptance, and relationship. In S. C. Hayes, V. M. Follette, & M. Linehan (Eds.), *Acceptance, mindfulness, and behavior change* (pp. 1–29). New York: Guilford.

Heesacker, R. S., & Neimeyer, G. J. (1990). Assessing object relations and social cognitive correlates of eating disorder. *Journal of Counseling Psychology, 37,* 419–426.

Herzog, D. B., & Delinsky, S. S. (2001). Classification of eating disorders. In R. H. Striegel-Moore & L. Smolak (Eds.), *Eating disorders: Innovative directions for research and practice* (pp. 31–50). Washington, DC: American Psychological Association.

Herzog, D. B., Hopkins, J. D., & Burns, C. D. (1993). A follow-up study of 33 subdiagnostic eating disordered women. *International Journal of Eating Disorders, 14,* 261–267.

Hilbert, A., & Tuschen-Caffier, B. (2004). Body image interventions in cognitive-behavioural therapy of binge-eating disorder: A component analysis. *Behaviour Research and Therapy, 42*(11), 1325–1339.

Hill, K., Bucuvalas, J., McClain, C., Kryscio, R., Martini, R., Alfaro, M., et al. (2000). Pilot study of growth hormone administration during the refeeding of malnourished anorexia nervosa patients. *Journal of Child and Adolescent Psychopharmacology, 10*(1), 3–8.

Hoek, H. W., & van Hoeken, D. (2003). Review of prevalence and incidence of eating disorders. *International Journal of Eating Disorders, 34,* 383–396.

Hong, G. K., & Ham, M. D. (2001). *Psychotherapy and counseling with Asian American clients: A practical guide.* Thousand Oaks, CA: Sage.

Hsu, L. K. G. (1996). Epidemiology of the eating disorders. *Psychiatric Clinics of North America, 19,* 681–700.

Hsu, L. K. G., & Lee, S. (1993). Is weight phobia always necessary for a diagnosis of anorexia nervosa? *American Journal of Psychiatry, 150,* 1466–1471.

Hudson, J. I., Hiripi, E., Pope, H. G., & Kessler, R. (2007). The prevalence and correlates of eating disorders in the national comorbidity survey replication. *Biological Psychiatry, 61*(3), 348–358.

Hudson, J., McElroy, S., Raymond, N., Crow, S., Keck, P., Carter, W., et al. (1998). Fluvoxamine in the treatment of binge-eating disorder: A multicenter placebo-controlled, double-blind trial. *American Journal of Psychiatry, 155*(12), 1756–1762.

Humphrey, L. L., & Stern, S. (1988). Object relations and the family system in bulimia: A theoretical integration. *Journal of Marital and Family Therapy, 14,* 337–350.

Huon, G. F., Mingyi, Q., & Oliver, K. (2002). A large-scale survey of eating disorder symptomatology among female adolescents in the People's Republic of China. *International Journal of Eating Disorders, 32,* 192–205.

Huon, G. F., Walton, C. J., & Lim, J. (1999). Dieting among adolescent girls in Beijing. *Eating Disorders, 7, 4,* 271–278.

Ishikawa, K. (1984). Eating disorder and fathering [in Japanese]. *Kikan Seishin Ryoho, 10,* 143–148.

Ishikawa, K., Iwata, Y., & Hirano, G. (1960). Studies on the symptoms and the pathogenesis of anorexia nervosa [in Japanese with English abstract]. *Japanese Journal of Psychiatry and Neurology, 62,* 1203–1221.

Jackson, L. A., Sullivan, L. A., & Rostker, R. (1988). Gender, gender role, and body image. *Sex Roles, 19*(7–8), 429–443.

Jennings, P. S. Forbes, D., McDermott, B., Juniper, S., & Hulse, G. (2006). Acculturation and eating disorders in Asian and Caucasian Australian adolescents. *Psychiatry and Clinical Neurosciences, 59,* 56–61.

Johnson, C., Lewis, C., Love, S., Lewis, L., & Stuckey, M. (1984). Incidence and correlates of bulimic behavior in a female high school population. *Journal of Youth and Adolescence, 13,* 15–26.

Jung, J., & Forbes, G. B. (2007). Body dissatisfaction and disordered eating among college women in China, South Korea, and the United States: Contrasting predictions from sociocultural and feminist theories. *Psychology of Women Quarterly, 31*(4), 381–393.

Katzman, M. A., & Lee, S. (1997). Beyond body image: The integration of feminist and transcultural theories in the understanding of self starvation. *International Journal of Eating Disorders, 22, 4,* 385–394.

Keel, P. K., & Herzog, D. B. (2004). Long-term outcome, course of illness, and mortality in anorexia nervosa, bulimia nervosa, and binge eating disorder. In T. D. Brewerton (Ed.), *Clinical handbook of eating disorders: an integrated approach* (pp. 97–116). New York: Dekker.

Keel, P. K., & Klump, K. L. (2003). Are eating disorders culture-bound syndromes? Implications for conceptualizing their etiology. *Psychological Bulletin, 129,* 747–769.

Keel, P. K., & Mitchell, J. E. (1997). Outcome in bulimia nervosa. *American Journal of Psychiatry, 154,* 313–321.

Kempa, M. L., & Thomas, A. J. (2000). Culturally sensitive assessment and treatment of eating disorders. *Eating Disorders, 8,* 17–30.

Kennedy, A., Templeton, L., Gandhi, A., & Gorzalka, B. (2004). Asian body image satisfaction: Ethnic and gender differences across Chinese, Indo-Asian, and European-descent students. *International Journal of Eating Disorders, 12,* 321–336.

Kenny, M. E., & Hart, K. (1992). Relationship between parental attachment and eating disorders in an inpatient and a college sample. *Journal of Counseling Psychology, 39,* 521–526.

King, M. B. (1993). Cultural aspects of eating disorders. *International Review of Psychiatry, 5,* 205–216.

Kiriike, N., Nagata, T., Tanaka, M., Nishiwaki, S., Takeuchi, N., & Kawakita, Y. (1988). Prevalence of binge-eating and bulimia among adolescent women in Japan. *Psychiatry Research, 26,* 163–169.

Klibanski, A., Biller, B. M, Schoenfeld, D. A. Herzog, D. B., & Saxe, V. C. (1995). The effects of estrogen administration on trabecular bone loss in young women with anorexia nervosa. *Journal of Clinical Endocrinology and Metabolism, 80,* 898–904.

Klump, K. L., & Culbert, K. M. (2007). Molecular genetic studies of eating disorders: Current status and future directions. *Current Directions in Psychological Science, 16,* 37–41.

Ko, C., & Cohen, H. (1998). Intraethnic comparison of eating attitudes in Native Koreans and Korean Americans using a Korean translation of the Eating Attitudes Test. *Journal of Nervous and Mental Disease, 186,* 10, 631–636.

Koide, R., & Hasegawa, M. (1992). Fantasies of being in a desperate situation as a source of conflict in eating disorders [in Japanese with English abstract]. *Shinsin Igaka, 32,* 471–478.

Kok, L. P., & Tian, C. S. (1994). Susceptibility of Singapore Chinese schoolgirls to anorexia nervosa—Part I (Psychological factors). *Singapore Medical Journal, 35,* 481–485.

Krueger, D. (1990). Developmental and psychodynamic perspectives on body-image change. In Cash, T. F. & Pruzinsky, T. (Eds.), *Body images: Development, deviance, and change* (pp. 255–271). New York: Guilford.

Kuboki, T., Nomura, S., Ide, M., Suematsu, H., & Araki, S. (1996). Epidemiological data on anorexia nervosa in Japan. *Psychiatry Research, 62,* 11–16.

Kwak, K. (2003). Adolescents and their parents: A review of intergenerational family relations of immigrant and non-immigrant families. *Human Development, 46,* 2–3, 15–136.

Lai, K. Y. (2000). Anorexia nervosa in Chinese adolescents: Does culture make a difference? *Journal of Adolescence, 23,* 561–568.

Lee, A. M., & Lee, S. (1996). Disordered eating and its psychosocial correlates among Chinese adolescent females in Hong Kong. *International Journal of Eating Disorders, 20,* 177–183.

Lee, C., & Zhan, G. (1998). Psychosocial status of children and youths. In L. C. Lee & N. W. S. Zane (Eds.), *Handbook of Asian American psychology.* Thousand Oaks, CA: Sage.

Lee, S. (1991). Anorexia nervosa in Hong Kong: A Chinese perspective. *Psychological Medicine, 21,* 3, 703–711.

Lee, S. (1993a). Fat phobic and non-fat phobic anorexia nervosa: A comparative study of 70 Chinese patients in Hong Kong. *Psychological Medicine, 23,* 999–1017.

Lee, S. (1993b). How abnormal is the desire for slimness? A survey of eating attitudes and behaviour among Chinese undergraduates in Hong Kong. *Psychological Medicine, 23,* 437–451.

Lee, S. (1995). Self-starvation in context: Towards a culturally sensitive understanding of anorexia nervosa. *Social Science and Medicine, 41*(1), 25–36.

Lee, S. (1998). Global modernity and eating disorders in Asia. *European Eating Disorders Review, 6*(3), 151–153.

Lee, S. (2001). Fat phobia in anorexia nervosa: Whose obsession is it? In M. Nasser, M. Katzman, & R. Gordon (Eds.), *Eating disorders and cultures in transition* (pp. 40–54). New York: Taylor & Francis.

Lee, S., Hsu, L. K., & Wing, Y. K. (1992). Bulimia nervosa in Hong Kong Chinese patients. *British Journal of Psychiatry, 161,* 545–551.

Lee, S., & Lee, A. M. (2000). Disordered eating in three communities of China: A comparative study of female high school students in Hong Kong, Shenzhen, and rural Hunan. *International Journal of Eating Disorders, 27, 3,* 317–327.

le Grange, D., Lock, J., & Dymek, M. (2003). Family-based therapy for adolescents with bulimia nervosa. *American Journal of Psychotherapy, 57*(2), 237–251.

le Grange, D., Stone, A. A., & Brownell, K. D. (1998). Eating disturbances in white and minority female dieters. *International Journal of Eating Disorders, 24,* 395–403.

Leong, F. T. (1986). Counseling and psychotherapy with Asian Americans: Review of the Literature. *Journal of Counseling Psychology, 33*(2), 196–206.

Linehan, M. (1993). *Skills training manual for treating borderline personality disorder.* New York: Guilford.

Littlewood, R. (1995). Psychopathology and personal agency: Modernity, culture change, and eating disorders in South Asian societies. *British Journal of Medical Psychology, 68*(1), 45–63.

Lock, J., le Grange, D., Agras, W. S., & Dare, C. (2001). *Treatment manual for anorexia nervosa: A family-based approach.* New York: Guilford.

Masterson, J. (1977). Primary anorexia nervosa. In P. Haitocollis (Ed.), *Borderline personality disorder* (pp. 475–494). New York: International University Press.

McCarthy, A. M. (1998). Paternal characteristics associated with disturbed father-daughter attachment and separation among women with eating disorder symptoms. *Dissertation Abstracts International, 59,* 1861.

McElroy, S., Arnold, L., Shapira, N., Keck, P., Jr., Rosenthal, N., Karim, M., et al. (2003). Topiramate in the treatment of binge eating disorder associated with obesity: A randomized, placebo-controlled trial. *American Journal of Psychiatry, 160*(2), 255.

McElroy, S., Casuto, L., Nelson, E., Lake, K., Soutullo, C., Keck, P., et al. (2000). Placebo-controlled trial of sertraline in the treatment of binge eating disorder. *American Journal of Psychiatry, 157*(6), 1004–1006.

Miller, K., Grieco, K., & Klibanski, A. (2005). Testosterone administration in women with anorexia nervosa. *Journal of Clinical Endocrinology and Metabolism, 90*(3), 1428–1433.

Minuchin, P. (1985). Families and individual development: Provocations from the field of family therapy. *Child Development, 56*(2), 289–302.

Minuchin, S. (1974). *Families and family therapy.* Oxford: Harvard University Press.

Minuchin, S. (1975). A conceptual model of psychosomatic illness in children: Family organization and family therapy. *Archives of General Psychiatry, 32, 8,* 1031–1038.

Mintz, L. B., & Betz, N. E. (1986). Sex differences in the nature, realism, and correlates of body image. *Sex Roles, 15*(3–4), 185–195.

Mintz, L. B., & Kashubeck, S. (1999). Body image and disordered eating among Asian American and Caucasian college students: An examination of race and gender differences. *Psychology of Women Quarterly, 23*(4), 781–796.

Mitchell, J. E., Agras, S., & Wonderlich, S. (2007). Treatment of bulimia nervosa: Where are we and where are we going? *International Journal of Eating Disorders, 40*(2), 95–101.

Mukai, T., Crago, M., & Shisslak, C. M. (1994). Eating attitudes and weight preoccupation among female high school students in Japan. *Journal of Child Psychology and Psychiatry, 35,* 677–688.

Murray, K., Pombo-Carril, M. G., & Bara-Carril, N. (2003). Factors determining uptake of a CD-ROM-based CBT self-help treatment for bulimia: Patient characteristics and subjective appraisals of self-help treatment. *European Eating Disorders Review, 113*(3), 246–260.

Nakamura, K., Hoshino, Y., Watanabe, A., Honda, K., Niwa, S., Tominaga, K., et al. (2000). Eating problems in female Japanese high school students: A prevalence study. *International Journal of Eating Disorders, 26,* 91–95.

National Institute for Clinical Excellence (NICE). (2004). *Eating disorders: Core interventions in the treatment and management of anorexia nervosa, bulimia nervosa, and related eating disorders* (Clinical Guideline No. 9). London: Author.

Nauta, H., Hospers, H., Jansen, A., & Kok, G. (2000). Cognitions in obese binge eaters and obese non-binge eaters. *Cognitive Therapy and Research, 24*(5), 521.

Nevo, S. (1985). Bulimic symptoms: Prevalence and ethnic differences among college women. *International Journal of Eating Disorders, 4,* 151–168.

Nevonen, L., & Broberg, A. (2006). A comparison of sequenced individual and group psychotherapy for patients with bulimia nervosa. *International Journal of Eating Disorders, 39*(2), 117–127.

Nielsen, S. (2001). Epidemiology and mortality of eating disorders. *Psychiatric Clinics of North America, 24,* 201–214.

Nogami, Y. (1997). Eating disorders in Japan: A review of the literature. *Psychiatry and Clinical Neuroscience, 51,* 339–346.

Ogden, J. (2002). *The psychology of eating.* Boston, MA: Blackwell.

Palmer, R., Birchall, H., McGrain, L., & Sullivan, V. (2002). Self-help for bulimic disorders: A randomised controlled trial comparing minimal guidance with face-to-face or telephone guidance. *British Journal of Psychiatry, 181,* 230–235.

Pate, J. E., Pumariega, A. J., Hester, C., & Garner, D. M. (1992). Cross-cultural patterns in eating disorders: A review. *Journal of the American Academy of Child and Adolescent Psychiatry, 31,* 802–809.

Patton, C. (1992). Fear of abandonment and binge eating: A subliminal psychodynamic activation investigation. *Journal of Nervous and Mental Disorders, 180,* 484–490.

Peterson, C., Mitchell, J., Engbloom, S., Nugent, S., Mussell, M., & Miller, J. (1998). Group cognitive-behavioral treatment of binge eating disorder: A comparison of therapist-led versus self-help formats. *International Journal of Eating Disorders, 24*(2), 125–136.

Phan, T., & Tylka, T. L. (2006). Exploring a model and moderators of disordered eating with Asian American college women. *Journal of Counseling Psychology, 53*(1), 36–47.

Phinney, J. S. (1989). Stages of ethnic identity development in minority group adolescents. *Journal of Early Adolescence, 9* (1–2), 34–49.

Pike, K. M., & Borovoy, A. (2004). The rise of eating disorders in Japan: Issues of culture and limitations of the model of "Westernization." *Culture, Medicine, and Psychiatry, 28,* 493–531.

Pike, K. M., & Mizushima, H. (2005). The clinical presentation of Japanese women with anorexia nervosa and bulimia nervosa: A study of the Eating Disorders Inventory-2. *International Journal of Eating Disorders, 37,* 26–31.

Pike, K. M., & Walsh, B. T. (1996). Ethnicity and eating disorders: Implications for incidence and treatment. *Psychopharmacology Bulletin, 32,* 265–274.

Pike, K., Walsh, B., Vitousek, K., Wilson, G., & Bauer, J. (2003). Cognitive behavior therapy in the posthospitalization treatment of anorexia nervosa. *American Journal of Psychiatry, 160*(11), 2046–2049.

Piran, N., Jasper, K., & Pinhas, L. (2004). Feminist therapy and eating disorders. In J. K. Thompson (Ed.), *Handbook of eating disorders* (pp. 263–278). Hoboken, NJ: Wiley.

Prince, R. (1985). The concept of culture-bound syndromes: Anorexia nervosa and brain-fag. *Social Science and Medicine, 21, 2,* 197–203.

Ritenbaugh, C., Shisslak, C. M., Teufel, N., & Leonard-Green, T. K. (1996). A cross-cultural review of eating disorders in regard to DSM-IV. In J. E. Mezzich, A. Kleinman, H. Fabrega, Jr., & D. L. Parron (Eds.), *Culture and psychiatric diagnosis: A DSM-IV perspective* (pp. 171–185). Washington, DC: American Psychiatric Press.

Robin, A., Siegel, P., Koepke, T., Moye, A., & Tice, S. (1994). Family therapy versus individual therapy for adolescent females with anorexia nervosa. *Journal of Developmental and Behavioral Pediatrics, 15*(2), 111–116.

Rodriguez, R., Marchand, E., Ng, J., & Stice, E. (2008). Effects of a cognitive dissonance-based eating disorder prevention program are similar for Asian American, Hispanic, and white participants. *International Journal of Eating Disorders, 41,* 618–625.

Romano, S., Halmi, K., Sarkar, N., Koke, S., & Lee, J. (2002). A placebo-controlled study of fluoxetine in continued treatment of bulimia nervosa after successful acute fluoxetine treatment. *American Journal of Psychiatry, 159*(1), 96–102.

Root, M. P. (1990a). Recovery and relapse in former bulimics. *Psychotherapy, 27*(3), 397–403.

Root, M. P. P. (1990b). Disordered eating in women of color. *Sex Roles, 22,* 525–535.

Roh Ryu, H., Lyle, R. M., & McCabe, G. P. (2003). Factors associated with weight concerns and unhealthy eating patterns among young Korean females. *Eating Disorders, 11,* 129–141.

Rorty, M., & Yager, J. R. (2000). Parental intrusiveness in adolescence recalled by women with a history of bulimia nervosa and comparison women. *International Journal of Eating Disorders, 28, 2,* 202–208.

Safer, D. L., Telch, C. F., & Agras, W. S. (2001). Dialectical behavior therapy for bulimia nervosa. *American Journal of Psychiatry, 158*(4), 632–634.

Salzman, J. P. (1997). Ambivalent attachment in female adolescents: Association with affective instability and eating disorders. *International Journal of Eating Disorders, 21*, 251–259.

Sands, T. (1998). Feminist counseling and female adolescents: Treatment strategies for depression. *Journal of Mental Health Counseling, 20*, 42–55.

Scholz, M., & Asen, E. (2001). Multiple family therapy with eating disordered adolescents: Concepts and preliminary results. *European Eating Disorders Review, 9*(1), 33–42.

Selvini-Palazzoli, M. (1974). *Self-starvation: From the intrapsychic to the transpersonal approach to anorexia nervosa.* London, UK: Chancer.

Selvini-Palazzoli, M. (1978). *Self-starving: From individual to family treatment of anorexia nervosa.* New York: Brunner Mazel.

Serfaty, M., Turkington, D., Heap, M., Ledsham, L., & Jolley, E. (1999). Cognitive therapy versus dietary counseling in the outpatient treatment of anorexia nervosa: Effects of the treatment phase. *European Eating Disorders Review, 7*(5), 334–350.

Sesan, R., & Katzman, M. (1998). Empowerment and the eating-disordered client. In I. B. Seu & M. C. Heenan (Eds.), *Feminism and psychotherapy: Reflections on contemporary theories and practices* (pp. 78–95). London: Sage.

Shaw, H., Ramirez, L., & Trost, A. (2004). Body image and eating disturbances across ethnic groups: More similarities than differences. *Psychology of Addictive Behaviors, 18*(1),12–18.

Sherwood, N., Jeffery, R., & Wing, R. (1999). Binge status as a predictor of weight loss treatment outcome. *International Journal of Obesity and Related Metabolic Disorders, 23*(5), 485–493 .

Shimosaka, K. (1961). Psychiatrische Studien uber Pubertats-magersucht (Anorexia nervosa) [in Japanese with German abstract]. *Japanese Journal of Psychiatry and Neurology 63*, 1041–1082.

Smith, D. E. (1995). Binge eating in ethnic minority groups. *Addictive Behaviors, 20*, 695–703.

Smolak, L., & Murnen, S. K. (2001). Gender and eating problems. In R. H. Striegel-Moore & L. Smolak (Eds.), *Eating disorders: Innovative directions in research and practice* (pp. 91–110). Washington, DC: American Psychological Association.

Smolak, L., & Striegel-Moore, R. H. (2001). Challenging the myth of the golden girl: Ethnicity and eating disorders. In R. H. Striegel-Moore & L. Smolak (Eds.), *Eating disorders: Innovative directions in research and practice* (pp. 111–132). Washington, DC: American Psychological Association.

Snow, J. T., & Harris, M. B. (1986). An analysis of weight and diet content in five women's interest magazines. *Journal of Obesity and Weight Regulation, 5*(4), 194–214.

Sodowsky, G. R., Kwan, K. K., & Pannu, R. (1995). Ethnic identity of Asians in the United States. In J. G. Ponterotto, J. M. Casas, L. A. Suzuki, & C. M. Alexander (Eds.), *Handbook of multicultural counseling* (pp. 123–154). Newbury Park, CA: Sage.

Stark-Wroblewski, K., Yanico, B. J., & Lupe, S. (2005). Acculturation, internalization of western appearance norms, and eating pathology among Japanese and Chinese international student women. *Psychology of Women Quarterly, 29*, 1, 38–46.

Stice, E. (1994). Review of the evidence for a sociocultural model of bulimia nervosa: An explanation of the mechanisms of action. *Clinical Psychology Review, 14*, 633–661.

Stice, E. (1999). Clinical implications of psychosocial research on bulimia nervosa and binge-eating disorder. *Journal of Clinical Psychology, 55*, 675–683.

Stice, E. (2001). A prospective test of the dual pathway model of bulimic pathology: Mediating effects of dieting and negative affect. *Journal of Abnormal Psychology, 110*, 124–135.

Stice, E., & Hoffman, E. (2004). Eating disorder prevention programs. In J. K. Thompson (Ed.), *Handbook of eating disorders and obesity* (pp. 33–57). Hoboken, NJ: Wiley.

Stice, E., & Shaw, H. (2002). Role of body dissatisfaction in the onset and maintenance of bulimic Journal of Psychosomatic Research pathology: A synthesis of research findings., 53, 985–993.

Striegel-Moore, R. H., & Bulik, C. M. (2007). Risk factors for eating disorders. *American Psychologist, 62*, 181–198.

Striegel-Moore, R. H., Silberstein, L. R., & Rodin, J. (1986).Toward an understanding of risk factors for bulimia. *American Psychologist, 41*, 246–263.

Strober, M., Freeman, R., & Morrell, W. (1997). The long-term course of severe anorexia nervosa in adolescents: survival analysis of recovery, relapse, and outcome predictors over 10–15 years in a prospective study. *International Journal of Eating Disorders, 22*(4), 339–360.

Sue, D. W., & Sue, S. (1987) Cultural factors in the clinical assessment of Asian Americans. *Journal of Consulting and Clinical Psychology, 55*(4), 479–487.

Sue, D. W., & Sue, D. (2003). Counseling Asian Americans. In *Counseling the culturally diverse: Theory and practice* (4th ed., pp. 327–342). New York: Wiley.

Takahashi, K. (1990). Are the key assumptions of the "Strange Situation" procedure universal? A view from Japanese research. *Human Development, 33*(2), 23–30.

Tasca, G. A., Balfour, L., Ritchie, K., & Bissada, H. (2007). The relationship between attachment scales and group therapy alliance growth differs by treatment type for women with binge-eating disorder. *Group Dynamics: Theory, Research, and Practice, 11*(1), 1–14.

Telch, C., Agras, W., & Linehan, M. (2001). Dialectical behavior therapy for binge eating disorder. *Journal of Consulting And Clinical Psychology, 69*(6), 1061–1065.

Thelen, M. H., Farmer, J., Wonderlich, S, & Smith, M. (1991). A revision of the Bulimia Test: The BULIT—R. *Psychological Assessment, 3,* 119–124.

Tomiyama, A. J., & Mann, T. (2008). Cultural factors in collegiate eating disorder pathology: When family culture clashes with individual culture. *Journal of American College Health, 57*(3), 309–313.

Tong, J., Miao, S. J., Wang, J., Zhang, J. J., Wu, H. M., Li, T., et al. (2005). Five cases of male eating disorders in Central China. *International Journal of Eating Disorders, 37,* 72–75.

Treasure, J., Todd, G., Brolly, M., Tiller, J., Nehmed, A., & Denman, F. (1995). A pilot study of a randomised trial of cognitive analytical therapy vs educational behavioral therapy for adult anorexia nervosa. *Behaviour Research and Therapy, 33*(4), 363–367 .

Tsai, G. (2000). Eating disorders in the Far East. *Eating and Weight Disorders, 5,* 183–197.

Tsukahara, M. & Shimosaka, K. (1994). Developmental psychopathology of eating disorders as viewed by fathers' attitude. *Seishin Ryoho, 20,* 420–421.

Uba, L. (1994). *Asian Americans: Personality patterns, identity, and mental health.* New York: Guilford.

U. S. Census Bureau. (2001). *Population by race only, race in combination only, race alone or in combination, and Hispanic or Latino origin, for the United Sates: 2000* [Data table]. Retrieved July 13, 2008, from the Population Division, Population Estimates Program: http://www.census.gov/population/cen2000/phc-t1/tab03.pdf

Vitousek, K., Watson, S., & Wilson, G. (1998). Enhancing motivation for change in treatment-resistant eating disorders. *Clinical Psychology Review, 18*(4), 391–420.

Warren, C. S., Gleaves, D. H., Cepeda-Benito, A., del Carmen Fernandez, M., & Rodriguez-Ruiz, S. (2005). Ethnicity as a protective factor against internalization of a thin ideal and body dissatisfaction. *International Journal of Eating Disorders, 37,* 3, 241–249.

White, M. I. (1993). *The material child: Coming of age in Japan and America.* New York: Free Press.

Wildes, J. E., Emery, R. E., & Simons, A. D. (2001). The roles of ethnicity and culture in the development of eating disturbance and body dissatisfaction: A meta-analytic review. *Clinical Psychology Review, 21,* 521–551.

Wilfley, D., Agras, W., Telch, C., Rossiter, E., Schneider, J., Cole, A., et al. (1993). Group cognitive-behavioral therapy and group interpersonal psychotherapy for the nonpurging bulimic individual: A controlled comparison. *Journal of Consulting and Clinical Psychology, 61*(2), 296–305.

Wilfley, D. E. (2002). Psychological treatment of binge eating disorder. In C. G. Fairburn & K. D. Brownell (Eds.), *Eating disorders and obesity: A comprehensive handbook* (2nd ed., pp. 350–353). New York: Guilford.

Williamson, D. A., Gleaves, D. H., & Stewart, T. M. (2005). Categorical versus dimensional models of eating disorders: An examination of the evidence. *International Journal of Eating Disorders, 37,* 1–10.

Wilson, G. T. (1989). The treatment of bulimia nervosa: A cognitive-social learning analysis. In A. J. Stunkard, & A. Baum (Eds.), *Eating, sleeping, and sex* (pp. 73–98). Hillsdale, NJ: Erlbaum.

Wilson, G. T., Grilo, C. M., & Vitousek, K. M. (2007). Psychological treatment of eating disorders. *American Psychologist, 62,* 199–216.

Wilson, G., & Pike, K. (2001). Eating disorders. In D. H. Barlow (Ed.), *Clinical handbook of psychological disorders: A step-by-step treatment manual* (3rd ed., pp. 332–375). New York: Guilford.

Wonderlich, S. A., Joiner, T. E., Jr., Keel, P. K., Williamson, D. A., & Crosby, R. D. (2007). Eating disorder diagnoses: Empirical approaches to classification. *American Psychologist, 62,* 167–180.

Wong, E. C., Kim, S. K., Zane, N. W., Kim, I. J., & Huang, J. S. (2003). Examining culturally based variables associated with ethnicity: Influences on credibility perceptions of empirically supported interventions. *Cultural Diversity and Ethnic Minority Psychology, 9*, 88–96.

Woodside, D. B., & Twose, R. (2004). Diagnostic issues in eating disorders: Historical perspectives and thoughts for the future. In T. D. Brewerton (Ed.), *Clinical handbook of eating disorders: An integrated approach* (pp. 1–20). New York: Dekker.

World Health Organization (1992). *International statistical classification of diseases and related health problems* (10th ed.) Geneva, Switzerland: Author. (ICD-10)

World Health Organization (2004). Appropriate body-mass index for Asian populations and its implications for policy and intervention strategies. *Lancet, 353*, 157–163.

Yager, J. (1982). Family issues in the pathogenesis of anorexia nervosa. *Psychosomatic Medicine, 44*(1), 43–60.

Yee, B. W. K., DeBaryshe, B. D., Yuen, S., Kim, S. Y., & McCubbin, H. I. (2007). Asian American and Pacific Islander families: Resiliency and life-span socialization in a cultural context. In F. T. L. Leong, A. Ebreo, L. Kinoshita, A. G. Inman, L. H. Yang, & M. Fu (Eds.), *Handbook of Asian American psychology* (2nd ed., pp. 69–86). Thousand Oaks, CA: Sage.

Zhang, A. Y., & Snowden, L. R. (1999). Ethnic characteristics of mental disorders in five U.S. communities. *Cultural Diversity and Ethnic Minority Psychology, 5*, 134–146.

| 12 |

SLEEP DISORDERS IN ASIANS

Donald M. Sesso, Allison V. Chan, and Clete A. Kushida

IDENTIFYING SLEEP DISORDERS IN ASIANS

Sleep occupies nearly a third of our lives. Thus, derangements of sleep can have a significant impact on one's longevity and quality of life. Poor sleep can be manifested by impaired cognitive, academic, or occupational performance. Patients with sleep disorders are predisposed to domestic, motor vehicle, or work-related accidents, which may result in serious injury or death. Furthermore, sleep disruption may result in neurobehavioral dysfunction and impaired social adjustment or mood disorders. In addition, sleep disorders may exacerbate or contribute to other psychiatric or medical conditions. In fact, both cardiopulmonary and neurologic morbidity are associated with disrupted sleep (He, Kryger, Zorick, et al., 1998; Dincer, O'Neill, 2006; Yaggi, Concato, Kernan, et al., 2005).

While there has been interest in sleep for well over a century, the past several decades have witnessed an explosion of research and investigation into the field of sleep medicine. Once perceived as an esoteric field in medicine, sleep is now recognized as a matter of public health and necessary for a healthy life. Sleep disorders are common in the general population. Consequently, the public is learning that impaired sleep can have health consequences similar to that of smoking, alcohol abuse, and poor diets.

A plethora of sleep disorders are now recognized. Certain disorders, such as obstructive sleep apnea (OSA) and insomnia have been well described in the literature. However, other sleep disorders and their pathophysiological mechanisms are poorly understood. In order to comprehend the presenting symptoms, pathophysiology, etiology, diagnosis, and treatment of these sleep disorders, a nosology or classification scheme was developed.

Published in 1979, the *Diagnostic Classification of Sleep and Arousal Disorders* was the first major classification scheme for sleep disorders. This allowed clinicians and researchers to differentiate between the disorders. The classification was based on presenting symptoms. Subsequently, this system has undergone many revisions. Currently, three major classification schemes are used for diagnosing and coding sleep disorders. They include the *Diagnostic and Statistical Manual of Mental Disorders* (*DSM-IV-TR*), the *International Classification of Diseases* (ICD), and the *International Classification of Sleep Disorders* (ICSD-2). These revisions allow classifying disorders by symptoms and pathophysiology where applicable. Essentially, the classification schemes identify eight major categories of sleep disorders. They include: (1) insomnias; (2) sleep-related breathing disorders; (3) hypersomnias not due to a sleep-related breathing disorder; (4) circadian rhythm sleep disorders; (5) parasomnias; (6) sleep-related movement disorders; (7) isolated symptoms, apparently normal variants, and unresolved issues; and (8) other sleep disorders (American Academy of Sleep Medicine, 2005; American Psychiatric Association [APA], 2000; Thorpy, 2005).

CURRENT *DSM* NOSOLOGY AND CRITERIA FOR SLEEP DISORDERS

Insomnia

Stated simply, sleep is defined as a reversible behavioral state of perceptual disengagement from and unresponsiveness to the environment. Insomnia is simply the disruption of normal sleep. The insomnias can be either primary or secondary. The *DSM-IV-TR* defines primary insomnia as difficulty initiating or maintaining sleep, or nonrestorative sleep, at least 3 times a week for at least 1 month despite adequate time and opportunity for sleep. This sleep disturbance or associated daytime fatigue causes clinically significant distress or impairment in social, occupational, or other important areas of functioning (APA, 2000). Secondary forms occur when the insomnia is a symptom of a mental or medical disorder, due to the physiologic effects of a substance (e.g., drug abuse, medications), or the result of another sleep disorder (American Academy of Sleep Medicine, 2005; APA, 2000; Doghramji, 2006).

There are six types of primary insomnia (Thorpy, 2005). Psychophysiologic insomnia is one of the more common manifestations of insomnia. It is characterized by a heightened state of arousal, both during the day and the night, with learned sleep-preventing associations that are present for at least one month (Hauri & Fisher, 1986). Patients associate the bedroom with activities other than sleep. This stimulation inhibits sleep and a preoccupation with the inability to sleep develops. Paradoxical insomnia is associated with complaints of little or no sleep. However, there is no objective evidence of sleep disturbance. In addition, these patients do not experience the degree of daytime impairment that would be expected by the lack of sleep reported (Salin-Pascual, Roehrs, Merlotti, et al., 1992). Adjustment sleep disorder is described as an insomnia that is associated with a specific stressor, which can be physical, physiologic, psychological, or environmental. Typically, the insomnia will resolve when the stressor is eliminated. The disorder usually lasts days to weeks. Inadequate sleep hygiene implies that certain behaviors may impede sleep and thus, modification of these behaviors may alleviate insomnia. Actions such as irregular wake and sleep onset times and performing stimulating activities before bedtime may cause insomnia. Moreover, ingesting certain substances before sleep, such as alcohol, caffeine, or cigarettes, is associated with poor sleep hygiene. However, it should be noted that these actions do not cause sleep disturbances in all patients (Silber, 2007). Idiopathic insomnia arises insidiously from childhood and will persist through adulthood without remission. There is no identifiable etiology (Hauri & Olmstead, 1980). Behavioral insomnia of childhood is divided into sleep-onset association disorder and limit-setting sleep disorder. Sleep-onset association disorder is characterized by a dependence on environmental stimuli to initiate sleep, including the presence of a bottle of milk or a lighted room. The limit-setting type is expressed as a child refusing to go to bed at an appropriate time because the parent has difficulty enforcing behaviors and expressing expectations. This insomnia resolves once the caretaker enforces limits on sleep times and behaviors (Gaylor, Goodlin-Jones, & Anders, 2001).

Insomnia is the most commonly reported sleep disorder in the industrialized world (Sateia, Doghramji, Hauri, et al., 2000). In fact, a Gallup poll performed in 1979 demonstrated that 95% of a randomly selected adult population complained of insomnia at some point in their lives (Gallup Organization, 1979). Fortunately, most of these events are transient and the insomnia will resolve when the causative factors are removed. Chronic insomnia, which is persistent and is associated with impaired daytime function, while common, is much less prevalent than transient symptoms. The reported prevalence of chronic insomnia varies widely.

Ohayon reported in 2002 that the prevalence of chronic insomnia ranged from 4.4% to 48% among a review of more than 50 epidemiological studies (Ohayon, 2002). This substantial variability is thought to be related to the authors' definition of insomnia. When the more stringent DSM-IV criteria for insomnia have been utilized, the estimated prevalence is significantly lower (Ohayon, 1997). The U.S. National Institutes of Health (NIH) State-of-the-Science Conference on Manifestations and Management of Chronic Insomnia in Adults reported that 30% of the adult population had complaints of sleep disruption, while 10% had symptoms that met the criteria for chronic insomnia (National Institutes of Health, 2005). Risk factors include female gender, advancing age, mental disorders, and chronic medical conditions.

Studies concerning the effect of race or ethnicity on the prevalence of insomnia have indicated that East Asians as a group are not at higher risk for insomnia. Consequently, East Asian ethnicity is not an independent risk factor for insomnia. Numerous studies have demonstrated that insomnia rates in Asia are comparable to that reported in Western countries. In 2002, an epidemiology study of Chinese adults in Hong Kong demonstrated that 11.9% of the study group complained of insomnia (R. Li, Wing, Ho, et al., 2002). Furthermore, Ohayon et al., found that 5% of a sample of South Korean adults met the DSM-IV criteria for insomnia diagnoses (Ohayon & Hong, 2002). Other studies have directly compared the prevalence and impact of insomnia among different Asian populations. One such study examined the rates of insomnia among Japanese, South Korean, and Taiwanese subjects. The prevalence was 4%, 9.9%, and 10.3% respectively (Nomura, Yamaoka, Nakao, et al., 2005). The Japanese have extensively published data on the epidemiology and effects on insomnia on their population. The outcomes and prevalence rates are similar to other Asian countries (Ishigooka, Suzuki, Isawa, et al., 1999; Yokoyama, Yasuhiko, Yoshitaka, et al., 2008).

Comparatively few studies contrast the prevalence of insomnia among Asian Americans versus East Asians. However, one such study describes the prevalence of insomnia in elderly Japanese American men residing in Hawaii to be comparable to that of other Asian and Caucasian populations (Barbar, Enright, Boyle, et al., 2000). While a majority of the data suggests that no significance exists, some others have noted an exception. A study evaluating elderly first-generation

Korean American immigrants noted a higher prevalence rate (Sok, 2008). Additionally, an ethnocultural study of insomnia in American adolescents indicated a slightly lower prevalence in Chinese Americans (Roberts, Roberts, & Chen, 2000).

These mixed results suggest that Asian ethnicity alone is not a risk factor for insomnia. Asians and Asian Americans seem to be equally as affected as Caucasian populations. The etiology of insomnia is multifactorial and is more likely related to age, gender, socioeconomic factors, and medical or psychiatric disorders. In addition, reported prevalence varied in part to the criteria utilized by investigators to define insomnia in these studies. It should be noted that an epidemiologic review of the prevalence of insomnia in Asians revealed the same at-risk populations that were noted in Western countries. Women, those with psychiatric and medical conditions, and the indigent are more susceptible to insomnia (R. Li, Wing, Ho, et al., 2002; Ohayon, Hong, 2002; Nomura, Yamaoka, Nakao, et al., 2005; Ishigooka, Suzuki, Isawa, et al., 1999; Yokoyama, Yasuhiko, Yoshitaka, et al., 2008; Barbar, Enright, Boyle, et al., 2000; Sok, 2008).

Applying the *DSM-IV* criteria to diagnose insomnia in Asian populations is sound. East Asians do not seem to be at higher risk of developing this disorder; however recognition of its presence may be underestimated. Despite similar prevalence rates, Asian subjects are less likely to seek treatment for this condition as compared to their Western counterparts (Ohayon & Hong, 2002). Clearly, treatment would be beneficial for these patients. Thus, an increased educational effort is needed for both patients and physicians.

Sleep-Related Breathing Disorders

Sleep-related breathing disorders (SRBD) include both obstructive sleep apnea and central sleep apnea. They are characterized by abnormal respiration during sleep. The *DSM-IV* criterion for SRBD is sleep disruption leading to excessive sleepiness that is judged to be due to a sleep-related breathing condition. Furthermore, this sleepiness should not be accounted for by another mental condition, medical illness, or substance abuse (APA, 2000). Any patient suspected of having this disorder requires a comprehensive history and physical examination. The history should focus on both nocturnal and diurnal symptoms, familial history of similar symptoms, and exacerbating factors (Chan & Kushida, 2007). Frequently, the patient's bed partner may provide invaluable information regarding sleep habits. A complete physical exam with vital signs and body mass index (BMI) should be performed on every patient. Specific attention is focused in the regions of the head and neck that have been well described as potential sites of upper airway obstruction, such as the nose, palate, and base of tongue (Rojewski, Schuller, Clark, et al., 1984). Polysomnography (PSG) remains the gold standard for diagnosing SRBD.

Obstructive sleep apnea (OSA) is due to a partial and/or complete repetitive collapse of the pharyngeal airway during sleep. This reduction of airway caliber may cause sleep fragmentation and subsequent behavioral derangements, such as excessive daytime sleepiness (EDS) or insomnia (Kales, Cadieux, Bixler, et al., 1985). Polysomnography is used to establish the diagnosis. A respiratory disturbance index (RDI) of greater than or equal to 5 per hour with symptoms, such as EDS, is considered confirmatory. The RDI refers to the combined number of apneas, hypopneas, or respiratory effort–related arousals (RERAs) that occur per hour of sleep. An apneic event is defined as the cessation of airflow for at least 10 seconds that occur with an electroencephalo-graphic (EEG) arousal and are accompanied by an oxygen desaturation, often at least 2% to 4%. The definition of hypopneas has been standardized by the American Academy of Sleep Medicine; most recognize it as a reduction in airflow of 30% or greater with a 4% or greater drop in oxygen saturation for at least 10 seconds. RERAs are events characterized by an increased inspiratory effort that coincides with an EEG arousal and do not meet the definition of an apnea or hypopnea (American Academy of Sleep Medicine, 2005).

An RDI of 5 to 15 abnormal respiratory events is considered mild OSA, between 15 and 30 events is moderate OSA, and greater than 30 events per hour of sleep is considered severe OSA. The diagnosis of OSA can also be established in the absence of symptoms; however the RDI should be equal to or greater than 15 abnormal events (American Academy of Sleep Medicine, 2005). Upper airway resistance syndrome (UARS) is within the continuum of SRBD. UARS is marked by increased respiratory effort during sleep with an RDI less than 5. Furthermore, a pre-ponderance of RERAs is noted on the PSG. Rarely will the oxygen desaturation levels fall below 90%. Patients with UARS do not typical complain of EDS. Yet, they may report a history of being fatigued that has impaired their activities of daily life.

Epidemiologic studies of the general population estimate that 2% to 5% of adults meet the criteria for OSA. These studies were collected from primarily Caucasian subjects (Bresnitz, Goldberg, & Kosinski, 1994; Olson, King, Hensley, et al., 1995). While prevalence rates have been much higher in certain reports, this is thought to be related to disparities in techniques used for monitoring sleep and variability in the criteria utilized for diagnosing OSA. The ratio of OSA in men compared to women is approximately two to one (Punjabi, 2008).

Obesity (BMI > $30kg/m^2$) and age greater than 65 years are the greatest risk factors in OSA. Epidemiologic studies performed in Western and Asian countries have consistently identified obesity as the strongest risk factor for OSA (Punjabi, 2008; Phillips, Cook, Schmitt, et al., 1989; Rajala, Partinen, Sane, et al., 1991). The Wisconsin Sleep Cohort Study demonstrated that obese patients had a 4-fold increase in the prevalence of OSA (Young, Palta, Dempsey, et al., 1993). Moreover, data from the Sleep Heart Healthy Study, among others indicated that an increase in body weight over time can accelerate the progression of OSA or lead to the development of more severe apnea (Newman, Foster, Givelber, et al., 2005; Peppard, Young, Palta, et al., 2000). With advancing age, the reported prevalence of OSA increases. Ancoli-Israel et al. found that 56% of women and 70% of men between the ages of 65 and 99 years had OSA defined as an apnea-hypopnea index (AHI) of at least 10 events per hour of sleep (Ancoli-Israel, Kripke, Klauber, et al., 1991). While this prevalence is higher than typically reported, it confirms subsequent studies that indicate advanced age as a risk factor for OSA.

A positive family history increases the risk for OSA by at least 2-fold. First-degree relatives of those with OSA are more prone to be at risk compared with first-degree relatives of those without the disorder. Furthermore, familial susceptibility to obstructive sleep apnea increases directly with the number of affected relatives. This genetic predisposition is likely related to inherited cranio-facial features and a familial history of obesity (Guilleminault, Partinen, Hollman, et al., 1995; Redline, Tishler, Tosteson, et al., 1995).

Certain craniofacial features have been identified that narrow the posterior airway space or increase the propensity of the pharyngeal airway to collapse during sleep. Physical findings such as an arched hard palate, an enlarged tongue or elongated soft palate, tonsillar hypertrophy, retrognathia, maxillary and mandibular retroposition, and an inferior positioned hyoid bone are associated with OSA in both adult and pediatric patients. A meta-analysis of studies investigating the craniofacial features that were associated with OSA found that mandibular body length had the strongest association (Miles, Vig, Weyant, et al., 1996). Differences in craniofacial morphology are noted among different racial groups, and this difference becomes quite important in the discussion of the prevalence of OSA in Asian populations.

Until recently, the majority of data available about the prevalence of OSA was based on Western groups. However, studies are continuously emerging regarding the prevalence of OSA in Asian populations. Interestingly, most of these studies indicate the occurrence of symptomatic and asymptomatic OSA in Asian patients is comparable to that documented in Caucasians. Punjabi's review of the epidemiology of OSA revealed a prevalence of 4.1% and 4.5% of Chinese and Korean men, respectively (Punjabi, 2008). In addition, several studies of Chinese subjects in Hong Kong demonstrated a prevalence rate of 4.1% in men and 2.1% in women (Lam, Lam, & Ip, 2007). Another prevalence study performed on 3,240 healthy Japanese subjects indicated an occurrence of 1.94% (Ohta, Okada, Kawakami, et al., 1993). Furthermore, the literature reviewing prevalence of OSA in Asian patients has consistently confirmed that obesity and male gender are risk factors for developing this syndrome, as found in Caucasian groups (Punjabi, 2008; Lam, Lam, & Ip, 2007; Ohta, Okada, Kawakami, et al., 1993).

Since obesity is considered a risk factor for OSA and Asians are less obese than Caucasians, one would expect the incidence of OSA to be less in Asians. However, this is not the case. Moreover, Asians tend to have a greater severity of illness, as indicated by a higher AHI, compared with Caucasians matched for BMI, gender, and age (Ong & Clerk, 1998; K. K. Li, Kushida, Powell, et al., 2000). Differences in craniofacial features are thought to contribute to these findings. Cephalometric analysis has identified a shortened cranial base, a narrower cranial base flexure and retrognathia in Asians. These studies of Chinese, Japanese, and Korean subjects found that this population has larger posterior airway spaces (PAS). Despite the larger PAS, Asians had more severe OSA. This would imply that cranial base dimensions may have a significant impact on the pathogenesis of OSA in Asians (K. K. Li, Kushida, Powell, et al., 2000; Lam, Ip, Tench, et al., 2005; Chen, Li, Li, et al., 2002).

The prevalence of OSA does not appear to differ in Asian Americans as compared to East Asians (Lam, Lam, & Ip, 2007; Ohta, Okada, Kawakami, et al., 1993; Ong & Clerk, 1998). However, as the incidence of obesity increases in the United States, Asian Americans may be at greater risk for OSA. In addition, minority groups tend to have poorer access to health care and the prevalence of OSA in Asian Americans may be underreported. More research is needed in this area.

Central sleep apnea is due to a loss of ventilatory effort that causes recurrent episodes of apnea (Guilleminault & Robinson, 1996). A central apnea is defined as a period of at least 10 seconds without airflow and the absence of ventilatory effort. As compared to obstructive apnea, the central apneas lack pharyngeal obstruction and subsequent ventilatory efforts against an occluded airway. Patients typically complain of EDS, insomnia, or difficulty breathing during sleep. Ideally, diagnosis is performed by a full-night PSG with esophageal pressure measurements. A central apnea index of greater than 5 events per hour of sleep is required for diagnosis.

Primary central sleep apnea is a disorder of unknown etiology. These patients are not hypercapnic (PCO_2 > 45 mmHg) and they usually have a PCO_2 that is less than 40 mmHg during wakefulness. Other central sleep apnea disorders have been described, and include Cheyne-Stokes breathing pattern and high-altitude periodic breathing pattern. Cheyne-Stokes breathing pattern is characterized by repeated central apneas and/or hypopneas (at least 10 events per hour of sleep) alternating with prolonged hyperpnea in which the tidal volume demonstrates a crescen-do-decrescendo pattern that is accompanied by frequent arousal from sleep and derangement of sleep structure. This pattern occurs in non-REM (NREM) sleep. Cheyne-Stokes breathing pattern is associated with congestive heart failure, cerebrovascular disorders, and renal failure. High-altitude periodic breathing disorder typically occurs at elevations greater than 7,600 meters. An ascent of at least 4,000 meters is required to make the diagnosis. This pattern is the result of acute mountain sickness. The cycle of breathing is marked by alternating apnea and hyperpnea. The cycle length is approximately 12 to 34 seconds. No ventilatory effort is noted during the periods of apnea (Thorpy, 2005; White, 2005).

Secondary central sleep apnea due to substance abuse has been well documented (Walker, Farney, Rhondeau, et al., 2007). It is most commonly associated with long-term opioid use. The class of medication causes respiratory depression by binding to the mu-receptors of the ventral medulla. Similar to the other central apneas, at least 5 events per hour of sleep must be documented on PSG.

The body of literature regarding the epidemiology of central sleep apnea is somewhat limited. Studies indicate that approximately 4% to 10% of patients that present to sleep laboratories have predominant central sleep apnea (Guilleminault, van de Hoed, & Mitler, 1978; DeBacker, 1995). Studies investigating symptomatic idiopathic central sleep apnea reveal that it is primarily found in middle-aged to older adults. However, younger patients have been identified. Guilleminault et al. have reported a strong male predominance; however, other studies have not supported this gender bias (American Academy of Sleep Medicine, 2005; Guilleminault, van de Hoed, & Mitler, 1978; DeBacker, 1995; Roehrs, Conway, Wittig, et al., 1985). Conversely, Cheyne-Stokes breathing pattern is predominantly seen in men older than 60 years (Sin, Fitzgerald, Parker, et al., 1999). In the setting of chronic congestive heart failure, a prevalence of 40% has been reported. Following stroke the prevalence is nearly 10% of patients (American Academy of Sleep Medicine, 2005; White, 2005). No studies specifically address an ethnic or inherited risk for developing central sleep apnea.

Current *DSM-IV* criteria for the diagnosis of SRBD in Asians have proven to be quite effective. This is largely due to the objective findings documented by PSG. However, it is troublesome that Asian patients have a greater severity of OSA as compared to Caucasians at time of diagnosis. Both patients and physicians need to forego the stereotypical image of an obese man as the classic patient with this disorder, especially given the fact that Asians have a lower incidence of obesity as compared to other populations. Perhaps screening patients at an earlier age may be more appropriate for Asian patients. Furthermore, a family history of SRBD and questions regarding sleep from both the patient and bed partner should be considered during routine physical examinations. Despite the numerous advancements in our understanding of SRBD, a majority of those affected remain undiagnosed. This may be related to the fact that the field of sleep medicine is still in the developmental stage in many Asian countries. As availability of these services increases, the prevalence of SRBD may increase as well (Punjabi, 2008; Lam, Lam, & Ip, 2007).

Hypersomnias Not Due to a Sleep-Related Breathing Disorder

The hypersomnias are a group of disorders in which the primary complaint is daytime sleepiness and the cause of the primary symptom is not disturbed sleep or misaligned circadian rhythms. The *DSM-IV* criteria for primary hypersomnia is excessive sleepiness that persists for at least 1 month (or less if recurrent) and is associated with significant impairment in social, occupational, or other important areas of functioning. Other sleep disorders can be present, but they first must be properly treated prior to establishing diagnoses in this category. Recurrent hypersomnia is characterized by periods of daytime sleepiness that last at least 3 days occurring several times a year for at least 2 years. Daytime sleepiness is defined as the inability to stay awake and alert during the major waking episodes of the day, resulting in unintended lapses into sleep (American Academy of Sleep Medicine, 2005; APA, 2000). The hypersomnias are categorized as: (1) narcolepsy with cataplexy, (2) narcolepsy without cataplexy, (3) narcolepsy due to a medical condition, (4) recurrent hypersomnia, (5) idiopathic hypersomnia with long sleep time, (6) recurrent hypersomnia without long sleep time, (7) behaviorally induced insufficient sleep syndrome, (8) hypersomnia due to a medical condition, (9) hypersomnia due to a drug or substance, (10) hypersomnia not due to substance or known physiological condition, and (11) physiological hypersomnia (American Academy of Sleep Medicine, 2005; APA, 2000).

Narcolepsy with cataplexy has certain diagnostic criteria. A patient should have EDS that occurs almost daily for at least 3 months. A definite history of cataplexy should be established. Cataplexy is defined as a sudden and transient loss of muscle tone that is triggered by strong emotions, such as anger or laughing. Consciousness is typically preserved at least at the beginning of the episode. In addition, the hypersomnia is not better explained by another sleep disorder, neurologic disorder, medical disorder, mental disorder, medication, or substance use disorder. The diagnosis of narcolepsy with cataplexy can be made based on clinical findings. However, a PSG (minimum of 6 hours sleep) followed by a multiple sleep latency test (MSLT) should be done for confirmation of the diagnosis. The mean sleep latency on MSLT should be less than or equal to 8 minutes, and 2 or more naps should demonstrate sleep-onset REM periods (SOREMPs). Alternatively, CSF hypocretin-1 levels may be drawn to confirm a diagnosis. A hypocretin-1 level less than or equal to 110 pg/mL or one-third of mean normal control values is diagnostic (American Academy of Sleep Medicine, 2005; Overeem, Mignot, van Dijk, et al., 2001).

Narcolepsy without cataplexy similarly requires a patient to experience EDS almost daily for at least 3 months. Clear-cut cataplexy is not present, but there are sleep paralysis and hypnagogic hallucinations. Contrary to narcolepsy with cataplexy, this diagnosis must be confirmed by a PSG followed by a MSLT. The polysomnographic and MSLT findings are the same as those required for the diagnosis of narcolepsy with cataplexy (American Academy of Sleep Medicine, 2005).

Narcolepsy due to a medical condition applies to patients with EDS who has a significant neurologic or medical disorder that accounts for this complaint. Narcolepsy must documented either clinically or polysomnographically. One of the following must be observed: a definite history of cataplexy, PSG and MSLT findings suggestive for narcolepsy or CSF hypocretin-1 levels less than 110 pg/mL. Parkinson's disease, multiple sclerosis, and Neiman-Pick type C disease are a few of the disorders that have been shown to produce secondary narcolepsy.

Recurrent hypersomnia or periodic hypersomnia is characterized by recurrent episodes of excessive sleepiness of 2 days' to 4 weeks' duration. These episodes occur once to 10 times a year. The patient has normal alertness, cognitive functioning, and behavior between attacks. The most described recurrent hypersomnia is Kleine-Levin syndrome (KLS). Yet, it is still rare, with only a few hundred cases reported in the literature. The male to female ratio for KLS is about 4:1. This syndrome is typified by sleepiness accompanied by hypersexuality, binge eating, or mood changes such as aggression and irritability. Menstrual-related hypersomnia is also a type of recurrent hypersomnia. This condition occurs within the first months after menarche. Excessive sleepiness is associated with the menstrual cycle. Symptoms usually last about a week and will resolve quickly at the time of menses (American Academy of Sleep Medicine, 2005; APA, 2000).

Idiopathic hypersomnia with long sleep time is marked by constant and excessive sleepiness with prolonged but unrefreshing naps, a prolonged major sleep episode, and great difficulty waking from sleep. A major sleep episode is defined as 10 or more hours of sleep. Typically, these sleep episodes last 12 to 14 hours. Sleep drunkenness or postawakening confusion is often reported. The diagnosis of idiopathic hypersomnia without long sleep time is reserved for patients with idiopathic hypersomnia who do not meet the criteria for hypersomnia with long sleep time. The main distinguishing feature is a normal or slightly prolonged sleep time that is less than 10 hours in duration. Unintended, nonrefreshing naps are common. The polysomnographic and MSLT findings are similar between these two types of hypersomnia with the exception of sleep time, and the narcolepsy criterion of 2 or more SOREMPs on the MSLT is not met in either condition (American Academy of Sleep Medicine, 2005; Billiard & Dauvilliers, 2001).

Behaviorally induced insufficient sleep syndrome occurs in patients who persistently deprive themselves of the necessary amount of sleep to maintain normal levels of wakefulness. However, when this habitual pattern of sleep deprivation is not maintained, they will sleep for a considerably longer amount of time. Often times a markedly extended sleep time will be noted on weekends and holidays as compared to weekdays. A therapeutic trial of extended sleep time may alleviate the symptoms. PSG is not initially required to establish a diagnosis. If implementing longer sleep time reverses the symptoms, than the diagnosis of behaviorally induced insufficient sleep syndrome can be made (American Academy of Sleep Medicine, 2005; APA, 2000).

Hypersomnia due to a medical condition is excessive sleepiness that is the direct result of a coexisting medical or neurological disorder. No cataplexy or any other diagnostic features of narcolepsy can be present to make this diagnosis. Parkinson's disease, head trauma, brain tumors, and hypothyroidism are associated with this form of hypersomnia. Likewise, hypersomnia due to a drug or substance is diagnosed when sleepiness is thought to be related to past or current use of drugs or alcohol. This category can be further subdivided into hypersomnia related to prescribed medications or abuse of street drugs. Opioids, stimulants, sedative-hypnotics and sedative anti-epileptics are commonly linked with this disorder (American Academy of Sleep Medicine, 2005; APA, 2000).

Hypersomnia not due to substance or known physiological condition is excessive sleepiness temporarily associated with a psychiatric disorder. These patients tend to be disproportionately fixated on their hypersomnia. Features of underlying psychiatric disorders are often apparent on evaluation. Mood disorders, conversion disorder, and schizoaffective disorder are linked to this hypersomnia. PSG demonstrates reduced sleep efficiency and increased frequency and duration of awakenings. Furthermore, variable, often normal sleep latencies are noted on MSLT (American Academy of Sleep Medicine, 2005; APA, 2000). Lastly, physiological or organic hypersomnia is diagnosed when a physiologic condition is believed to be the etiology of the complaint. In addition, the clinical and MSLT findings are consistent with hypersomnia, but these findings do not meet the criteria for another hypersomnia disorder.

Narcolepsy with cataplexy affects approximately 20 to 50 people per 100,000 of the United States and Western European populations (Longstreth, Koepsell, Ton, et al., 2007; Silber, Krahn, Olson, et al., 2002). Many of the early studies reported a higher occurrence of narcolepsy. However these studies frequently employed less sound methodologies for diagnosis. More recently, as stricter screening criteria are used, the prevalence rates of narcolepsy with cataplexy have been lower and more consistent with the previously mentioned rate (Longstreth, Koepsell, Ton, et al., 2007). Both sexes are affected, however males have a slightly higher preponderance of 1.4:1 (Longstreth, Koepsell, Ton, et al., 2007; Silber, Krahn, Olson, et al., 2002). The tendency for narcolepsy to have a familial tendency has long been recognized (Mignot, 1998; Guilleminault, Mignot, & Grumet, 1989; Chen, Fong, Lam, et al., 2007).

The prevalence of narcolepsy without cataplexy is more uncertain. This is likely due to the fact that patients without cataplexy are more likely to be undiagnosed. Cases of narcolepsy without cataplexy comprise 20% to 50% of narcolepsy cases (Mignot, Hayduk, Black, et al., 1997). A study of patients in Olmsted County, Minnesota, found incidence rate of 1.37 per 100,000 persons for narcolepsy with or without cataplexy (Silber, Krahn, Olson, et al., 2002). This was comparable to the rate of patients with narcolepsy-cataplexy and suggests a significant prevalence for narcolepsy without cataplexy in the general population.

Epidemiologic studies for narcolepsy with cataplexy have been performed in different countries throughout Asia. Notably, there is an increased prevalence of this disorder among the Japanese people in contrast to other Eastern Asian and Western groups. Two studies in Japan have reported a prevalence rate of 0.16% and 0.18% (Honda, 1997; Tashiro, Kanbayashi, Iijima, et al., 1992). Others have suggested that the design of these studies could account for the higher prevalence rates. For example, these studies did not use PSG to confirm the diagnosis of narcolepsy. However, it is widely accepted that Japanese ethnicity is associated with a greater risk of developing narcolepsy with cataplexy (American Academy of Sleep Medicine, 2005). As in Europe and North America, a genetic link for narcolepsy has been identified in the Japanese population (Mignot, Lin, Rogers, et al., 2001).

In 2002, Wing et al. reported the prevalence of narcolepsy in Southern China to be 0.034%. In this study strict epidemiological methodologies were used to diagnose narcolepsy. Patients identified by a screening questionnaire subsequently underwent clinical, polysomnographic, and human leukocyte antigen (HLA) testing for confirmation (Wing, Li, Lam, et al., 2002). Other population studies of Chinese subjects have demonstrated similar rates of prevalence. In addition, the frequency of narcolepsy in first-degree relatives and the association of HLA DQB1*0602 with this disorder in the Chinese is comparable to Caucasian populations (Chen, Fong, Lam, et al., 2007). Utilizing similar diagnostic criteria, the prevalence of narcolepsy with cataplexy was determined to be 0.015% in Korean adolescents (Shin, Yoon, Han, et al., 2008). With the exception of the Japanese studies, these results confirm that the prevalence rate of narcolepsy among Eastern Asians is comparable to the rates for other populations.

While the literature does not reveal studies that directly compare the prevalence of narcolepsy between Eastern Asians and Asian Americans, certain inferences can be made from the available data. Although the study populations are small, Asian Americans have a similar presentation and prevalence of narcolepsy when compared to Eastern Asians and other ethnic groups (Okun, Lin, Pelin, et al., 2002).

The current *DSM-IV* nosology for this group of disorders appears to be applicable to Asian populations. However, several diagnostic tools used to determine inclusion into this group of disorders may be flawed. Two studies of narcolepsy in Chinese subjects identified testing deficiencies that may underestimate the actual prevalence of narcolepsy. First, the subjective questionnaire measurements, Epworth Sleepiness Scale and Ullanlinna Narcolepsy Scale, were unable to detect the presence of narcolepsy spectrum disorders among relatives of affected patients. Furthermore, the presence of two or more sleep-onset REM periods (SOREMPs) on MSLT in Chinese-Taiwanese patients is not sufficient to identify narcolepsy in these patients (Chen, Fong, Lam, et al., 2007).

Circadian Rhythm Sleep Disorders

The circadian rhythm sleep disorders share a common feature in that there is a persistent or recurrent misalignment between an individual's own (endogenous) circadian sleep-wake cycle from the pattern that is considered the societal norm. In other words, the patient cannot sleep when sleep is required or expected. Optimal sleep requires that the desired sleep time should be synchronous with the timing of the circadian rhythm of sleep and wake propensity. The diagnostic criterion for this group of disorders requires that the misalignment of circadian rhythms leads to insomnia, excessive daytime sleepiness, or both. In addition, the sleep disturbance is associated with significant impairment in social, occupational, or other important areas of functioning. Moreover, the sleep disturbance cannot be better explained by another sleep disorder, mental disorder, medical disorder, or the result of a substance. Although the basic pathophysiology of these disorders is an alteration of the endogenous circadian rhythms, maladaptive behaviors and environmental influences can be contributing factors as well. The circadian rhythm sleep disorders include: (1) delayed sleep-phase type, (2) advanced sleep-phase type, (3) free-running type, (4) irregular sleep-wake type, (5) shift work sleep type, (6) jet lag type, (7) circadian rhythm sleep disorder due to a medical condition, (8) other circadian rhythm sleep disturbances due to a drug or substance, and (9) other circadian rhythm sleep disorders (American Academy of Sleep Medicine, 2005; APA, 2000; Reid & Zee, 2005).

The delayed sleep phase disorder is characterized by a delay in sleep-wake times by at least two hours as compared to normal subjects. Affected patients complain of the inability to fall asleep or awake at a desired and socially acceptable time. Typically, these patients have difficulty initiating sleep and prefer later wake-up times. However, when allowed to follow their preferred schedule, patients exhibit normal sleep quality and duration. Diagnostic criteria also require that a sleep log or actigraphy monitoring for a minimum of seven days demonstrates a habitual delay in the timing of sleep. Attempts to fall asleep at earlier times are usually unsuccessful (American Academy of Sleep Medicine, 2005; APA, 2000; Reid & Zee, 2005).

Conversely, the advanced sleep phase disorder is marked by an advance in the phase of the major sleep period in relation to the desired sleep time and wake-up time. Patients complain of a chronic inability to stay awake and to remain asleep at the desired and socially accepted times. This disorder often manifests as early evening sleepiness, early sleep onset, and spontaneous early morning awakening. If patients are allowed to maintain this advanced schedule, they will have normal quality and duration of sleep. Sleep logs or actigraphy monitoring for a minimum of seven days will demonstrate a recurrent pattern of an advance in the timing of sleep typically between 6 p.m. and 9 p.m. (American Academy of Sleep Medicine, 2005).

Circadian rhythm sleep disorder, free-running type, occurs because the intrinsic circadian pacemaker is not entrained to a 24-hour period or is "free running" with a non-24-hour period (usually longer). Insomnia or excessive sleepiness can result due to the abnormal synchronization between the 24-hour light-dark cycle and the endogenous circadian rhythms. Sleep patterns can be variable, so sleep logs should be maintained for more than 7 days in order to establish this pattern (American Academy of Sleep Medicine, 2005). Most individuals with this nonentrained disorder are blind, and as a result of their blindness, there is a lack of photic input to the circadian pacemaker (Sack, Lewy, Blood, et al., 1992).

The irregular sleep-wake type disorder is characterized by a lack of a clearly defined circadian rhythm of sleep and wakefulness. Sleep logs indicate a variable pattern of sleep and wake periods throughout a 24-hour cycle. Although total sleep time in a 24-hour period is normal, these patients complain of chronic fatigue, insomnia or both. Lack of exposure to activity, light, and social schedules, particularly in institutionalized elderly, may be predisposing factors (American Academy of Sleep Medicine, 2005; Pollack & Stokes, 1997).

The criteria for the diagnosis of shift work sleep disorder are insomnia or excessive sleepiness that is temporally associated with a work schedule that overlaps the usual time for sleep. Furthermore, these symptoms must be present for at least one month. This disorder is most commonly reported with night or early morning shifts. Total sleep time is shortened by one to four hours in these patients. This disorder can occur despite attempts to optimize environmental conditions for sleep (American Academy of Sleep Medicine, 2005; APA, 2000). Besides fatigue, alertness can be seriously impaired. This has significant implications for occupational performance and safety (Akerstedt, 2003).

Jet lag disorder is related to a temporary mismatch between the timing of the sleep-wake cycle generated by the endogenous circadian clock and that of the sleep-wake cycle required by travel to a different time zone. Diagnostic criteria require that this transmeridian jet travel across two time zones causes insomnia or EDS. Moreover, there should be impairment of daytime function, general malaise, or somatic complaints within two days after travel (American Academy of Sleep Medicine, 2005). The direction of travel and the number of time zones crossed affect the severity of symptoms. Eastward travel, requiring advancing sleep-wake hours, is usually more problematic than westward travel.

Circadian rhythm sleep disorder due to a medical condition results in an aberrant sleep-wake cycle that produces EDS or insomnia. An underlying medical or neurological disorder primarily accounts for this altered sleep-wake cycle. Parkinson's disease, dementia, and hepatic encephalopathy are common culprits of this disorder. Circadian rhythm sleep disorder due to a drug or substance is self-explanatory. Alcohol, street drugs, and prescribed medications are included within this group. Lastly, other circadian rhythm sleep disorder (unspecified) is diagnosed when the patient's symptoms meet the criteria described previously (insomnia or EDS). In addition, this misalignment of the sleep-wake cycle cannot be better explained by another type of circadian rhythm sleep disorder or be the result of a drug or substance (American Academy of Sleep Medicine, 2005; APA, 2000).

Estimates of the prevalence of delayed sleep phase type (DSPT) vary widely. The revised International Classification of Sleep Disorders (ICSD-2) states that approximately 10% of patients with chronic insomnia who present to sleep clinics have DSPT (American Academy of Sleep Medicine, 2005). A recent study of middle-aged subjects found the prevalence of subjective complaints of DSPT-like symptoms was 3.1% (Ando, Kripke, & Ancoli-Israel, 2002). However, a study of Norwegian subjects found an occurrence rate of 0.17% (Schrader, Bovim, & Sand, 1993). The discrepancies between these results could be explained by the different study methodologies employed by the researchers. While the actual prevalence of DSPT in the general population is uncertain, it is clear that adolescents are more likely to be affected by this disorder. The reported prevalence in adolescents is from 7% to 16% (Pelayo, Thorpy, & Govinski, 1988; Regestein & Monk, 1995). Both genders are equally affected.

The prevalence of advanced sleep phase type (ASPT) in the general population is also scarcely noted in the literature. However, ASPT is thought to be less common than DSPT with a reported prevalence of 1% of middle-aged adults (Ando, Kripke, & Ancoli-Israel, 1995). Contrary to DSPT, the presence of this disorder seems to increase with age. No gender predilection has been observed.

It is estimated that 20% of the workforce in industrialized nations is employed in jobs that require shift work. Thus, the prevalence of shift work sleep disorder is directly proportional to the percentage of the population that is involved in shift work. Estimates suggest the prevalence of shift work sleep disorder to be 2% to 5% (American Academy of Sleep Medicine, 2005; Akerstedt, 2003)

Based on a review of the literature, Asian ethnicity does not appear to be a risk factor for DSPT in adults. A study of the prevalence of DSPT in Japanese adults found that 0.13% of the study population was affected by this disorder (Yazaki, Shirakawa, Okawa, et al., 1999). Similar to Western nations, Eastern Asian adolescents are more affected than adults. Studies of adolescents in Hong Kong and Taiwan indicate a similar prevalence rate to Caucasian subjects (Chung & Cheung, 2008; Gau, Soong, & Merikangas, 2004). However, studies that have evaluated preadolescents have noted a disturbing trend in Asian children. For example, a study comparing preadolescent children in the United States and China found that the Chinese students slept one hour less per night. Furthermore, the Chinese subjects were more likely to experience daytime sleepiness and other sleep problems (Liu, Liu, Owens, et al., 2005). The literature also suggests that Korean preadolescents and adolescents have a higher prevalence of later onset sleep and sleep deprivation as compared to other Eastern Asian and Western populations. Yang et al., stated that Korean children do not get adequate sleep and they have profound discrepancies in their sleep-wake cycles between school and weekend nights. In fact, this study indicated that the Korean children had 100 minutes less of sleep time than that of their American peers. This sleep time was also significantly less than the reported sleep time for Japanese and Chinese children (Yang, Kim, Patel, et al., 2005).

Epidemiologic studies of shift work sleep disorder and other circadian rhythm disorders indicate that Eastern Asian or Asian Americans are not at an increased risk of developing these disorders (Doi, 2005). Rather, their prevalence rates are similar and most likely related to other etiologic factors besides ethnicity.

Current *DSM-IV* nosology for diagnosing circadian rhythm sleep disorders may be flawed in identifying this disorder in Asians. As compared to the other sleep disorders, the current system may underestimate this disorder, as demonstrated in the study of sleep-wake patterns in Korean adolescents (Yang, Kim, Patel, et al., 2005). Diagnosis requires a misalignment of endogenous circadian rhythms from the pattern that is considered the social norm. Furthermore, the patient must complain of EDS that significantly impacts the quality of life. This is problematic in Korean culture, since these patients are less likely to complain of EDS or fatigue. In addition, delaying or limiting sleep time may not be considered abnormal behavior. In this subgroup, total sleep time should be considered in the diagnostic criteria. A better diagnostic system may allow for early intervention and a potential paradigm shift regarding healthy sleep habits.

Parasomnias

Parasomnias are events that occur as one falls asleep, is asleep, or has an arousal from sleep. They are classified into disorders of arousal (from NREM sleep), those usually associated with REM sleep, and others. Disorders of arousal from NREM sleep include confusional arousals, sleepwalking, and sleep terrors. The parasomnias usually associated with REM sleep include REM sleep behavior disorder (RBD), recurrent isolated sleep paralysis, and nightmare disorder. A discussion of other less classical parasomnias, including sleep related dissociative disorders, sleep enuresis, sleep related groaning (catathrenia), exploding head syndrome, sleep related hallucinations, sleep related eating disorder, unspecified parasomnias, and those due to a drug or medical condition, is beyond the scope of this chapter (American Academy of Sleep Medicine, 2005; APA, 2000).

A confusional arousal is confused behavior or mentation during sleep or after an arousal from sleep. Classically, this phenomenon occurs out of slow wave sleep, which predominates in the first third of the night; however, this disorder can also occur when an individual is awakened from sleep in the morning. There is a blunted response to questions, slow speech, impaired mentation with retrograde and anterograde amnesia, and disorientation to place and time. Over a period of minutes to hours, one's behavior may be inappropriate, resistive, or violent; it may be simple or complex (Mahowald & Cramer Bornemann, 2005).

Sleepwalking occurs as an arousal out of slow wave sleep and consists of walking while judgment is impaired and consciousness is altered. Events typically occur in the first third of the night. The individual may sit upright and appear confused, ambulate, or bolt out of bed. While sleepwalking the person usually has a blank, staring face and is relatively unresponsive to the efforts of others to communicate with him or her. It may be challenging to awaken the sleepwalker, he or she may appear confused upon arousal, he or she may manifest amnesia for the event, his or her behavior may be inappropriate or dangerous, or he or she may engage in routine behavior at an inappropriate time. Within several minutes after awakening from the sleepwalking episode, there is no impairment of mental activity or behavior. *DSM-IV* diagnostic criteria also require that this disorder results in significant impairment of social, occupational, or other important areas of functioning (APA, 2000).

Diagnosis of sleep terror is defined as an arousal from slow wave sleep with a hallmark scream or cry and behavioral and autonomic nervous system manifestations of fear. Skin flushing, diaphoresis, increased muscle tone, tachypnea, tachycardia, and mydriasis may occur. It can be difficult to awaken the individual. If he or she does wake up, the sleepwalker is confused and amnestic. Their behavior may be violent (APA, 2000).

RBD is diagnosed on polysomnography when the individual is in REM sleep but manifests atonia with elevated submental tone or EMG twitching. In reporting the episodes to a clinician, the patient with RBD describes behavior that is violent, caused injury, or was disruptive. No evidence of seizure or other explanation is apparent in RBD.

Recurrent isolated sleep paralysis is an inability to move the limbs and trunk as one falls asleep or awakens from sleep. The events are brief, lasting only a few seconds or minutes; they may occur only once in a lifetime or multiple times a year. There is no other supporting evidence of narcolepsy in these individuals. Being touched or spoken to may terminate the event. Consciousness is preserved, and respiration is normal (American Academy of Sleep Medicine, 2005).

Nightmare disorder involves waking up with clear recollection of a dream. The individual may be anxious, fearful, sad, or angry, but not confused. There may be difficulty returning to sleep. The nightmare occurs in the latter half of the sleep period (APA, 2000).

The prevalence of sleepwalking in children ranges from 1% to 17% peaking at 8 to 12 years of age. There is no significant sex difference in childhood sleepwalking. The reported prevalence of sleepwalking in adults is 4% (Hublin, Kaprio, Partinen, et al., 1997; Ohayon, Guilleminault, Priest, et al., 1999; Klackenberg, 1982). In adults, sleepwalking associated with violence or injury is more common in men. Genetic factors and familial patterns appear to exert an influence on the prevalence of this disorder. The rate of childhood sleepwalking is 60% if both parents are affected. In fact, twin studies have implicated genetic factors in 65% of cases of sleepwalking (Hublin, Kaprio, Partinen, et al., 1997). Genetic factors appear to play a role in sleep terrors as well. The reported prevalence of sleep terrors is 1% to 6.5% in children and 2.2% in adults (Simonds & Parraga, 1982).

RBD has a strong male predilection. This disorder typically emerges after the age of 50 years. The exact prevalence of this disorder is unknown; however a recent survey estimated the prevalence to be 0.5% of the population (Ohayon, Caulet, & Priest, 1997). An overwhelming risk factor appears to be an underlying neurologic condition, particularly Parkinsonism.

Nightmares are more prevalent in childhood with 30% to 90% of this group admitting to occasional nightmares. Furthermore, 10% to 50% of children aged 3 to 5 years have nightmares severe enough to disturb their parents. The prevalence decreases in adulthood. However, a majority of the general population will recall an occasional nightmare. Estimates suggest the prevalence of nightmare disorder in the adult population is 2% to 8% (American Academy of Sleep Medicine, 2005; Nielsen & Zadra, 2005).

Eastern Asian populations are not at an increased risk for the development of a parasomnia as compared to Western populations. The epidemiology of these disorders are similar and confirms previously know risk factors, specifically age, gender, genetics, and neurologic conditions (Gau & Soong, 1995). However, there is not a wealth of data examining these disorders in Asian populations. Conversely, studies examining the health of Vietnamese immigrants in the Unites States demonstrated that the Vietnamese Americans had a higher incidence of nightmares, depression, and stress (Tran, 1993). In addition, many of these immigrants suffer from post-traumatic stress disorder (PTSD) suffered in childhood in their native country. Since PTSD is strongly associated with nightmares, the incidence of nightmare disorder may be higher in this population.

The *DSM-IV* criteria for diagnosis of parasomnia are valid in Asians. Rather, it is the screening evaluations and awareness of this disorder, in at risk groups, which needs to be improved.

Sleep Related Movement Disorders

Sleep related movement disorders are characterized by relatively simple movements that disturb sleep. Nocturnal sleep disturbance or complaints of EDS are required to make these diagnoses (American Academy of Sleep Medicine, 2005). There are several types of disorders within this category; however this discussion will focus on restless leg syndrome (RLS).

According to the revised International Classification of Sleep Disorders (ICSD-2), RLS is a sensorimotor disorder in which the key component is an irresistible urge to move the legs (American Academy of Sleep Medicine, 2005). For centuries, this sleep-related movement disorder has been recognized. However, it was not until 1945 that Ekbom named this phenomenon and detailed its characteristics (Ekbom, 1945). The International Restless Legs Syndrome Study Group (IRLSSG) has further standardized the definition (Allen, Picchietti, Hening, et al., 2003).

Four criteria define RLS. The first is an overwhelming desire to move the legs, but patients may also have an unpleasant and uncomfortable feeling in the legs. The arms may also be involved. Patients have described the sensation as a creeping or tingling feeling. Next, this urge to move or the uncomfortable feelings occur or are exacerbated when the individual is sedentary. When one is physically immobile or cognitively inactive, the restless legs sensations are noticeable. Third, moving, walking, and stretching alleviate the symptom, either entirely or partially; however, the feeling returns upon cessation of such activity. Finally, patients appreciate this disorder in the evening more so than during the day.

Epidemiologic studies initially estimated that about 5% to 15% of Western adult populations had symptoms of RLS (Lavigne & Montplaisir, 1994; Phillips, Young, Finn, et al., 2000). But more recent studies, which required the presence of all four diagnostic criteria of RLS, demonstrated that the actual prevalence of this disorder is 7% to 10% of the adult population (Rothdach, Trenkwalder, Haberstock, et al., 2000; Ulfberg, Nystrom, Carter, et al., 2001; Ulfber, Nystrom, Carter, et al., 2001; Allen, Walters, Montplaisir, et al., 2005; Berger, Luedemann, Trenkwalder, et al., 2004). Older age and female gender were identified as risk factors.

It appears that the prevalence of RLS in Asian populations is lower than in Caucasian populations. A self-administered questionnaire conducted among 4,612 Japanese individuals examined for symptoms suggestive of RLS and periodic limb movement disorder (PLMD) found that 3% of women aged 20–29 years old had symptoms suggestive of RLS and PLMD, whereas 7% of women aged 50–59 answered affirmatively to the questionnaire. In contrast to American and European studies, Japanese men appeared to have a higher prevalence of RLS than women, and the men had no positive correlation with age. It should be emphasized that this study did not inquire about RLS alone, nor were the 4 diagnostic criteria considered requisite for a positive answer (Kageyama, Kabuto, Nitta, et al., 2000).

When a study in Singapore applied the IRLSSG criteria, the prevalence of RLS in the younger cohorts was found to be 0.1% and 0.6% in the older cohorts (Tan, Seah, See, et al., 2001). A study of 5,000 Korean adults showed that 3.9% met the criteria for definite RLS and 3.6% had probable RLS; the prevalence of RLS was more prevalent in Korean women (4.4%) than in Korean men (3.3%) (Cho, Shin, Yun, et al., 2008).

Although about 80% of patients with RLS demonstrate PLMD on polysomnography, PLMD has been observed in multiple other conditions, including Huntington's chorea, amyotrophic lateral sclerosis, chronic myelopathies, stiff man syndrome, uremia, and sleep apnea. Periodic limb movements are repetitive, highly stereotyped movements that occur during sleep. Classically, they involve extension of the great toe and may also occur with partial hip, knee, and ankle flexion.

Standardization of the diagnostic criteria for RLS established by the IRLSSG has provided a reliable, reproducible system that is applicable to all populations. Thus, these guidelines for the diagnosis of RLS in Asian populations are valid. One criterion included in the diagnosis is the sensory component of an unpleasant sensation in the leg. In several studies it was observed that some patients did not perceive this sensory component, which may lead to a false negative response. This was found in both European and Asian studies. Therefore, the current diagnostic criteria are appropriate and effective in identifying this disorder in Asians. However, the epidemiologic studies of RLS in Asians confirmed a common theme noted in the study of most sleep disorders in this population (Cho, Shin, Yun, et al., 2008; J. Kim, Choi, Shin, et al., 2005). Namely that RLS is underdiagnosed in Asians and those that are affected are less likely to seek treatment as compared to Western populations.

Isolated Symptoms, Apparently Normal Variants, and Other Sleep Disorders

This section will briefly discuss these two categories of sleep disorders. Within the rubric of isolated symptoms, apparently normal variants includes: long sleeper and short sleeper. There are other disorders within this group; however they are beyond the scope of this chapter. The common theme of these disorders is symptoms that lie at the borderline between normal and abnormal sleep. Long sleeper refers to patients who sleep more than 10 hours a day. In children this has to be modified to sleep that exceed age appropriate sleep times. EDS occurs when the patient fails to get this amount of sleep. Conversely, a short sleeper typically sleeps less than 5 hours a day. Simple snoring is included within this group if there is no association with insomnia or EDS. Furthermore, snoring associated with OSA in not included within this diagnosis. Long sleep time affects approximately 1.5% of the population. Short sleep has been noted in 3.6% to 4.3% of the population (American Academy of Sleep Medicine, 2005; National Sleep Foundation, 2003). The prevalence of short sleepers and long sleepers is similar in Asian populations. Although, epidemiologic population-based studies in Asian groups is quite limited (Utsugi, Saijo, Yoshioka, et al., 2005).

Other sleep disorders refer to those diagnoses that do not fit within the criteria assigned to the other sleep disorders previously discussed. Two of these disorders are other physiologic (organic) sleep disorder and environmental sleep disorder. The former term refers to a disorder that is related to a physiologic or medical condition that has yet to be determined. The latter is diagnosed when environmental factors lead to insomnia or EDS (American Academy of Sleep Medicine, 2005). The prevalence of these disorders is unknown.

The diagnostic criteria used to confirm long sleepers and short sleep is objective. Thus, this method is suitable for use in Asian populations. In addition, diagnosis of other sleep disorders is somewhat vague, and no definitive criteria have been established for any population. Essentially, they are diagnoses of exclusion.

PERSPECTIVES ON THE CAUSES OF SLEEP DISORDERS IN ASIANS

Insomnia

Insomnia can be described as a state of hyperarousal. This heightened level of arousal can interfere with the initiation or maintenance of sleep. Biological, psychological, and social models have been proposed as potential etiologies of this disorder. A review of these models indicates that insomnia is not likely to be defined by a single factor. Rather, this disorder is complex and related to multiple influences (genetic, behavioral, and cognitive).

Both genetic and neuroendocrine factors have been implicated as biologic models for the development of insomnia. With the exception of fatal familial insomnia, little is known about the specific genes that are potentially involved in this disorder. However, many studies have asserted a genetic vulnerability for insomnia (Beaulieu-Bonneau, LeBlanc, Mérette, et al., 2007; Watson, Goldberg, Arguelles, et al., 2006). One such study reported that 48.8% of its subjects determined to have insomnia had a first-degree relative that was affected by this disorder (Yves, Morin, Cervena, et al., 2003). Asian ethnicity does not increase genetic susceptibility to insomnia.

Activation of the hypothalamic-pituitary-adrenal (HPA) axis has been suggested as a potential neuroendocrine etiology of insomnia. This model proposes that acute stress stimulates the HPA axis and the sympathetic nervous system resulting in the release of cortisol and epinephrine. Elevated levels of cortisol, adrenocorticotropic hormone and epinephrine have been documented in patients with insomnia. However, it is unclear if these neuroendocrine findings cause insomnia or if they are the results of chronic insomnia (Perlis, Smith, & Pigeon, 2005). Consequently, this model alone does not fully explain the etiology of insomnia. These findings have not been studied in Asian populations.

Potential psychological etiologies of insomnia are the cognitive and behavioral models. The primary tenet of the cognitive model is that worry or rumination causes a state of hyperarousal that interferes with sleep. Worry and rumination can predispose one to insomnia and furthermore they can precipitate and perpetuate this disorder. Those individuals who are prone to these tendencies are more apt to react to life stressors. Furthermore, these patients are less able to effectively cope with mild stressors as compared to people who do not have high trait levels of cognitive arousal. The behavioral model of insomnia describes certain behaviors that are incompatible with sleep. This theory is supported, in part, due to the fact that many insomnia treatment modalities are aimed at modifying behaviors that are not conducive to sleep (Perlis, Smith, & Pigeon, 2005). Both the poor sleep hygiene model and the Spielman model have been proposed as behavioral sources of insomnia. Spielman's model postulates that acute insomnia is the consequence of life stressors and the presence of high trait levels for worry or rumination. In addition, the chronic form of insomnia develops as a result of maladaptive coping strategies (Spielman, Caruso, & Glovinsky, 1987).

Psychological models of insomnia have been well studied in Asian populations. While ethnicity does not increase the predisposition for traits that are associated with insomnia, life stressors in Asian groups have been implicated in behaviors associated with insomnia. In particular, work related stress and the drive to excel in the workplace have been identified as significant sources of insomnia (Utsugi, Saijo, Yoshioka, et al., 2005). The impacts of a stressful lifestyle and behaviors that are not conducive to sleep have been demonstrated in Asian adolescents and adults. In fact, children experience similar stress to perform in school as adults do in the workplace. Kaneita et al. found that insomnia in Japanese adolescents is common and is related to behaviors intended to succeed in school (Kaneita, Ohida, Osaki, et al., 2006). This model of insomnia applies quite well to both Eastern Asian and Asian American populations. The majority of studies have been performed in Japanese subjects. Most likely based on the fact that Japan has been an industrialized nation for many years, the effects of work stress have been well documented. As the other Asian countries become more industrialized, similar work related stress and insomnia would be expected.

The concept of a psychosocial model as an etiology for insomnia certainly fits well in an attempt to understand this disorder in Asians. Asia is becoming more industrialized, and this is fundamentally changing the social structures of these countries. More emphasis is placed on performance in school and work. Asian cultures often link achievement at work or school with personal identity. Thus, sleep becomes less important in the pursuit of success. Behaviors that are detrimental to sleep such as long work hours and early wake times are rewarded. Consequently, the current societal norms regarding sleep and work must be reevaluated. Furthermore, unemployment, lower socioeconomic status, physical inactivity, alcohol consumption, poor interpersonal relationships, and marital status are social risk factors associated with insomnia (R. Li, Wing, Ho, et al., 2002; K. Kim, Uchiyama, Okawa, et al., 2000; Tachibana, Izumi, Honda, et al., 1996). While these factors are present in all populations, it is likely to be more relevant to Asian American immigrant populations. This group is more likely to experience poverty, divorce, weak support systems, substance abuse, psychiatric disorders, and difficulties acclimating to a new culture and environment (Tran, 1993). Two studies have examined the sleep patterns of Korean Americans and Japanese Americans and found that difficulties in adjusting to a new social culture alone could precipitate insomnia (Barbar, Enright, Boyle, et al., 2000; Sok, 2008). Thus, this social model fits well in defining the etiology of insomnia in both Eastern Asians and Asian Americans. The most striking weakness appears to be the lack of education regarding the prevalence of this disorder in this population. Further effort is needed in identifying at-risk patients and more importantly assisting these patients in seeking treatment.

Sleep-Related Breathing Disorders

The etiology of primary central sleep apnea is unknown. However, various etiologic models have been proposed for OSA. The biologic basis for this disorder is related to excess body weight, anatomical abnormalities, genetic factors, and decreased neuromotor tone of the upper airway. It has long been recognized that obesity is the strongest risk factor for OSA (Young, Palta, Dempsey, et al., 1993; Young, Peppard, & Gottlieb, 2002). Central obesity, large neck circumference, and enlarged pharyngeal fat pads can result from excessive weight and contribute to airway collapse. Clearly, the anatomic hypothesis for this disorder is extensively supported in the literature. Craniofacial morphology affects both the bony and soft tissue structures of the pharyngeal airway. Certain abnormalities are known to predispose patients to OSA, particularly in Asians, by reducing upper airway patency. Namely, mandibular retrognathia, a shortened cranial base, and a narrow nasion-sella-basion angle have been associated with OSA in Asians (Lam, Ip, Tench, et al., 2005; Schwab, 2003; Schwab, Pasirstein, Pierson, et al., 2003). Genetic studies have lagged behind those of other common medical disorders, however recent literature provides an undeniable observation that the development of OSA is related to genetic and familial factors. In fact, the heritability of OSA in first-degree relatives of affected patients is estimated to by 35% to 40% (Redline, 2005). Furthermore, genetics can influence body weight, craniofacial morphology, and ventilatory control mechanisms, which may enhance one's susceptibility to OSA (Redline & Tishler, 2000; Arens & Marcus, 2004). Thus, development of OSA is unlikely to be related to single loci, but rather due to a multifactorial genetic influence. Lastly, decreased neuromotor tone of the pharyngeal musculature has been implicated as a biologic etiology of OSA. While this mechanism is not clearly understood, it is hypothesized that OSA patients may have decreased neuromotor tone of the upper airway muscles during sleep, which restricts airway patency (D'Avanzo, 1997).

Social factors play a role in the etiology of OSA. Alcohol and tobacco use are known to have a detrimental effect on sleep. These substances can precipitate or exacerbate SRBD. The prevalence of alcohol abuse in Asians is generally less common as compared to Caucasians. Yet, immigrant Asian American groups may be at greater risk for substance abuse due to psychological and social stressors. Lamentably, there is a critical shortage of culturally appropriate treatment and intervention programs as the prevalence of substance misuse increases in these populations (Wetter, Young, Bidwell, et al., 1994). Smokers have an odds ratio that is 4-fold greater than those who never smoke for having at least moderate OSA (Yang, Fan, Tan, et al., 1999). This is a major public health concern for Asian populations, especially China. China is the world's largest producer and consumer of tobacco products. The prevalence of smoking continues to rise in China as do the associated health risks (Choi, Rankin, Stewart, et al., 2008). Another worrisome trend is the prevalence of smoking in Asian American immigrants. Southeast Asian immigrants appear to be the most at risk group. A study of acculturation in these immigrants revealed that acculturated men had a reduced risk of smoking, while acculturated women were more likely to smoke than traditional women (Wu, Zhou, Tao, et al., 2002). Immediate smoking cessation and education initiatives are needed to eliminate this completely preventable risk factor.

Lastly, a discussion of the etiological models of OSA would be incomplete without further examining the impact of obesity on Asian populations. The biologic basis for the link between obesity and OSA has been previously mentioned. However, psychological and social etiologic models may exist as well. It is noted that Asians have a lower prevalence of obesity than Americans. Yet, the prevalence of obesity is steadily increasing in Asia. This is probably directly related to social changes in the populations. China is the prime example of how social changes are influencing a higher prevalence of obesity and OSA. In Beijing, the average BMI of both adults and children has significantly increased over the past ten years. This has coincided with emergence of China as a world financial power and an urbanization of its previous agrarian population. The rise of the middle class and unparalleled economic growth has fundamentally changed the Chinese lifestyle and increased this population's susceptibility to obesity and OSA (Wu, Zhou, Tao, et al., 2002; Ke-You & Da-Wei, 2001).

Hypersomnias Not Due to a Sleep-Related Breathing Disorder

The etiology of narcolepsy with cataplexy is best explained by a biologic model. Genetic, autoimmune, environmental, and familial modes of transmission have been suggested. The tendency for narcolepsy to have a familial tendency has long been recognized (Mignot, 1998; Guilleminault, Mignot, & Grumet, 1989; Chen, Fong, Lam, et al., 2007). A review of the literature indicates the familial risk of first-degree relatives for narcolepsy is 10–280 times higher than the prevalence in the general population (Chen, Fong, Lam, et al., 2007). A similar prevalence was noted by Mignot, who described a 1% to 2% risk for the development of narcolepsy-cataplexy in first-degree relatives (Mignot, 1998). In recent decades, the identification of human leukocyte antigen (HLA) DQB1*0602 in narcolepsy-cataplexy patients has supported a genetic mode of transmission for this disorder. It has been hypothesized that the genetic contribution of HLA DQB1*0602 increases susceptibility in the Japanese population. In fact, 6% of DQB1*0602 homozygotes in Japan could have narcolepsy-cataplexy as compared to only 0.6% in Caucasians (Mignot, Lin, Rogers, et al., 2001). However, genetic factors other than HLA-DQ are thought to be involved in narcolepsy predisposition. For example, genetic studies of Japanese subjects further demonstrated a potentially susceptible gene for narcolepsy-cataplexy on 4q13–23 (Nakayama, Miura, Honda, et al., 2000). An association with tumor necrosis factor-α polymorphism has also been suggested (Wieczorek, Gencik, Rujescu, et al., 2003).

Genetic factors alone cannot explain the biologic etiology of narcolepsy-cataplexy. An autoimmune pathophysiologic mechanism has been asserted as well. An absence or diminished levels of the neuropeptide hypocretin has been observed in narcoleptic patients. Thus, it is hypothesized that an autoimmune alteration of hypocretin-containing cells within the hypothalamus could account for this finding. Environmental factors such as unspecified viral illnesses, head trauma, sustained sleep deprivation, and inflammatory disorders are thought to be potential sources for suppressing hypocretin production (Nishino, Ripley, Overeem, et al., 2000; Mignot, Lammers, Ripley, et al., 2002). Although a single biological model cannot fully explain the etiology of narcolepsy, it provides the most plausible etiology of this disorder in Asian and Caucasian populations. Psychological and social models are not applicable to this disorder.

However, the etiology of behaviorally induced insufficient sleep syndrome (BIISS) can be linked to psychological and social models. Similar to insomnia, this disorder can be precipitated by work-related or social pressure to delay sleep even though the need for sleep is high. A study of Japanese patients with EDS found that 7.1% of these patients met the criteria for BIISS. These models are quite appropriate in Asian populations as societal and cultural norms often expect personal achievement, often at the expense of sleep. Unfortunately, Asian cultures are less likely to perceive insufficient sleep or fatigue as a serious problem. Rather, it is often viewed as an expected consequence of efforts needed to succeed in society. These behaviors are not benign. Besides impaired personal relationships and cognitive function, these patients with BIISS are 22% more likely to be involved in accidents or near-miss accidents (Komada, Inoue, Hayashida, et al., 2007).

Circadian Rhythm Sleep Disorders

Biological or genetic models have been suggested as an etiology for delayed and advanced sleep phase type. Alterations in the circadian clock genes hPer3 and hPer2 have been associated with DSPT and ASPT disorders respectively (American Academy of Sleep Medicine, 2005). The genetic influence on the development of these disorders is poorly understood, and no genetic predisposition is noted in Asian populations.

Psychosocial models of the etiology of these disorders best explain their occurrence in Asian populations. This includes cultural, economic, parental, and environmental pressures that can alter or shift circadian rhythms. For example, Korean society has a strong tradition of Confucianism, in which academic success is linked to family honor and personal identity. Consequently, a strong emphasis is placed on education, and performance on college entrance examinations is paramount. Thus, delayed or restricted sleep time may not be perceived as contrary to the societal norm by Korean students. In addition, they are less likely to complain of fatigue, insomnia, or EDS, as these symptoms may be perceived as normal. Furthermore, Korean parents do not tend to impose strict sleep times on their children if they are engaged in schoolwork. Moreover, Asian countries typically have earlier school start times as compared to Western societies (Liu, Liu, Owens, et al., 2005; Yang, Kim, Patel, et al., 2005). Carskadon et al. found that these early start times directly conflict with normal circadian rhythms of children (Carskadon, Wolfson, Acebo, et al., 1998). Besides academic pressures, as Internet access and television have become more accessible to Asian children, this has resulted in additional environmental stimuli that disrupt sleep. Similar findings have been documented in Chinese and Japanese subjects.

These social models for circadian rhythm sleep disorders in children have been confirmed for shift work disorder in adult Asians. Essentially, the same pressures to succeed in school will translate to the workplace. This disorder is more prevalent in industrialized nations, where shift work is more common.

Parasomnias

The exact mechanism of the parasomnias is unknown; however genetic factors clearly contribute to the etiology of this disorder. Sleepwalking, sleep terrors, and confusional arousals are associated with a genetic susceptibility. The HLA DQB1 gene has been linked to sleepwalking (Lecendreux, Bassetti, Dauvilliers, et al., 2003). Other biological mechanisms that may contribute to these disorders are sleep inertia and sleep state instability. Furthermore, these disorders of arousal may be triggered by different sleep disorders (OSA), medications, pregnancy, menstruation, hypothyroidism, or other hormonal factors. However, none of these etiologies can fully account for the prevalence of the parasomnias. Asians do not appear to have an increased biological susceptibility to these disorders as compared to other groups.

Psychological and social models contribute to the etiology of the parasomnias as well. Sleep deprivation and emotional and physical stress are known to evoke these disorders. However, social factors unique to Asian cultures do not predispose individuals belonging to these cultures to the parasomnias. It would be intuitive to assume that since sleep deprivation is common in Asia then these disorders should be more prevalent in Asian populations. Yet, epidemiologic studies have failed to confirm this assumption.

However, these psychosocial models may be more appropriate when applied to Asian American groups. Vietnamese immigrants are known to be more likely to suffer from PTSD and nightmares (Tran, 1993). In addition immigrants are more likely to have lower socioeconomic status, poorer health, and less access to health care, which can further predispose one to stress and PTSD. Simply attempting to acclimate to unfamiliar surroundings can be an etiology of the parasomnias. Regrettably, this group tends to lack the social and family support systems to cope with these eliciting factors.

Sleep Related Movement Disorders—Restless Leg Syndrome

The etiology of RLS is best explained by a biological model. RLS can be primary or secondary. Primary RLS most likely has an autosomal dominant mode of inheritance and a heritability of about 50%. Although no gene mutation has been established, five gene loci have been mapped in primary RLS to chromosomes 12q12–21 (RLS1), 14q13–21 (RLS2), 9p24–22 (RLS3), 2q33 (RLS4), and 20p13 (RLS5) (Desautels, Turecki, Montplaisir, et al., 2001; Bonati, Ferini-Strambi, Aridon, et al., 2003; Chen, Ondo, Rao, et al., 2004; Pichler, Marroni, Volpato, et al., 2006; Levchenko, Provost, Montplaisir, et al., 2006), and PLMS have been linked to chromosome 6p. Pharmacologic studies have suggested a possible endogenous opiate system dysfunction as a potential etiology of RLS, however no concrete evidence has been found to support this hypothesis (Montplaisir, Lorrain, & Godbout, 1991).

RLS can be secondary to other medical conditions, psychiatric disorders, and medications. Iron deficiency, in which the ferritin is less than 50 ng/ml, peripheral neuropathy, radiculopathy, renal failure, pregnancy (typically in the third trimester and associated with folate or iron deficiency), heart disease, hypertension, rheumatoid arthritis, and fibromyalgia are all associated with secondary RLS. Depression, anxiety, and attention deficit hyperactivity disorder are psychiatric conditions that occur with RLS. Medications that have been associated with this disorder include antipsychotics, antidepressants (excluding bupropion), antihistamines, and dopamine blocking agents (like neuroleptics, metoclopramide, and antiemetics).

The current method of defining the etiology of RLS is applicable to Asian populations. No identifiable psychological or social etiology has been defined in the literature. However, little is known about the etiology of this disorder, and further research is needed in this area. It appears that Asians tend be less affected by this disorder. However, the question remains if there is a protective mechanism associated with Asian ethnicity, or is RLS simply under reported in this group.

TREATING SLEEP DISORDERS IN ASIANS

Insomnia

The biological treatment for insomnia entails pharmacological therapies. Although sleep aids may be beneficial in the acute setting, there is the concern for dependency and eventual lack of efficacy for chronic cases. Thus, psychological treatment modalities should be explored by the clinician when confronted with insomnia in their practice.

Flurazepam and quazepam are long-acting benzodiazepines approved by the Food and Drug Administration for insomnia, but their risks of cognitive deficits and daytime somnolence preclude their use in general practice. An intermediate-acting benzodiazepine, like temazepam, can also result in EDS. Improvement in insomnia without the associated risk of tolerance has been achieved with an intermediate-acting nonbenzodiazepine benzodiazepine-receptor agonist called eszopiclone, although patients have reported an unpleasant taste and morning drowsiness (Krystal, Walsh, Laska, et al., 2003). Sleep maintenance insomnia has also shown response to controlled-release zolpidem. Sleep onset insomnia may respond to zolpidem (a nonbenzodiazepine benzo-diazepine-receptor agonist) and triazolam, both of which are short-acting. Somnambulism has been reported with zolpidem (Morgenthaler & Silber, 2002). Anterograde amnesia and rebound insomnia upon withdrawal of triazolam have both been noted with this benzodiazepine. Zaleplon is an ultrashort-acting nonbenzodiazepine benzodiazepine-receptor agonist used for sleep onset insomnia. Since its half-life is 1 hour, a patient may be able to take a dose halfway through the night to treat sleep maintenance insomnia as long as they can devote another 4 hours to sleep (Walsh, Pollak, Scharf, et al., 2000). Mild sleep onset insomnia may respond to ramelteon, a melatonin MT1- and MT2-receptor agonist.

Clinicians have used sedating antidepressants for treatment of primary insomnia. Although less effective than zolpidem, trazodone is often prescribed but can cause hypotension and priapism in men. Amitriptyline, nortriptyline, and doxepin are all tricyclic antidepressants that have been associated with weight gain, daytime sleepiness, cardiac arrhythmias, dry mouth, and postural hypotension.

Patients also have access to over-the-counter sleep aids. Melatonin, diphenhydramine, and the herbal remedy valerian root have been used in the treatment of insomnia. The deleterious effects of alcohol on sleep have been well documented. However, Kaneita et al. found that Japanese subjects who had difficulty maintaining sleep were more apt to use alcohol as a sleep aid than hypnotic medication (Kaneita, Uchiyama, Takemura, et al., 2007). This exposes a trend in Asian populations concerning a lack of education regarding sleep disorders and a reluctance to seek appropriate treatment.

The psychological approach used in the treatment of insomnia involved cognitive behavioral therapy (CBT). The components of CBT include cognitive therapy, sleep-hygiene education, stimulus-control therapy, sleep-restriction therapy, and relaxation therapy. Not all patients necessarily need to implement each component; the therapy is tailored to the individual. Identifying incorrect beliefs about sleep is the core of cognitive therapy (Hauri, 1991). Sleep-hygiene education involves creating an environment conducive to sleep, e.g., a cool temperature and absence of noise and light. Patients are counseled about maintaining regular exercise (but not too close to bedtime) and avoiding caffeine, nicotine, and alcohol. One hour before bedtime, they are advised to relax with activities that are soothing and refrain from watching TV, using the computer, and playing video games. Once they are in bed, they should refrain from watching the clock. To break the conditioned response that the bedroom is associated with wakefulness, stimulus control is implemented. If the patient feels that they are unable to fall asleep in what feels like a reasonable amount of time (approximately 15 minutes), they should get of bed, leave the bedroom, and engage in a quiet activity. For those patients who spend an excessive amount of time in bed, sleep-restriction therapy is utilized. Patients are advised to limit their time in bed (but not less than 5 hours). They maintain a regular bedtime (but do not force themselves into bed at that time if they are not sleepy) and rise time (no matter how little sleep they obtained the previous night) on weekdays and weekends. Over time, the patient will demonstrate increased sleep efficiency with this schedule and can gradually increase their time in bed (by no more than 15 minutes a night). Relaxation therapy comprises both a mental and a physical component. The former entails hypnosis, imagery training, and meditation. The former involves muscle relaxation or biofeedback. This model of treatment is quite appropriate for Asians. In fact, a study examined the cultural compatibility of CBT initially developed in Caucasian populations with that of Chinese values. This study found that a new indigenized therapy was not needed; rather simple structural changes would suffice. Furthermore, the authors proposed that Chinese patients may benefit from challenging their irrational cognitions that are bound up in their strict adherence to social norms (Hodges & Oei, 2007). As stated previously, identifying incorrect beliefs is at the core of CBT.

The social approach to insomnia is supportive of the psychological techniques. If a spouse snores, this could impair the sleep of the patient. The snoring should be evaluated and treated by a physician in order to prevent the couple from sleeping separately, which could be divisive to their marriage. The spouse should also be supportive of the insomniac's needs; for example, they should not insist on watching TV in the bedroom at night when their partner is trying to sleep. The spouse and other family members should encourage the patient to implement CBT.

One social issue that should also be addressed is any economic factors that may be motivating the insomniac to maintain an unproductive sleep schedule. A fear of lack of productivity or an overwhelming sense of responsibility to provide financial support for one's family should be addressed.

In conclusion, insomnia can be a debilitating medical problem with a multitude of etiologies. Recognizing the precipitating and perpetuating factors will be important in management. Although a multitude of pharmacological therapies are available, CBT should be incorporated into the treatment plan.

Sleep-Related Breathing Disorders

Biological modalities are the mainstay of treatment of SRBD. Currently, continuous positive airway pressure (CPAP) is the preferred first-line method of treatment of OSA and the standard to which other modalities are compared. The efficacy of CPAP has clearly been demonstrated and proper use of this device can alleviate the pathophysiological and neurobehavioral sequelae associated with OSA (Sullivan, Issa, Berthon-Jones, et al., 1981; Ballestar, Badia, Hernandez, et al.,

1999). The main challenge physicians encounter with this treatment is patient noncompliance. One key to successful use of CPAP is finding the right interface. A poor fitting mask may make CPAP intolerable. In addition, nasal congestion can be addressed by providing heated humidification. Nonetheless, it is essential for the sleep specialist to regularly follow-up with their patients. This allows the patient to disclose any source of dissatisfaction with their CPAP device or interface. Attentive care of a patient is likely to improve CPAP compliance.

Patient compliance with CPAP varies in the literature depending on the criteria used to define compliance. However, the reported rate of CPAP compliance in Asian patients with OSA has been reported to be about 70% (Hui, Chan, Choy, et al., 2000). This rate is similar to that reported among Caucasians. Yet, compliance with CPAP in Asia is effected by economic and social factors as well. In many Asian countries, the health care systems will not pay for CPAP devices. Thus, patients must finance their treatment themselves, and this may be a deterrent to CPAP use (Lam, Lam, & Ip, 2007).

Surgery is another treatment option, especially for the subset of patients that struggle to comply with CPAP therapy. The aim of surgical treatment is to alleviate upper airway obstruction and its associated neurobehavioral symptoms and morbidities. No longer is a 50% reduction in the AHI deemed acceptable. Rather, the objective is to treat to cure (normalization of respiratory events and elimination of hypoxemia) and to achieve the results typically obtained by CPAP therapy. Upper airway obstruction can occur at the nose, palate, and base of tongue. Often, multilevel obstruction can occur. One must be willing to treat all areas of obstruction in order to achieve a cure. Surgeons have a variety of procedures available within their armamentarium to treat OSA. Selecting the appropriate surgery for a patient can be challenging. However, Riley and Powell have created a two-phase surgical protocol as a logically directed plan to treat the specific areas of upper airway obstruction. This protocol has a success rate of greater than 90% (Sesso, Powell, Riley, et al., 2007). A review of the literature has shown similar outcomes in Asian patients. In particular, studies have demonstrated an improved quality of life in pediatric Asian patients with OSA who underwent adenotonsillectomy (Ye, Li, Liu, et al., 2007). Furthermore, Asian patients may have more access to surgery as it may be covered by national health programs. This treatment modality also accounts for the specific craniofacial anatomical features that predispose Asians to OSA. Thus, surgery can be directed to these anatomical sites.

Oral appliances are an alternative method to treat OSA. The current recommendation from the American Academy of Sleep Medicine is that these devices are only indicated in patients with mild to moderate OSA who cannot tolerate CPAP (Kushida, Morganthaler, Littner, et al., 2006). The most common device is the mandibular repositioning device. Essentially, this device advances the mandible forward to prevent the tongue base from occluding the posterior airway space. The effectiveness of these devices has been measured in Asian populations. A study of Chinese subjects with mild to moderate OSA indicated that they had response rates similar to those in Caucasians (Sam, Lam, Ooi, et al., 2006; Gotsopoulos, Chen, Qian, et al., 2002). Similarly, the cost of these devices and limited access to dental care may limit the availability of oral appliances in less developed Asian countries.

Behavioral modification has been employed in the treatment of OSA. Treatment may consist of weight loss, avoidance of alcohol and sedating medications, and manipulation of body position during sleep. Rarely, are these methods curative, however they can be beneficial

(Guilleminault, 1989; Cartwright, Lloyd, Lilie, et al., 1985). This model of therapy may prove to be beneficial in Asian groups as the incidence of obesity continues to rise. Furthermore, these measures are simple to perform and should be available to a patient of any socioeconomic class.

Although no social model of treatment exists, changes in societal views in Asian countries may improve diagnosis and subsequent treatment. Despite advances in the field of sleep medicine, a majority of those affected with OSA remain undiagnosed. Thus, improved education is required as is access to sleep medicine centers.

Treatment of central sleep apnea is primarily based on a biological model. This model is similar for both Asian and Caucasian populations. Bilevel positive pressure ventilation (BPAP) is an effective therapeutic choice. This has been demonstrated in Japanese patients with Cheyne-Stokes respiration (Kasai, Narui, Dohi, et al., 2005). Additional low-flow oxygen may be beneficial as well. However, the exact mechanism of action in which oxygen improves central apnea is not clear. Furthermore, idiopathic central sleep apnea may respond to acetazolamide administration. Acetazolamide is a carbonic anhydrase inhibitor that causes a metabolic acidosis and leads to a decrease in the frequency of central apneas with an improvement in hypersomnolence. The choice of treatment should be tailored to the specific cause of ventilatory instability (Chan & Kushida, 2007).

Hypersomnias Not Due to a Sleep-Related Breathing Disorder

This section will focus on the treatment of narcolepsy with cataplexy. Narcolepsy is incurable and therefore requires lifelong treatment. The biological method of treating this disorder relies primarily on pharmacologic therapy, although there is a role for behavioral therapy. Most patients require several medications to control both the daytime sleepiness and the cataplexy. The goal of treatment is to control the narcoleptic symptoms and allow the patient to maintain an active life, while limiting side effects and tolerance to medications.

Stimulants, such as dextroamphetamine and methylphenidate, were traditionally used to treat EDS. These medications are effective in improving somnolence, however they have no effect on cataplexy. Significant adverse effects associated with these medications include headaches, irritability, insomnia, gastrointestinal upset, and cardiovascular stimulation. A small risk of addiction exists. Drug tolerance can occur. Recently, modafinil has become the first-line treatment of EDS in most patients. Modafinil is chemically unrelated to the stimulants and is not associated with rebound hypersomnolence as are the CNS stimulants. Modafinil's exact mechanism of action is unknown; however it acts in part on the histaminergic system. The main benefit of this drug is its relative lack of side effects. Modafinil has no blood pressure effects and is not addictive (Black & Guilleminault, 2001).

Sodium oxybate (GHB) is a naturally occurring metabolite of the human nervous system found primarily in the basal ganglia and hypothalamus. This medication is also effective in the treatment of EDS in narcoleptic patients. In addition, sodium oxybate has proven to have a beneficial effect on cataplexy (Thorpy, 2007). The mechanism of action is related to the inhibition of several neurotransmitters, including dopamine, GABA, and glutamate. Furthermore, sodium oxybate has been found to reduce nocturnal awakenings, increase stages 3 and 4 sleep, and consolidate

REM sleep periods. As mentioned, this medication significantly reduces cataplexy without the development of tolerance. It also has the benefit of no rebound cataplexy upon sudden cessation of treatment. Side effects are typically mild and consist of nausea, vomiting, enuresis, and dizziness. In fact, patients tend to prefer this drug to other anticataplectic drugs because of the milder side effects (Xyrem® International Study Group, 2005). Its potential for abuse restricts its availability through a centralized pharmacy.

Classically, the tricyclic antidepressants (TCAs) and the selective serotonin reuptake inhibitors (SSRIs) have been used to manage cataplexy. While effective, use of the TCAs is often limited by significant atropinic adverse effects. The TCAs can cause sexual dysfunction, tachycardia, dry mouth, urinary retention, and constipation. The SSRIs (fluoxetine) are more commonly used to treat cataplexy due to less adverse reactions. Similar to the TCAs, the SSRIs block presynaptic neurotransmitter reuptake, but with greater specificity for serotonin. Sexual dysfunction can be associated with these medications as well. Like the TCAs, abruptly discontinuing these medications can result in severe rebound cataplexy. Atypical antidepressants, such as venlafaxine have also been reported to successfully treat cataplexy (Xyrem® International Study Group, 2005).

Behavioral approaches to the treatment of narcolepsy-cataplexy are typically insufficient to effectively manage the symptoms of this disorder. However, they can be beneficial for certain patients. Strategies include maintaining regular sleep times, avoiding heavy meals and alcohol intake, and strategically timed naps. Furthermore, patients can be referred to support groups (Narcolepsy Network) to enhance their social support systems. In addition, career counseling is important for patients and their employers. This would include avoiding shift work and driving. Employers must be educated that scheduled 15-minute naps every 4 hours may improve the employee's productivity.

Current biological treatments of narcolepsy-cataplexy are effective in Asian populations. However, greater efforts must be made in Asian populations for the acceptance of social and behavioral treatments. This would include increased awareness and education of employers and expanded access to support groups.

Circadian Rhythm Sleep Disorders

The biological approach to treating circadian rhythm sleep disorders (CRSDs) involves pharmacology. Vitamin B12, benzodiazepines, lithium, monoamine oxidase inhibitors, and tricyclic antidepressants have been shown to affect biological rhythms (Okawa, Mishima, Nanami, et al., 1990; Turek & Losee-Olsen, 1987; Hallonquist, Goldberg, & Brandes, 1986). Secreted by the pineal gland, melatonin is coupled to the sleep-wake cycle and the circadian cortisol rhythm. Biological rhythms appear to be influenced by exogenous melatonin (Sack, Lewy, Blood, et al., 1992). However, patients should be informed that the prescription of melatonin is off-label.

CRSDs may respond to a psychological approach comprising phototherapy. Bright light of 2,500 lux or more can advance the sleep-wake cycle when administered in the morning or delay the sleep-wake cycle if provided at night (Czeisler, Kronauer, Allen, et al., 1989). The light should be applied indirectly to avoid eye strain. Another potential adverse effect is headache. Mania has also been induced in bipolar patients (Schwitzer, Neudorfer, Blecha, et al., 1990). The timing and duration of phototherapy is critical.

Social factors regarding treatment of CRSDs imply familial encouragement and economic interests. Compliance with daily light exposure may be significantly easier if the entire family supports this exercise. Economically, the patient must be able to afford the time to engage in light therapy.

The biological treatment of CRSDs is similar in Asian and Western populations. Thus, the current biological approach is applicable to Asians. However, the social treatment approach may be lacking in Asian populations. As previously noted, Yang et al. reported that Korean children were significantly more likely to be sleep deprived, as compared to Eastern Asian and Western populations. Moreover, it was reported that Korean parents were less likely to enforce strict bedtimes on their children as compared to Western parents. Korean parents are willing to accept the poor sleep habits if the child is pursing academic interests (Yang, Kim, Patel, et al., 2005). Consequently, greater efforts must be made to educate Asian populations about the negative sequelae of poor sleep. This may require a shift in cultural norms and practices. However, education is essential if one expects to change a group's behaviors.

Parasomnias

Psychological and social approaches are often the treatments of choice for disorders of arousal from non-REM sleep. In fact, education of the patient, bed partner, and family remains the cornerstone of treatment. The family must learn to properly care for patients during these events. For instance, patients should not be awakened during events. Rather, they should be safely guided back to bed. In addition, the home can be made safe by removing potentially dangerous objects, locking doors, and placing gates on stairs. Patients should be advised to limit potential sources of arousal. Furthermore, drugs, alcohol, sleep deprivation, and exercise in the evening should be avoided. Psychotherapy, hypnosis, behavioral therapy, progressive relaxation, and stress management are effective long-term treatment protocols (Mahowald & Cramer Bornemann, 2005; Vaughn & D'Cruz O'Neill, 2007).

Pharmacologic or biological treatment is necessary when symptoms cannot be controlled by other means or if the patient becomes extremely disruptive or dangerous. Low dose benzodiazepines and tricyclic antidepressants may reduce arousals. In select cases, trazodone and paroxetine may be efficacious in limiting arousal events (Balon, 1994; Lillywhite, Wilson, & Nutt, 1994).

Treatment of RBD is aimed at preventing violent behaviors. Pharmacologic therapy remains the mainstay of treatment. The benzodiazepines are highly effective in suppressing these problematic events, and may improve the condition by reducing the amounts of slow-wave sleep and heightening the arousal threshold. In fact, clonazepam has a reported efficacy of greater than 90% (Schenck & Mahowald, 1990). Typically, an initial dose of 0.5 mg is administered at bedtime. Melatonin, dopamine agonists, and donepezil may be utilized as well.

It should be noted that pharmacologic therapy is not foolproof. Patients may need time to respond to therapy. Furthermore, certain medications may be ineffective, or a patient can be noncompliant. Therefore, both social and behavioral therapies have a role in treatment. Education is imperative to create a safe environment for sleep. Bed partners should sleep in a different room until the patient's violent behaviors are controlled and any potentially dangerous objects should be removed from the bedroom.

The treatment of Eastern Asians and Asian Americans is identical to that of other populations. Ethnicity does not alter treatment protocols. Consequently, current therapies are applicable to Asians. However, access to care may be different. In particular, at-risk populations, such as the poor and immigrants, may have limited means to seek treatment. While a search for different treatment options in Asians may not be warranted, certainly the availability of treatment must be expanded.

Sleep Related Movement Disorders—Restless Leg Syndrome

The treatment of RLS often requires multiple modalities. Biological, psychological, and social approaches are utilized in controlling the symptoms associated with this disorder. The biological model is utilized to identify potential secondary causes of RLS and administer pharmacologic therapy. If there is a secondary cause of RLS that can be treated (e.g., iron replacement in cases of ferritin deficiency), clinicians should address this issue. Otherwise, first-line treatment for RLS includes dopaminergic agents. Nonergot preparations, including pramipexole and ropinorole, have received FDA-approval in patients with RLS. For those patients who fail to respond to first-line agents, an anticonvulsant, such as gabapentin, may be considered. Benzodiazepines, such as clonazepam and diazepam, are second-line treatment. Methadone, oxycodone, and codeine are opioids that can be considered to treat patients with RLS.

Nonpharmacologic treatment of RLS involves consideration of elimination of all precipitants of RLS, including antipsychotics, antidepressants, antihistamines, and dopamine blocking agents. Furthermore, patients should be counseled to refrain from nicotine, alcohol, and caffeine. Good sleep hygiene should be practiced by all patients with RLS. Clinicians should emphasize the importance of maintaining regular sleep and wake times (during not only week nights but also weekends), limiting one's activity in bed to sleep and intimacy, and engaging in relaxing activities before bedtime.

Behavioral interventions may be helpful in addressing restless leg complaints. A cold shower, brief walk in the evening, and limb massage may provide relief. Patients should be cautioned against engaging in excessive exercise, which can precipitate RLS. Weight management should be encouraged.

Family and community support are also useful for patients with RLS. The RLS Foundation (www.rls.org) is an advocacy organization for these patients. The American Academy of Sleep Medicine, the National Sleep Foundation, the National Center for Sleep Disorders Research, and WeMove are other sources of information.

Asian ethnicity does not alter the current treatment paradigm for RLS. Similar to other populations, a combined behavioral, pharmacologic, and social treatment program is necessary for a successful outcome. Fortunately, a plethora of publications and research is emerging in regard to this disorder. In addition, a strong support network has been established improving patients access to care.

CONCLUSION

Sleep disorders and excessive fatigue are pervasive in modern society. Unfortunately, shifts in cultural norms have continued to negatively impact normal, healthy sleep patterns. Often times, depriving oneself of sleep in order to achieve success at work or in school is worn as a "badge of honor." While most of the epidemiologic data on sleep disorders was initially performed on Western societies, similar trends have been noted in Asian populations. Clearly, the neurobehavioral derangements and medical morbidity associated with sleep disorders has been well established. Despite this wealth of information, a substantial percentage of patients with a sleep disorder are undiagnosed.

Current treatment paradigms for the diagnosis, classification, and treatment of sleep disorders are essentially applicable to Eastern Asian and Asian American populations. Since the field of sleep medicine is relatively novel to many Asian countries, more research is needed to determine if new modalities may be effective for these subgroups of patients. However, a common theme noted throughout the literature review was a need for better awareness and education regarding sleep disorders in Asian groups. Consequently, sleep disorders are likely underdiagnosed in Asia. Certain cultural norms, school schedules and work practices unique to Asia likely impair sleep. Commonly, fatigue is perceived as a normal consequence of daily life. In fact, seeking treatment for fatigue may even be considered a sign of weakness. This trend of sleep deprivation is particularly alarming among Asian schoolchildren. These findings highlight the need to educate patients about the magnitude of sleep disorders and its detrimental effects on society. Physicians as well as patients need to be more aware of harmful sleep patterns. As a matter of public health it is imperative to promote public awareness regarding sleep disorders and to invest more resources toward diagnosis and treatment. Hopefully, as the field of sleep medicine continues to expand in Asia and access to sleep centers improves, more patients will receive the appropriate treatment.

REFERENCES

Akerstedt, T. (2003). Shift work and disturbed sleep/wakefulness. *Occupational Medicine, 53*(2), 89–94.

Allen, R. P., Picchietti, D., Hening, W., et al. (2003). Restless legs syndrome: Diagnostic criteria, special considerations, and epidemiology. A report from the restless legs syndrome diagnosis and epidemiology workshop at the National Institutes of Health. *Sleep Medicine, 4*(2), 101–119.

Allen, R. P., Walters, A. S., Montplaisir, J., et al. (2005). Restless legs syndrome prevalence and impact: REST general population study. *Archives of Internal Medicine, 165*(11), 1286–1292.

American Academy of Sleep Medicine. (2005). *International classification of sleep disorders* (2nd ed.). Westchester, IL: Author.

American Psychiatric Association (APA). (2000). *Diagnostic and statistical manual of mental disorders* (4th ed., text rev.) Washington, DC: Author.

Ancoli-Israel, S., Kripke, D. F., Klauber, M. R., et al. (1991). Sleep-disordered breathing in community-dwelling elderly. *Sleep, 14*(6), 486–495.

Ando, K., Kripke, D. F., & Ancoli-Israel, S. (1995). Estimated prevalence of delayed and advanced sleep phase syndromes. *Sleep Research, 24,* 509.

Ando, K., Kripke, D. F., & Ancoli-Israel, S. (2002). Delayed and advanced sleep phase symptoms. *Israel Journal of Psychiatry and Related Sciences, 39*(1), 11–18.

Arens, R., & Marcus, C. L. (2004). Pathophysiology of upper airway obstruction: A developmental perspective. *Sleep, 27*(5), 997–1019.

Ballestar, E., Badia, J. R., Hernandez, L., et al. (1999). Evidence of the effectiveness of CPAP in the treatment of sleep apnea/hypopnea syndrome. *American Journal of Respiratory and Critical Care Medicine, 159*(5 Pt 1), 495–501.

Balon, R. (1994). Sleep terror disorder and insomnia treated with trazodone. *Annals of Clinical Psychiatry, 6*(3), 161–163.

Barbar, S. I., Enright, P. L., Boyle, P., et al. (2000). Sleep disturbances and their correlates in elderly Japanese American men residing in Hawaii. *Journals of Gerontology. Series A, Biological Sciences and Medical Sciences, 55*(7), 406–411.

Beaulieu-Bonneau, S., LeBlanc, M., Mérette, C., et al. (2007). Family history of insomnia in a population-based sample. *Sleep, 30*(12), 1739–1745.

Berger, K., Luedemann, J., Trenkwalder, C., et al. (2004). Sex and the risk of restless legs syndrome in the general population. *Archives of Internal Medicine, 164*(2), 196–202.

Billiard, M., & Dauvilliers, Y. (2001). Idiopathic hypersomnia. *Sleep Medicine Reviews, 5*(5), 349–358.

Black, J., & Guilleminault, C. (2001). Medications for the treatment of narcolepsy. *Expert Opinion on Emerging Drugs, 6*(2), 239–247.

Bonati, M. T., Ferini-Strambi, L., Aridon, P., et al. (2003). Autosomal dominant restless legs syndrome maps on chromosome 14q. *Brain, 126*(Pt 6), 1485–1492.

Bresnitz, E. A., Goldberg, R., & Kosinski, R. M. (1994). Epidemiology of obstructive sleep apnea. *Epidemiologic Reviews, 16*(2), 210–227.

Carskadon, M. A., Wolfson, A. R., Acebo, C., et al. (1998). Adolescent sleep pattern, circadian timing, and sleepiness at a transition to early school days. *Sleep, 21*(8), 871–881.

Cartwright, R. D., Lloyd, S., Lilie, J., et al. (1985). Sleep position training as treatment for sleep apnea syndrome: A preliminary study. *Sleep, 8*(2), 87–94.

Chan, A., & Kushida, C. A. (2007). Sleep-disordered breathing. *Continuum: Lifelong Learning in Neurology, 13*(3), 139–152.

Chen, L., Fong, S. Y., Lam, C. W., et al. (2007). The familial risk and HLA susceptibility among narcolepsy patients in Hong Kong Chinese. *Sleep, 30*(7), 851–858.

Chen, N. H., Li, K. K., Li, S. Y., et al. (2002). Airway assessment by volumetric computed tomography in snorers and subjects with obstructive sleep apnea in a Far-East Asian population (Chinese). *Laryngoscope, 112*(4), 721–726.

Chen, S., Ondo, W. G., Rao, S., et al. (2004). Genomewide linkage scan identifies a novel susceptibility locus for restless legs syndrome on chromosome 9p. *American Journal of Human Genetics, 74*(5), 876–885.

Cho, Y. W., Shin, W. C., Yun, C. H., et al. (2008). Epidemiology of restless legs syndrome in Korean adults. *Sleep, 31*(2), 219–223.

Choi, S., Rankin, S., Stewart, A., et al. (2008). Effects of acculturation on smoking behavior in Asian Americans: A meta-analysis. *Journal of Cardiovascular Nursing, 23*(1), 67–73.

Chung, K. F., & Cheung, M. M. (2008). Sleep-wake patterns and sleep disturbance among Hong Kong Chinese adolescents. *Sleep, 31*(2), 185–194.

Czeisler, C. A., Kronauer, R. E., Allen, J. S., et al. (1989). Bright light induction of strong (type 0) resetting of the human pacemaker. *Science, 244*(4910), 1328–1333.

D'Avanzo, C. E. (1997). Southeast Asians: Asian-Pacific Americans at risk for substance misuse. *Substance Use and Misuse, 32*(7–8), 829–848.

DeBacker, W. A. (1995). Central sleep apnoea, pathogenesis and treatment: An overview and perspective. *European Respiratory Journal, 8*(8), 1372–1383.

Desautels, A., Turecki, G., Montplaisir, J., et al. (2001). Identification of a major susceptibility locus for restless legs syndrome on chromosome 12q. *American Journal of Human Genetics, 69*(6), 1266–1270.

Dincer, H. E., & O'Neill, W. (2006). Deleterious effects of sleep-disordered breathing on the heart and vascular system. *Respiration, 73*(1), 124–130.

Doghramji, P. (2006). Insomnia—a clinical perspective. In: Richardson, G. (Ed.), *Update on the science, diagnosis, and management of insomnia* (pp. 21–43). London: Royal Society of Medicine Press.

Doi, Y. (2005). An epidemiologic review on occupational sleep research among Japanese workers. *Industrial Health, 43*(1), 3–10.

Ekbom, K. A. (1945). Restless legs. *Acta Medica Scandinavica, 158*(Suppl):1–124.

Gallup Organization. (1979). *The Gallup study of sleeping habits*. Princeton, NJ: Author.

Gau, S. F., & Soong, W. T. (1995). Sleep problems of junior high school students in Taipei. *Sleep, 18*(8), 667–673.

Gau, S. S., Soong, W. T., & Merikangas, K. R. (2004). Correlates of sleep-wake patterns among children and young adolescents in Taiwan. *Sleep, 27*(3), 512–519.

Gaylor, E. E., Goodlin-Jones, B. L., & Anders, T. F. (2001). Classification of young children's sleep problems: A pilot study. *Journal of the American Academy of Child and Adolescent Psychiatry, 40*(1), 61–67.

Gotsopoulos, H., Chen, C., Qian, J., et al. (2002). Oral appliance therapy improves symptoms in obstructive sleep apnea syndrome: A randomized, controlled trial. *American Journal of Respiratory and Critical Care Medicine, 166*(5), 743–748.

Guilleminault, C. (1989). Weight loss in sleep apnea. *Chest, 96*(3), 703–704.

Guilleminault, C., Mignot, E., & Grumet, F. C. (1989). Familial patterns of narcolepsy. *Lancet, 2*(8676), 1376–1379.

Guilleminault, C., Partinen, M., Hollman, K., et al. (1995). Familial aggregates in obstructive sleep apnea syndrome. *Chest, 107*(6), 1545–1551.

Guilleminault, C., & Robinson, A. (1996). Central sleep apnea. *Neurologic Clinics, 14*(3), 611–628.

Guilleminault, C., van de Hoed, J., & Mitler, M. (1978). Clinical overview of the sleep apnea syndromes. In C. Guilleminault, & W. Dement (Eds.), *Sleep apnea syndromes* (pp. 1–11). New York: Liss.

Hallonquist, J. D., Goldberg, M. A., & Brandes, J. S. (1986). Affective disorders and circadian rhythms. *Canadian Journal of Psychiatry, 31*(3), 259–272.

Hauri, P. J. (1991). Sleep hygiene, relaxation therapy, and cognitive interventions. In P. J. Hauri, (Ed.), *Case studies in insomnia* (pp. 65–84). New York: Plenum.

Hauri, P., & Fisher, J. (1986). Persistent psychophysiologic (learned) insomnia. *Sleep, 9*(1), 38–53.

Hauri, P., & Olmstead, E. (1980). Childhood-onset insomnia. *Sleep, 3*(1), 59–65.

He, J., Kryger, M., Zorick, T., et al. (1998). Mortality and apnea index in obstructive sleep apnea: Experience in 385 male patients. *Chest, 94*(1), 9–14.

Hodges, J., & Oei, T. P. (2007). Would Confucius benefit from psychotherapy? The compatibility of cognitive behaviour therapy and Chinese values. *Behaviour Research and Therapy, 45*(5), 901–914.

Honda, Y. (1997). Consensus of narcolepsy, cataplexy, and sleep life among teenagers in Fujisawa City. *Sleep Research, 8*, 191.

Hublin, C., Kaprio, J., Partinen, M., et al. (1997). Prevalence and genetics of sleepwalking: A population-based twin study. *Neurology, 48*(1), 177–181.

Hui, D. S., Chan, J. K., Choy, D. K., et al. (2000). Effects of augmented continuous positive airway pressure education and support on compliance and outcome in a Chinese population. *Chest, 117*(5), 1410–1416.

Ishigooka, J., Suzuki, M., Isawa, S., et al. (1999). Epidemiological study on sleep habits and insomnia of new outpatients visiting general hospitals in Japan. *Psychiatry and Clinical Neurosciences, 53*(2), 515–522

Kageyama, T., Kabuto, M., Nitta, H., et al. (2000). Prevalences of periodic limb movement-like and restless legs-like symptoms among Japanese adults. *Psychiatry and Clinical Neurosciences, 54*(3), 296–298.

Kales, A., Cadieux, R. J., Bixler, E. O., et al. (1985). Severe obstructive sleep apnea: I. Onset, clinical course, and characteristics. *Journal of Chronic Diseases, 38*(5), 419–425.

Kaneita, Y., Ohida, T., Osaki, Y., et al. (2006). Insomnia among Japanese adolescents: A nationwide representative survey. *Sleep, 29*(12), 1543–1550.

Kaneita, Y., Uchiyama, M., Takemura, S., et al. (2007). Use of alcohol and hypnotic medication as aids to sleep among the Japanese general population. *Sleep Medicine, 8*(7–8), 723–732.

Kasai, T., Narui, K., Dohi, T., et al. (2005). Efficacy of nasal bi-level positive airway pressure in congestive heart failure patients with Cheyne-Stokes respiration and central sleep apnea. *Circulation Journal, 69*(8), 913–921.

Ke-You, G., & Da-Wei, F. (2001). The magnitude and trends of under- and over-nutrition in Asian countries. *Biomedical and Environmental Sciences, 14*(1–2), 53–60.

Kim, J., Choi, C., Shin, K., et al. (2005). Prevalence of restless legs syndrome and associated factors in the Korean adult population: The Korean Health and Genome Study. *Psychiatry and Clinical Neurosciences, 59*(3), 350–353.

Kim, K., Uchiyama, M., Okawa, M., et al. (2000). An epidemiologic study of insomnia among the Japanese general population. *Sleep, 23*(1), 41–47.

Klackenberg, G. (1982). Somnambulism in childhood—Prevalence, course, and behavioral correlations: A prospective longitudinal study (6–16 years). *Acta Paediatrica Scandinavica, 71*(3), 495–499.

Komada, Y., Inoue, Y., Hayashida, K., et al. (2007, November 2). Clinical significance and correlates of behaviorally induced insufficient sleep syndrome. *Sleep Medicine*, [Epub ahead of print].

Krystal, A. D., Walsh, J. K., Laska, E., et al. (2003). Sustained efficacy of eszopiclone over 6 months of nightly treatment: Results of a randomized, double-blind, placebo-controlled study in adults with chronic insomnia. *Sleep, 26*(7), 793–799.

Kushida, C. A., Morganthaler, T. I., Littner, M. R., et al. (2006). Practice parameters for the treatment of snoring and obstructive sleep apnea with oral appliances: An update for 2005. *Sleep, 29*(2), 240–243.

Lam, B., Ip, M. S., Tench, E., et al. (2005). Craniofacial profile in Asian and white subjects with obstructive sleep apnoea. *Thorax, 60*(6), 504–510.

Lam, B., Lam, D. C., & Ip, M. S. (2007). Obstructive sleep apnoea in Asia. *International Journal of Tuberculosis and Lung Disease, 11*(1), 2–11.

Lavigne, G. J., & Montplaisir, J. Y. (1994). Restless legs syndrome and sleep bruxism: Prevalence and association among Canadians. *Sleep, 17*(8), 739–743.

Lecendreux, M., Bassetti, C., Dauvilliers, Y., et al. (2003). HLA and genetic susceptibility to sleepwalking. *Molecular Psychiatry, 8*(1), 114–117.

Levchenko, A., Provost, S., Montplaisir, J. Y., et al. (2006). A novel autosomal dominant restless legs syndrome locus maps to chromosome 20p13. *Neurology, 67*(5), 900–901.

Li, K. K., Kushida, C., Powell, N. B., et al. (2000). Obstructive sleep apnea syndrome: A comparison between Far-East Asian and white men. *Laryngoscope, 110*(10 Pt 1), 1689–1693.

Li, R., Wing, Y. K., Ho, S. C., et al. (2002). Gender differences in insomnia: A study in the Hong Kong Chinese population. *Journal of Psychosomatic Research, 53*(1), 601–609.

Lillywhite, A. R., Wilson, S. J., & Nutt, D. J. (1994). Successful treatment of night terrors and somnambulism with paroxetine. *British Journal of Psychiatry, 164*(4), 551–554.

Liu, X., Liu, L., Owens, J. A., et al. (2005). Sleep patterns and sleep problems among schoolchildren in the United States and China. *Pediatrics, 115*(1 Suppl), 241–249.

Longstreth, W. T., Koepsell, T. D., Ton, T. G., et al. (2007). The epidemiology of narcolepsy. *Sleep, 30*(1), 13–26.

Mahowald, M. W., & Cramer Bornemann, M. A. (2005). NREM sleep-arousal parasomnias. In M. H. Kryger, T. Roth, & W. C. Dement (Eds.), *Principles and practices of sleep medicine* (4th ed., pp. 889–896). Philadelphia: Elsevier Saunders.

Mignot, E. (1998). Genetic and familial aspects of narcolepsy. *Neurology, 50*(2 Suppl 1), S16–S21.

Mignot, E., Hayduk, R., Black, J., et al. (1997). HLA DQB1'0602 is associated with cataplexy in 509 narcoleptic patients. *Sleep, 20*(11), 1012–1020.

Mignot, E., Lammers, G. J., Ripley, B., et al. (2002). The role of cerebrospinal fluid hypocretin measurement in the diagnosis of narcolepsy and other hypersomnias. *Archives of Neurology, 59*(10), 1553–1562.

Mignot, E., Lin, L., Rogers, W., et al. (2001). Complex HLA-DR and -DQ interactions confer risk of narcolepsy-cataplexy in three ethnic groups. *American Journal of Human Genetics, 68*(3), 686–699.

Miles, P. G., Vig, P. S., Weyant, R. J., et al. (1996). Craniofacial structure and obstructive sleep apnea syndrome: A qualitative analysis and meta-analysis of the literature. *American Journal of Orthodontics and Dentofacial Orthopedics, 109*(2), 163–172.

Montplaisir, J., Lorrain, D., & Godbout, R. (1991). Restless legs syndrome and periodic leg movements in sleep: The primary role of dopaminergic mechanism. *European Neurology, 31*(1), 41–43.

Morgenthaler, T. I., & Silber, M. H. (2002). Amnestic sleep-related eating disorder associated with zolpidem. *Sleep Medicine, 3*(4), 323–327.

Nakayama, J., Miura, M., Honda, M., et al. (2000). Linkage of human narcolepsy with HLA association to chromosome 4q13-q21. *Genomics, 65*(1), 84–86.

National Institutes of Health. (2005, June 13–15). NIH State-of-the-Science Conference on Manifestations and Management of Chronic Insomnia in Adults. *NIH Consensus and State-of-the-Science Statements, 22,* 1–30.

National Sleep Foundation. (2003). *Sleep in America poll*. Washington, DC: Author.

Newman, A. B., Foster, G., Givelber, R., et al. (2005). Progression and regression of sleep-disordered breathing with changes in weight: The Sleep Heart Health Study. *Archives of Internal Medicine, 165*(20), 2408–2413.

Nielsen, T. A., & Zadra, A. (2005). Nightmares and other common dream disturbances. In M. H. Kryger, T. Roth, & W. C. Dement (Eds.), *Principles and practices of sleep medicine* (4th ed., pp. 926–935). Philadelphia: Elsevier Saunders.

Nishino, S., Ripley, B., Overeem, S., et al. (2000). Hypocretin (orexin) deficiency in human narcolepsy. *Lancet, 355*(9197), 39–40.

Nomura, K., Yamaoka, K., Nakao, M., et al. (2005). Impact of insomnia on individual health dissatisfaction in Japan, South Korea, and Taiwan. *Sleep, 28*(10), 1328–1332.

Ohayon, M. M. (1997). Prevalence of DSM-IV diagnostic criteria of insomnia: Distinguishing insomnia related to mental disorders from sleep disorders. *Journal of Psychiatric Research, 31*(3), 333–346.

Ohayon, M. M. (2002). Epidemiology of insomnia: What we know and what we still need to learn. *Sleep Medicine Reviews, 6*(2), 97–111.

Ohayon, M. M., Caulet, M., & Priest, R. G. (1997). Violent behavior during sleep. *Journal of Clinical Psychiatry, 58*(8), 369–376.

Ohayon, M. M., & Hong, S. C. (2002). Prevalence of insomnia and associated factors in South Korea. *Journal of Psychosomatic Research, 53*(1), 593–600.

Ohayon, M., Guilleminault, C., Priest, R. G., et al. (1999). Night terrors, sleepwalking, and confusional arousal in the general population: Their frequency and relationship to other sleep and mental disorders. *Psychiatry, 60*(4), 268–276.

Ohta, Y., Okada, T., Kawakami, Y., et al. (1993). Prevalence of risk factors for sleep apnea in Japan: a preliminary report. *Sleep, 16*(Suppl), S6–S7.

Okawa, M., Mishima, K., Nanami, T., et al. (1990). Vitamin B12 treatment for sleep-wake rhythm disorders. *Sleep, 13*(1), 15–23.

Okun, M. L., Lin, L., Pelin, Z., et al. (2002). Clinical aspects of narcolepsy-cataplexy across ethnic groups. *Sleep, 25*(1), 27–35.

Olson, L. G., King, M. T., Hensley, M. J., et al. (1995). A community study of snoring and sleep-disordered breathing: Prevalence. *American Journal of Respiratory and Critical Care Medicine, 152*(2), 711–716.

Ong, K. C., & Clerk, A. A. (1998). Comparison of the severity of sleep-disordered breathing in Asian and Caucasian patients seen at a sleep disorders center. *Respiratory Medicine, 92*(2), 843–848.

Overeem, S., Mignot, E., van Dijk, J. G., et al. (2001). Narcolepsy: Clinical features, new pathophysiologic insights, and future perspectives. *Journal of Clinical Neurophysiology, 18*(2), 78–105.

Pelayo, R., Thorpy, M. J., & Govinski, P. (1988). Prevalence of delayed sleep phase syndrome among adolescents. *Sleep Research, 17*(1), 392.

Peppard, P. E., Young, T., Palta, M., et al. (2000). Longitudinal study of moderate weight change and sleep-disordered breathing. *Journal of the American Medical Association, 284*(23), 3015–3021.

Perlis, M. L., Smith, M. T., & Pigeon, W. R. (2005). Etiology and pathophysiology of insomnia. In M. H. Kryger, T. Roth, & W. C. Dement (Eds.), *Principles and practices of sleep medicine* (4th ed., pp. 714–725). Philadelphia: Elsevier Saunders.

Phillips, B., Cook, Y., Schmitt, F., et al. (1989). Sleep apnea: Prevalence of risk factors in the general population. *Southern Medical Journal, 82*(9), 1090–1092.

Phillips, B., Young, T., Finn, L., et al. (2000). Epidemiology of restless legs syndrome in adults. *Archives of Internal Medicine, 160*(14), 2137–2141.

Pichler, I., Marroni, F., Volpato, C. B., et al. (2006). Linkage analysis identifies a novel locus for restless legs syndrome on chromosome 2q in a South Tyrolean population isolate. *American Journal of Human Genetics, 79*(4), 716–723.

Pollack, C., & Stokes, P. (1997). Circadian rest-activity rhythms in demented and non-demented older community residents and their caregivers. *Journal of the American Geriatrics Society, 45*(4), 446–452.

Punjabi, N. M. (2008). The epidemiology of adult obstructive sleep apnea. *Proceedings of the American Thoracic Society, 5*(2), 136–143.

Rajala, R. M., Partinen, M., Sane, T., et al. (1991). Obstructive sleep apnoea in morbidly obese patients. *Journal of Internal Medicine, 230*(2), 125–129.

Redline, S. (2005). Genetics of obstructive sleep apnea. In M. H. Kryger, T. Roth, & W. C. Dement (Eds.), *Principles and practices of sleep medicine* (4th ed., pp. 1013–1022). Philadelphia: Elsevier Saunders.

Redline, S., & Tishler, P. V. (2000). The genetics of sleep apnea. *Sleep Medicine Reviews, 4*(6), 583–602.

Redline, S., Tishler, P. V., Tosteson, T. D., et al. (1995). The familial aggregation of obstructive sleep apnea. *American Journal of Respiratory and Critical Care Medicine, 151*(3 Pt 1), 682–687.

Regestein, Q. R., & Monk, T. H. (1995). Delayed sleep phase syndrome: A review of its clinical aspects. *American Journal of Psychiatry, 152*(4), 602–608.

Reid, K. J., & Zee, P. C. (2005). Circadian disorders of the sleep-wake cycle. In M. H. Kryger, T. Roth, & W. C. Dement (Eds.), *Principles and practices of sleep medicine* (4th ed., pp. 691–701). Philadelphia: Elsevier Saunders.

Roberts, R. E., Roberts, C. R., & Chen, I. G. (2000). Ethnocultural differences in sleep complaints among adolescents. *Journal of Nervous and Mental Disease, 188*(4), 222–229.

Roehrs, T., Conway, W., Wittig, R., et al. (1985). Sleep-wake complaints in patients with sleep-related respiratory disturbances. *American Review of Respiratory Disease, 132*(3), 520–523.

Rojewski, T. E., Schuller, D. E., Clark, R. W., et al. (1984). Videoendoscopic determination of the mechanism of obstruction in obstructive sleep apnea. *Otolaryngology and Head and Neck Surgery, 92*(2), 127–131.

Rothdach, A. J., Trenkwalder, C., Haberstock, J., et al. (2000). Prevalence and risk factors of RLS in an elderly population: The MEMO study; Memory and Morbidity in Augsburg Elderly. *Neurology, 54*(5), 1064–1068.

Sack, R. J., Lewy, A. J., Blood, M. L., et al. (1992). Circadian rhythm abnormalities in totally blind people: Incidence and clinical significance. *Journal of Clinical Endocrinology and Metabolism, 75*(1), 127–134.

Salin-Pascual, R. J., Roehrs, T. A., Merlotti, L. A., et al. (1992). Long-term study of the sleep of insomnia patients with sleep state misperception and other insomnia patients. *American Journal of Psychiatry, 149*(7), 904–908.

Sam, K., Lam, B., Ooi, C. G., et al. (2006). Effect of a non-adjustable oral appliance on upper airway morphology in obstructive sleep apnoea. *Respiratory Medicine, 100*(5), 897–902.

Sateia, M. J., Doghramji, K., Hauri, P., et al. (2000). Evaluation of chronic insomnia: An American Academy of Sleep Medicine review. *Sleep, 23*(2), 243–308.

Schenck, C. H., & Mahowald, M. W. (1990). Polysomnographic, neurologic, psychiatric, and clinical outcome report on 70 consecutive cases with REM sleep behavior disorder (RBD): Sustained clonazepam efficacy in 89.5% of 57 treated patients. *Cleveland Clinic Journal of Medicine, 57*(Suppl), S9–S23.

Schrader, H., Bovim, G.,& Sand, T. (1993). The prevalence of delayed and advanced sleep phase syndromes. *Journal of Sleep Research, 2*(1), 51–55.

Schwab, R. J. (2003). Pro: Sleep apnea is an anatomic disorder. *American Journal of Respiratory and Critical Care Medicine, 168*(3), 270–271; discussion 273.

Schwab, R. J., Pasirstein, M., Pierson, R., et al. (2003). Identification of upper airway anatomic risk factors for obstructive sleep apnea with volumetric magnetic resonance imaging. *American Journal of Respiratory and Critical Care Medicine, 168*(5), 522–530.

Schwitzer, J., Neudorfer, C., Blecha, H. G., et al. (1990). Mania as a side effect of phototherapy. *Biological Psychiatry, 28*(6), 532–534.

Sesso, D. M., Powell, N. B., Riley, R. W., et al. (2007). Upper airway surgery in the adult. In C. A. Kushida (Ed.), *Obstructive sleep apnea: Diagnosis and treatment* (pp. 191–215). New York: Informa Healthcare.

Shin, Y. K., Yoon, I. Y., Han, E. K., et al. (2008). Prevalence of narcolepsy-cataplexy in Korean adolescents. *Acta Neurologica Scandinavica, 117*(4), 273–278.

Silber, M. H. (2007). Insomnia. *Continuum: Lifelong Learning in Neurology, 13*(3), 85–100.

Silber, M. H., Krahn, L. E., Olson, E. J., et al. (2002). The epidemiology of narcolepsy in Olmstead County, Minnesota: A population-based study. *Sleep, 25*(2), 197–202.

Simonds, J., & Parraga, H. (1982). Prevalence of sleep disorders and sleep behaviors in children and adolescents. *Journal of the American Academy of Child and Adolescent Psychiatry, 21*(4), 383–388.

Sin, D. D., Fitzgerald, F., Parker, J. D., et al. (1999). Risk factors for central and obstructive sleep apnea in 450 men and women with congestive heart failure. *American Journal of Respiratory and Critical Care Medicine, 160*(4), 1101–1106.

Sok, S. R. (2008). Sleep patterns and insomnia management in Korean-American older adult immigrants. *Journal of Clinical Nursing, 17*(1), 135–143.

Spielman, A., Caruso, L., & Glovinsky, P. (1987). A behavioral perspective on insomnia treatment. *Psychiatric Clinics of North America, 10*(4), 541–553.

Sullivan, C. E., Issa, F. G., Berthon-Jones, M., et al. (1981). Reversal of obstructive sleep apnea by continuous positive airway pressure applied through the nares. *Lancet, 1*(8225), 862–865.

Tachibana, H., Izumi, T., Honda, S., et al. (1996). A study of the impact of occupational and domestic factors on insomnia among industrial workers of a manufacturing company in Japan. *Occupational Medicine, 46*(3), 221–227.

Tan, E. K., Seah, A., See, S. J., et al. (2001). Restless legs syndrome in an Asian population: A study in Singapore. *Movement Disorders, 16*(3), 577–579.

Tashiro, T., Kanbayashi, T., Iijima, S., et al. (1992). An epidemiological study of narcolepsy in Japanese. *Journal of Sleep Research, 1*(Suppl 1), 228.

Thorpy, M. J. (2005). Classification of sleep disorders. In M. H. Kryger, T. Roth, & W. C. Dement (Eds.), *Principles and practices of sleep medicine* (4th ed., pp. 615–625). Philadelphia: Elsevier Saunders.

Thorpy, M. J. (2007). Narcolepsy. *Continuum: Lifelong Learning in Neurology, 13*(3), 101–114.

Tran, T. V. (1993). Psychological traumas and depression in a sample of Vietnamese people in the United States. *Health and Social Work, 18*(3), 184–194.

Turek, F. W., & Losee-Olsen, S. (1987). Entrainment of the circadian activity rhythm to the light-dark cycle can be altered by short-acting benzodiazepine, triazolam. *Journal of Biological Rhythms, 2*(4), 249–260.

Ulfber, J., Nystrom, B., Carter, N., et al. (2001). Restless legs syndrome among working-aged women. *European Neurology, 46*(1), 17–19.

Ulfberg, J., Nystrom, B., Carter, N., et al. (2001). Prevalence of restless legs syndrome among men aged 18 to 64 years: An association with somatic disease and neuropsychiatric symptoms. *Movement Disorders, 16*(6), 1159–1163.

Utsugi, M., Saijo, Y., Yoshioka, E., et al. (2005). Relationships of occupational stress to insomnia and short sleep in Japanese workers. *Sleep, 28*(6), 728–735.

Utsugi, M., Saijo, Y., Yoshioka, E., et al. (2005). Relationships of occupational stress to insomnia and short sleep in Japanese workers. *Sleep, 28*(6), 728–735.

Vaughn, B. V., D'Cruz O'Neill. (2007). Parasomnias and other nocturnal events. *Continuum: Lifelong Learning in Neurology, 13*(3), 225–247.

Walker, J. M., Farney, R. J., Rhondeau, S. M., et al. (2007). Chronic opioid use is a risk factor for the development of central sleep apnea and ataxic breathing. *Journal of Clinical Sleep Medicine, 3*(5), 455–461.

Walsh, J. K., Pollak, C. P., Scharf, M. B., et al. (2000). Lack of residual sedation following middle-of-the-night zaleplon administration in sleep maintenance insomnia. *Clinical Neuropharmacology, 23*(1), 17–21.

Watson, N. F., Goldberg, J., Arguelles, L., et al. (2006). Genetic and environmental influences on insomnia, daytime sleepiness, and obesity in twins. *Sleep, 29*(5), 645–649.

Wetter, D. W., Young, T. B., Bidwell, T. R., et al. (1994). Smoking as a risk factor for sleep-disordered breathing. *Archives of Internal Medicine, 154*(19), 2219–2224.

White, D. P. (2005). Central sleep apnea. In M. H. Kryger, T. Roth, & W. C. Dement (Eds.), *Principles and practices of sleep medicine* (4th ed., pp. 969–982). Philadelphia: Elsevier Saunders.

Wieczorek, S., Gencik, M., Rujescu, D., et al. (2003). TNFA promoter polymorphisms and narcolepsy. *Tissue Antigens, 61*(6), 437–442.

Wing, Y. K., Li, R. H., Lam, C. W., et al. (2002). The prevalence of narcolepsy among Chinese in Hong Kong. *Annals of Neurology, 51*(5), 578–584.

Wu, Y., Zhou, B., Tao, S., et al. (2002). Prevalence of overweight and obesity in Chinese middle-aged populations: Current status and trend of development. *Zhonghua Liu Xing Bing Xue Za Zhi, 23*(1), 11–15.

Xyrem® International Study Group. (2005). A double-blind, placebo-controlled study demonstrates sodium oxybate is effective for the treatment of cataplexy: A double-blind, placebo-controlled study in 228 patients. *Sleep Medicine, 6*(5), 415–421.

Yaggi, H. K., Concato, J., Kernan, W. N., et al. (2005). Obstructive sleep apnea as a risk factor for stroke and death. *New England Journal of Medicine, 353*(19), 2034–2041.

Yang, C. K., Kim, J. K., Patel, S. R., et al. (2005). Age-related changes in sleep/wake patterns among Korean teenagers. *Pediatrics,115*(1 Suppl), 250–256.

Yang, G., Fan, L., Tan, J., et al. (1999). Smoking in China: Findings of the (1996). National Prevalence Survey. *Journal of the American Medical Association, 282*(13), 1247–1253.

Yazaki, M., Shirakawa, S., Okawa, M., et al. (1999). Demography of sleep disturbances associated with circadian rhythm disorders in Japan. *Psychiatry and Clinical Neurosciences, 53*(2), 267–268.

Ye, J., Li, Y., Liu, H., et al. (2007). Impact of adenotonsillectomy on quality of life in children with sleep disordered breathing. *Lin Chung Er Bi Yan Hou Tou Jing Wai Ke Za Zhi, 21*(6), 254–258.

Yokoyama, E., Yasuhiko, S., Yoshitaka, K., et al. (2008). Association between subjective well-being and sleep among the elderly in Japan. *Sleep Medicine, 9*(2), 157–164.

Young, T., Palta, M., Dempsey, J., et al. (1993). The occurrence of sleep-disordered breathing among middle-aged adults. *New England Journal of Medicine, 32*(17), 1230–1235.

Young, T., Peppard, P. E., & Gottlieb, D. J. (2002). Epidemiology of obstructive sleep apnea: A population health perspective. *American Journal of Respiratory and Critical Care Medicine, 165*(9), 1217–1239.

Yves, E., Morin, C., Cervena, K., et al. (2003). Family studies in insomnia. *Sleep, 26*, A304.

| 13 |

ADJUSTMENT DISORDERS
IN ASIANS

Kevin M. Chun and Jeanette Hsu

Empirical data on the nature and treatment of adjustment disorder for diverse Asian populations is somewhat cursory given their underrepresentation in psychopathology research. Complicating matters, the *DSM* diagnosis of adjustment disorders has received relatively scant attention in the mental health literature; thus, pressing questions concerning its clinical markers and assessment, and even its very existence as a valid and reliable diagnostic category, remain unresolved. Nonetheless, stress and coping studies provide some insights to the types of stressors precipitating psychological distress and heightening risk for adjustment problems among Asians. The preponderance of these studies focuses on Asian American rather than East Asian groups, with specific attention to psychological responses to acculturation and ethnic minority stressors. *DSM-IV-TR* or ICD-10 diagnoses of adjustment disorders are rarely the foci of this body of research, but are nonetheless inferred mostly by measures of nonspecific psychological distress, general depressive and anxiety symptoms, and psychosocial dysfunction.

IDENTIFYING ADJUSTMENT DISORDERS
IN ASIANS

Current DSM Nosology and Criteria for Adjustment Disorders

Current *DSM-IV-TR* nosology outlines five major diagnostic criteria for adjustment disorders. The first criterion specifies the onset of "emotional or behavioral symptoms" within a 3-month period following an "identifiable stressor" that is specified on Axis IV. The second criterion defines these symptoms or behaviors as being clinically significant evidenced by "marked distress" exceeding normative responses to the identifiable stressor, or significant social and occupational functioning deficits. To facilitate differential diagnosis, the third criterion requires that the "stress-related disturbance" does not meet the diagnostic criteria for any other Axis I disorder and is not an "exacerbation" of an Axis I or II disorder that preexists the observed symptoms in question. The fourth criterion specifies that the observed symptoms are not representative of bereavement, while the fifth and final criterion stipulates that symptoms do not extend beyond an additional six months following the termination of the stressor or its consequences. Clinicians are required to include an "acute" (disturbance lasting less than six months) or "chronic" (disturbance lasting six months or longer) designation with their diagnosis of adjustment disorder, and to note its subtype based on the most predominant symptom presentation. Subtypes are categorized by the preponderance of depressed mood, anxiety, mixed anxiety and depressed mood, disturbance of conduct, or mixed disturbance of emotions and conduct. Clinicians can opt for an "unspecified" categorization if most of the symptoms fall outside the parameters of these subtypes.

Published epidemiological data on the prevalence of adjustment disorders in Asian American and East Asian communities is scarce; widely referenced prevalence studies such as the Epidemiological Catchment Area Studies (Robins & Regier, 1991) and the National Comorbidity Survey (Kessler et al., 1994) did not have sufficient numbers of Asian American participants to generate meaningful estimates of psychopathology for the diverse cross-sections in this population (S. Sue & Chu, 2003). Also, the few large-scale prevalence studies of Asian Americans, most notably the National Latino and Asian American Study (Alegria et al., 2004) and the Chinese American Psychiatric Epidemiological Study (S. Sue et al., 1995; Takeuchi et al., 1998), have primarily reported on more severe psychopathology. Nonetheless, findings from the few studies on adjustment disorders for East Asians and Asian Americans indicate that rates are equivalent to or well above the 5–20% range that is reported for mental health outpatients in the *DSM-IV*. Among a patient sample of adult East Asian Indians admitted for suicidal behavior, approximately 24% of females and 23% of males were diagnosed with *DSM-IV* adjustment disorder (Parkar, Dawani, & Weiss, 2008). In a descriptive study of school refusal for a small outpatient sample of primary and junior high school students in Japan, 36% met *DSM-IV* criteria for adjustment disorder in response to stressors to succeed academically and strict school discipline (Iwamoto & Yoshida, 1997). In a study of psychiatric disorders in a Hmong refugee community in the United States, approximately 30% met *DSM-III* criteria for adjustment disorder, with the majority evidencing the depressed mood subtype (Westermeyer, 1988). The author of this latter study noted however that "refugee adjustment syndrome" or "refugee acculturation phenomenon" were perhaps more accurate clinical descriptors than adjustment disorder for their Hmong participants because their symptoms were more chronic and their functional impairment more varied than what is specified in the *DSM-III*. In sum, prevalence rates of adjustment disorder in East Asian and Asian American communities remain speculative at best given the paucity of empirical data on this topic.

Strengths, Weaknesses, and Alternatives in Applying Current Nosology and Diagnostic Criteria for Identifying Adjustment Disorders in Asians

Despite the lack of research on the *DSM-IV-TR* diagnosis of adjustment disorders for East Asians and Asian Americans, this diagnostic category can still serve as a valuable clinical tool to evaluate and treat cultural adjustment and adaptation problems for the subgroup of immigrants in these populations. Yeung and Chang (2002) illustrated the utility of this diagnostic category in capturing the broad and pervasive effects of acculturation stress on psychosocial adjustment for a first-generation Taiwanese immigrant father and his family in the United States. In this case study, multiple and cumulative acculturation stressors—including English-language difficulties, intergenerational conflict, status inconsistency, and financial strain—contributed to family dysfunction and an incident of child physical abuse. In their case formulation, Yeung and Chang utilized the diagnosis of adjustment disorder with disturbance of conduct, in conjunction with V-codes for acculturation, occupational, and parent-child relational problems to effectively convey the extent and nature of cultural adjustment problems for this immigrant father. This type of case formulation underscores that acculturation stressors are often cumulative and interrelated (Chun, Marin, & Balls Organista, 2003), and that both individual and family level clinical interventions are indicated for recently arrived Asian immigrants (Chun, 2006). Lastly, the "specific culture, age, and gender features" noted for adjustment disorders in the *DSM-IV-TR* highlight the cultural context of stress and adjustment. This is especially pertinent in determining whether distress is excessive and stress responses are maladaptive for diverse Asian groups. Important cultural variations in symptom expression can complicate attempts to assess severity of distress among Asians. For instance, Asian individuals socialized around interdependent self-construals and a collectivistic social orientation may be reluctant to openly express distress or "ego-focused" emotions (e.g., anger and depression) that are perceived to threaten or upset social relations (Chun, Eastman, Wang, & Sue, 1998). Consequently, underreporting or even denial of distress may occur during intake and therapy sessions. In addition, cultural stigma attached to certain stressors (e.g., divorce, intimate partner violence) can complicate attempts to comprehend their nature and impact on daily functioning for certain Asian individuals. Again, a particular strength of *DSM-IV-TR* nosology is that it compels clinicians to address such cultural considerations in their assessment and diagnosis of adjustment disorder.

Still, the very existence of adjustment disorder as a diagnostic entity has been called into question since its initial entry in the *DSM-II* as "adjustment reaction" (Bisson & Sakhuja, 2006). Much of the criticism centers on its diffuse clinical markers, contributing to its dubious reputation as a "catch-all" or "waste basket" diagnostic category for nonspecific psychological distress (Andreasen & Wasek, 1980; Fabrega, Mezzich, & Mezzich, 1987). Of particular concern are two so-called "border disputes" associated with this disorder: (1) difficulties exist in distinguishing the broad range of symptoms of this disorder from normative responses to stressors, and (2) core symptoms of adjustment disorder overlap with those of other disorders, although both the *DSM-IV* and ICD-10 specify that other Axis I or II disorders should first be considered or ruled out even when an identifiable stressor precedes presenting symptoms (Casey, Dowrick, & Wilkinson, 2001). In regard to this latter point, some researchers speculate whether adjustment disorder is more accurately viewed as a "subthreshold" category of major psychological disorders (Carta, Balestrieri, Murru, & Hardoy, 2009; Casey, 2009), including as a "stress-response syndrome" related to posttraumatic stress disorder (Laughame, van der Watt, & Janca, 2009). Researchers have likewise noted that adjustment disorder symptoms overlap with psychosomatic syndromes, eliciting further questions about its diagnostic utility for medical patients (Grassi et al., 2007). Despite these concerns, empirical data on this disorder, though limited, supports its inclusion as a distinct psychiatric disorder in the *DSM* characterized by predominantly depressive symptoms following marital and family problems (Despland, Monod, & Ferrero, 1995).

PERSPECTIVES ON THE CAUSES OF ADJUSTMENT DISORDERS IN ASIANS

Critical Appraisal of Major Etiological Models of Adjustment Disorders

Although genetic risk factors for adjustment disorders have been implicated in a few studies, biological models of this mental illness are scarce (Gur, Hermesh, Laufer, Gogol, & Gross-Isseroff, 2005), and cultural variations in biological risk factors for Asians have not been studied. However, certain aspects of psychological and social models are particularly relevant in determining whether certain segments of Asian populations are more susceptible to this disorder. As noted in this book, psychological models include cognitive and behavioral risk factors underlying psychopathology, while social models include family, interpersonal, cultural, political, and economic risk factors. Two specific risk factors—acculturation stressors and ethnic minority stressors—are pertinent to both psychological and social models in this regard and warrant special attention for Asians.

In the context of a psychological model, acculturation stressors create adjustment difficulties when new Asian immigrants face demands to acquire or learn new behavior skills or cultural competencies (e.g., demands to acquire a new language and communication skills), and demands to make cognitive shifts in their cultural value orientation (e.g., demands to acquire new cultural values and attitudes). Adjustment difficulties are especially likely when the new cultural behaviors and values are incongruent or conflict with the behavioral norms and value system of an immigrant's culture of origin. From the perspective of a social model, family factors such as family relations and family structure affect Asian immigrants' responses to acculturation stressors, potentially heightening or lowering risk for adjustment difficulties. Asian American immigrants also encounter ethnic minority stressors, which are additional social risk factors for psychological maladjustment. Experiences of racial and socioeconomic stratification in the United States, manifested by economic hardship, limited social mobility, and racial discrimination and prejudice, have been implicated in experiences of heightened psychological distress and poorer adjustment for Asian American groups (Balls Organista, Marin, & Chun, 2010).

Before discussing at length the nature of acculturation and ethnic minority stressors and their relationship to adjustment problems for Asians, two important caveats are in order. First, these two classes of stressors rarely, if at all, are linked to a formal *DSM-IV-TR* diagnosis of adjustment disorder in the research literature. Nonetheless, studies clearly show that both stressors are salient risk factors for psychosocial dysfunction and marked psychological distress, which are core features of adjustment disorder. Second, although acculturation and ethnic minority stressors affect Asian populations around the globe, the extant psychological literature on these stressors focuses on Asian American rather than East Asian study samples. This trend in the literature reflects the long and complicated history of racial and immigration stressors confronting Asian Americans in the United States. Thus, the following discussion spotlights acculturation and ethnic minority stressors as salient risk factors for adjustment problems among Asian Americans manifested by psychological distress and psychosocial dysfunction.

Acculturation Stressors and Adjustment

The construct of acculturation has received considerable attention in mental health research over the past two decades in response to the growing influx of new Asian immigrant groups to the United States, particularly from China, the Philippines, India, and Southeast Asia. Comprehending the nature of cultural adaptation and adjustment lies at the forefront of this research enterprise. Although there is a lack of consensus on the operational definition of acculturation, much of the acculturation literature acknowledges that it fundamentally involves a process of adjusting and adapting to a new cultural context over a sustained time period, which can lead to experiences of acculturative stress and related adjustment problems. For the purposes of this chapter, acculturation is defined as:

A dynamic and multidimensional process of adaptation and adjustment that occurs with sustained contact between distinct cultures. It involves different degrees and instances of cultural learning, maintenance, and synthesis that are contingent on individual, group, and environmental factors. Acculturation is dynamic because it is a continuous and fluctuating process, and it is multidimensional because it transpires across multiple indices of psychosocial functioning (Chun, 2007; Marin, Balls Organista, & Chun, 2003).

This definition of acculturation proposes that the process of learning new cultural behaviors and values in a novel cultural setting, maintaining or preserving cultural behaviors and values from one's culture of origin, and synthesizing or integrating cultural behaviors and values from a new cultural setting with those in one's culture of origin, are potentially stressful experiences affecting multiple domains of individual and family functioning. Also embedded in this definition is the notion that risk for adjustment disorders during acculturation is shaped by individual attributes and skills, group and family dynamics and relations, and the presence of ecological demands and coping resources.

Among the broad array of acculturation stressors that have been identified for recently arrived Asian American immigrant groups, perhaps the most salient stressor is low English language proficiency. Among Chinese Americans, the largest Asian American immigrant group in the United States, nearly 80% of adults aged 25 years or older primarily speak Chinese at home, and almost 50% report low to problematic English-speaking abilities (Shinagawa & Kim, 2008). Studies indicate that low English-language proficiency is one of the most robust predictors of anxiety and depressive symptoms for Asian American immigrants (Chun, Eastman, Wang, & Sue, 1998). For instance, among a college sample of Chinese, Vietnamese, Filipino, Korean, Japanese, and Hmong American students, English-language competence proved to be the strongest predictor of adjustment than any other acculturation domain, supporting its function as a primary conduit for the exchange and sharing of cultural information (Kang, 2006). English language difficulties have also been tied to social isolation and loneliness for elderly Asian American immigrants with limited physical mobility (Iwamasa & Sorocco, 2007), in addition to problems in seeking employment and achieving upward socioeconomic mobility, and restricted access to coping resources such as government subsidies and health care (Balls Organista, Marin, & Chun, 2010). In short, English-language difficulties have pervasive and cumulative negative effects on daily functioning that consequently heighten risk for adjustment disorders.

Conflicting cultural norms, beliefs, and values have likewise been widely discussed as pressing acculturation stressors for Asian American immigrants. Such acculturation stressors arise when Asian American immigrants socialized to collectivistic values, norms, and beliefs in their respective home countries are confronted by a predominant and conflicting individualistic social orientation in the United States. There has been considerable discussion on the myriad manifestations of conflicting collectivistic and individualistic cultural orientations in the social, family, and occupational lives of new Asian American immigrants. In the case of public displays of emotion, Asian collectivistic norms encourage monitoring certain negative or ego-focused emotions (e.g., anger, sadness) in social or public settings in the interest of protecting social relations and minimizing loss of face (Markus & Kitayama, 1991). However, this collectivistic norm may be incompatible with individualistic norms in America favoring overt and direct emotional expression in social, work, and therapy settings (D. W. Sue & Sue, 2007). Pertinent to adjustment disorders is the inherent stress associated with learning such seemingly counterintuitive and contraindicated individualistic norms, coupled with demands to determine when and how to apply them appropriately across different social contexts.

Pressures to adopt a new culture can result in chronic adjustment problems. A community based survey found that it took over a decade for non-English-speaking Vietnamese adult immigrants and refugees to adjust to their new American cultural setting (Tran, Manalo, & Nguyen, 2007). In a similar vein, other community-based studies reported that acculturation stressors are pervasive and cumulative in the daily lives of Asian American immigrants. Data from the Chinese American Psychiatric Epidemiological Study (CAPES) focusing on Chinese American adults in Los Angeles revealed that pressures to adjust to a new culture were akin to experiencing multiple daily hassles, which are more closely linked to self-reported psychological distress than life events (Mak, Chen, Wong, & Zane, 2005). Additional research indicates that cultural adjustment problems for Asian American immigrants are exacerbated by co-occurring racial discrimination, resulting in "bicultural stress" and related depressive symptoms and lowered optimism (Romero, Carvajal, Valle, & Orduña, 2007). Although there is an overall trend of heightened risk for adjustment problems with exposure to acculturation stressors, research findings can be mixed. Inconsistent findings are often tied to unresolved conceptual and measurement issues in acculturation research, including widespread use of self-report acculturation measures that do not sufficiently assess the multidimensional and dynamic properties of this construct (Chun, Morera, Andal, & Skewes, 2007). Notwithstanding, important contextual variables such as social and family environments in which acculturation transpires are often overlooked, further obscuring acculturation effects on adjustment (Chun & Akutsu, 2003). Also, proxy variables (e.g., years of residency in the United States, country of origin, and generational status) are often exclusively used to assess acculturation levels even though they might be distal or too far removed from the actual process of cultural adjustment and adaptation to render meaningful data (Chun, 2007). Problems in utilizing proxy variables to examine acculturation effects on adjustment were demonstrated in a study of predominantly Chinese, Vietnamese, Japanese, Taiwanese, and Korean American college students (Hwang & Ting, 2008). In this study, degree of acculturation stress was a more accurate and proximal predictor of adjustment problems and psychological distress than acculturation levels.

Researchers have also noted that mixed or inconsistent findings for acculturation effects on adjustment reflect the complex and multifaceted nature of this relationship. For Chinese American adults, acculturation can have a "paradoxical relationship" with adjustment; greater acculturation has been positively associated with both depressive symptoms and socioeconomic status, the latter of which is typically associated with better mental health (Shen & Takeuchi, 2001). A number of mediating and moderating variables contributes to added variations in adjustment patterns during acculturation. The acculturation mode of marginalization has been associated with depressive symptoms for Korean, Chinese, and Japanese American parents and their adolescent offspring (S. Y. Kim, Gonzales, Stroh, & Wang, 2006) while an acculturation mode of integration or biculturalism has been found to promote positive cultural adjustment for Chinese and Korean American older adult immigrants (S. T. Wong, Yoo, & Stewart, 2006). Additionally, certain personality traits or characteristics potentially mediate acculturation stress and its effects on adjustment. For Chinese American and South Asian Indian adult immigrants, high socioeconomic status and "John Henryism," or a predisposition for high effort coping when faced with difficult psychosocial and environmental barriers, may guard against stress and promote more positive health perceptions (Haritatos, Mahalingam, & James, 2007). Among Taiwanese international college students, extroverted traits are linked to more positive feelings about living and studying in the United States and better overall adjustment (Ying & Han, 2006). Lastly, social support buffers against acculturation stress for Korean and South Asian Indian American immigrant adolescents (Thomas & Choi, 2006) and for foreign-born Korean American adult immigrants (M. T. Kim, Han, Shin, Kim, & Lee, 2005). For older adult Korean American immigrants living with their spouses, their adult children may still serve as a primary source of social support (Han, Kim, Lee, Pistulka & Kim, 2007). Lastly, greater social support combined with a sense of mastery, or the belief in one's capability to overcome life adversities, predicts greater happiness and less dysphoria for Korean American adult immigrants (Shin, Han, & Kim, 2007).

Special Consideration of Family Acculturation Stressors and Family Adjustment Issues

Asian American family acculturation stressors also increase risk for adjustment disorders. There are a number of compelling reasons to examine the family context of acculturation stress and adjustment for Asian American immigrants. Acculturation is likely to be a family rather than an individual experience because new Asian American immigrants tend to live in multigenerational family households upon resettling in the United States. Also, new Asian American immigrants may hold collectivistic norms, interdependent self-construals, and certain Confucian cultural values that make their families and home environment central to their daily lives and psychosocial adjustment. To fully comprehend psychosocial adjustment to acculturation stressors, the nature of Asian American family environments, dynamics, and relations must therefore be carefully considered.

Much of the literature on family acculturation and related adjustment problems focuses on the parent-child, couple, and sibling subsystems. For the parent-child subsystem, studies have primarily focused on intergenerational conflict stemming from differential rates of acculturation; U.S.-born Asian American youth are more likely to adopt new American cultural values and beliefs that conflict with the traditional Asian values held by their first-generation immigrant parents and older family members (E. Lee, 1997). Although researchers have cautioned that "traditional Asian values" are often narrowly construed and may not be entirely relevant to Asian American populations, particularly for those born in the United States (Okazaki, Lee, & Sue, 2007), studies with Asian American parent-child dyads have reported intergenerational conflict over differing cultural beliefs and expectations for dating and marriage, academic and career choices, filial piety and fulfillment of family duties, and adherence to patrilineal family hierarchies (Fuligni,1998; Tsai-Chae & Nagata, 2008; Yee, DeBaryshe, Yuen, Kim, & McCubbin, 2007; Ying, 1999). Moreover, such cultural value differences can last well into late adolescence and adulthood (R. M. Lee, Su, & Yoshida, 2005; Mui & Kang, 2006) and can be a stronger predictor of perceived parent-child conflict than differences in cultural behaviors (i.e., differences in language, affiliation with members of the same ethnicity, participation in ethnic activities) (Tsai-Chae & Nagata, 2008). Emotional distancing and communication problems are other key processes underlying intergenerational differences and resultant parent-child relationship problems (Hwang, 2006). Weakening of affective ties between parents and their offspring is especially likely for those immigrant families who face significant economic hardship requiring parents to maintain demanding work schedules that keep them away from their children (Yeh, Kim, Pituc & Atkins, 2008). Among Vietnamese and Cambodian adolescents, weak bonds stemming from conflict and value differences with their immigrant parents predict a number of self-reported problem behaviors such as being arrested, carrying a weapon to school, running away from home, and hurting others (Choi, He, & Harachi, 2008). Likewise, Chinese and Southeast Asian American teens are more likely to associate with delinquent peers and engage in violent behaviors when reporting heightened differences with their immigrant parents (Le & Stockdale, 2008).

Adjustment problems related to parent-child role reversals have also received considerable attention in the literature. This phenomenon is most pertinent to less acculturated first-generation, monolingual Asian American immigrant parents and their more acculturated second-generation offspring who possess greater bicultural competencies. A reversal in family duties and responsibilities occurs as second-generation children are expected to serve as their family's primary liaisons and translators in their new cultural settings, which can last well into their adulthood. Weighty family responsibilities assigned to second-generation children can include managing family finances, acting as translators for family members, supporting younger siblings' educational and career goals, and managing other day-to-day family activities. Not surprisingly, second-generation Asian Americans who are placed in these demanding family roles can be high-risk candidates for adjustment problems (Nguyen & Huang, 2007).

Studies have also highlighted a number of mediators and moderators of acculturation effects on parent-child adjustment. In South Asian Indian families, risk for parent-child conflict is affected by the acculturation mode of immigrant parents, with separation or marginalization modes posing the highest risk (Farver, Bhadha & Narang, 2002). Similarly, for Chinese American parents and their adolescent offspring, a shared or mutual bicultural orientation appears to lower risk for adolescent depressive symptoms (Weaver & Kim, 2008). Lastly, Asian American college students from foreign-born families report more family conflict than those from U.S.-born families

(R. M. Lee, Choe, Kim & Ngo, 2000), and Hmong American college students who blame themselves for family conflict report more distress and adjustment problems (Su, Lee, & Vang 2005).

Asian American couples also experience a distinct set of acculturation stressors and adjustment issues. Of particular note is the phenomenon of shifting gender roles between Asian American wives and husbands as a function of differential rates of acculturation. Researchers have noted a general trend of first-generation Asian American immigrant women acculturating at a faster rate than their first-generation husbands when entering the workforce to meet new socioeconomic demands in the United States (Chun & Akutsu, 2003; Gupta, 2005). Asian American women who learn new gender role attitudes and beliefs in their new job settings and achieve greater earning potential than their husbands may seek expanded roles in household and financial decision-making. Conversely, their first-generation husbands may experience "status inconsistency" or downward social mobility if their educational and occupational skills are not transferable to the U.S. job market. A poignant example of this was witnessed for a Vietnamese male refugee who was a high-ranking commanding officer in the South Vietnamese army with considerable responsibilities and high social status, but soon found himself unemployed and unable to recoup his occupational prestige in the United States (Chun, Akutsu, & Abueg, 1994). Consequently, he reported depressive symptoms, loss of face, and shame in his inability to provide for his family as the head of his household as he had once done in his native country. Marital conflict and health problems may occur with shifting gender roles (Karasz, 2005) and, in the worst case scenario, risk for intimate partner violence may increase. Intimate partner violence is more likely if husbands struggle to maintain traditional patriarchal gender norms and have been exposed to high levels of premigration violence as witnessed for traumatized Southeast Vietnamese refugees. Risk also increases if wives are linguistically isolated, separated from family and social support networks following migration, lack economic resources to escape abusive households with their children, fear loss of face and cultural stigma associated with separation or divorce, and maintain certain cultural values that compel them to endure their suffering in their roles as wife, mother, and daughter-in-law (e.g., "gaman" in the Japanese culture) (Ho, 1990; I. J. Kim, Lau, & Chang, 2007).

Finally, acculturation adjustment issues for Asian American sibling subsystems are receiving growing attention. A qualitative study of Korean and Vietnamese American second-generation siblings (Pyke, 2005) reported distinct acculturation patterns and relationship problems based on birth-order, which can plausibly extend into adulthood. Specifically, older siblings in this study were more likely to hold traditional values while their younger siblings tended to be more assimilated. Older siblings consequently viewed their younger siblings as "black sheep" because they failed to uphold traditional values and family practices, while younger siblings perceived their older siblings as "generational traitors" because they coalesced with their immigrant parents on enforcing cultural and family traditions. Still, sibling conflict is not an absolute outcome of acculturation; instead, research shows that older siblings may serve as stewards and guardians of their younger siblings in their role as cultural brokers (Chun, 2006). Evaluating risk for adjustment problems associated with cultural brokering and with other family acculturation demands requires careful consideration of the developmental tasks and abilities of family members, availability of coping resources (e.g., peer and family support), and distinct adjustment demands across different family ecologies (Chun & Akutsu, 2009).

Ethnic Minority Stressors and Adjustment

Ethnic minority status confers restricted access to society's wealth and resources based on historical ethnic and racial hierarchies established by the dominant group. For Asian Americans and other ethnic minority groups, restricted access to capital and economic resources, comprehensive health care, safe and affordable housing, quality education, and employment opportunities create chronically stressful life circumstances that compromise psychosocial adjustment and health (Balls Organista, Marin, & Chun, 2010). Other forms of racism and discrimination associated with ethnic minority status, including encountering the Model Minority Stereotype, overt racial denigration, and "racial microaggressions" increase risk for adjustment problems.

In assessing risk for adjustment problems from economic stress, it is important to consider that perceived or subjective impression of financial hardship can be a stronger predictor of psychological functioning than traditional socioeconomic indicators like per capita and household income (Barrera, Caples, & Tein, 2001). Also, the broad and multifaceted impact of economic stress on numerous spheres of daily functioning must be evaluated. Impoverished Asian American families, for instance, are more likely to reside in stressful, densely populated metropolitan settings (Reeves & Bennett 2003) and face restricted educational and career resources and opportunities (Hsia & Peng, 1998; S. J. Lee & Kumishiro, 2005).

Racial stressors have been well documented in the Asian American psychology literature, with special attention afforded to stress incurred from the "Model Minority" stereotype. This historical stereotype, which casts Asian Americans as a uniformly well adjusted and successful racial group, was propagated in the popular media in the 1960s to sustain racial stratification and justify social disparities between ethnic minorities (Yu, 2001). Although casting Asian Americans as exemplars of educational and occupational achievement may appear to be laudatory or even benign, studies have shown that it places considerable pressure on those who cannot live up this idealized racial stereotype (F. Wong & Halgin, 2006; Tseng, Chao, & Padmawidjaja, 2007) and obscures the distinct mental health, educational, and social service needs of Asian Americans (Leong et al., 2007).

Psychological sequelae to more generalized forms of racism have likewise been reported for Asian Americans. Perceived discrimination, in conjunction with low social standing, heightened risk for parent-to-child abuse for a predominantly Chinese, Vietnamese, and Filipino American sample in the National Latino and Asian American Study (Lau, Takeuchi, & Alegria, 2006). Data from this national study also indicated that Asian Americans may be more susceptible to cardiovascular and respiratory problems and experiences of physical pain with greater exposure to discrimination, and that Filipino Americans are at particular risk for health problems associated with racism-related stress (Gee, Spencer, Chen, & Takeuchi, 2007). Greater exposure to discrimination has also been linked to more psychiatric symptoms and a more than 2-fold increase in smoking for an ethnically diverse, predominantly female adult sample (6% self-identifying Asian American) (Landrine, Klonoff, Corral, Fernandez, & Roesch, 2006). Finally, in a diverse sample of Asian American college students mostly of Chinese, Korean, Taiwanese, and Asian Indian descent, the experience of racism-related stress was related to lowered self-esteem (Liang & Fassinger, 2008).

Adjustment to "racial microaggressions" against Asian Americans and other ethnic minority groups is receiving growing attention in the mental health literature. According to D. W. Sue and colleagues (2007), racial microaggressions are stunning racial insults or "put downs" that are automatically and unconsciously directed toward ethnic minorities. After conducting in-depth interviews with a small group of self-identified Asian American adults, D. W. Sue et al. (2007) identified several types of racial microaggressions aimed at Asian Americans: automatically being viewed as foreigners and intellectually gifted, having others invalidate or deny one's experiences of discrimination, exoticization of Asian American women, invalidation of interethnic differences between Asians, denigration or stigmatization of Asian cultural values and communication styles, experiencing second-class citizenship, and being overlooked or ignored in social groups. Sue and his colleagues asserted that unlike overt racist acts, the cumulative, unexpected, and subtle nature of these racial microaggressions make them potentially more harmful to adjustment and health.

Still, a number of protective factors can buffer the deleterious effects of racism-related stress on adjustment. For English-proficient Vietnamese American college students, a sense of coherence or perceiving life as being comprehensible, manageable, and meaningful guards against depression from perceived racial discrimination (Lam, 2007). Other research shows a more complex relationship between perceived discrimination and adjustment. In a diverse Asian American college student sample (over 75% were of Chinese or Filipino ancestry), social support in the form of explicit discussions with family, friends, and mentors about race resulted in greater sensitivity to and reporting of racism (Alvarez, Juang, & Liang, 2006). A later study with another diverse Asian American college student sample (over 75% similarly reporting Chinese or Filipino ancestry), found an important caveat to these seemingly protective effects of social support; Asian American male participants actually experienced more racism-related stress if they sought social support to cope with racial microaggressions (Liang, Alvarez, Juang, & Liang, 2007). The authors of this study surmised that certain types of social support may actually exacerbate racism-related stress by encouraging avoidance behaviors or by invalidating experiences of racism. Thus, these authors cautioned mental health professionals and researchers to inquire about the nature of the social support to accurately assess whether it potentially buffers against or contributes to racism-related adjustment problems.

Effects of ethnic and racial identity on psychological responses to racism-related stress are equally complex. A strong ethnic identity may unexpectedly compound the negative effects of perceived racial discrimination on adjustment. In one study, U.S.-born Asian American college students asked to imagine instances of racial discrimination reported lower well-being if they strongly identified with their ethnic group and took pride in their ethnic group membership (Yoo & Lee, 2005). The researchers of this study hypothesized that those with stronger ethnic identities might be more sensitive and take greater offense to racial discrimination than those with weaker ethnic identification. These researchers also proposed that U.S.-born Asian Americans might be more sensitive to perceived discrimination because they grew up in this country and thus have a greater stake in being a member of American society. Other researchers have noted that the mediating effects of ethnic identity are not uniform because the meaning and nature of ethnic identity formation and development changes across the life span (Yip, Gee, & Takeuchi, 2008), while others assert that certain components of ethnic identity might be more salient than others when predicting psychological adjustment to discrimination. In this latter regard, affective components of ethnic identity, such as having emotional pride and a strong sense of belonging to one's ethnic group, may intensify depression for Korean American adults who perceive high levels of discrimination (R. M. Lee, 2005). Finally, studies with diverse Asian American samples show that reported levels of racism-related stress can vary by racial identity status, with "dissonance" (holding ambivalent or conflicted racial and cultural attitudes toward one's own racial group and toward whites) and "immersion" (immersion in and idealization of one's own race and culture while rejecting and holding negative attitudes about dominant society) statuses potentially generating high stress (Chen, LePhuoc, Guzmán, Rude, & Dodd, 2006). Multiracial individuals may adjust to racism-related stress in qualitatively different ways given their chronic exposure to racial stressors and social marginalization within and outside of Asian American communities (Choi, Harachi, Gillmore, & Catalano, 2006).

Strengths, Weaknesses, and Alternatives in Applying Current Etiological Models of Adjustment Disorders to Asians

Both psychological and social models offer important insights to the significance of acculturation and ethnic minority stressors to adjustment for Asian Americans. In regard to acculturation stressors, a notable strength of the psychological model is its emphasis on the acquisition and development of new cultural behaviors, skills, and competencies (most notably English-language proficiencies) for positive adjustment outcomes. In this context, mental health interventions aimed at promoting cultural adaptation among new Asian American immigrant groups should incorporate bicultural skills training. S. Sue (2003) indicated however that acquiring new cultural behaviors or skills can buffer against acculturation stress insofar as they match the unique characteristics of one's ecological niche or cultural environment. Positive adjustment may require new Asian American immigrants to acquire English-language skills in certain locales although this may not hold true for those relocating to ethnic enclaves where English is not the primary language. Hence, adjustment to acculturation stressors should not be exclusively evaluated by the acquisition rate of new cultural skills and behaviors per se, but rather by the degree of their "environmental match" or relevance to the cultural settings of interest. The social model also serves as a helpful referent to understand family adjustment to acculturation stressors. Specifically, this model spotlights family relations and dynamics as key influences on family acculturation and adjustment patterns, which are highly relevant to many Asian American immigrants whose family lives are central to their daily functioning.

In regard to adjustment to ethnic minority stressors, the psychological model provides a helpful conceptual framework to understand its cognitive dimensions, which again has important treatment interventions from a cognitive-behavioral perspective. Specifically, this model suggests that adjustment to racism-related stressors is influenced by how Asian Americans cognitively interpret or frame them. Granted that altering one's cognitions about racism-related stressors does not fully resolve their resultant problems, it might nonetheless help strengthen one's sense of self-efficacy and agency to cope with such stressors. Finally, a social model likewise provides helpful insights to adjustment to ethnic minority stressors; its emphasis on cultural, political, and socio-economic risk factors illuminates the pervasive and historical effects of racial stratification and social marginalization on psychological adjustment in Asian American communities. As such, the social model serves as an important reminder that attempts to effectively mitigate ethnic minority stress necessitate macro-level interventions through public policy and the law conjoint with individual level interventions like therapy and counseling services.

A major limitation of both the psychological and social models is that studies have yet to fully articulate the nature of acculturation and ethnic minority stressors and how they potentially heighten stress and precipitate adjustment problems. For ethnic minority stressors, it is unclear whether adjustment difficulties result from stress of actual incidents of discrimination or from the emotional toll of remaining hypervigilant to guard against them (Lau, Takeuchi, Alegria, 2006). In regard to acculturation stressors, a set of interrelated conceptual and measurement issues in acculturation research must be resolved before their relationship to adjustment can be elucidated (Chun, Balls Organista, Marin, 2003). One major issue lies in the narrow and vague ways in which acculturation is conceptualized in research, obscuring its multidimensional and dynamic properties and complex linkages with adjustment. In related fashion, an overreliance on proxy measures of acculturation, such as birthplace or country of origin and years of residency in the United States, makes it difficult to identify the potential effects of more proximal acculturation domains (e.g., sense of belonging to one's new cultural setting, perceived self-efficacy in adjusting to a new culture) on adjustment. The context in which acculturation and resultant stress transpire, and the relative salience or importance of different acculturation domains and their potential interactive effects on adjustment, also require further exploration. Complicating matters, acculturation and adjustment studies are typically based on college student convenience samples, thus data on the psychological adjustment of low-SES, monolingual Asian American immigrant families in the community remain scarce. Assessing risk for adjustment disorder for diverse Asian American clients thus requires in-depth inquiries of their acculturation and ethnic minority experiences as indicated in a comprehensive intake interview. This can include assessing Asian American clients' immigration history, pre- and post-migration cultural environments, family context of acculturation, bicultural competencies, and access to coping resources and social support networks in domestic and transnational arenas (Chun & Akutsu, 2009).

TREATING ADJUSTMENT DISORDERS IN ASIANS

As discussed earlier in this chapter, the diagnostic category of adjustment disorder (AD) suffers from a lack of consensus about its construct validity and a lack of behavioral or operational criteria. Given such controversies over the validity and reliability of this diagnosis, it is not surprising that little treatment outcome research exists to guide clinicians in formulating appropriate or optimal treatments for this disorder (Azocar & Greenwood, 2007). In addition, some research suggests that treatments for adjustment disorder may differ depending on whether the symptoms are a response to acute or chronic stressors, and which subtypes are presented (e.g., with depressed mood, with anxious mood, with disturbance of conduct). Finally, some researchers assert that adjustment disorder is a subclinical syndrome that may "[serve] as a marker for serious and life-threatening symptoms … and the future occurrence of other major mental disorders" (Strain et al., 1998, p. 148). Indeed, future randomized clinical trials to determine the evidence-based treatments for adjustment disorder will need to grapple with these controversies and dilemmas. In the meantime, we present some guidelines for thoughtfully determining treatment strategies likely to be effective for treating adjustment disorders in Asian Americans.

Culturally sensitive assessment forms the basis of determining an appropriate diagnosis and the most effective treatment for Asian Americans presenting with adjustment difficulties or any other form of psychological distress. In addition to building and establishing rapport with clients and obtaining an initial description of the presenting problem in the client's own words, it is important to conduct a multidimensional assessment, taking into account various dimensions of the clients' lived experiences, including their ethnic identity development, acculturation levels, generational status, socioeconomic status, religious and spiritual beliefs, sexual orientation, and family influences (Kinoshita & Hsu, 2007; Hays, 2001). Acculturation levels in particular may impact clients' willingness to engage in specialty mental health services versus alternative or indigenous services (Meyer et al., 2009). The client's strengths and coping skills should also be assessed. Since Asians may adhere to a more holistic view of mind and body and collectivist values, conducting a biopsychosocial assessment would be consistent with Asian cultural beliefs about health and illness and the importance of family and community in one's overall adjustment and well-being. Within this biopsychosocial perspective, somatic symptoms reported by Asian clients can be understood as culturally acceptable expressions of psychological distress. Using collateral sources such as family members and community members can provide additional vital information about a client's psychological and social adjustment. However, even if such collateral sources are unavailable, the individual and the presenting problem must be understood in the context of the client's family and community and associated health beliefs, values, resources, and coping strategies (Kinoshita & Hsu, 2007). Finally, depending on the acculturation level of the client, communicating an understanding of and integrating traditional Asian healing practices into mental health treatment may prove effective for some Asian clients by helping to strengthen the therapeutic alliance (Iwamasa, Hsia, & Hinton, 2006; Park & Bernstein, 2008).

Critical Appraisal of Major Treatment Approaches for Adjustment Disorders

Biological Approaches to Treatment

Despite a lack of clear guidelines or treatment standards, psychopharmacological agents constitute the main biological treatment for adjustment disorder and its attendant symptoms. Research on psychopharmacological interventions in Asians have not specifically examined treatment of adjustment disorders, but instead primarily focus on psychotropic treatment of more severe mental illness, such as schizophrenia, psychoses, and bipolar disorder. The bulk of this literature suggests that the pharmacokinetics of these medications may differ in Asians (Lin, Poland, Smith, & Strickland, 1991) and that lower dosages are often recommended. Additional research on the effects of psychotropic medications with Southeast Asian refugees, such as Cambodians with a history of trauma and diagnoses of PTSD and depression (Kinzie & Edeki, 1998; Kroll et al., 1990), suggest that nonadherence with medication regimens can be significant, presenting challenges to studying effective pharmacological treatments with these Asian groups.

In a study of utilization of the AD diagnosis and subsequent pharmacological treatment in university teaching hospitals in the United States, Canada, and Australia, Strain et al. (1998) found that the AD diagnosis was made in 12% of patients, with an additional 10.6% receiving AD as a "rule-out" diagnosis. AD subtypes with anxious or depressed mood were the most commonly diagnosed. This finding supports the results of a previous study showing 14.8% of psychiatric outpatients with adjustment disorder (Samuelian et al., 1994), with the most frequently diagnosed subtypes being anxious mood followed by depressed mood, with physical complaints, and with mixed emotional features. One study of 229 Chinese American private practice clients (Lin, 1998) also found that 14.85% of clients were diagnosed with adjustment disorders. In the study by Strain et al. (1998), the rates of prescription of anxiolytics and antidepressants were at "rates indistinguishable from those for other Axis I and II diagnoses" (p. 147). In the absence of standards of practice for treatment of adjustment disorders, prescribing physicians appear to target the symptoms of anxiety or depressed mood with anxiolytics and antidepressants rather than the diagnosis per se.

Prescribing physicians may need to be guided by the existing literature on psychopharmacological treatment of anxiety and depressed mood in Asian populations. Several recent studies have examined the use of psychotropic medications for treatment of symptoms of anxiety or depression among East Asians. One study investigated the treatment of the culture-bound syndrome Taijin-Kyofu-Sho ("anthropophobia") in three cases in Japan (Kobayashi et al., 2003). Taijin-Kyofu-Sho shows psychopathological similarities with social phobia, depression, and obsessive-compulsive disorder, though an emic view of this culturally distinct disorder suggests that shame and low self-esteem in Japanese culture contribute to fear of distressing others in interpersonal interactions. Kobayashi et al. (2003) found that use of paroxetine, a commonly prescribed selective serotonin reuptake inhibitor (SSRI) altered phobic and obsessive thought patterns, suggesting treatment effectiveness in the two cases showing neurotic rather than psychotic symptoms. Another study conducted in Korea of 190 patients with major depressive disorder (Pae et al., 2007) also found that paroxetine significantly reduced symptoms of MDD in this East Asian population. Kwong et al. (1999) also examined the use of fluoxetine, another common SSRI, in the treatment of 460 patients with depression or dysthymia from seven Asian countries. This study also provided support for the safe and effective use of fluoxetine in the treatment of depressive symptoms in Asians. A recent study compared the use of duloxetine and paroxetine in a predominantly Asian patient sample from three Asian countries and Brazil (P. Lee et al., 2007). Results from this study supported the use of the newer SSRI, duloxetine, for safe and effective treatment of emotional and physical symptoms of major depressive disorder in this sample.

A few recent studies have also examined the use of psychotropic medications in Asian American patient samples. For example, Roy-Byrne et al. (2005) conducted a pooled analysis of 14,875 adults who participated in 104 clinical trials investigating the effectiveness of paroxetine. Analyses by ethnic group, including Asian Americans, showed no significant differences in medication response or tolerability, leading researchers to conclude that paroxetine is an effective treatment of anxiety and depression for ethnic minority populations.

Despite strong evidence that some psychotropic medications may be effective for treatment of symptoms of anxiety and depression in Asians, they may be reluctant to use them. Gonzalez et al. (2010) recently examined a nationally representative sample of Asian Americans and non-Latino whites meeting criteria for 12-month depressive and anxiety disorders. They found that Asian Americans were significantly less likely to report antidepressant use in the past year compared to non-Latino whites, which could not be explained by mental health need or access to mental health care. This finding is supported by another population-based study using data from the Multi-Ethnic Study of Atherosclerosis (Delaney et al., 2009), which found that "the lowest utilization of antidepressant drugs in the United States is among persons of Asian ethnic origin" (p. 7).

Roy-Byrne et al. (2005) suggest that these disparities in psychotropic medication utilization are possibly due to Asian Americans' negative attitudes toward these medications and their illness and treatment beliefs. According to Givens et al. (2007), compared to African Americans and white Americans, Asian/Pacific Islanders and Hispanics were more likely to view medications as addictive, less likely to see depression as biologically based, and more likely to see counseling as effective in treating depression. Overall, Asian/Pacific Islanders in this study preferred counseling to medications for treatment of depression. These study results thus indicate that Asian Americans may prefer psychosocial approaches over psychotropics to treat adjustment disorders with depressed or anxious mood.

An earlier study by Bokan and Campbell (1984) documenting treatment of a Laotian refugee suffering from psychotic depression showed that combining a traditional, culturally appropriate healing ceremony with antidepressant medication contributed to greater adherence to medication and a more positive outcome at one-year follow-up. This finding may likely hold for less acculturated individuals, not only because of their beliefs in traditional healing practices, but also because they may view their treatment providers as being more credible when offering culturally consistent treatments (e.g., S. Sue & Zane, 1987).

Finally, a more recent study by Otto et al. (2003) treated a pharmacotherapy-refractory group of Cambodian women suffering from war-related PTSD with a combination of sertraline, another common SSRI, and cognitive behavioral therapy (CBT) using a culturally and linguistically modified treatment protocol including information, exposure, and cognitive restructuring. Group CBT in combination with sertraline "provided substantial additional benefit" (p. 1274) compared to sertraline alone in the reduction of PTSD and associated symptoms. The results of this study thus support the use of a cultural-specific version of CBT to facilitate adjustment among traumatized Asian refugee populations.

In summary, psychotropic medications appear to effectively treat depressive and anxiety symptoms for Asians although they might view these treatments with skepticism. Reluctance to use medications may be due to a lack of cultural sensitivity in the prescription of these medications, lack of credibility earned by treatment providers, or lack of consistency with Asian clients' cultural health beliefs. Asians may perceive the causes of their psychological symptoms to be psychosocial, and perhaps even more so when diagnosed with an adjustment disorder in which a psychosocial stressor is readily identifiable. Given that research on the use of psychotropic medications for adjustment disorders "remains without consensus or guidelines" (Strain et al., 1998, p. 147) for any population, including Asians, we strongly recommend that treatment providers consider psychosocial treatment approaches as the first line of treatment. Psychotropic medications should be cautiously considered for the most acculturated individuals or only in combination with psychosocial treatments such as CBT, traditional healing practices, or other treatment approaches described later in this chapter.

Psychological Approaches to Treatment

As discussed earlier in the chapter, salient psychosocial stressors that may precipitate adjustment problems or disorders in Asian Americans include acculturation and ethnic minority stressors. Distress related to health problems (e.g., diagnoses of illness, onset of disability) is also pertinent to adjustment difficulties in light of Asians' holistic view of mind and body. Psychological interventions addressing these problems of adjustment should be time-limited and problem-focused, with an active, directive therapy style (D. W. Sue & Sue, 2007; Iwamasa, Hsia, & Hinton, 2006). While there is limited available evidence on empirically supported psychotherapies for Asians (Nagayama Hall & Eap, 2007; Hwang, Lin, Cheung & Wood, 2006; Voss Horrell, 2008), the consensus in the literature is that problem-focused treatment approaches such as cognitive therapy (CT) or cognitive behavioral therapy (CBT) are more consistent with the expectations of Asians seeking therapy for a specific problem, and that a long-term, insight-oriented approach would not be favored by this population. Furthermore, because adjustment disorders by definition rarely persist for more than 6 months, a short-term treatment approach is indicated. In addition, given that family and community are particularly important to Asians, the presenting problem must also be understood in the context of the cultural beliefs and values of the client's family and community (E. Lee, 1996; Tien & Olson, 2003). Although an exhaustive review of the treatment literature for Asian populations is beyond the scope of this chapter, ten general treatment guidelines and strategies come to the fore when treating adjustment problems and disorders.

Kinoshita and Hsu (2007) outlined the following general treatment considerations for working with Asian Americans:

1. Therapist self-awareness of own personal history and cultural heritage, which may influence a therapist's personal biases, values, assumptions, and worldview (Hays, 2001)
2. Increased and early self-disclosure in the service of making a personal, contextualized, and meaningful connection with the client
3. Acknowledgment and understanding of cultural factors (including sociopolitical history, immigration experiences, and current sociocultural context of the client's ethnic group) that may influence the client's presenting problem or expression of psychological distress
4. Attention to nonverbal behaviors and different communication styles
5. Focusing on client strengths and cultural assets, not deficits
6. Understanding the importance of the family in Asian American culture
7. Avoiding psychological jargon and terminology
8. Conveying respect and compassion for the client's lived experiences
9. Gaining further culture-specific knowledge and utilizing culturally sensitive interventions
10. Seeking consultation from cultural "experts" whenever needed

With regard to acculturation stressors, ethnic minority stressors, and health-related stressors that may precipitate adjustment problems for Asian Americans, it is important to assess and acknowledge the strengths and functioning of the individual prior to the onset of the acute stressor. A primary goal of psychosocial treatment approaches is to return individuals to their previous level of functioning as quickly as possible. The therapist should discuss and explain the process and goals of therapy with their clients. Therapists and clients should then engage in collaborative goal-setting and an agreement about how to achieve those goals in a short period of time. Park and Bernstein (2008) also advocate that therapists educate clients about the expected process and outcomes of psychotherapy, paying special attention to shame and loss of face associated with seeking mental health treatment. Intervention strategies that may be useful to address these problems include psychoeducation about adjustment problems and about psychotherapy, teaching adaptive bicultural coping skills, cognitive behavioral approaches such as behavioral activation and cognitive challenging, cultural values clarification for ethnic identity issues, and mind-body interventions such as relaxation training, exercise, meditation, and yoga. Social approaches such as family therapy, self-help/support groups, and community resources are discussed in the next section.

An excellent review of CBT with Chinese American clients (Hwang, Lin, Cheung, & Wood, 2006) describes key therapeutic principles for adapting CBT to meet their needs. These principles support the use of "directed, structured, task-oriented and symptom-focused" (p. 295) treatments; psychoeducation to teach clients about therapy, therapist and client roles, and expectations for therapy; including family members in treatment whenever possible; and integrating cultural strengths and healing practices into the client's treatment plan. They describe the concept of "cultural bridging," whereby CBT concepts and principles are reframed using cultural strengths and beliefs, making important connections to clients' underlying schemas. For example, reframing cognitive flexibility and emotion regulation in Taoist concepts of acceptance, or suggesting that relaxation training or cognitive restructuring help balance one's *qi*. Hwang et al. (2006) also suggest that Chinese American clients may need more time and practice to express their emotions in therapy, and may believe that it is more morally virtuous to avoid or suppress their true feelings. They recommend that these cultural beliefs be acknowledged while encouraging clients to challenge these beliefs through cognitive restructuring. The authors further assert that, while somatic symptoms may be initially presented when seeking treatment for depression, Chinese American clients who become more comfortable with therapy will then start to express other affective and cognitive symptoms. This strongly suggests that, in treatment for adjustment disorders, somatic symptoms in Asian clients can be addressed first, serving as an effective therapeutic gateway for further treatment addressing psychological and emotional issues.

Additional examples of cultural adaptations to existing types of treatments include psychoeducation and teaching culturally appropriate communication skills to Asian American family members presenting with adjustment difficulties related to acculturation differences. A study by Crane et al. (2005) found that large differences in acculturation between Chinese American parents and children and low family functioning was positively related to adolescent adjustment problems, specifically depression and delinquency. Among other recommendations, the authors describe the importance of educating both parents and adolescents about acculturation, emphasizing that cultural conflicts are normative for immigrant families when resettling in a new culture. They recommend that therapists help parents and adolescents to understand that some of their relationship conflicts may be due to acculturation differences. This externalizing of relationship conflicts may foster further discussion of parents' culturally based expectations and adolescents' experiences living in American society, helping parents and adolescents gain greater perspective and understanding of each other and themselves (Crane et al., 2005). Another study reported positive outcomes resulting from improving communication between an elderly Chinese parent and a more acculturated adult child serving as a caregiver (Wang & Gallagher-Thompson, 2005). In this case study, the middle-aged adult Chinese American daughter was encouraged to increase and practice respectful communication with her elderly father when discussing care of her elderly mother with dementia. Both these studies underscore the importance of considering cultural family dynamics when working with Asian American individuals. Therapy with individuals must take into account the role of the individual in the family and balance the cultural value of family harmony with the more Western values of independence and assertiveness. Hwang et al. (2006) and other Asian American researchers have described the utility of encouraging "codeswitching" or bicultural adaptation among clients trying to reconcile acculturation conflicts and negotiate different cultural settings (e.g., school/work settings and home/family settings).

Other recent studies (Otto & Hinton, 2006; Hinton & Otto, 2006) also demonstrate how CBT can be successfully adapted for Southeast Asian refugees suffering from trauma and anxiety-related symptoms. For example, Otto and Hinton (2006) provided treatment services in Cambodian, offered group treatment in a local Buddhist temple, used concepts from Cambodian culture as often as possible to explain core treatment concepts, and integrated an understanding of culture-specific interpretations of anxiety symptoms into their treatment protocol. As an example of recognizing the sociopolitical history of their treatment sample, they also took into account the past traumatizing experiences of Cambodian trauma survivors in indoctrination sessions by the Khmer Rouge regime; thus, the researchers designed the group treatment to avoid a "classroom"-like feel. Otto and Hinton effectively utilized relaxation training in their treatment protocol, linking this strategy to mindfulness practices taught in Buddhist temples. This study suggests that milder forms of anxiety such as adjustment disorders with anxious mood can be effectively treated with culturally modified cognitive-behavioral approaches, including relaxation training linked to culturally consistent mindfulness practices.

Similar principles apply when working from a health psychology perspective with Asian clients. Stressors such as the onset of an illness or disability or exacerbation of a chronic condition can also trigger adjustment problems in any population. For Asian Americans, contextual factors such as prejudice and discrimination, immigration and acculturative stress, linguistic problems or isolation, and restricted access to societal resources including adequate health care and safe living environments can contribute to significant health disparities (Ebreo, Shiraishi, Leung, & Yi, 2007). Therefore, in addition to modifying behavioral risk factors such as reducing tobacco use, lowering blood cholesterol levels, and increasing exercise, interventions aimed at reducing stress can have significant impact on cardiac risk factors such as high blood pressure. According to Ebreo et al. (2007), past studies suggest that "cultural stress and recent immigration were among the possible reasons for high blood pressure" (p. 312).

Few empirical studies have examined the impact of illness or disability as a stressor in Asian populations. Ebreo et al. (2007) report that, anecdotally, some Asians may view illness and disability as a result of "fate," and therefore believe that there is little they can do to prevent negative health outcomes. In addition, some Asians may see illness and disability as shameful (Ebreo et al., 2007), leading to denial of their condition or delay in seeking appropriate medical care. In psychotherapeutic interactions, it is important to explore culturally derived beliefs about health and illness, acknowledge and integrate traditional healing practices such as herbal medicine or acupuncture (Nagayama Hall & Eap, 2007), and involve the individual and family members in discussion of perspectives on illness, treatment, and expectations about family roles. Behavioral medicine interventions such as psychoeducation, motivational interviewing, relaxation training, and teaching and encouraging behavioral lifestyle changes may reduce individuals' health risks, morbidity, and mortality. In addition, psychotherapeutic approaches addressing symptoms of anxiety and depression in response to illness and disability can have positive impacts on physical health and overall well-being.

With regard to family roles, discussion of expectations of caregiving is important for both the well-being of the ill or disabled individual and the caregiver (Wang & Gallagher-Thompson, 2005). Although research on Asian American family caregiving stress is scarce, cultural beliefs of filial piety, mutual obligations to family members, and the value of emotional stoicism to preserve family harmony (E. Lee, 1996) may increase expectations for family members to serve as caregivers to the detriment of the caregiver's own well-being. Research findings suggest that practical problem-solving strategies, increasing communication between family members, and encouraging caregivers to seek support and practical assistance from outside the family may be helpful and effective in reducing caregiver stress and adjustment problems (Wang & Gallagher-Thompson, 2005). A recent study by Gallagher-Thompson et al. (2010) explored whether a culturally tailored CBT skill training program delivered via DVD to Chinese American dementia caregivers mitigated caregiver stress and depressive symptoms. The results showed that the caregivers randomly assigned to the CBT skills group reported increased positive affect (though no change in negative depressive symptoms), less stress related to patient behaviors, and greater belief in their caregiving effectiveness, compared to those caregivers randomly assigned to a general educational DVD on dementia. Future development of such culturally tailored evidence-based intervention strategies are clearly needed in the treatment of this source of stress and subsequent adjustment difficulties among Asian Americans.

Social Approaches to Treatment

In most Asian cultures heavily influenced by Confucianism, the family is the primary social unit rather than the individual as in most Western cultures (E. Lee, 1996; Tien & Olson, 2003). When working with an Asian American client with adjustment problems or disorders, therapists need to understand the client's family's cultural and immigration context, involve the family in understanding the family member's distress, and utilize family therapy when possible. Structural family therapy, in particular, appears to be culturally consistent with Confucian-based beliefs in the executive functions of parents and the proper roles of different family members (Tien & Olson, 2003; J. M. Kim, 2003). However, it is recommended that rather than reinforcing obedience, proper conduct, and restriction of individual family members in service to family harmony, therapists should invite Asian American families to seek a new form of family harmony that takes into account acculturation and adaptation to American society and culture (Tien & Olson, 2003). Such interventions can be implemented in individual and family systems-oriented therapy with some or all family members present.

Guidelines for family therapy with Asian American families (E. Lee, 1996) include establishing initial cultural credibility by addressing and hearing elders' (usually parents') perspectives on the presenting problem first, educating the family on the role of the therapist and expectations for therapy, then providing psychoeducation about the presenting problem. Typically, Asian American families first seek help from relatives and friends, other community members, or even physicians prior to seeking mental health treatment. Thus, normalizing adjustment problems as expected reactions to significant stressors will help reduce their cultural stigma. At the same time, mobilizing parents' obligations to seek help to preserve family harmony and promote successful adaptation among their children, can effectively engage Asian American families in treatment. As in individual treatment, mutual goal-setting and a practical, problem-solving style, particularly for adjustment disorders, would be received positively by Asian American clients. Family therapists can then help facilitate the expression of other family members' experiences in order to enhance mutual understanding and communication among all family members. Additional interventions within family therapy may include skills-focused training and practice such as communication training, problem-solving strategies, conflict-resolution techniques, and behavioral management skills (E. Lee, 1996).

As described earlier in this chapter, intergenerational family conflict can result from differential acculturation rates between family members leading to family adjustment problems. Some individual treatments addressing family acculturation problems were discussed earlier, focusing on psychoeducation of parents and children (Crane et al., 2005). In addition to individual and family interventions, Crane et al. also recommend that bilingual education programs on the acculturation process for Asian American families be placed in schools and community centers to reduce stigma in seeking mental health treatment. One such community-based prevention program is the Strengthening of Intergenerational/Intercultural Ties in Immigrant Chinese American Families (SITICAF) (Ying, 1999). This 8-week, 2-hour-per-week, program was developed for first-generation, immigrant Chinese American parents of school-age children, and offered in Mandarin. The curriculum focuses on educating parents about the cross-cultural encounters their children regularly engage in, increasing their awareness of their children's ethnic identity formation, improving their cross-cultural parenting skills, and helping them better cope with the stress of parenting in a culturally different context. Given the normative experience of acculturative stress for individuals and acculturation conflicts in immigrant Asian American families, this community-based, early intervention program serves as a model for addressing family acculturation and adjustment problems.

As emphasized earlier, therapists working with Asian American individuals and families should explore and underscore cultural and community strengths and resources. In a review of stress and coping among Asian Americans, Inman and Yeh (2007) discussed the importance of coping styles that value interdependence and social support among Asian Americans, including social support from family members, peers (especially racially and ethnically similar individuals), and religious and spiritual leaders. In particular, the use of indigenous healers often integrates all these supportive networks (Inman & Yeh, 2007). Therapists addressing adjustment disorders in Asian Americans should integrate traditional healers and healing practices in the treatment plan, as well as encourage increased social connections with culturally similar individuals and groups.

Support groups may also be an effective intervention with some Asian American individuals, if Asian Americans can overcome the stigma and possible feelings of shame around seeking help outside the family. One recent study examined the development of a confidential online support group designed to reduce stigma and shame as barriers to help-seeking and provide support to Asian American male college students coping with ethnic identity issues (Chang, Yeh, & Krumboltz, 2001). Results from this study showed that online support group members "felt supported by the other members of the group, felt the discussion topics generated by the moderator as well as by other group members were relevant to their concerns, and felt comfortable in and connected to the group" (p. 325). Group members found the website convenient and accessible. It appeared that the group structure addressed some common barriers to treatment related to cultural factors, such as shame, stigma, and inconvenience, and was a potentially effective vehicle for psychoeducation, support, and counseling for Asian Americans.

Finally, given that many of the psychosocial stressors faced by Asian Americans are related to a lack of societal resources, connecting Asian American clients with various community agencies and nonprofit organizations offering instrumental support can be an important feature of an overall treatment plan for adjustment disorders. These may include working with community agencies that provide pro bono legal assistance with immigration and citizenship, ESL instruction, adult education, domestic violence counseling, food banks, housing assistance, elder respite care, "meals on wheels," credit and loan counseling, and other social services.

Strengths, Weaknesses, and Alternatives in Applying Current Treatment Approaches for Adjustment Disorders to Asians

In summary, the literature on treatment of adjustment disorders in general lacks consensus and, in the case of Asians, it is nearly nonexistent. Research on evidence-based treatments for Asians suffering from psychological distress, depressive and anxiety symptoms is also somewhat minimal. However, guidelines for individual and family treatment of Asian Americans show strong consensus in the literature, and much can be adapted for brief treatments of adjustment disorders that are by definition limited in time and severity. Clearly, additional research including randomized clinical trials and case studies need to be conducted to determine the most effective, evidence-based treatment for Asians suffering from adjustment disorders. The heterogeneity of the Asian population will continue to present challenges for researchers, as will the reluctance of less acculturated Asian individuals to participate in mental health research. The literature is also limited in that the relatively few treatment studies in existence mainly focus on Chinese American samples, with little to no treatment guidelines for other Asian populations. In the absence of convincing empirical evidence for specific treatment approaches for adjustment disorders, clinicians must continue to rely on their own clinical judgment in applying existing treatment approaches for their Asian clients. Finally, it is crucial that clinicians comprehensively assess for adjustment disorders among Asian groups because treatment of this disorder can potentially prevent later occurrences of more serious mental disorders (Strain et al., 1998; Kaminski & Garber, 2002).

CONCLUSION

Comprehending the nature and prevalence of adjustment disorder among Asians can be a daunting task given insufficient empirical data on this disorder and the long-standing issue of "benign neglect" of Asian populations in the general mental health literature. Although pressing questions concerning the validity and reliability of this *DSM-IV-TR* diagnostic category have yet to be resolved, its' *utility* as a clinical tool for case formulation and treatment of Asian clients should be seriously considered. This is perhaps most pertinent to clinical evaluations of acculturation and ethnic minority stressors and their well-documented pervasive effects on psychological adjustment across Asian American groups. As indicated by Asian American mental health research, psychological responses to these two classes of stressors can include nonspecific forms of psychological distress, general depressive and anxiety symptoms, and behavioral maladjustment that warrant clinical attention, but do not indicate severe psychopathology. In such cases, a *DSM-IV-TR* diagnosis of adjustment disorder may be appropriate, especially when a range of V-codes can effectively convey the extent and nature of these stressors in Asian Americans' daily lives. Future clinical research should more comprehensively articulate the etiology of this disorder in Asian groups, and provide clearer clinical markers for differential diagnosis with other anxiety and mood disorders. Such research would provide a stronger foundation for further study of biological, psychological, and social models of treatment that directly target this disorder. Although there is growing consensus on culturally appropriate psychological and social approaches to treating Asian American clients, promising cognitive behavioral and family interventions to mitigate acculturative and racism-related stress still require extensive testing in clinical trials with diverse Asian samples. Improved understanding of the triggers, development, and course of adjustment disorders and more data on evidence-based treatments will help to improve mental health and adjustment outcomes for East Asian and Asian American populations.

AUTHORS' NOTE

We thank Ivan Wu, USF Psychology Research Assistant, for his assistance with this book chapter.

REFERENCES

Alvarez, A. N., Juang, L., & Liang, C. T. H. (2006). Asian Americans and racism: When bad things happen to "model minorities." *Cultural Diversity and Ethnic Minority Psychology, 12*(3), 477–492.

Alegria, M., Takeuchi, D., Canino, G., Duan, N., Shrout, P., Meng, X. L. et al. (2004). Considering context, place and culture: the National Latino and Asian American Study. *International Journal of Methods in Psychiatric Research, 13*(4), 208–220.

Andreasen, N. C., & Wasek, P. (1980). Adjustment disorders in adolescents and adults. *Archives of General Psychiatry, 37,* 1166–1170.

Azocar, F., & Greenwood, G. L. (2007). Service use for patients with adjustment disorder and short term treatment: A brief report. *Internet Journal of Mental Health, 4.*

Balls Organista, P., Marin, G., & Chun, K. M. (2010). *The psychology of ethnic groups in the U.S.* Thousand Oaks, CA: Sage.

Barrera, M., Jr., Caples, H., & Tein, J. Y. (2001). The psychological sense of economic hardship: Measurement models, validity, and cross-ethnic equivalence for urban families. *American Journal of Community Psychology, 29*(3), 493–517.

Bisson, J. I., & Sakhuja, D. (2006). Adjustment disorders. *Psychiatry, 5*(7), 240–242.

Bokan, J. A., & Campbell, W. (1984). Indigenous psychotherapy in the treatment of a Laotian refugee. *Hospital and Community Psychiatry, 35,* 281–282.

Carta, M. G., Balestrieri, M., Murru, A., & Hardoy, M. C. (2009). Adjustment disorder: Epidemiology, diagnosis, and treatment. *Clinical Practice and Epidemiology in Mental Health, 5,* 1–15.

Casey, P. (2009). Adjustment disorder: Epidemiology, diagnosis, and treatment. *CNS Drugs, 23* (11), 927–938.

Casey, P., Dowrick, C., & Wilkinson, G. (2001). Adjustment disorders: Fault line in the psychiatric glossary. *British Journal of Psychiatry, 179,* 479–481.

Chang, T., Yeh, C. J., & Krumboltz, J. D. (2001). Process and outcome evaluation of an on-line support group for Asian American male college students. *Journal of Counseling Psychology, 48,* 319–329.

Chen, G. A., LePhuoc, P., Guzmán, M. R., Rude, S. S., & Dodd, B. G. (2006). Exploring Asian American racial identity. *Cultural Diversity and Ethnic Minority Psychology, 12*(3), 461–476.

Choi, Y., Harachi, T. W., Gillmore, M. R., & Catalano, R. F. (2006). Are multiracial adolescents at greater risk? Comparisons of rates, patterns, and correlates of substance use and violence between monoracial and multiracial adolescents. *American Journal of Orthopsychiatry, 76*(1), 86–97.

Choi, Y., He, M., & Harachi, T. W. (2008). Intergenerational cultural dissonance, parent-child conflict and bonding, and youth problem behaviors among Vietnamese and Cambodian immigrant families. *Journal of Youth and Adolescence, 37*(1), 85–96.

Chun, K. M. (2006). Conceptual and measurement issues in family acculturation research. In M. H. Bornstein & L. R. Cote (Eds.), *Acculturation and parent child relationships: measurement and development* (pp. 63–78). Mahwah, NJ: Erlbaum.

Chun, K. M. (2007, August). Understanding the nature and process of acculturation: Preliminary findings from two community-based studies of Chinese Americans in San Francisco. In F. T. L. Leong (Chair), *To change or not to change: Current research on acculturation among Asian Americans.* Symposium conducted at the 115th Annual Convention of the American Psychological Association, San Francisco, CA.

Chun, K. M., & Akutsu, P. D. (2003). Acculturation processes among ethnic minority families. In K. M. Chun, P. Balls Organista, & G. Marin (Eds.), *Acculturation: Advances in theory, measurement, and applied research* (pp. 95–119). Washington, DC: American Psychological Association.

Chun, K. M. & Akutsu, P. D. (2009). Assessing acculturation in Asian American immigrant and refugee families: guidelines for mental health practitioners. In N. H. Trinh, Y. Rho, F. Lu, & K. M. Sanders (Eds.), *Handbook of mental health and acculturation in Asian American families* (pp. 99–122). Totowa, NJ: Humana Press.

Chun, K. M., Akutsu, P. D., & Abueg, F. R. (1994, November). *A study of Southeast Asian veterans of the Vietnam War.* Poster session presented at the 28th annual convention of the Association for Advancement of Behavior Therapy, San Diego, CA.

Chun, K. M., Morera. O., Andal, J., & Skewes, M. (2007). Conducting research with diverse Asian American groups. In F. T. L. Leong, A. G. Inman, A. Ebreo, L. Yang, L. Kinoshita, & M. Fu (Eds.), *Handbook of Asian American psychology* (2nd ed., pp. 47–65). Thousand Oaks, CA: Sage.

Chun, K. M., Balls Organista, P., & Marin, G. (Eds.). (2003). *Acculturation: Advances in theory, measurement, and applied research.* Washington, DC: American Psychological Association.

Chun, K. M., Eastman, K., Wang, G., & Sue, S. (1998). Psychopathology. In N. W. S. Zane & L. Lee (Eds.), *Handbook of Asian American psychology* (1st ed., pp. 457–483). Thousand Oaks, CA: Sage.

Crane, D. R., Ngai, S. W., Larson, J. H., & Hafen, M. (2005). The influence of family functioning and parent-adolescent acculturation on North American Chinese adolescent outcomes. *Family Relations, 54,* 400–410.

Delaney, J. A. C., Oddson, B. E., McClelland, R. L., & Psaty, B. M. (2009). Estimating ethnic differences in self-reported new use of antidepressant medications: Results from the multi-ethnic study of atherosclerosis. *Pharmacoepidemiology and Drug Safety, 18*(7), 545–553.

Despland, J. N., Monod, L., & Ferrero, F. (1995). Clinical relevance of adjustment disorder in DSM-III-R and DSM-IV. *Comprehensive Psychiatry, 36*(6), 454–460.

Ebreo, A., Shiraishi, Y., Leung, P., & Yi, J. K. (2007). Health psychology and Asian Pacific Islanders: Learning from cardiovascular disease. In F. T. L. Leong, A. G. Inman, A. Ebreo, L. H. Yang, L. Kinoshita, & M. Fu (Eds.), *Handbook of Asian American psychology* (pp. 303–322). Thousand Oaks, CA: Sage.

Fabrega H., Mezzich J. E., & Mezzich A. C. (1987). Adjustment disorder as a marginal or transitional illness category in DSM-III. *Archives of General Psychiatry, 44,* 567–572.

Farver, J. A. M., Bhadha, B. R., & Narang, S. K. (2002). Acculturation and psychological functioning in Asian Indian adolescents. *Social Development, 11*(1), 11–29.

Fuligni, A. J. (1998). Authority, autonomy, parent-adolescent conflict and cohesion: a study of adolescents from Mexican, Chinese, Filipino, and European backgrounds. *Developmental Psychology, 34,* 782–792.

Gallagher-Thompson, D., Wang, P. C., Liu, W., Cheung, V., Peng, R., China, D., et al. (2010). Effectiveness of a psychoeducational skill training DVD program to reduce stress in Chinese American dementia caregivers: Results of a preliminary study. *Aging and Mental Health, 14*(3), 263–273.

Gee, G. C., Spencer, M. S., Chen, J., & Takeuchi, D. (2007). A nationwide study of discrimination and chronic health conditions among Asian Americans. *American Journal of Public Health, 97*(7), 1275–1282.

Givens, J. L., Houston, T. K., Van Voorhees, B. W., Ford, D. E., & Cooper, L. A. (2007). Ethnicity and preferences for depression treatment. *General Hospital Psychiatry, 29,* 182–191.

Gonzalez, H. M., Tarraf, W., West, B. T., Chan, D., Miranda, P. Y., & Leong, F. T. (2010). Research article: Antidepressant use among Asians in the United States. *Depression and Anxiety, 27*(1), 46–55.

Grassi, L., Mangelli L., Giovanni A. F., Grandi S., Ottolini, F., Porcelli, P., et al. (2007). Psychosomatic characterization of adjustment disorders in the medical setting: Some suggestions for DSM-V. *Journal of Affective Disorders, 101,* 251–254.

Gupta, R. (2005). Acculturation and marital problems among South Asian immigrants: Implications for practitioners. *Clinical Gerontologist, 29*(1), 71–77.

Gur, S., Hermesh, H., Laufer, N., Gogol, M., & Gross-Isseroff, R. (2005). Adjustment disorder: A review of diagnostic pitfalls. *Israel Medical Association Journal, 7,* 726–731.

Han, H. R., Kim, M., Lee, H. B., Pistulka, G., & Kim, K. B. (2007). Correlates of depression in the Korean American elderly: Focusing on personal resources of social support. *Journal of Cultural Gerontology, 22,* 115–127.

Haritatos, J., Mahalingam, R., & James, S. A. (2007). John Henryism, self-reported physical health indicators, and the mediating role of perceived stress among high socio-economic status Asian immigrants. *Social Science and Medicine, 64,* 1192–1203.

Hays, P. A. (2001). *Addressing cultural complexities in practice: A framework for clinicians.* Washington, DC: American Psychological Association.

Hinton, D. E., & Otto, M. W. (2006). Symptom presentation and symptom meaning among traumatized Cambodian refugees: Relevance to a somatically-focused cognitive-behavioral therapy. *Cognitive and Behavioral Practice, 13,* 249–260.

Ho, C. K. (1990). An analysis of domestic violence in Asian American communities: A multicultural approach to counseling. *Women and Therapy, 9,* 129–150.

Hsia, J., & Peng, S. S. (1998). Academic achievement and performance. In N. W. S. Zane & L. Lee(Eds.), *Handbook of Asian American psychology* (1st ed., pp. 325–357). Thousand Oaks, CA: Sage.

Hwang, W. C. (2006). Acculturative family distancing: Theory, research, and clinical practice. *Psychotherapy, 43*(4), 397–409.

Hwang, W. C., Lin, K. M., Cheung, F., & Wood, J. J. (2006). Cognitive-behavioral therapy with Chinese Americans: Research, theory, and clinical practice. *Cognitive and Behavioral Practice, 13,* 293–303.

Hwang, W. C., & Ting, J. Y. (2008). Disaggregating the effects of acculturation and acculturative stress on the mental health of Asian Americans. *Cultural Diversity and Ethnic Minority Psychology, 14*(2), 147–154.

Inman, A. G., & Yeh, C. J. (2007). Asian American stress and coping. In F. T. L. Leong, A. G. Inman, A. Ebreo, L. H. Yang, L. Kinoshita, & M. Fu (Eds.), *Handbook of Asian American psychology* (pp. 323–340). Thousand Oaks, CA: Sage.

Iwamasa, G. Y., Hsia, C., & Hinton, D. (2006). Cognitive-behavioral therapy with Asian Americans. In A. Hays and G. Y. Iwamasa (Eds.), *Culturally responsive cognitive-behavioral therapy: Assessment, practice, and supervision* (pp. 117–140). Washington, DC: American Psychological Association.

Iwamasa, G. Y., & Sorocco, K. H. (2007). The psychology of Asian American older adults. In F. T. L. Leong, A. G. Inman, A. Ebreo, L. Yang, L. Kinoshita, & M. Fu (Eds.), *Handbook of Asian American psychology* (2nd ed., pp. 213–226). Thousand Oaks, CA: Sage.

Iwamoto, S., & Yoshida, K. (1997). School refusal in Japan: The recent dramatic increase in incidence is a cause for concern. *Social Behavior and Personality, 25*(4), 315–320.

Kaminski, K., & Garber, J. (2002). Depressive spectrum disorders in high-risk adolescents: Episode duration and predictors of time to recovery. *Journal of the American Academy of Child and Adolescent Psychiatry, 41,* 410–418.

Kang, S. M. (2006). Measurement of acculturation, scale formats, and language competence: Their implications for adjustment. *Journal of Cross-Cultural Psychology, 37*(6), 669–693.

Karasz, A. (2005). Marriage, depression, and illness: Sociosomatic models in a South Asian immigrant community. *Psychology and Developing Societies, 17*(2), 161–180.

Kessler, R. C., McGonagle, K. A., Zhao, S., Nelson, C. B., Hughes, M., Eshelman, S., et al. (1994) Lifetime and 12-month prevalence of DSM-III-R disorders in the United States. *Archives of General Psychiatry, 51,* 8–19.

Kim, I. J., & Lau, A. S., & Chang, D. F. (2007). Family violence among Asian Americans. In F. T. L. Leong, A. G. Inman, A. Ebreo, L. H. Yang, L. Kinoshita, & M. Fu (Eds.), *Handbook of Asian American psychology* (pp. 363–378). Thousand Oaks, CA: Sage.

Kim, J. M. (2003). Structural family therapy and its implications for the Asian American family. *Family Journal, 11,* 388–392.

Kim, M. T., Han, H. R., Shin, H. S., Kim, K. B., & Lee, H. B. (2005). Factors associated with depression experience of immigrant populations: A study of Korean immigrants. *Archives of Psychiatric Nursing, 19*(5), 217–225.

Kim, S. Y., Gonzales, N. A., Stroh, K., & Wang, J. J.-L. (2006). Parent-child cultural marginalization and depressive symptoms in Asian American family members. *Journal of Community Psychology, 34*(2), 167–182.

Kinoshita, L. M., & Hsu, J. (2007). Assessment of Asian Americans: Fundamental issues and clinical applications. In F. T. L. Leong, A. G. Inman, A. Ebreo, L. H. Yang, L. Kinoshita, & M. Fu (Eds.), *Handbook of Asian American Psychology* (pp. 409–428). Thousand Oaks, CA: Sage.

Kinzie, J. D., & Edeki, T. (1998). Ethnicity and psychopharmacology: The experience of Southeast Asians. In S. O. Okpaku (Ed.), *Clinical methods in transcultural psychiatry* (pp. 171–190), Washington, DC: American Psychiatric Association.

Kobayashi, N., Kurauchi, S., Sawamura, T., Shigemura, J., Sano, S. Y., & Nomura, S. (2003). The effect of paroxetine on taijinkyofusho: A report of three cases. *Psychiatry: Interpersonal and Biological Processes, 66,* 262–267.

Kroll, J., Linde, P., Habenicht, M., Chan, S., Yang, M., Souvannasoth, L., et al. (1990). Medication compliance, antidepressant levels, and side effects in Southeast Asian patients. *Journal of Clinical Psychopharmacology, 10,* 279–283.

Kwong, K., Fung, M. C., Wu, H., Plewes, J., & Judge, R. (1999). Meta-analysis of safety of fluoxetine in Asian patients. In J. M. Herrera, W. B. Lawson, & J. J. Sramek (Eds.), *Cross cultural psychiatry* (pp. 221–238). New York: Wiley.

Lam, B. T. (2007). Impact of perceived racial discrimination and collective self-esteem on psychological distress among Vietnamese-American college students: Sense of coherence as mediator. *American Journal of Orthopsychiatry, 77*(3), 370–376

Landrine, H., Klonoff, E. A., Corral, I., Fernandez, S., & Roesch, S. (2006). Conceptualizing and measuring ethnic discrimination in health research. *Journal of Behavioral Medicine, 29*(1), 79–94.

Lau, A. S., Takeuchi, D. T., & Alegria, M. (2006). Parent-to-child aggression among Asian American parents: Culture, context, and vulnerability. *Journal of Marriage and Family, 68*(5), 1261–1275.

Laughame, J., van der Watt, G., & Janca, A. (2009). It is too early for adjusting the adjustment disorder category. *Current Opinion in Psychiatry, 22*(1), 50–54.

Le, T. N., & Stockdale, G. (2008). Acculturative dissonance, ethnic identity, and youth violence. *Clinical Diversity and Ethnic Minority Psychology, 14*(1), 1–9.

Lee, E. (1996). Asian American families. In M. McGoldrick, J. Giordano, & J. K. Pearce (Eds.), *Ethnicity and family therapy,* (pp. 227–248). New York: Guilford.

Lee, E. (1997). Overview: The assessment and treatment of Asian American families. In E. Lee (Ed.), *Working with Asian Americans: A guide for clinicians* (pp. 3–36). New York: Guilford.

Lee, P., Shu, L., Xu, X., Wang, C. Y., Lee, M. S., Liu, C. Y., et al. (2007). Once-daily duloxetine 60mg in the treatment of major depressive disorder: Multicenter, double-blind, randomized, paroxetine-controlled, non-inferiority trial in China, Korea, Taiwan, and Brazil. *Psychiatry and Clinical Neurosciences, 61,* 295–307.

Lee, R. M. (2005). Resilience against discrimination: ethnic identity and other-group orientation as protective factors for Korean Americans. *Journal of Counseling Psychology, 52,* 36–44.

Lee, R. M., Choe, J., Kim, G., & Ngo, V. (2000). Construction of the Asian American family conflicts scale. *Journal of Counseling Psychology, 47*(2), 211–222.

Lee, R. M., Su, J., & Yoshida, E. (2005). Coping with intergenerational family conflict among Asian American college students. *Journal of Counseling Psychology, 52*(3), 389–399.

Lee, S. J., & Kumishiro, K. K. (2005). A report on the status of Asian Americans and Pacific Islanders in education: Beyond the "model minority" stereotype. Washington, DC: National Education Association.

Leong, F. T. L., Inman, A. G., Ebreo, A., Yang, L., Kinoshita, L., & Fu, M. (Eds.). (2007). *Handbook of Asian American psychology* (2nd ed.). Thousand Oaks, CA: Sage.

Liang, C. T. H., Alvarez, A. N., Juang, L. P., & Liang, M. X. (2007). The role of coping in the relationship between perceived racism and racism-related stress for Asian Americans: Gender differences. *Journal of Counseling Psychology, 54*(2), 132–141.

Liang, C. T. H., & Fassinger, R. E. (2008). The role of collective self-esteem for Asian Americans experiencing racism-related stress: A test of moderator and mediator hypotheses. *Cultural Diversity and Ethnic Minority Psychology, 14*(1), 19–28.

Lin, J. C. H. (1998). Descriptive characteristics and length of psychotherapy of Chinese American clients seen in private practice. *Professional Psychology: Research and Practice, 29,* 571–573.

Lin, K. M., Poland, R. E., Smith, M. W., & Strickland, T. L. (1991). Pharmacokinetic and other related factors affecting psychotropic responses in Asians. *Psychopharmacology Bulletin, 27,* 427–439.

Mak, W. W. S., Chen, S. X., Wong, E. C., & Zane, N. W. S. (2005). A psychosocial model of stress-distress relationship among Chinese Americans. *Journal of Social and Clinical Psychology, 24*(3), 422–444.

Marin, G., Balls Organista, P., & Chun, K. M. (2003). Acculturation research: Current issues and findings. In G. Bernal, J. E. Trimble, F. T. L. Leong, & A. K. Burlew (Eds.), *Handbook of racial and ethnic minority psychology* (pp 208–219). Thousand Oaks, CA: Sage.

Markus, H. R., & Kitayama, S. (1991). Culture and the self: implications for cognition, emotion, and motivation. *Psychological Review, 98*(2). 224–253.

Meyer, O. L., Zane, N., Cho, Y. I., & Takeuchi, D. (2009). Use of specialty mental health services by Asian Americans with psychiatric disorders. *Journal of Consulting and Clinical Psychology, 77*(5), 1000–1005.

Mui, A. C., & Kang, S. Y. (2006). Acculturation stress and depression among Asian immigrant elders. *National Association of Social Workers, 51*(3), 243–255.

Nagayama Hall, G. C., & Eap, S. (2007). Empirically supported therapies for Asian Americans. In F. T. L. Leong, A. G. Inman, A. Ebreo, L. H. Yang, L. Kinoshita, & M. Fu (Eds.), *Handbook of Asian American psychology* (pp. 449–467). Thousand Oaks, CA: Sage.

Nguyen, L., & Huang, L. N. (2007). Understanding Asian American youth development: A social ecological perspective. In F. T. L. Leong, A. G. Inman, A. Ebreo, L. H. Yang, L. Kinoshita, & M. Fu (Eds.), *Handbook of Asian American psychology* (pp. 87–104). Thousand Oaks, CA: Sage.

Okazaki, S., Lee, R. M., & Sue, S. (2007). Theoretical and conceptual models: Toward Asian Americanist psychology. In F. T. L. Leong, A. G. Inman, A. Ebreo, L. Yang, L. Kinoshita, & M. Fu (Eds.), *Handbook of Asian American psychology* (2nd ed., pp. 29–46). Thousand Oaks, CA: Sage.

Otto, M. W., & Hinton, D. (2006). Modifying exposure-based CBT for Cambodian refugees with posttraumatic stress disorder. *Cognitive and Behavioral Practice, 13,* 261–270.

Otto, M. W., Hinton, D., Korbly, N. B., Chea, A., Ba, P., Gershuny, B. S., et al. (2003). Treatment of pharmacotherapy-refractory posttraumatic stress disorder among Cambodian refugees: A pilot study of combination treatment with cognitive-behavior therapy vs. sertraline alone. *Behaviour Research and Therapy, 41,* 1271–1276.

Pae, C., Bahk, W., Jon, D., Lee, S., Yoon, B., & Min, K. J. (2007). Effectiveness and tolerability of paroxetine controlled release (CR) in the treatment of major depressive disorder: An open-label, prospective, multi-center trial in Korea. *Human Psychopharmacology: Clinical and Experimental, 22*, 351–359.

Park, S-Y, & Bernstein, K. S. (2008). Depression and Korean American immigrants. *Archives of Psychiatric Nursing, 2*(1), 12–19.

Parkar, S. R., Dawani, V., & Weiss, M. G. (2008). Gender, suicide, and the sociocultural context of deliberate self-harm in an urban general hospital in Mumbai, India. *Culture, Medicine, and Psychiatry, 32*, 492–515.

Pyke, K. (2005). "Generational deserters" and "black sheep": Acculturative differences among siblings in Asian immigrant families. *Journal of Family Issues, 26*(4), 491–517.

Reeves, T., & Bennett, C. (2003). *The Asian and Pacific Islander population in the United States: March 2002* (Current Population Reports, P20–540).Washington, DC: U.S. Census Bureau.

Robins, L., & Regier, D. A. (1991). *Psychiatric disorders in America: The epidemiologic catchment area study*. New York: Free Press.

Romero, A. J., Carvajal, S. C., Valle, F., & Orduña, M. (2007). Adolescent bicultural stress and its impact on mental well-being among Latinos, Asian Americans, and European Americans. *Journal of Community Psychology, 35*(4), 519–534.

Roy-Byrne, P. P., Perera, P., Pitts, C. D., & Christi, J. A. (2005). Paroxetine response and tolerability among ethnic minority patients with mood or anxiety disorders: A pooled analysis. *Journal of Clinical Psychiatry, 66*, 1228–1233.

Samuelian, J. C., Charlot, V., Derynck, F., & Roullon, F. (1994). Troubles de l'adaptation: a propos d'une enquete epidemiologique. *Encéphale, 20*, 755–765.

Shen, B.-J., & Takeuchi, D. T. (2001). A structural model of acculturation and mental health status among Chinese Americans. *American Journal of Community Psychology, 29*(3), 387–418.

Shin, H. S., Han, H. R., & Kim, M. T. (2007). Predictors of psychological well-being amongst Korean immigrants to the United States: A structured interview survey. *International Journal of Nursing Studies, 44*, 415–426.

Shinagawa, L. H., & Kim, D. Y. (2008). *A portrait of Chinese Americans* (1st ed.).Washington, DC: Organization of Chinese Americans and the University of Maryland.

Strain, J. J., Smith, G. C., Hammer, J. S., McKenzie, D. P., Blumenfield, M., Muskin, P., et al. (1998). Adjustment disorder: A multisite study of its utilization and interventions in the consultation-liaison psychiatry setting. *General Hospital Psychiatry, 20*, 139–149.

Su, J., Lee, R. M., & Vang, S. (2005). Intergenerational family conflict and coping among Hmong American college students. *Journal of Counseling Psychology, 52*(4), 482–489.

Sue, D. W., Bucceri, J., Lin, A. I., Nadal, K. L., & Torino, G. C. (2007). Racial microaggressions and the Asian American experience. *Cultural Diversity and Ethnic Minority Psychology,13*(1), 72–81.

Sue, D. W., & Sue, S. (2007). *Counseling the culturally diverse: Theory and practice* (5th ed.). New York: Wiley.

Sue, S. (2003). Foreword. In K. M. Chun, P. Balls Organista, & G. Marin (Eds.), *Acculturation: Advances in theory, measurement, and applied research* (pp. xvii–xxi). Washington, DC: American Psychological Association.

Sue, S., & Chu, J. Y. (2003). The mental health of ethnic minority groups: Challenges posed by the supplement to the surgeon general's report on mental health. *Culture, Medicine, and Psychiatry, 27*, 447–465.

Sue, S., Sue, D. W., Sue, L., & Takeuchi, D. T. (1995) Psychopathology among Asian Americans: A model minority? *Cultural Diversity and Mental Health, 1*, 39–54.

Sue, S., & Zane, N. (1987). The role of culture and cultural techniques in psychotherapy: A critique and reformulation. *American Psychologist, 42*, 37–45.

Takeuchi, D. T., Chung, R. C., Lin, K. M., Shen, H., Kurasaki, K., Chun, C., et al. (1998). Lifetime and twelve-month prevalence rates of major depressive episodes and dysthymia among Chinese Americans in Los Angeles. *American Journal of Psychiatry, 155*, 1407–1414.

Thomas, M., & Choi, J. B. (2006). Acculturative stress and social support among Korean and Indian immigrant adolescents in the United States. *Journal of Sociology and Social Welfare, 33*(2), 123–143.

Tien, L., & Olson, K. (2003) Confucian past, conflicted present: Working with Asian American families. In L. B. Silverstein & T. J. Goodrich (Eds.), *Feminist family therapy: Empowerment in social context* (pp. 135–146). Washington, DC: American Psychological Association.

Tran, T. V., Manalo, V., & Nguyen, V. T. D. (2007). Nonlinear relationship between length of residence and depression in a community-based sample of Vietnamese Americans. *International Journal of Social Psychiatry, 53*(1), 85–94.

Tsai-Chae, A. H., & Nagata, D. K. (2008). Asian values and perceptions of intergenerational family conflict among Asian American students. *Cultural Diversity and Ethnic Minority Psychology, 14*(3), 205–214.

Tseng, V., Chao, R. K., & Padmawidjaja, I. A. (2007). Asian Americans' educational experiences. In F. T. L. Leong, A. G. Inman, A. Ebreo, L. Yang, L. Kinoshita, & M. Fu (Eds.), *Handbook of Asian American psychology* (2nd ed., pp. 105–124). Thousand Oaks, CA: Sage.

Voss Horrell, S. C. (2008). Effectiveness of cognitive-behavioral therapy with adult ethnic minority clients: A review. *Professional Psychology: Research and Practice, 39*, 160–168.

Wang, P.-C., & Gallagher-Thompson, D. (2005). Resolution of intergenerational conflict in a Chinese female dementia caregiver: A case study using cognitive/behavioral methods. *Clinical Gerontologist, 28*(3), 91–94.

Weaver, S. R., & Kim, S. Y. (2008). A person-centered approach to studying the linkages among parent-child differences in cultural orientation, supportive parenting, and adolescent depressive symptoms in Chinese American families. *Journal of Youth and Adolescence, 37*(1), 36–49.

Westermeyer, J. (1988). DSM-III psychiatric disorders among Hmong refugees in the United States: A point prevalence study. *American Journal of Psychiatry, 50*, 181–183.

Wong, F., & Halgin, R. (2006). The "model minority": Bane or blessing for Asian Americans? *Journal of Multicultural Counseling and Development, 34*(1), 38–49.

Wong, S. T., Yoo, G. J., & Stewart, A. L. (2006). The changing meaning of family support among older Chinese and Korean immigrants. *Journals of Gerontology, 61B*(1), S4–S9.

Yee, B. W. K., DeBaryshe, B. D., Yuen, S., Kim, S. Y., & McCubbin, H. I. (2007). Asian American and Pacific Islander families: Resiliency, and life-span socialization in context. In F. T. L. Leong, A. G. Inman, A. Ebreo, L. Yang, L. Kinoshita, & M. Fu (Eds.), *Handbook of Asian American psychology* (2nd ed., pp. 69–86). Thousand Oaks, CA: Sage.

Yeh, C. J., Kim, A. B., Pituc, S. T., & Atkins, M. (2008). Poverty, loss, and resilience: The story of Chinese immigrant youth. *Journal of Counseling Psychology, 55*(1), 34–48.

Yeung, A. S., & Chang, D. F. (2002). Adjustment disorder: Intergenerational conflict in a Chinese immigrant family. *Culture, Medicine, and Psychiatry, 26*(4), 509–525.

Ying, Y. W. (1999). Strengthening intergenerational/intercultural ties in migrant families: A new intervention for parents. *Journal of Community Psychology, 27*, 89–96.

Ying, Y. W., & Han, M. (2006). The contribution of personality, acculturative stressors, and social affiliation to adjustment: A longitudinal study of Taiwanese students in the United States. *International Journal of Intercultural Relations, 30*, 623–635.

Yip, T., Gee, G. C., & Takeuchi, D. T. (2008). Racial discrimination and psychological distress: The impact of ethnic identity and age among immigrant and United States-born Asian adults. *Developmental Psychology, 44*(3), 787–800.

Yoo, H. C., & Lee, R. M. (2005). Ethnic identity and approach-type coping as moderators of the racial discrimination/well-being relation in Asian Americans. *Journal of Counseling Psychology, 52*(4), 497–506.

Yu, H. (2001). *Thinking Orientals: migration, contact, and exoticism in modern America.* New York: Oxford University Press.

| 14 |

PERSONALITY DISORDERS
IN ASIANS

ANDREW G. RYDER, JESSICA DERE, JIAN YANG,
AND KENNETH FUNG

INTRODUCTION

Working with personality disorders (PDs) and working with culture in context each present challenges for researcher and clinician alike. As personality and culture are deeply intertwined, to the point where they can be said to constitute one another (Markus, 2004), working with both multiplies the difficulties. Complicating matters further, the cultural and cross-cultural research database for PDs is limited, whether for Asians or for other ethnocultural groups. A final obstacle is the diagnostic status of PDs; not only are there long-standing controversies in the literature about how PDs can best be categorized, but also there are questions about whether they should even be considered categories at all. Indeed, there is a high likelihood that the PD system in *DSM*-5 will be radically changed from previous editions, incorporating a proposed new dimensional system for pathological personality traits. To address these concerns, this review begins with the PDs as currently defined in *DSM-IV*, presenting issues of identification, etiology, and treatment in Asian populations, while also providing a culturally based critique and discussion of alternatives. As much as possible, the review is evidence-based, although the state of the literature at times requires speculation informed by clinical and cultural experience.

Before turning to the research literature, we should briefly define "Asian" and "Western," the two broad and heterogeneous cultural groups that are contrasted throughout much of this chapter. Our definitions are provisional by necessity, driven as much by the needs of the chapter and the provenance of most available literature as by the features of the cultural groups themselves. Our use of "Asian" is considerably more limited than the vast continent implied by the term. We focus on people whose origins are in societies shaped in part by Confucian cultural values, and on those people who either live in these societies or who trace their origins to them. Thus, we are referring primarily to China (including Hong Kong and Taiwan), Japan, and Korea; to a lesser extent Southeast Asia and the Pacific Islands; and not societies further west, such as the Indian subcontinent or the Middle East. By "Western," meanwhile, we are referring to those societies based or rooted in Europe and the people who reside in these societies with European cultural origins. Here, we mainly focus on Euro-Americans and Euro-Canadians, as dictated by the available data and our own experience.

IDENTIFYING PERSONALITY DISORDERS IN ASIANS

Current DSM Nosology and Criteria for Personality Disorders

PDs are among the most common mental disorders (Skodol et al., 2002) and they exact a heavy cost on the sufferer and society, not least on the mental health system (Bender et al., 2001). DSM-IV provides a general definition of PDs as pervasive, inflexible, maladaptive, and enduring expressions of personality that cause significant impairment or distress and that deviate from cultural expectations (APA, 2000). This last criterion requires that clinicians have sufficient knowledge of what these cultural expectations might be. There is considerable controversy regarding the best ways to conceptualize PDs as a class and to make distinctions among specific PDs (e.g., Widiger & Trull, 2007). Nonetheless, we will begin by reviewing briefly the PDs as defined in DSM-IV, before turning our attention to the prevalence and features of PDs in Asian populations.

Personality Disorders in DSM-IV

DSM-IV includes specific descriptive diagnostic criteria for 10 PDs, forming three broad clusters based on their similarities. Cluster A, the odd-eccentric cluster, includes paranoid, schizoid, and schizotypal PDs. Paranoid PD is characterized by a consistent pattern of distrust; there is a tendency to assume that others will deliberately be exploitative, harmful, or deceptive, and to read hidden intentions behind innocuous statements. Schizoid PD is characterized by a tendency to be indifferent to pleasure or to social relationships, with blunted emotional expression and lack of engagement with interests or with other people. Schizotypal PD is characterized by ideas of reference, odd beliefs, preoccupations with the paranormal, bodily illusions, and sensory alterations, all symptoms that resemble mild forms of the positive symptoms observed in schizophrenia. In addition, presentations can include mild forms of negative symptoms, such as social awkwardness and constricted affect.

Cluster B, the dramatic-erratic cluster, consists of antisocial, borderline, histrionic, and narcissistic PDs. Antisocial PD refers to a pervasive pattern of irresponsibility and disregard for others that begins as childhood conduct disorder, and includes impulsiveness, irritability, aggression, manipulativeness, and lack of remorse at having hurt or mistreated others. Borderline PD is characterized by disturbances in identity and emotion regulation, including features such as rapid affective shifts, impulsivity, interpersonal chaos, transient psychosis, feelings of emptiness, and lack of a clear sense of self (Trull, Stepp, & Solhan, 2006). ICD-10 has a similar construct called emotionally unstable PD, with borderline and impulsive subtypes; the latter emphasizes impulsivity without the disturbances in personal identity and interpersonal relations. Histrionic PD, with origins in writings on "hysteria," is characterized by dramatic emotions, attention-seeking, seductiveness, and the denial of anger (Horowitz, 1991). Finally, narcissistic PD is characterized by a sense of entitlement, extreme self-importance, arrogance, and grandiosity (Westen & Shedler, 1999), due either to unusually rigid high self-esteem or to a fragile high self-esteem protecting a vulnerable interior (Cain, Pincus, & Ansell, 2008).

Cluster C, the anxious-fearful cluster, includes avoidant, dependent, and obsessive-compulsive PDs. Avoidant PD was distinguished from schizoid PD by Millon (1981), who argued that there are some people who avoid or are uncomfortable in social situations, are hypersensitive to criticism or perceived rejection, and yet long for close relationships. Such people may engage in a more general avoidance of new experiences and strong emotions, including positive emotions (Taylor, Laposa, & Alden, 2004). There may be some overlap with social anxiety disorder, especially of the generalized subtype (Schneier et al., 2004). Dependent PD is characterized by a pervasive need to be protected and cared for, with strong beliefs that it is necessary to rely heavily on other people for advice or reassurance. Finally, obsessive-compulsive PD is characterized by needs for order, perfection, morality, and control, accompanied by emotional constriction and a preoccupation with minor details. The relationship between obsessive-compulsive PD and obsessive-compulsive disorder remains to be clarified, with some studies showing elevated OCPD among OCD populations (Coles et al., 2008; Eisen et al., 2006). ICD-10 avoids the appearance of overlap by using the term anankastic PD.

Prevalence of DSM-IV Personality Disorders in Asians

Research on the prevalence of PDs in Asians is limited by the small number of studies directly comparing different societies. Recent work by Y. Huang and colleagues (2009) using data from the World Health Organization's Mental Health Surveys collected in 13 countries marks an important exception. Using 33 screening questions from the International Personality Disorder Examination, the researchers were able to present prevalence estimates for the three *DSM-IV* PD clusters. At the American site, estimates for Clusters A, B, and C were 4.0%, 2.0%, and 4.2%, respectively, with 7.6% meeting criteria for any PD; comparable figures at the Chinese site were 3.1%, 1.3%, and 1.4%, respectively, with 4.1% meeting criteria for any PD. The difference for Cluster C PDs is particularly striking, with these diagnoses being three times more common in the United States. Moreover, whereas 6.6% of the participants in China had sought treatment for PD in the previous year, 37.3% in the United States had done so.

B. Huang and colleagues (2006) studied 12-month prevalence and co-occurrence of substance use, mood, anxiety, and several PDs (paranoid, schizoid, antisocial, histrionic, avoidant, dependent, and obsessive-compulsive PDs) in the United States. The study was conducted on a representative sample of 43,093 participants, analyzed within several major ethnic blocs. There was a 10.1% rate of any PD in the Asian group, significantly lower than the white (14.6%), black (16.6%), Native American (24.1%), and Hispanic (14.0%) groups. Although Asian respondents also had low over-all rates of substance use disorders, the co-occurrence of substance use and personality disorders was significantly higher in the Asian group, compared to the white, black, and Native American groups. This finding is consistent with the idea that behaviors that are both unusual and destructive in a given cultural context may serve as useful warning signs of PD.

C. K. Lee and colleagues (1990) reported prevalence rates for antisocial PD in both urban and rural South Korea, in the context of a study largely focusing on Axis I psychopathology. Whereas most of these disorders were more common in the rural sample, antisocial PD had a rate of only 0.98% in the rural sample compared with 2.08% in the urban sample. Compton and colleagues (2005) studied rates of antisocial PD in the United States using data from the National Epidemiologic Survey on Alcohol and Related Conditions. They found an overall rate, across all ethnic blocs, of 3.6%, with Asian participants having a significantly lower rate than white partici-pants (OR = 0.4). Grant and colleagues (2008) used data from the same project to study U.S. rates of borderline PD. They found a lifetime prevalence of 5.9%, with a rate of 3.4% among Asians. Although rates of borderline PD were somewhat higher in women as compared with men overall, Asian women had significantly lower odds of a diagnosis, with a rate of 2.5%.

Features of DSM-IV Personality Disorders in Asians

Sato and colleagues (1993, 1997) studied PDs in a sample of 96 Japanese outpatients with nonbipo-lar depression. The four most common PD diagnoses were, in turn, avoidant, obsessive-compulsive, narcissistic, and dependent PDs. The authors argued that diagnostic rates were generally in the range reported in similar Western studies except narcissistic and schizoid PDs, which had higher rates in Japan. Although the authors raise the issue of whether cultural differences might lead to higher rates of certain PDs, or to problems with the validity of specific PD criteria, they do not elaborate. Importantly, they also found that patients with one or more PD diagnoses had signifi-cantly worse outcome after four months of antidepressant pharmacotherapy, compared to patients with no PD diagnosis; the effect was much stronger in cases with two or more PDs (Sato, Sakado, & Sato, 1993).

A handful of Asian studies have focused specifically on borderline PD, most of them in Japan. Moriya and colleagues (1993) published a preliminary report on 85 female outpatients aged 18 to 30, 32 of whom met criteria for borderline PD based on structured interview. These patients had similar rates of depression, anger, and self-mutilating behaviors; lower rates of substance abuse; and higher rates of derealization and depersonalization as compared with findings from similar studies conducted in the United States. The authors also observed that a greater number of these patients lived with their parents as compared with similar Euro-American samples from previ-ous studies. They concluded that although there were some minor differences requiring further investigation, borderline PD can be identified in Japanese clinical samples. Ikuta and colleagues (1994) followed up with a direct comparison of 19 Japanese and 33 American female outpatients diagnosed with borderline PD. Their conclusion was much stronger: "differences in borderline psychopathology between the samples were minimal. In other words, it is clear that there are borderline patients in Japan whose psychopathology is basically identical to that of American borderline patients" (p. 385). Note that this statement was based entirely on symptom presentation. Other aspects of psychopathology, such as etiology, treatment response, outcome, and so on, were not considered; neither was the cultural meaning of the symptoms or the context in which they were experienced.

Yoshida and colleagues (2006) identified 72 patients in Japan with borderline PD based on retrospective chart diagnosis and successfully contacted 19 of these former patients for questionnaire-based testing. Five of the original group of 72 patients had committed suicide, a rate similar to that reported in North America. The authors reported a link between overinvolvement in family relationships and poorer outcome, similar to previous U.S. findings but, like Moriya and colleagues (1993), they also found that the Japanese patients were more likely to live with their parents, consistent with common practice in many Asian cultural contexts. Also in Japan, Machizawa-Summers (2007) compared 45 psychiatric outpatients with borderline PD to 45 psychiatric outpatients with Axis I psychopathology and no PD. Patients in the borderline PD group reported experiencing higher levels of: physical, emotional, and sexual abuse; physical and emotional neglect; paternal and maternal overprotectiveness; and lack of care. Emotional abuse, emotional neglect, and paternal overprotectiveness were significant independent predictors of borderline PD diagnosis.

Much less work on borderline PD has been conducted in China, likely because the diagnosis has not been incorporated into the Chinese Classification of Mental Disorders, currently in its third revision (CCMD-3; Chinese Society of Psychiatry, 2001). Instead, CCMD-3 includes a category for impulsive PD similar to the impulsive subtype of emotionally unstable PD (i.e., lacking the interpersonal and identity disturbances of borderline PD). Zhong and Leung (2007) note that the few published studies in the Chinese literature suggest that borderline PD, "is a valid clinical diagnostic category among the Chinese population and deserves more research attention" (p. 79). At the same time, they suggest that certain culturally inappropriate criteria would have to be changed, providing "fear of abandonment" and "chronic feelings of emptiness" as examples. S. Lee (2001) reports that the CCMD-3 committee had been reluctant to include borderline PD due to fears of creating social problems by medicalizing impulsivity and emotional instability. Interestingly, whereas *DSM-IV* states that about 75% of borderline PD patients are female, CCMD-3 points out that more than 60% of impulsive PD patients are male. It is not clear at present whether this variation is due to culturally shaped differences in the underlying pathology, or whether impulsive PD criteria describes a group that differs in important ways from borderline PD criteria.

Assessment of DSM-IV Personality Disorders in Asians

X. Huang, Ling, Yang, and Dou (2007) evaluated the Personality Disorders Questionnaire (PDQ-4+; Hyler, 1994), a self-report questionnaire designed to screen for PDs, in a sample of 4,811 college students. They conclude that the instrument, widely used in China, has adequate psychometric properties, and report differences in specific PDs according to a range of demographic variables. Notably, the borderline PD scale is elevated in women, as in the United States and unlike the demographic profile of impulsive PD in CCMD-3. Yang and colleagues (2000) examined the properties of the PDQ-4+ in a sample of 1926 Chinese psychiatric patients, 525 of whom also were administered the Personality Disorder Interview (PDI-IV; Widiger, Mangine, Corbitt, Ellis, & Thomas, 1995). Like Huang and colleagues (2007), they concluded that the Chinese version of the PDQ-4+ has psychometric properties comparable to results obtained in Western countries. The individual PDQ-4+ scales only had modest agreement with their PDI-IV counterparts, attributable in part to having much higher sensitivity than specificity. In other words, as in Western studies (Bagby & Farvolden, 2004), the questionnaire screening measure leads to much higher estimates of PD and PD severity as compared to the corresponding interview measure.

This discrepancy was apparent in a South Korean study of 585 young men sampled from the general population, more than two-thirds of whom were identified as having one or more PDs on the PDQ-4+ (Ha, Kim, Abbey, & Kim, 2007). Although the authors do not comment in detail about this high rate, they do state that self-report measures of PD should be used for screening purposes rather than for diagnosis. They also administered the Temperament and Character Inventory (TCI; Cloninger, Svrakic, & Przybeck, 1993) and found that low self-directedness was the strongest predictor of the presence of PD.

Osone and Takahashi (2003) investigated the psychometric properties of both the self-report screen and interview instruments of the Structured Clinical Interview for DSM-IV, Axis II (SCID-II; First, Gibbon, Spitzer, Williams, & Benjamin, 1997). They administered both instruments to 120 Japanese psychiatric outpatients, repeating the procedure 12 months after the initial interview. As in other studies, the questionnaire had adequate psychometric properties for screening purposes but had a high rate of false positives. The interview had excellent test-retest reliability, attributed by the authors to the use of a single experienced rater who established good rapport with the patients to reduce defensiveness. Based on the interview, 48% and 42% of the sample fulfilled criteria for any PD at Time 1 and Time 2, respectively; obsessive-compulsive and avoidant PDs were the most frequently diagnosed.

Strengths, Weaknesses, and Alternatives in Applying Current Nosology and Diagnostic Criteria for Identifying Personality Disorders in Asians

Limitations of the literature. Many of the major weaknesses found in the current literature on PDs in Asians are attributable to the lack of empirical research. It is difficult to draw conclusions about psychopathology when most of the relevant work focuses on base rates and the psychometric properties of commonly used instruments. Before issuing a general call for more research, however, we believe it is important to look more closely at other weaknesses in the Asian PD literature, and in the PD literature more generally. The studies reviewed here usually do not consider the influence of language and cultural context on the experience and expression of PD symptoms, typical of the PD literature as a whole. That PDs are universal syndromes composed of universal symptoms is taken for granted, rather than serving as a hypothesis. Most of the reviewed studies proceed with translated versions of Western instruments, and most of them briefly describe the use of the translation/back-translation method to maximize translation fidelity. Although the result may be reasonable from a semantic point of view, concerns should remain about the meaning of the constructs measured—both the individual symptoms and their corresponding syndromes. Significant cultural variations exist in such varied domains as self-concept, emotional expressivity, and interpersonal relationships. Examination of various *DSM-IV* PD criteria suggests that caution is required when applying this system across different cultural groups.

For example, two of the diagnostic criteria for dependent personality disorder are, "has difficulty expressing disagreement with others because of fear of loss of support or approval," and, "needs others to assume responsibility for most major areas of his or her life" (APA, 2000, p. 725). However, these traits may be normative rather than pathological in Asian contexts, and therefore carry a significantly different meaning than originally intended. In collectivistic cultural contexts that are interdependent or hierarchical, such as many Asian contexts, it can be damaging for individuals to express disagreement, due to interpersonal concerns about social harmony and status hierarchies. It is also not uncommon in many Asian communities for adults, especially when unmarried, to live with their parents, who may strongly influence or even make decisions for their adult child. This highlights the importance of recognizing the degree to which so-called dependent behaviors are appropriate within an individual's sociocultural context. Successfully doing so, however, requires a clinician who is sufficiently aware of the patient's cultural world and the ways in which it may differ from the clinician's own. Unfortunately, little help in this regard is provided by the existing literature, where there is minimal consideration of the cultural meaning associated with PD criteria.

Examples such as the one above highlight the need to recognize cultural context when interpreting and applying diagnostic criteria, as well as the potential for substantial variations in meaning for the same symptom in different cultural contexts. Translation methods that only emphasize literal or semantic equivalence do not address these crucial issues. Although there is no such thing as "perfect" equivalence of meaning across cultures, careful attention to content validity can help move a given research project in the right direction. It is from such efforts that culturally grounded hypotheses often emerge. Cross-cultural measurement techniques to establish structural and item equivalence (e.g., van de Vijver & Leung, 1997) can further support these efforts when datasets of reasonable size are collected. If individual symptoms carry the same meaning across cultures, we would expect them to interrelate in similar ways (structural equivalence) and to have similar patterns of association with syndrome severity (item equivalence). This approach requires that data be collected from multiple cultural contexts and then compared, which comes with its own difficulties. Nonetheless, it is vastly preferable to adapting an instrument developed in a different cultural context and then arguing that finding broadly similar diagnostic rates is evidence of equivalence, let alone universality.

Returning to the example of dependent personality disorder, it might be the case that another criterion, "Urgently seeks another relationship as a source of care and support when a close relationship ends," would be a particularly unusual, and perhaps unnecessary, response by people who are deeply embedded in an interdependent social network. If so, we would expect a much lower correlation between this criterion and "difficulty expressing disagreement." Moreover, the two criteria would have very different relations with the overall diagnosis: "difficulty expressing disagreement" would need to reach higher levels in Asian cultural contexts compared to Euro-American contexts before indicating psychopathology; the reverse might hold for, "urgently seeks another relationship". Finally, both criteria may need to be discarded for more culturally meaningful alternatives.

Theoretical writing on the centrality of culture to the study of PDs is at present far ahead of, and barely reflected in, the existing empirical database. Alarcón (1996) argues that cultural contextualization is even more important for the PDs than for other forms of psychopathology, given that the nature of personality itself is at least in part shaped by culture and the local context. In contrast, most of the studies reviewed spend very little time describing the cultural context in which the research took place. S. Lee (2001) notes that substantial cultural differences involving the PD criteria and descriptions in *DSM-IV* and CCMD-3 are not surprising given that these disorders, "vary according to the culture-specific conceptions of personhood" (p. 427). Acknowledgment and exploration of these differences would be welcome in the empirical PD literature; direct investigation of their effects would be ideal.

Most of the existing literature of PDs in Asian populations takes an etic approach, where the universality of existing categories or dimensions is assumed. Supposedly universal PD categories, when studied in different cultural groups, are implicitly or explicitly compared to the normative group—Western Europeans and Euro-Americans—among whom these categories were first constructed. This approach does allow for cross-cultural differences to emerge, but at a surface level; PDs might differ in their base-rates, their descriptive features, or their impact on functioning depending on the population being studied, but the categories themselves remain intact. The emic perspective, in contrast, anticipates that cross-cultural differences in complex phenomena such as PDs likely go much deeper—different symptoms, different core concerns, even different constructs altogether.

We do not believe that PDs necessarily must be entirely emic phenomena, and indeed we suspect that PDs likely have both emic and etic characteristics. Our concern is rather that the quantitative literature on PDs in Asian (and other) cultural groups assumes universality. Potential cultural influences are not studied, and often are not even mentioned. In the absence of an Asian PD literature that considers the possibility of important differences, we present here a series of lay concepts that have emerged from work with Asian patients. Rather than seeing these lay descriptions as incontrovertible evidence of cultural difference, we hope they serve as vivid examples of the potential for such difference and as a starting-point for future research. We begin with Asian personality norms and ideals from which PDs would be seen to deviate, organized according to the major philosophical traditions that have deeply influenced East Asian societies. Then, we consider descriptions of pathological personality traits, organized according to descriptive similarity. These lay descriptions emphasize Chinese descriptions, given our clinical and research experience, supplemented where possible by Japanese and Korean examples.

Lay Concepts of Ideal Personality

It is instructive to consider the many differences in the structure and content of Asian personality in light of the philosophical and cultural traditions that have deeply influenced people who trace their background to this part of the world. Although there are a number of Asian philosophical schools, three broad traditions have had widespread influence: Confucianism, Daoism, and Buddhism. There are many specific points on which these perspectives disagree, but there is a tendency across them to tolerate differences and even to entertain paradoxes. What they do have in common is an emphasis on acceptance, interpersonal relatedness, and respect for the natural order. Importantly for our purposes, they represent a significant departure from Western ideals of individuation and mastery, providing a richly detailed alternative conception of "normal"—the standard against which PDs in Asian societies should ultimately be compared.

Since 500 B.C.E., the Analects of Confucius have profoundly influenced Asian societies, especially China, through an emphasis on harmony and the maintenance of the social order as overarching principles (DeBary & Bloom, 1999; Tseng et al., 2005). Society was conceived as hierarchical, with people at a higher station showing benevolence and concern for those at a lower station in return for their devotion and deference. At the individual level, Confucius advocated moderation between extremes of behavior. The upright person, or Junzhi, therefore behaves temperately and respects the social hierarchy; the person of bad character, or Xiaoren, places an inappropriate value on the self. The Junzhi is more concerned with justice, morality, and the welfare of society than he or she is with self-interest and personal gain. Interpersonally, the Junzhi is able to get along well with others, adhering to moral and ethical values without imposing them on other people (Confucius, 1979).

In contrast to the Confucian emphasis on self-cultivation through discipline, learning, and practice, Daoism emphasizes self-cultivation through purification of the heart, which is best achieved through nonstriving (DeBary & Bloom, 1999; Tseng et al., 2005). The wise person, according to Daoism, may refrain from action, *wu wei*, or may act with genuineness, spontaneity, selfless, unconditional love, self-subordination, and noncompetitiveness: "So the wise man acts, but does not possess; accomplishes but lays claim to no credit. If he accomplishes a task, achieves an aim, he does not wish to reveal himself as better than others. So he seems to claim no credit. He seems to have no wish to appear superior, no desire to display excellence" (Lao-Tzu, 1963, ch. 77).

Buddhism is the third major philosophical tradition to deeply influence Asian societies, at the core of Buddhism lie the "Four Noble Truths": (1) life means suffering; (2) the origin of suffering is attachment; (3) the cessation of suffering is attainable; and (4) there is a path to the cessation of suffering. From a psychological point of view, attachment includes attachment to thoughts, emotions, wishes, and even seemingly given ideas such as the self. The "Eightfold Path" to the cessation of suffering includes both the attainment of wisdom and proper ethical living, along with the cultivation of mindfulness and concentration (DeBary & Bloom, 1999). Valued personality characteristics are those that help a person along the eightfold path, and that further develop through following this path; for example, the capacity to resist the pull of anger or desire. A state to strive for, influenced by Buddhist beliefs, is to become less attached to one's ideas and emotions and to be able to see all things lightly and dispassionately. Another important Buddhist concept impacting on Asian people is the karmic law of cause and effect, including beliefs about reincarnation. Some Asian people may attribute their current difficulties in life, including current interpersonal problems, to past life transgressions or past life relationships. These beliefs may also serve as motivation toward righteous behaviors for good karma, to achieve enlightenment, or to reduce suffering when reincarnated.

The prominence and general acceptance of these different strains of thought have varied with time. For example, Confucianism was denigrated by the Chinese government during the Qin dynasty, and again during the Cultural Revolution. European and American cultural values have also influenced Asian societies since the beginning of the colonial era, a process that has only accelerated with globalization. Furthermore, there is a long history of emigration from these societies to North America and Western Europe. Immigrants have found various ways of negotiating heritage and mainstream cultural identities, with implications for personality and self-concept (Ryder, Alden, & Paulhus, 2000). At times, these various forces have worked in concert to bring about striking changes—the influences of Chinese communism and Western ideals have both worked against the traditional patriarchal structure of Confucianism. More often, there are conflicts between various traditional and modern value systems. Therefore, these brief descriptions of philosophical influences must be read as potential contributors to, rather than determinants of, the shape of personality in Asian populations, providing alternative perspectives that can continue to inform both researchers and clinicians.

Lay Concepts of Problematic Personality

Norms of healthy emotional functioning are profoundly shaped by culture. Whereas Euro-American cultural norms often advocate the "pursuit of happiness" as the best way of reaching an ideal emotional state, the preferred emotional state can be described in Chinese as, 心平氣和 "both heart and *qi* at peace," in contrast to being 煩 "agitated or disturbed." Abnormality is conceived in terms of imbalance, as excessive tendency toward any emotional state. In short, Euro-American cultural norms emphasize the promotion of positive affect whereas Asian cultural norms emphasize either low-arousal positive affective states (Tsai, 2007) or moderation and balance of affective states. One consequence may be a tendency to communicate, or even to experience, emotional distress with an emphasis on somatic symptoms rather than psychological symptoms (see also Chapter 9). Somatic symptoms may be seen as socially less disruptive compared with psychological symptoms, especially when describing one's experience to a people with whom one does not have a relationship. Recent cross-cultural depression research has confirmed higher levels of somatic symptom reporting in China, and there is evidence linking this pattern to a cultural tendency to deemphasize the importance of reflecting on inner emotional states or communicating these states to others (Parker, Cheah, & Roy, 2001; Parker, Gladstone, & Chee, 2001; Ryder et al., 2008).

In Chinese, there are numerous expressions to describe people who tend toward certain extreme emotional reactions, reflecting the tendency to value a balanced emotional life. Angry people, for example, are described as 脾氣暴躁, having a problematic "*qi* of the spleen," in reference to concepts from traditional Chinese medicine (TCM); similarly, chronic fearfulness is sometimes referred to as 膽小, "a small gallbladder." Excessive sadness and anxiety are frowned upon, whereas the tendency to be quietly content is described as 開朗, "open like clear weather." The Korean folk category of *hwa byung* ("fire illness")—believed to be caused by unresolved suppressed anger and possibly a variant of mood disorder—has increasingly become a focus of clinical attention in work with Koreans (e.g., Kim, Kim, & Kelly, 2006), suggesting a particular concern with problematic anger. While impulsively acting on one's emotions is often tolerated and sometimes celebrated in the West, doing so is considered a character weakness in Asian societies. Emotional stability is valued; a person who has mood swings is described as 喜怒无常 ("joy and anger never stable") or 情緒化 ("overly emotional").

Many, if not all, PDs involve marked impairment in relating to others. In Chinese, people who have difficulty in this domain are said to have poor Ren Yuan, which may be attributed to external forces such as fate or destiny or to a person's own personality. Numerous expressions describe people who lack compassion and who tend to offend, even oppress, other people. Such people might be described as 鐵石心腸 "having heart and intestines made of steel and stone," or as 橫行霸道 "walking sideways to block other people's paths by force." While a lack of empathy and compassion might map onto Western ideas of narcissim, antisociality and psychopathy, there is comparatively greater devaluing of independence relative to dependence in Chinese in general; in contrast, *DSM-IV* pathologizes the latter (dependent PD) but not the former. People who insist on their own ideas are described as unnecessarily stubborn, 死牛一邊頸 "like a dead cow with a twisted neck and unable to turn." Having the ability to advocate one's perspective and to debate with others is a hallmark of intellectual maturity in Western contexts, but may be seen as disruptive and detrimental to learning in Asian societies (Tweed & Lehman, 2002).

It follows that overconfidence, boastfulness, and grandiosity are viewed very negatively within traditional Chinese culture—similar to narcissistic PD, but with a much lower tolerance threshold before such behaviors are seen as pathological. Maintaining one's "face" and the good impressions of others is important, but being excessively concerned with these issues can be seen as selfish. Instead, it is preferable to focus one's concern on helping others to maintain their face and act in a humble and self-effacing manner. People in a well-functioning in-group focus on helping each other make a good impression, rather than on projecting a good impression themselves. In this way, harmony is maintained. Similar concerns can be identified in Japanese and Korean cultural contexts (e.g., Hamamura & Heine, 2007).

Although the ideal Asian interpersonal style is not necessarily characterized by traits traditionally associated with Western extraversion (e.g., assertiveness, confidence), an emphasis is nonetheless placed on social engagement over withdrawal. Social avoidance and isolation are pathologized, similar to schizoid or avoidant PDs, but especially when the isolation is from family. Studies of social avoidance in China and Japan (Dinnel, Kleinknecht, & Tanaka-Matsumi, 2002; A. Y. Zhang, Yu, Draguns, Zhang, & Tang, 2000) suggest that a major component of the underlying anxiety is a fear of causing discomfort to others and thereby disrupting social harmony. Although this concern is not absent in North America (Rector, Kocovski, & Ryder, 2006), it is less central than are fears of displaying an inadequate self and of being rejected, as in *DSM*-based descriptions of social phobia. This distinction raises the possibility that some PDs may share similar behavioral manifestations (e.g., nervousness in social situations) but with different underlying rationales.

In China, there are descriptions of patients who become afraid that they are giving away secrets and past transgressions through subtle social cues that they cannot control (A. Y. Zhang et al., 2000). In Japan, social avoidance due to a fear of giving offense is known as Taijin-Kyofu-Sho and includes the themes that one is inadvertently and inappropriately giving away too much about the self, leading others to feel uncomfortable. At the extreme, there are reports of debilitating concerns about the impact of one's gaze or one's body odor, concerns that might be deemed delusional in North America (Cousins, 1990). A rapidly growing problem in Japan is a condition of extreme isolation, often following a shameful failure experience, known as *hikikomori* (Watts, 2002). Such individuals may isolate themselves, even from close family, for many years. Little is known about this phenomenon beyond anecdotes, but the chronicity combined with onset in adolescence or early adulthood suggests PD.

PERSPECTIVES ON THE CAUSES OF PERSONALITY DISORDERS IN ASIANS

The discussion above includes an overview of some of the personality traits seen as undesirable within Asian cultural contexts. Whether undesirable or even maladaptive traits necessarily equate to "pathology" or treatable entities depends on one's philosophical and theoretical orientation. As we turn to various perspectives on cause, we are reminded again that the category of PD is fraught with uncertainty—there are increasingly mainstream concerns about whether PDs constitute valid diagnostic entities at all, in Western societies or anywhere else. PDs have been criticized for their poor interrater reliability, questionable validity, high levels of conceptual and empirical overlap, and failure to adequately categorize the surprising number of patients who meet criteria for PD-NOS without fitting into any of the existing categories (Clark et al., 1997; Livesley, 1998). Indeed, the assumption that PDs are even categories at all has increasingly been called into question (Clark & Watson, 1999; Ryder et al., 2002).

There is growing support for the idea that personality pathology has a replicable dimensional structure that can be integrated with the literature on "normal" personality (Costa & Widiger, 2002; Widiger & Trull, 2007). The following section therefore includes a detailed consideration of the approach that has thus far received the most empirical attention. Successful adoption of such a model has the potential to link long-separated literatures on normal and abnormal personality, and would substantially alter the research agenda for the cross-cultural study of PDs. Nonetheless, we would do well to remember that the use of dimensional models does not negate the problems and complexities with defining "pathology" or the danger of conflating undesirable sociocultural values with pathology (Wakefield, 2008).

Critical Appraisal of Major Etiological Models of Personality Disorders

Biological Models

The first biological models of PD etiology came from the early psychiatric taxonomists, who observed that the relatives of patients with schizophrenia would often show personality traits that appeared to be attenuated symptoms (Oldham, Skodol, & Bender, 2009). Behavioral genetic research on the heritability of schizotypal PD continues to show evidence of this link (e.g., Lenzenweger, 1998; Torgersen et al., 2000). For example, Torgersen (1984) found that 7 of 21 identical twins of schizophrenia patients met criteria for schizotypal PD, whereas only 1 of 23 fraternal twins did so. Adoption studies, meanwhile, have demonstrated that antisocial PD has both genetic and environmental roots; for example, Cadoret and colleagues (1995) found that adult adoptees are four times more likely to have problems with aggression if their biological parent has been arrested for antisocial behavior, but also are three times more likely to have these problems if it is their adoptive parent who has been arrested. Finally, behavior genetic research on borderline PD has had more success showing high heritability for specific components rather than for the diagnosis as a whole (Oldham et al., 2009).

Several biological models have attempted to link PDs and their features to specific neurobiological systems. The most widely researched effort is Cloninger's (1998) seven-factor model of personality, which includes four dimensions of "temperament," each linked to one or two neurotransmitter systems: novelty-seeking (dopamine), harm avoidance (serotonin), reward dependence (norepinephrine and serotonin), and persistence (glutamate and serotonin). Broadly speaking, Cluster A PDs are linked to low reward dependence, Cluster B PDs to high novelty-seeking, and Cluster C PDs to high harm avoidance (Oldham et al., 2009). Although different in their specifications, models by Siever and Davis (1991) and by Depue and colleagues (Depue & Collins, 1999; Depue & Lenzenweger, 2001) represent broadly similar attempts to develop models in which PD-relevant traits can be mapped in the brain.

Psychological Models

Psychoanalytic theorists were the first to develop psychological models of PDs, doing so originally using classical notions of conflict and defense. There has been increasing appreciation in recent years, by psychoanalysts and also by other PD researchers, that these patients also have problems with temperament and attachment. Oldham and colleagues (2009) argue that PDs have five features that are important from a psychodynamic point of view: (1) they are patterns rather than distinct symptoms; (2) they exist on a continuum from health to pathology; (3) character style is orthogonal to level of disturbance; (4) they involve implicit and explicit processes; and (5) they are deeply entrenched, often serve multiple functions, and are resistant to change. Kernberg (1984) has described a detailed model of PD in which personality organization ranges along a continuum encompassing healthy, neurotic, borderline, and psychotic levels of functioning. Borderline PD patients are seen as having trouble constructing a coherent identity, most often placing them at the borderline level of functioning; many narcissistic PD patients, in contrast, function at a higher level in that their inflated and thereby distorted identity retains coherence.

A major alternative to psychodynamically based psychological models comes from the social learning tradition, an amalgamation of behavioral and cognitive theories that has only recently been applied to PDs (Oldham et al., 2009). Patients with PDs misinterpret information, develop pathological self-schemas, attend to information in biased ways, and encode information in biased ways. For example, a patient with paranoid PD might selectively look for evidence of threat and interpret ambiguous social interactions as evidence of attack. Beck and colleagues (2003) have linked PDs to particular cognitive schemas that organize and perpetuate patterns of bias. Building on this approach, Young and colleagues (2003) have hearkened back to psychodynamic thinking by introducing the idea of early maladaptive schemas, which tend to be particularly pervasive and affect-laden relative to schemas consisting mainly of automatic thoughts and underlying assumptions. They describe cognitive processes involving schema maintenance, avoidance, and compensation, processes that lead to the development and maintenance of pathological schemas.

Social Models

Many of the psychological models of PD include social elements, usually interpersonal, in which people with PDs interpret the behaviors of others and in turn behave in ways that impact on others. Systems theorists have gone further, describing ways in which the behavior of PD patients actually elicits particular responses from others, actively feeding a pathological interpersonal cycle. Benjamin (1993) provides a modern example of such an approach, integrating interpersonal and object-relations theories. In this approach, children learn to respond to others by acting like them, eliciting familiar behaviors from them, and treating others as they have been treated. Over time, this learning process leads to different ways of behaving with others, which Benjamin codes on three interpersonal circles: how one acts toward another, how one interprets the actions of another, and how one views the self. Each of these circles contrasts "love" versus "hate" on one axis and "enmeshment" versus "differentiation" on the other. PDs and their specific criteria have been described according to this interpersonal system.

The Five-Factor Model of Personality as an Integrative Approach

While the various models of PD all potentially have something to contribute to our understanding of PDs in Asians, most of them lack research in this population. The five-factor model of personality (FFM), by contrast, has a vast research literature that can be brought to bear on Asian PDs. Arguably, many of the flaws in the current PD system could be addressed through a dimensional approach, not least the considerable heterogeneity within each PD category combined with the number of clearly disordered people who fall in the gaps between these categories (Livesley, 1998; Ryder et al., 2002; Widiger & Trull, 2007). Moreover, the move toward a dimensional system for *DSM-5* has been driven at least in part by research linking the FFM to specific PDs, and it is likely that whatever system ends up being adopted will at least be influenced by, and linked to, the FFM (Costa & Widiger, 2002; Widiger & Mullins-Sweatt, 2009). While generally conceived as a psychological theory of personality, the FFM can be seen as an integrative approach—the traits have received more behavioral genetics attention than have the PDs, and their interpersonal implications have been studied extensively.

The FFM has its origins in a decades-long effort to find a core set of traits that could provide a common language for the field. Allport and Odbert (1936) began this process by proposing the lexical hypothesis that important concepts for describing individual differences in personality would be encoded in the natural language used by laypeople. The application of modern factor analytic techniques to trait adjectives has consistently pointed to a five-factor structure, often referred to as the Big Five (John & Srivastava, 1998). McCrae and Costa (1985) originally proposed a three-factor model, with neuroticism (N), extraversion (E), and openness (O) as primary dimensions. Comparisons of this model with scales from the lexical tradition showed that N, E, and O captured three of the lexical factors. Two additional lexical factors—agreeableness (A) and conscientiousness (C)—were not well defined. As a result, Costa and McCrae (1985) developed the NEO Personality Inventory (NEO PI) to measure N, E, O, A, and C.

Although there is widespread agreement among trait psychologists about the centrality of the five factors, there is less of a consensus on whether we should expect to see similar distributions of traits across different cultural groups. McCrae (2001, 2002) notes that there is good evidence for the reliability and factorial validity of the NEO PI-R across a wide range of cultural and linguistic groups. A study of college students in 50 countries using the peer-rating version of the NEO PI-R demonstrated that highly similar factor structures emerge across all samples (McCrae et al., 2005). Moreover, country-level factor analyses, in which country means are treated as single observations, also yield the five-factor structure (McCrae, 2001, 2002). An index of country distance using all five factors is modestly correlated with genetic distance between countries (Allik, 2005). Twin studies of the FFM have shown moderate heritability for all five domains as well as unique heritability for most of the facets; notably, the same studies show little evidence of the shared environment effects that would result from cultural influence (Jang et al., 1998; Loehlin, 1992).

Strengths, Weaknesses, and Alternatives in Applying Current Etiological Models of Personality Disorders to Asians

Applicability of the FFM to Asian Contexts

Rather than simply validating the NEO PI-R across cultural groups, any attempt to apply the FFM to Asians requires evidence that the approach can be used to predict the same external variables in different ethnocultural groups. Looking at research on Asian samples, there is evidence for good interjudge agreement in Hong Kong (Yik, Bond, & Paulhus, 1998) and self-spouse agreement in Koreans studying in the United States (Spirrison & Choi, 1998). The NEO PI-R domains relate similarly to life satisfaction in Hong Kong and the United States (Kwan, Bond, & Singelis, 1997), and to the overall pattern of momentary affect ratings in Japan and Canada (Yik et al., 2002). McCrae and colleagues (1998) showed mean differences between Hong Kong Chinese and Euro-Canadian samples, suggesting lower levels of imaginative fantasy, need for variety, liberalism, and optimism among the Chinese. They interpreted these results as consistent with portrayals of Chinese culture as conservative and pragmatic.

Although some of the above findings are promising for the application of the FFM to Asian cultural groups, the possibility remains that the use of a single instrument in various translations is to some extent imposing a particular structure, akin to the problems already described for PD instruments. After all, the NEO PI-R was developed in the United States for the purpose of comprehensively measuring the FFM. Failure to replicate its structure in other countries would be strong evidence against the FFM; consistent replication is promising, but not definitive. Indeed, Church (2000) notes that many other Western-developed instruments that carve up the personality space in quite different ways have also shown a replicable structure across different cultural groups. For example, the structure of the Temperament and Character Inventory (TCI) has been replicated among Japanese (Tomita et al., 2000) and Malaysian Chinese (Parker, Cheah, & Parker, 2003) samples.

These last findings notwithstanding, efforts to link observed trait differences with consensus impressions of different cultures have not been particularly successful. McCrae (2001) presented lists of countries, each rank-ordered by an FFM domain, to eight prominent cross-cultural psychologists and asked them to identify the domain used to organize the list. The experts only performed at the level of chance and reported that they found the task difficult. Church and Katigbak (2002) asked 43 "bicultural judges" who had spent considerable time living in both the Philippines and the United States whether Filipinos or Americans would score higher on a particular trait. Although there was a high degree of interjudge agreement, the responses did not correspond with mean NEO PI-R profiles. Finally, Terracciano and colleagues (2005) asked respondents in 49 countries to rate a typical person from their own country and found a low correspondence between mean profiles based on ethnic self-stereotypes and actual mean profiles previously obtained from each country. The authors interpreted the results as evidence that there is little validity to these stereotypes, although Heine, Buchtel, and Norenzayan (2008) found that country-level self-stereotypes of conscientiousness are considerably better predictors of external criterion variables than are aggregate self- or peer-report ratings.

When the lexical approach was originally proposed, one of its stated advantages was the freedom of trait adjectives from the theoretical commitments of specific researchers. Rather than importing instruments designed to optimize a given structure, some research teams have repeated the lexical procedure in a variety of languages. Yang and Bond (1990) used a set of personality descriptors extracted from Chinese written sources, together with an established set of translated English descriptors, and asked Taiwanese students to rate six target people using this combined set. Although five dimensions emerged from factor analysis of the Chinese descriptors, only two of them had a one-to-one correspondence with FFM domains. Church, Reyes, Katigbak, and Grimm (1997) asked Filipino students to rate themselves on 622 personally trait and evaluative adjectives. A seven-factor solution was identified containing the lexical Big Five, with N split into two factors and with negative evaluative terms loading on a separate factor. Hahn, Lee, and Ashton (1999) asked Korean students to rate themselves on the 406 most commonly used Korean trait adjectives along with translated markers of the lexical Big Five. Factor analysis of the Korean adjectives yielded four factors corresponding to N, E, A, and C; forcing a fifth factor yielded a dimension corresponding to the intellectual aspects of O.

An alternative approach, one that often grows out of initial lexical work, is the development of indigenous personality instruments. The CPAI (F. M. Cheung et al., 1996) was developed in Hong Kong and Mainland China to measure personality and psychopathology in Chinese cultural contexts using both emic and etic constructs. Emic concepts were derived from reviews of novels, proverbs, informal surveys, and reviews of the psychological literature on Chinese personality. Factor analysis of the personality scales in a large standardization sample yielded four factors, including one originally called Chinese tradition, later relabeled interpersonal relatedness (IR). In a separate study of Chinese students, joint factor-analysis with the NEO PI-R supported a six-factor solution, with N, E, O, A, C, and IR each emerging as separate factors; there were no NEO PI-R scales on IR and no CPAI scales on O. Individual scales on the IR factor were moderately related to, but not redundant with, the FFM factors either independently or in combination (F. M. Cheung et al., 2001). J. Zhang and Bond (1998) found that specific components of the IR domain predicted endorsement of filial piety, an important value in Chinese societies, over and above the contributions of the FFM.

Many studies have shown difficulties in identifying a separate and reliable O domain in Asian samples. Low reliabilities for O scales have been found in Chinese students (McCrae, Costa, & Yik, 1996; F. M. Cheung et al., 2001), Filipino students (Katigbak, Church, Guanzon-Lapeña, Carlota, & del Pilar, 2002), Malay students (Mastor, Jin, & Cooper, 2000), and Chinese patients (Yang et al., 1999), for the domains and especially for some of the individual facets of the NEO PI-R. Indeed, Leung and colleagues (1997) reported confirmatory factor analyses using individual NEO PI-R items, and found that the facet scales measuring openness to actions and values were particularly problematic. Yang and Bond (1990) did not identify a single Chinese etic factor corresponding to O in their lexical study, and previous efforts to develop Chinese indigenous personality instruments have never yielded a clear O factor (P. C. Cheung et al., 1992; Yik & Bond, 1993). Neither the QZPS from Mainland China nor the PKP from the Philippines include subscales that correlate with O (Katigbak et al., 2002; Wang et al., 2005).

Applicability of Fixed Personality Traits to Asian Contexts

The results summarized above argue against the simple adoption of the FFM in Asian societies, leading immediately to thoughts of possible alternatives. One might modify the FFM, or emphasize those aspects that do clearly replicate. Alternatively, one might look for another trait theory—perhaps one of the biological approaches to personality and PD that are more clearly based on genetic and neuroscience research. More fundamental, however, is the extent to which a trait approach to personality should be taken as the best way, or the sole way, to conceive of personality in Asian societies. As we shall see, cultural psychologists have raised serious questions about the assumption of more-or-less fixed personality traits and whether this assumption holds equally true in different cultural contexts. Given that many approaches to PD emphasize fixedness, we can expect this debate to have implications for cross-cultural analysis of PDs as well regardless of which system is ultimately adopted for *DSM-5*.

That an interpersonal relatedness factor might emerge more strongly and consistently in Asian samples dovetails with several other lines of cultural psychology research. Markus and Kitayama (1991) reviewed the literature on the self-concept in the United States and Japan, contrasting the former's emphasis on the independent self-concept with the latter's emphasis on interdependent self-concept. Whereas the independent self is a separate entity grounded in and focused on internal traits, the interdependent self is grounded in roles and in relationships with others, a distinction that resembles the distinction between individualistic and collectivistic cultural values. The considerable empirical literature that followed publication of this review established that these differences in the self-concept have implications for emotional, motivational, cognitive, and even perceptual processes (see reviews by Markus & Kitayama, 1991; Nisbett, Peng, Choi, & Norenzayan, 2001; Heine, 2007).

One finding is that people in Asian cultural contexts generally have a much weaker motivation to pursue psychological elevation of their self-esteem as compared with people in Western cultural contexts. A meta-analysis of cross-cultural comparisons shows a robust difference across a variety of samples and methodologies, and a second meta-analysis of within-culture self-enhancing biases shows a large effect in Western samples and no effect in Asian samples (Heine & Hamamura, 2007). Moreover, the pursuit of self-esteem may actually be less beneficial in Asian cultural contexts, where self-esteem is not as strongly correlated with subjective well-being on the one hand (Diener & Diener, 1995; Kwan, Bond, & Singelis, 1997) or depression on the other (Heine & Lehman, 1999). These findings challenge long-held beliefs in social psychology about the centrality of self-esteem and the universality of the biases and distortions that help maintain it. They also have potentially important—and at present, all but unexplored—clinical ramifications.

In self-evaluation research, Asian respondents are more likely to take the perspective of an external evaluator as compared with Western respondents, who attend more to internal standards (for a review, see Cohen, Hoshino-Browne, & Leung, 2007). This tendency has been linked to the Asian concern for maintaining "face" and even has implications for memory and perception. For example, there is evidence that Asian, compared to Western, individuals are more likely to remember themselves from a third-person perspective when thinking back to times when they were the center of attention (Cohen & Gunz, 2002), and they perform better on tasks where they have to take the visual perspective of another person (Wu & Keysar, 2007).

There are also established cross-cultural differences in the beliefs that people have about the nature of abilities, talents, and skills. Several questionnaire studies have demonstrated that Asian students are more likely to perceive school performance as based on effort compared with Western students (for a review, see Heine & Buchtel, 2009). An experimental study with Japanese and American students demonstrated a tendency to emphasize either effort or ability, respectively, unless primed to think otherwise (Heine et al., 2001). To the extent that people who favor ability over effort directly link success and failure link to deep and relatively unchangeable aspects of the self, it is not surprising that Western people, much more than Asian people, would be motivated to engage in various biases to avoid focusing on actual or potential failure.

Finally, cross-cultural variation in self-enhancing motivations can be linked to cultural differences in tolerance for contradiction (Peng & Nisbett, 1999). Asian respondents are more likely to endorse opposing propositions when describing their personalities (Choi & Choi, 2002), current emotional state (Bagozzi, Wong, & Yi, 1999), self-esteem (Spencer-Rodgers, Peng, Wang, & Hou, 2004), and behavior across situations (Suh, 2002). This tendency, referred to as naive dialecticism (Peng & Nisbett, 1999), would lead to moderate views of the self with a greater tolerance for seeing the self as having both positive and negative characteristics. In contrast, Euro-Americans generally report self-views that are massively positive (Heine et al., 1999). Indeed, there is evidence to suggest that high self-esteem is maintained in part by the ability to maintain a view of the self that is both positive and consistent (Campbell et al., 1996).

If traits are less influential and less useful to Asian as compared with Western people, we would predict that the spontaneous self-descriptions of the former might contain fewer trait adjectives. In the Twenty Statements Test (Kuhn & McPartland, 1954), participants are asked to complete 20 sentences starting with "I am ... " On the whole, individuals from Asian cultural contexts tend to list fewer pure psychological attributes as compared with individuals from Western cultural contexts, instead preferring to describe themselves according to roles and/or concrete personal descriptors (see Heine & Buchtel, 2009). Cousins (1989) demonstrated, in samples of Japanese and American students, that this cross-cultural difference disappears when respondents are provided situational contexts to frame the open-ended statements. It may be that Asian people use trait terms to describe themselves in context more often than they use them to describe themselves in the abstract.

There is evidence to suggest that Asian individuals do report a wider range of personality variation depending on context. Suh (2002) asked Korean and American participants to provide self-reports of personality "in general," as well as with four specified types of person (e.g., "with a close friend"). The consistency among these five ratings was much lower among Korean participants as compared with American participants. Moreover, self-consistency positively predicted subjective well-being and positive ratings from others among American participants, but not Korean participants. English and Chen (2007) also asked Asian- and Euro-American participants to rate their personality in reference to different relationship contexts, but in this case repeated the task after intervals of several months. Results showed less cross-situational consistency in Asian Americans as compared with Euro-Americans, but the two groups demonstrated the same consistency over time within each situational context. The researchers concluded that trait consistency in Asian people, rather than being absent, depends on the interpersonal context (see also Kashima et al., 2004).

In an eight-country study of lay beliefs about personality (Church et al., 2006), American and Euro-Australian participants strongly endorsed ideas consistent with the traditional view of personality traits, such as the belief that traits are good predictors of behavior across different situations. Asian-Australian, Japanese, Chinese-Malaysian, Malay, Filipino (and also Mexican) participants, in contrast, were much more likely to state that social roles or responsibilities are better predictors of behavior. The finding that Asian newspapers are less likely to provide personality trait information as compared with Western newspapers (Morris & Peng, 1994) may reflect, as well as reinforce, these different lay beliefs.

Tentative Conclusions

Several approaches to PDs take a trait approach to personality, one that might reflect a Western tendency to see the self as relatively fixed and separated from context. While the research reviewed above does not invalidate personality traits in Asian contexts, it suggests that the importance of traits as compared with more situationally based factors may be relatively less than in Western contexts. We should therefore be cautious when applying existing theories of personality, or of PD, to Asian societies, or indeed to many other parts of the world. Unfortunately, we are again hampered here by the lack of research testing specific etiological models of PD in Asian contexts, a problem worsened by the plethora of different theories available. More theoretically driven research would be invaluable here, and such research should include a greater attention to social and contextual factors than is usual. As well, we would hope that the increased focus on these ingredients of PD would not only take place in Asian studies but would also inform other PD researchers, enriching the main body of literature on personality pathology.

TREATING PERSONALITY DISORDERS IN ASIANS

Researchers continue to struggle with how best to define both normal and problematic personality. This section will focus on exploring a clinical approach to assessing and treating PDs in Asian people, which may also have implications for the definition and understanding of PDs in general, across a range of cultural groups. Approaches to culturally competent care generally emphasize two intersecting domains of competence. Generic cultural competence encompasses the attitudes, knowledge, and skills necessary to work effectively across different cultures, whereas specific cultural competence includes the specialized knowledge and skills needed to work effectively with a particular cultural group (Lo & Fung, 2003). One framework for the former is to attend to and address cultural issues throughout the process of clinical intervention. Heuristically, this can be divided into five phases: pre-engagement; engagement; assessment; diagnosis and formulation; and treatment.

We begin with a brief summary of the first four phases, before moving on to a more detailed coverage of treatment.

Pre-Engagement and Engagement

Even before the clinician meets the patient, there are multiple pre-engagement cultural factors that may impact the later phases of treatment. In particular, culture shapes one's values and ideals, including the conceptions of ideal, normative, or deviant personalities, as discussed earlier. Engagement begins with the coming together of the clinician and patient, and the process of forming a therapeutic relationship. Building a mutual, trusting, and collaborative relationship helps clinicians to obtain information from patients, facilitates patients' commitment to move in a positive direction, enhances adherence to pharmacotherapy, and is crucial to success in psychotherapy. Establishing such a relationship can be particularly challenging for patients with PDs.

For Asian immigrants in Western settings, language barriers and cultural factors may further complicate engagement. One approach that may help to facilitate engagement is linguistic and cultural matching between therapist and patient (Sue, 1998). The patient may feel more comfortable and open in discussing his or her issues with the clinician, and it may be easier for clinicians to empathically see the world from the patient's perspective. Within any Asian cultural group, however, factors such as gender, class, and subcultures may be very important considerations in considering a patient-therapist "match." For example, among the Chinese, some patients may carry preconceived ideas or strong opinions about Chinese individuals from different parts of the world, such as Mainland China, Hong Kong, and Taiwan. In addition to practical considerations such as spoken dialect, different geographical origins may influence trust. Similarly, trust can be an issue between Northern and Southern Vietnamese, or Northern and Southern Koreans. For more conservative Asian patients, a gender difference between patient and therapist may interfere with the patient's comfort in discussing certain personal issues, such as intimate relationships.

Often, establishing a cultural and linguistic match is not feasible for patients from Asian immigrant communities. Further, some patients may prefer a therapist from outside of their cultural group, especially if they feel that those sharing their cultural values will judge them negatively. Under such circumstances, a clinician from a different cultural background may need to acquire skills in working with an interpreter. As well, when working cross-culturally, it is paramount for the clinician to examine his or her own attitudes and judgments regarding the patient's cultural group. A cultural consultant may be needed to fill in knowledge gaps.

Assessment

As patients with PDs often lack insight into their maladaptive personality traits, it is uncommon for personality problems to be identified as a "chief complaint." Instead, depression, anxiety, somatic complaints such as pain or insomnia, and stress related to impaired functioning, such as work or interpersonal problems, often compel patients to seek treatment. Alternatively, patients may present for treatment at the urging of family members, or even be brought in by family members.

Since PDs are, by definition, long-standing problems, they are often described by the patient, family members, or other informants as simply representing the way the patient has always been. The gathering of information depends on the specific therapist's orientation, the patient's clinical problems, and intended treatment goals. It is often crucial to interview family members or other informants to get a collateral history from various perspectives. Since situational, psychosocial, and cultural issues may confound the diagnosis, it is important to have a longitudinal assessment before a conclusive diagnosis is made.

In specialized clinics, structured interview, self-report, or clinician-administered questionnaires may be used to assess personality disorders. There are several limitations to the use of these instruments, however, namely: (1) need for training in administration and interpretation; (2) inflexibility of the instruments regarding, for example, length and required literacy level; (3) small evidence base to support cultural applicability and validity, especially for translated versions; and (4) unclear applicability to clinical treatment, especially in Asian populations. Additional tools might be administered depending on the clinician's theoretical orientation, but at present most such instruments suffer from similar problems.

Diagnosis and Formulation

The rationale underlying "diagnosis" is based on the biomedical model, in which the ultimate goal is to understand a pathological entity's etiology and pathophysiology; from this perspective, diagnosis has the potential to explicate symptoms, inform treatment, and predict outcome. As reviewed earlier, however, there are numerous questions about the validity of a categorical approach to PDs even for North American and European people. Regardless, even if a fully dimensional approach is eventually adopted, clinicians will still need to make some binary diagnostic decisions—most importantly, whether or not a constellation of personality traits is causing sufficient impairment to warrant treatment.

Regardless of the diagnostic approach, the act of making a diagnosis—the act of identifying personality pathology—has implications of which clinicians need to be aware. PD diagnoses are highly stigmatizing; for the Chinese, both the concept and the words used to describe it carry connotations of moral deficit. Diagnosis often leads to labeling, which in turn can decrease appreciation for individual differences among patients categorized under a common label. Moreover, unless properly framed, diagnosis tends to attribute blame to the individual rather than highlighting the interactions between the individual and his or her sociocultural environment, current stressors, and life history.

Rather than emphasizing diagnostic labels for personality disorders, clinicians may consider placing greater focus on the clinical formulation of their patients. A formulation is an explanation of why a client has encountered his or her identified problems. For example, the therapist may try to make a meaningful link between past events and present functioning, and between hypothesized psychological structures or processes and manifest symptoms. This process allows clinicians to collaboratively set goals and treatment plans with their patients and to make predictions about treatment course and patients' future behaviors. Individual case formulation is an iterative process, and formulated hypotheses can be validated or invalidated as new evidence emerges in working with the patient. Both the formulation and the resulting plan of treatment need to be informed by considerations of culture.

Critical Appraisal of Major Treatment Approaches for Personality Disorders

Biological Approaches

Currently, medications used for the treatment of PDs target individual symptoms rather than diagnostic categories. Most of this work has focused on borderline PD (Oldham et al., 2001; Paris, 2008; Tyrer & Bateman, 2004). For example, affective dysregulation such as depressed mood with intense anger may be effectively treated with a selective serotonin reuptake inhibitor (SSRI) or serotonin-norepinephrine reuptake inhibitor (SNRI) (Paris, 2008). The effectiveness of escitalopram, in particular, has been established in Chinese psychiatric patients (Mao et al., 2008). SSRIs or SNRIs can also be used to help decrease anticipatory anxiety or social avoidance, alone or in combination with benzodiazepines or anticonvulsants such as gabapentin (Kasper, Stein, Loft, & Nil, 2005; Pande, Davidson, & Jefferson, 1999; Seedat & Stein, 2004). For patients exhibiting mood swings, mood stabilizers may also be tried (Frankenburg & Zanarini, 2002). If behavior control problems are more severe (e.g., impulsive aggression, self-mutilation, or other impulsive self-damaging behavior), a low-dose neuroleptic can be added (Zanarini & Frankenburg, 2001). Low doses of neuroleptics are also beneficial for the psychosis-like or dissociative symptoms associated with schizotypal or borderline PDs (Koenigsberg et al., 2003; Rocca, Marchiaro, Cocuzza, & Bogetto, 2002; Koenigsberg et al., 2003).

Herbs and plants from TCM may be more acceptable to some patients with Asian backgrounds, due to their alleged lower incidence of side effects. Experiencing, or even just anticipating, fewer side effects can markedly improve treatment adherence. Recently, Miyaoka and colleagues (2008) reported that Yi-gan san (YGS), a Chinese compound herbal medication, may be a safe and effective treatment for symptoms associated with borderline PD. They conducted a 12-week open-label pilot study with YGS on 20 women diagnosed with borderline PD according to DSM-IV criteria. Highly significant improvement was demonstrated on a variety of clinical assessment scales. Although YGS appears promising, double-blind randomized control trials will be needed to further examine its efficacy.

Psychological Approaches

Psychoanalysis and the various psychodynamic approaches have been introduced to, and used clinically by, psychologists and psychiatrists in many Asian countries, including China, Japan, and Korea. There is a lack of research on the effectiveness of this approach for treating PDs in Asian patients, although practitioners have written about the need to adapt techniques for patients with this background. Some of the underlying assumptions and basic constructs, however, may require further cultural consideration. For example, Mahler's description of child development as proceeding toward individuation, as well as Winnicott's emphasis on a true self versus a false self formed under the influence of social pressures, express ideals of Western individualism. Similarly, self-psychology's emphasis on the reparation of the self seems contradictory to Buddhism's goal of no-self.

To address some of these issues, psychoanalysts who are also students and practitioners of Zen Buddhism have written about how psychoanalysis may be compatible or even thoughtfully integrated with Buddhist teachings (Epstein, 1995; Magid, 2001). Although most practitioners are unlikely to integrate culturally specific Buddhist concepts into their work, there are some technical adjustments that should be considered when using conventional approaches with Asian patients. In formulating the goals of treatment, the clinician may need to consider the tendency to value individualism in psychodynamic therapies. Some patients may benefit from a more cohesive sense of independent self, while others may benefit from relinquishing their investment in the independent self.

In terms of process, emotional self-control and the ability to manage one's own emotional problems to maintain social harmony are valued in Asian culture (Atkinson & Gim, 1989; Shen & Alden, 2006). Attempts to conceal emotional distress and negative personal information may lead to avoidance during exploration of intrapsychic phenomena. Before a trusting relationship is established, the therapist should be cautious when encouraging patients to reveal their inner world, as Asian patients may be quite concerned about how they are perceived and judged by others. Therefore, confrontation should be carefully used, as not allowing an Asian patient to "save face" may result in a treatment-ending failure. Transference and countertransference need to be examined in cultural context, including ways in which the self and relationships are perceived in Asian culture.

Despite limited available evidence supporting the efficacy of cognitive behavior therapy (CBT) in Asia, there has been a steady increase in its popularity in Asian countries (Hodges & Oei, 2007). Luk and colleagues (1991) demonstrated that group CBT improved psychiatric symptoms, capacity to cope with problems, and increased social activities for Chinese clients with a variety of mental disorders, including 12 patients with PDs. A recent randomized wait-list control study has shown that group CBT for Chinese people with depression in Hong Kong is effective in reducing depression and increasing adaptive coping skills (Wong, 2008).

Some features of CBT may be more compatible with Asian values and preferences as compared with psychodynamic psychotherapies (Chen & Davenport, 2005; Hodges & Oei, 2007). Patients with an Asian cultural background will often favor a logical, rational, and directive counseling style over a reflective, affect-focused, and nondirective one (Atkinson, 1978). An approach based on education and problem resolution, with didactic instruction and homework assignments, appears to be consistent with Asian, particularly Confucian, emphases on learning and education. There are, nonetheless, recommendations to modify traditional CBT to improve its fit to Asian populations (Chen & Davenport, 2005; Hwang et al., 2006; Shen et al., 2006).

For Asian patients, the role of the therapist may be cast as a teacher with its embedded cultural meanings, which has both advantages and disadvantages. The teacher role is likely to be more familiar than that of "therapist," readily commanding respect and increasing receptivity to new ways of thinking and behaving. On the other hand, the consequence may also be to make the expression of disagreement more difficult, undermining the goal of collaborative empiricism in CBT and interfering with the full development of a therapeutic relationship. Psychoeducation about the importance of the patient's role can increase the patient's active participation in therapy, and diminish this power differential. Nevertheless, there may be a need for the therapist to negotiate and accept to an extent the role and responsibility of an expert, a teacher, and a parental figure with Asian patients.

Many Asian patients are able to grasp the model of CBT, but some may find it difficult to access their automatic thoughts or to distinguish them from emotions. As well, there can be reluctance to focus on negative thoughts and emotions due to beliefs that negativity may adversely affect their physical and mental health. When automatic thoughts are captured and challenged, some patients may argue that doing so is akin to deluding oneself in order to feel better. Further, Asian patients may have some culturally specific core beliefs, which can have adaptive features as well as consistency with their heritage culture; for example, "If I say no, I am a selfish person," or, "I must take care of others before myself" (Shen et al., 2006). Shen and colleagues (2006) also found that homework completion can be a problem, with patients preferring handouts to doing homework themselves. The use of self-report homework techniques, such as the thought record, often appear quite foreign and nonintuitive to many Asian patients, especially those with less education or less exposure to Western culture. Although various techniques to increase homework compliance can be tried, the therapist should flexibly design homework that is better suited for their particular patients.

The recent emergence of the so-called third wave of CBT is a significant development in the treatment of PDs. Developed independently of one another, they are designed for difficult-to-treat patients who do not respond well to traditional CBT. Third-wave CBT approaches include: dialectical behavior therapy, designed originally for borderline PD (Linehan, 1993); mindfulness-based cognitive therapy, which targets prevention of depressive relapse in individuals with chronic and recurrent depression (Segal, Williams, & Teasdale, 2002); and Acceptance and Commitment Therapy (ACT; Hayes, Strosahl, & Wilson, 2003). Although these approaches vary substantially from one another, there is a shared emphasis on mindfulness and acceptance, rather than changing dysfunctional thoughts as in CBT. The therapist and patient are encouraged to find ways to balance these tendencies rather than seeing them in opposition, thereby benefiting from both approaches.

Mindfulness, acceptance, and dialectical thinking are consistent in many ways with Asian cultural beliefs, especially those of Buddhism—a connection not lost on the developers of these approaches. Nonetheless, conceptual and technical challenges remain, not least the lack of an evidence base for the use of these treatments in Asian populations. Moreover, the continued emphasis on freely chosen individual values, divorced from the consideration of the demands made by family and other important people, can be especially difficult for some patients with Asian cultural backgrounds. The ideal of an equal relationship between patient and therapist, as well as the emotional intensity of the therapeutic relationship, can pose challenges for some patients who have more traditional role expectations for themselves and their therapists. Patients with PDs may find it particularly difficult to negotiate the therapeutic relationship when it does not conform to expectations.

Social Approaches

In conducting sessions with couples or families with an Asian background, the stigma of being involved with mental health treatment is often encountered as the first barrier. Further, due to strong cultural beliefs about keeping problems within the family, there may be considerable reluctance to disclose problems. The hierarchy of power within the family may further inhibit individual members from disclosing their feelings; challenging this hierarchy is difficult without risking a failure of empathy and loss of face for the patient or patients involved. Strong alliance building, psychoeducation, and normalization about the process are crucial to engage the couple or family. One approach is to focus on validating the roles and collective motivation of family members in the beginning and consider interviewing, and even intervening with, subunits of the family in addition to working with everyone.

At the same time, due to the interconnectedness of many Asian families, the patient or their family members may want a lot more family involvement, even in individual assessment or psychotherapy. Indeed, family members may sometimes wish to sit in on sessions. Some are very eager to supply collateral information, verbally or through written notes—and at times may conceal that they are doing so from the patient. These expectations require the clinician to be flexible in working with both the patient and his or her family, while at the same time balancing ethical and therapeutic issues. Prospective patients from an Asian cultural background often have more reservations about participating in couples or group therapy due to stigma, wanting to save face, reluctance to share personal information with "outsiders," and anxiety about speaking up or not speaking up in a group. Psychoeducation and a group structure that takes these factors into account can help to alleviate some of these fears. Once they have decided to participate, Asian participants will often gradually disclose more personal information as group cohesion builds and as they feel that the other group members are "insiders." On the other hand, they will sometimes use concrete, demonstrable behaviors to promote group cohesion, such as talking about things unrelated to therapy before or after the session starts, buying small items for other group members, or bringing in food to share on special occasions and on the last session of time-limited groups. There is also a strong cultural expectation for the group facilitator to fulfill the role of a teacher.

Strengths, Weaknesses, and Alternatives in Applying Current Treatment Approaches for Personality Disorders to Asians

Acceptability of Treatment

If a particular treatment does not make sense to the intended recipient, the likelihood of success can be utterly compromised. Such an outcome is particularly likely when moving treatment approaches across cultural boundaries, as patient and therapist might have very different views of how a given problem should be treated. One potential advantage of various CBT approaches is that there is now some evidence that they can be packaged in a way that makes more sense, and is more culturally acceptable, to Asian patients. Shen, Alden, Söchting, and Tsang (2006) describe a group CBT approach for Cantonese-speaking Chinese patients with depression. Many modifications to the standard protocol had to be made; for example, to capture specific depression constructs in Cantonese or to adapt cognitive modification strategies to address culture-syntonic beliefs about social relationships. Nonetheless, once these changes were made, the result was a treatment package that was seen as acceptable, appropriate, and well suited to patients' problems.

Attention to the Therapeutic Relationship

There is now a wealth of evidence that the quality of the relationship between patient and therapist is central to the success of psychological treatments. Often referred to as "nonspecific factors," suggesting effects left over after specific theory-driven interventions, the therapeutic alliance is an essential component of change. For individuals with PDs, however, the therapeutic relationship can also be fraught with complexity; for example, the patient's perception might be polarized into extremes of idealization and devaluation. In therapeutic relationships where therapist and patient come from different ethnocultural backgrounds, it is usually possible for them to identify common ground based on other shared identities or through reflecting on common elements of their human experience, an essential element of rapport building. Given the importance of interpersonal relationships in Asian cultural contexts, we should expect that these factors should at least be as important as in Western contexts, if not more so.

As the therapeutic relationship is also a genuine human relationship, it offers a chance for corrective emotional experiences where the patient learns that not all relationships have to follow a long-standing pattern. This experience can be powerful for people with PDs, whose symptoms are most often interpersonally disruptive and who likely have had difficult interpersonal relationships for many years. In addition, patients have the opportunity to learn more about human relationships and interpersonal skills through the therapeutic relationship. The challenge when carrying out treatment across cultural barriers is that therapist and patient might be operating under different interpersonal and social rules. Making the genuine attempt to overcome these limitations, while acknowledging that they cannot always be avoided, may be an important part of managing intercultural therapies.

Attention to Change Processes

In many therapies, one of the goals is to induce change through the patients achieving a different way of perceiving and understanding themselves or the world. Such examples include acquisition of insights from interpretations in psychodynamic therapy; ways of thinking more rationally in CBT; or ways of thinking more dialectically in DBT or ACT. These changes may result from the therapist actively advising and teaching, or by the patients reflecting on their own experiences as guided by the therapist. Though such interventions can be powerful, they are often tricky once one begins to take culture into account. When considering the specific content of an intervention, one must keep in mind that norms about the "correct" way of thinking, feeling, or behaving are themselves deeply rooted in cultural values. Secondly, it is unclear whether the best approach is to engage in direct teaching versus allowing self-discovery, a tension that exists in the general psychotherapy literature as well as having implications for patients from Asian backgrounds. Some patients might respond well to indirect methods of reflective or guided discovery, such as through meditation, analogies, or parables. Using culturally specific proverbs as a shorthand way of changing perceptions is one possible strategy. Other patients, in contrast, might benefit from a more direct approach, including explicit advice from the therapist.

Patients from an Asian background have ways of describing the experience of feeling better after emotionally intense sessions, akin to the English-language idiom, "letting off some steam."

For example, patients might state that their *qi* is no longer suppressed or they might report an easing of emotional or bodily discomfort. Due to the emphasis on family harmony, many patients are able to share their emotions more easily with a therapist once the requisite therapeutic alliance is in place. The expression, experience, and description of emotions are often embedded with physical sensations, including pain, discomfort, burning sensation, movements of *qi*, and so on. Rather than pathologizing this process as somatization or alexithymia, this tendency may alternatively be viewed as a richer and more holistic description of the totality of emotional experience. In fact, a useful technique to intensify affect in the session is to have the patient attend to these somatic sensations as they occur. Expression of intense emotions is not always helpful, particularly when the emotions are expressed in a repetitive way that traps the patient as a victim of his or her past, a tendency often observed in patients with PDs. Emotional expression is much more effective when it is brought into the present moment in therapy, where changes can occur.

CONCLUSIONS

Working with PDs can represent a significant clinical challenge, as can providing culturally competent care. Doing both at the same time is particularly difficult, especially as culture and personality are deeply intertwined with one another. The responsible clinician who wishes to proceed in an evidence-based manner is further hindered by the lack of research in this area, especially research that is grounded in cultural context. A final problem lies in the uncertainty over the structural organization of PDs themselves, in that categorical PDs as described by *DSM-IV-TR* may not even represent the best way of capturing problematic personality traits. So we conclude in part with a call for more research on PDs in various Asian cultural contexts, particularly research that takes these contexts into account. Although some of this research will likely rely on current PD categories, we look forward also to work that will avoid the problems with the current system, either by focusing on specific problem areas (e.g., impulsivity, dysphoria) or underlying dimensional traits.

The literature on "normal" personality variation in Asian samples can help to clarify issues that are currently unexplored in the Asian PD literature. There is a seeming correspondence between findings from the trait literature and more emic descriptions of normal or ideal personality. Moreover, the structural differences that apparently characterize Asian and Western samples fit with these emic descriptions. The domain of interpersonal relatedness emerges more readily and clearly in Asian samples, paralleling the importance of sensitivity to and connectedness with others in Asian cultural contexts. Similarly, the domain of openness-to-experience emerges more readily and clearly in Western samples, paralleling the importance of creativity and personal exploration in Western cultural contexts. Even the greater difficulty in identifying cross-situationally invariant personality traits in Asian samples fits with the idea that people from Asian cultural backgrounds are more likely to modify their behavior to fit the interpersonal context, and to be favored for doing so. The impact of cross-cultural differences in the "traitedness" of behavior on PDs—often described as fixed and invariant, to the point of rigidity—remains unexplored.

Clinicians will of course be called on to continue treating Asian patients with PDs, often cross-culturally, in the absence of solid research. To fill this gap, we have provided suggestions for this work that are consistent with the research that does exist, that emerge from an understanding of culturally specific aspects of personality, and that are informed by clinical work with Asian patients, especially Asian patients with PDs. These suggestions fall far short of being a manual, or even a checklist, of how to work with these patients; not least, since ultimately one treats individual patients rather than demographic groups. Our goal is rather to provide the clinician with additional possibilities to consider while working with Asian patients who display problematic personality traits, both in terms of understanding what is observed as well as deciding how to proceed. So, in the spirit of the Asian perspectives discussed throughout this chapter, the tension between research and clinical work can be expressed dialectically: we accept the limits of our current knowledge and proceed to give the best care we can with the tools available; we anticipate new research to expand that knowledge and improve care while accepting that our knowledge can never be complete.

REFERENCES

Alarcón, R. D. (1996). Personality disorders and culture in the DSM-IV: A critique. *Journal of Personality Disorders, 10,* 260–270.

Allik, J. (2005). Personality dimensions across cultures. *Journal of Personality Disorders, 19,* 212–232.

Allport, G. W., & Odbert, H. S. (1936). Trait-names: A psycho-lexical study. *Psychological Monographs: General and Applied, 47,* 171–220. (1, Whole No. 211).

American Psychiatric Association. (2000). *Diagnostic and statistical manual of mental disorders* (4th ed., text rev.). Washington, DC: Author.

Atkinson, D. R. (1978). Effects of counselor race and counseling approach on Asian Americans' perceptions of counselor credibility and utility. *Journal of Counseling Psychology, 25,* 76–82.

Atkinson, D. R., & Gim, R. H. (1989). Asian-American cultural identity and attitudes toward mental health services. *Journal of Counseling Psychology, 36,* 209–212.

Bagby, R. M., & Farvolden, P. (2004). The Personality Diagnostic Questionnaire-4 (PDQ-4). In M. J. Hilsenroth, & D. L. Segal (Eds.), *Comprehensive handbook of psychological assessment: Vol. 2. Personality assessment* (pp. 122–133). Hoboken, NJ: Wiley.

Bagozzi, R., Wong, N., & Yi, Y. (1999). The role of culture and gender in the relationship between positive and negative affect. *Cognition and Emotion, 13,* 641–672.

Beck, A. T., Freeman, A., Davis, D. D., et al. (2003). *Cognitive therapy of personality disorders* (2nd ed.). New York: Guilford.

Bender, D. S., Dolan, R. T., Skodol, A. E., Sanislow, C. A., Dyck, I. R., McGlashan, T. H., et al. (2001). Treatment utilization by patients with personality disorders. *American Journal of Psychiatry, 158,* 295–302.

Benjamin, L. (1993). *Interpersonal diagnosis and treatment of personality disorders.* New York: Guilford.

Cadoret, R. J., Yates, W. R., Troughton, E., et al. (1995). Genetic-environmental interaction in the genesis of aggressively and conduct disorders. *Archives of General Psychiatry, 52,* 916–924.

Cain, N. M., Pincus, A. L., & Ansell, E. B. (2008). Narcissism at the crossroads: Phenotypic description of pathological narcissism across clinical theory, social/personality psychology, and psychiatric diagnosis. *Clinical Psychology Review, 28,* 638–656.

Campbell, J. D., Trapnell, P. D., Heine, S. J., Katz, I. M., Lavallee, L. F., & Lehman, D. R. (1996). Self-concept clarity: Measurement, personality correlates, and cultural boundaries. *Journal of Personality and Social Psychology, 70,* 141–156.

Chen, S. W, & Davenport, D. (2005). Cognitive behavior therapy with Chinese American clients: Cautions and modifications. *Psychotherapy: Theory, Research, Practice, Training, 42,* 101–110.

Cheung, P. C., Conger, A. J., Hau, K.-T., Lew, W. J. F., & Lau, S. (1992). Development of the Multi-Trait Personality Inventory (MTPI): Comparison among four Chinese populations. *Journal of Personality Assessment, 59,* 528–551.

Cheung, F. M., Leung, K., Fan, R. M., Song, W.-Z., Zhang, J.-X., & Zhang, J.-S. (1996). Development of the Chinese Personality Assessment Inventory. *Journal of Cross-Cultural Psychology, 27,* 181–199.

Cheung, F. M., Leung, K., Zhang, J.-X., Sun, H.-F., Gan, Y.-Q., Song, W.-Z., et al. (2001). Indigenous Chinese personality constructs: Is the Five-Factor Model complete? *Journal of Cross-Cultural Psychology, 32,* 407–433.

Chinese Society of Psychiatry. (2001). *Chinese classification and diagnostic criteria of mental disorders* [in Chinese] (3rd ed.). Jinan: Shandong Science and Technology Press.

Choi, I., & Choi, Y. (2002). Culture and self-concept flexibility. *Personality and Social Psychology Bulletin, 28,* 1508–1517.

Church, A. T. (2000). Culture and personality: Toward an integrated cultural trait psychology. *Journal of Personality, 68,* 651–703.

Church, A. T., & Katigbak, M. S. (2002). The five-factor model in the Philippines: Investigating trait structure and levels across cultures. In R. R. McCrae & J. Allik (Eds.), *Five-factor model of personality across cultures* (pp. 129–154). New York: Kluwer Academic/Plenum.

Church, A. T., Katigbak, M. S., Del Prado, A. M., Ortiz, F. A., Mastor, K. A., Harumi, Y., et al. (2006). Implicit theories and self-perceptions of traitedness across cultures: Toward integration of cultural and trait psychology perspectives. *Journal of Cross-Cultural Psychology, 37,* 694–716.

Church, A. T., Reyes, J. A. S., Katigbak, M. S., & Grimm, S. D. (1997). Filipino personality structure and the Big Five model: A lexical approach. *Journal of Personality, 65,* 477–528.

Clark, L. A., Livesley, W. J., & Morey, L. (1997). Personality disorder assessment: The challenge of construct validity. *Journal of Personality Disorders, 11,* 205–231.

Clark, L. A., & Watson, D. (1999). Personality, disorder, and personality disorder: Towards a more rational conceptualization. *Journal of Personality Disorders, 13,* 142–151.

Cloninger, C. R. (1998). The genetics and psychobiology of the seven-factor model of personality. In K. R. Silk (Ed.), *Biology of personality disorders* (pp. 63–92). Washington, DC: American Psychiatric Press.

Cloninger, C. R, Svrakic, D. M, & Przybeck, T. R. (1993). A psychobiological model of temperament and character. *Archives of General Psychiatry, 50,* 975–990.

Cohen, D., & Gunz, A. (2002). As seen by the other…: Perspectives on the self in the memories and emotional perceptions of Easterners and Westerners. *Psychological Science, 13,* 55–59.

Cohen, D., Hoshino-Browne, E., & Leung, A. (2007). Culture and the structure of personal experience. In M. P. Zanna (Ed.), *Advances in experimental social psychology* (vol. 39, pp. 1–67). San Diego: Academic.

Coles, M. E., Pinto, A., Mancebo, M. C., Rasmussen, S. A., & Eisen, J. L. (2008). OCD with comorbid OCPD: A subtype of OCD? *Journal of Psychiatric Research, 42,* 289–296.

Compton, W. M., Conway, K. P., Stinson, F. S., Colliver, J. D., & Grant, B. F. (2005). Prevalence, correlates, and comorbidity of DSM-IV antisocial personality syndromes and alcohol and specific drug use disorders in the United States: Results from the national epidemiologic survey on alcohol and related conditions. *Journal of Clinical Psychiatry, 66,* 677–685.

Confucius. (1979). *Confucius: The analects* (D. C. Lau, Trans.). London: Penguin.

Costa, P. T., Jr., & McCrae, R. R. (1985). *The NEO Personality Inventory manual.* Odessa, FL: Psychological Assessment Resources.

Costa, P. T., Jr., & Widiger, T. A. (Eds.). (2002). Personality disorders and the five-factor model of personality (2nd ed.). Washington, DC: American Psychological Association.

Cousins, S. D. (1989). Culture and self-perception in Japan and the United States. *Journal of Personality and Social Psychology, 56,* 124–131.

Cousins, S. D. (1990). Culture and social phobia in Japan and the United States. Ph.D. dissertation, University of Michigan.

DeBary, W. T., & Bloom, I. (1999). *Sources of Chinese tradition* (2nd ed.). New York: Columbia University Press.

Depue, R., & Collins, P. (1999). Neurobiology of the structure of personality: Dopamine, facilitation of incentive motivation, and extraversion. *Behavioral and Brain Sciences, 22,* 491–569.

Depue, R., & Lenzenweger, M. (2001). A neurobehavioral dimensional model. In J. Livesley (Ed.), *Handbook of personality disorders: Theory, research, and treatment* (pp. 136–176). New York: Guilford.

Diener, E., & Diener, M. (1995). Cross-cultural correlates of life satisfaction and self-esteem. *Journal of Personality and Social Psychology, 68,* 653–663.

Dinnel, D. L., Kleinknecht, R. A., & Tanaka-Matsumi, J. (2002). A cross-cultural comparison of social phobia symptoms. *Journal of Psychopathology and Behavioral Assessment, 42,* 75–84.

Eisen, J. L., Coles, M. E., Shea, M. T., Pagano, M. E., Stout, R. L., Yen, S., et al. (2006). Clarifying the convergence between obsessive compulsive personality disorder criteria and obsessive compulsive disorder. *Journal of Personality Disorders, 20,* 294–305.

English, T., & Chen, S. (2007). Culture and self-concept stability: Consistency across and within contexts among Asian Americans and European Americans. *Journal of Personality and Social Psychology, 93,* 478–490.

Epstein, M. (1995). *Thoughts without a thinker: Psychotherapy from a Buddhist perspective.* New York: MJF Books.

First, M.B., Gibbon, M., Spitzer, R.L., Williams, J.B.W., Benjamin, L.S., & First, M.B. (1997). *Structured Clinical Interview for DSM-IV Axis II Personality Disorders (SCID-II).* Washington, DC: American Psychiatric Press.

Frankenburg, F. R., & Zanarini, M. C. (2002). Divalproex sodium treatment of women with borderline personality disorder and bipolar II disorder: A double-blind placebo-controlled pilot study. *Journal of Clinical Psychiatry, 63,* 442–446.

Grant, B. F., Chou, S. P., Goldstein, R. B., Huang, B., Stinson, F. S., Saha, T. D., et al. (2008). Prevalence, correlates, disability, and comorbidity of DSM-IV borderline personality disorder: results from the Wave 2 National Epidemiologic Survey on Alcohol and Related Conditions. *Journal of Clinical Psychiatry, 69,* 533–545.

Ha, J. H., Kim, E. J., Abbey, S. E., & Kim, T.-S. (2007). Relationship between personality disorder symptoms and temperament in the young male general population of South Korea. *Psychiatry and Clinical Neurosciences, 61,* 59–66.

Hahn, D.-W., Lee, K., & Ashton, M. C. (1999). A factor analysis of the most frequently used Korean personality trait adjectives. *European Journal of Personality, 13,* 261–282.

Hamamura, T., & Heine, S. J. (2007). The role of self-criticism in self-improvement and face maintenance among Japanese. In E. C. Chang (Ed.), *Self-criticism and self-enhancement: Theory, research, and clinical implications* (pp. 105–122). Washington, DC: American Psychological Association.

Hayes, S. C., Strosahl, K. D., & Wilson, K. G. (2003). *Acceptance and commitment therapy: An experiential approach to behavior change.* New York: Guilford.

Heine, S. J. (2007). Constructing good selves in Japan and North America. In R. M. Sorrentino, D. Cohen, J. M. Olson, & M. P. Zanna (Eds.), *Cultural and social behaviour: The Ontario Symposium* (Vol. 10, pp. 95–116). Mahwah, NJ: Erlbaum.

Heine, S. J., & Buchtel, E. E. (2009). Personality: The universal and the culturally specific. *Annual Review of Psychology, 60,* 369–394.

Heine, S. J., Buchtel, E. E., & Norenzayan, A. (2008). What do cross-national comparisons of personality traits tell us? The case of conscientiousness. *Psychological Science, 19,* 309–313.

Heine, S. J., & Hamamura, T. (2007). In search of East Asian self-enhancement. *Personality and Social Psychology Review, 11,* 1–24.

Heine, S. J., Kitayama, S., Lehman, D. R., Takata, T., Ide, E., Leung, C., et al. (2001). Divergent consequences of success and failure in Japan and North America: An investigation of self-improving motivations and malleable selves. *Journal of Personality and Social Psychology, 81,* 599–615.

Heine, S. J., & Lehman, D. R. (1999). Culture, self-discrepancies, and self-satisfaction. *Personality and Social Psychology Bulletin, 25,* 915–925.

Heine, S. J., Lehman, D. R., Markus, H. R., & Kitayama, S. (1999). Is there a universal need for positive self-regard? *Psychological Review, 106,* 766–794.

Hodges, J., & Oei, T. P. S. (2007). Would Confucius benefit from psychotherapy? The compatibility of cognitive behavior therapy and Chinese values. *Behaviour Research and Therapy, 45,* 901–914.

Horowitz, M. J. (1991). *Hysterical personality style and the histrionic personality disorder.* Northvale, NJ: Aronson.

Huang, B., Grant, B. F., Dawson, D. A., Stinson, F. S., Chou, S. P., Tulshi, D. S., et al. (2006). Race-ethnicity and the prevalence and co-occurrence of Diagnostic and Statistical Manual of Mental Disorders, Fourth Edition, alcohol and drug use disorders and Axis I and II disorders: United States, 2001–2002. *Comprehensive Psychiatry, 47,* 252–257.

Huang, X., Ling, H., Yang, B., & Dou, G. (2007). Screening of personality disorders among Chinese college students by personality diagnostic questionnaire-4+. *Journal of Personality Disorders, 21,* 448–454.

Huang, Y., Kotov, R., De Girolamo, G., Preti, A., Angermeyer, M., Benjet, C., et al. (2009). DSM–IV personality disorders in the WHO World Mental Health Surveys. *British Journal of Psychiatry, 195,* 46–53.

Hwang, W. C., Wood, J. J, Lin, K. M., & Cheung, F. (2006) Cognitive-behavioral therapy with Chinese Americans: Research, theory, and clinical Practice. *Cognitive and Behavioral Practice, 13,* 293–303.

Hyler, S. E. (1994). *Personality Diagnostic Questionnaire-4.* New York: New York State Psychiatry Institute.

Ikuta, N., Zanarini, M. C., Minakawa, K., & Miyake, Y. (1994). Comparison of American and Japanese outpatients with borderline personality disorder. *Comprehensive Psychiatry, 35,* 382–385.

Jang, K. L., Angleitner, A., Riemann, R., McCrae, R. R., & Livesley, W. J. (1998). Heritability of facet-level traits in a cross-cultural twin sample: Support for a hierarchical model of personality. *Journal of Personality and Social Psychology, 74,* 1556–1565.

John, O. P., &, Srivastava, S. (1998). The Big Five trait taxonomy: History, measurement, and theoretical perspectives. In L. A. Pervin, & O. P. John (Eds.), *Handbook of personality: Theory and research* (2nd ed., pp. 102–138). New York: Guilford.

Kashima, Y., Kashima, E., Farsides, T., Kim, U., Strack, F., Werth, L., et al. (2004). Culture and context-sensitive self: The amount and meaning of context-sensitivity of phenomenal self differ across cultures. *Self and Identity, 3,* 125–141.

Kasper, S., Stein, D. J., Loft, H., & Nil, R. (2005). Escitalopram in the treatment of social anxiety disorder. *British Journal of Psychiatry, 186,* 222–226.

Katigbak, M. S., Church, T. A., Guanzon-Lapeña, M. A., Carlota, A. J., & del Pilar, G. H. (2002). Are indigenous personality dimensions culture specific? Philippine inventories and the Five-Factor Model. *Journal of Personality and Social Psychology, 82,* 89–101.

Kernberg, O. F. (1984). *Severe personality disorders: Psychotherapeutic strategies.* New Haven, CT: Yale University Press.

Kim, I. J., Kim, L. I., & Kelly, J. G. (2006). Developing cultural competence in working with Korean immigrant families. *Journal of Community Psychology, 34,* 149–165.

Koenigsberg, H. W., Reynolds, D., Goodman, M., New, A. S., Mitropoulou, V., Trestman, R. L., et al. (2003). Risperidone in the treatment of schizotypal personality disorder. *Journal of Clinical Psychiatry, 64,* 628–634.

Kuhn, M. H., & McPartland, T. S. (1954). An empirical investigation of self-attitudes. *American Sociological Review, 19,* 68–76.

Kwan, V. S. Y., Bond, M. H., & Singelis, T. M. (1997). Pancultural explanations for life satisfaction: Adding relationship harmony to self-esteem. *Journal of Personality and Social Psychology, 73,* 1038–1051.

Lao-Tzu. (1963). *Tao Te Ching* (D. C. Lau, Trans.). London: Penguin.

Lee, C. K., Kwak, Y. S., Yamamoto, J., Rhee, H., Kim, Y. S., Han, J. H., et al. (1990). Psychiatric epidemiology in Korea: Part II. Urban and rural differences. *Journal of Nervous and Mental Disease, 178,* 247–252.

Lee, S. (2001). From diversity to unity: The classification of mental disorders in 21st-century China. *Psychiatric Clinics of North America, 24,* 421–431.

Lenzenweger, M. (1998). Schizotypy and schizotypic psychopathology. In M. Lenzenweger & R. Dworkin (Eds.), *Origins and development of schizophrenia: Advances in experimental psychopathology* (pp 93–122). Washington, DC: American Psychological Association.

Leung, K., Cheung, F. M., Zhang, J. X., Song, W. Z., & Xie, D. (1997). The Five Factor model of personality in China. In K. Leung, Y. Kashima, U. Kim, & S. Yamaguchi (Eds.), *Progress in Asian social psychology* (Vol. 1, pp. 231–244). Singapore: Wiley.

Linehan, M. M. (1993). *Cognitive-behavioral treatment for borderline personality disorder.* New York: Guilford.

Livesley, W. J. (1998). Suggestions for a framework for an empirically based classification of personality disorder. *Canadian Journal of Psychiatry/La Revue Canadienne de Psychiatrie, 43,* 137–147.

Lo, H., & Fung, K. P. (2003). Culturally competent psychotherapy. *Canadian Journal of Psychiatry, 48,* 161–170.

Loehlin, J. C. (1992). *Genes and environment in personality development.* Newbury Park, CA: Sage.

Luk, S. L., Kwan, C. S. F., Hui, J. M. C., Bacon-Shone, J., Tsang, A. K. T., Leung, A. C., & Tang, K. K. M. (1991). Cognitive-behavioural group therapy for Hong Kong Chinese adults with mental health problems. *Australian and New Zealand Journal of Psychiatry, 25,* 524–534.

Machizawa-Summers, S. (2007). Childhood trauma and parental bonding among Japanese female patients with borderline personality disorder. *International Journal of Psychology, 42,* 265–273.

Magid, B. (2001). *Ordinary mind: Exploring the common ground of Zen and psychotherapy.* Boston: Wisdom Publications.

Mao, P. X., Tang, F. L., Jiang, F., Shu, L., Gu, X., Li, M., et al. (2008). Escitalopram in major depressive disorder: A multicenter, randomized, double-blind, fixed-dose, parallel trial in a Chinese population. *Depression and Anxiety, 25,* 46–54.

Markus, H. R. (2004). Culture and personality: Brief for an arranged marriage. *Journal of Research in Personality, 38,* 75–83.

Markus, H. R., & Kitayama, S. (1991). Culture and the self: Implications for cognition, emotion, and motivation. *Psychological Review, 98,* 224–253.

Mastor, K. A., Jin, P., & Cooper, M. (2000). Malay culture and personality. *American Behavioral Scientist, 44,* 95–111.

McCrae, R. R. (2001). Trait psychology and culture: Exploring intercultural comparisons. *Journal of Personality, 69,* 819–846.

McCrae, R. R. (2002). NEO-PI-R data from 36 cultures: Further intercultural comparisons. In R. R. McCrae & J. Allik (Eds.), *The five-factor model of personality across cultures* (pp. 105–125). New York: Kluwer Academic/Plenum.

McCrae, R. R., & Costa, P. T., Jr. (1985). Openness to experience. In R. Hogan & W. H. Jones (Eds.), *Perspectives in personality* (Vol. 1, pp. 145–172). Greenwich, CT: JAI Press.

McCrae, R.R., Costa, P.T., Jr., & Yik, M. S. M. (1996). Universal aspects of Chinese personality structure. In M. H. Bond (Ed.), *The handbook of Chinese psychology* (pp. 189–207). Hong Kong: Oxford University Press.

McCrae, R. R., Terracciano, A., & 79 members of the Personality Profiles of Cultures Project. (2005). Personality profiles of cultures: Aggregate personality traits. *Journal of Personality and Social Psychology, 89,* 407–425.

McCrae, R. R., Yik, M. S. M., Trapnell, P. D., Bond, M. H., & Paulhus, D. L. (1998). Interpreting personality profiles across cultures: Bilingual, acculturation, and peer rating studies of Chinese undergraduates. *Journal of Personality and Social Psychology, 74,* 1041–1055.

Millon, T. (1981). *Disorders of personality. DSM-III: Axis II.* New York: Wiley.

Miyaoka, T., Furuya, M., Yasuda, H., Hayashia, M., Inagaki, T., & Horiguchi, J. (2008). Yi-gan san for the treatment of borderline personality disorder: An open-label study. *Progress in Neuro-Psychopharmacology and Biological Psychiatry, 32,* 150–154.

Moriya, N., Miyake, Y., Minakawa, K., & Ikuta, N. (1993). Diagnosis and clinical features of borderline personality disorder in the East and West: A preliminary report. *Comprehensive Psychiatry, 34,* 418–423.

Morris, M., & Peng, K. (1994). Culture and cause: American and Chinese attributions for social and physical events. *Journal of Personality and Social Psychology, 67,* 949–971.

Nisbett, R. E., Peng, K., Choi, I., & Norenzayan, A. (2001). Culture and systems of thoughts: Holistic versus analytic cognition. *Psychological Review, 108,* 291–310.

Oldham, J. M., Gabbard, G. O., Goin, M. K., Gunderson, J., Soloff, P., Spiegel, D., et al. (2001). Practice guideline for the treatment of borderline personality disorder. *American Journal of Psychiatry, 158,* 1–52.

Oldham, J. M., Skodol, A. E., & Bender, D. S. (2009). *Essentials of personality disorders.* Washington, DC: American Psychiatric Publishing.

Osone, A., & Takahashi, S. (2003). Twelve month test-retest reliability of a Japanese version of the Structured Clinical Interview for DSM-IV Personality Disorders. *Psychiatry and Clinical Neurosciences, 57,* 532–538.

Pande, A. C., Davidson, J. R., & Jefferson, J. W. (1999). Treatment of social phobia with gabapentin: A placebo-controlled study. *Journal of Clinical Psychopharmacology, 19,* 341–348.

Paris, J. (2008). An evidence-based approach to managing suicidal behaviour in patients with BPD. *Social Work in Mental Health, 6,* 99–108.

Parker, G., Cheah, Y. C., & Parker, K. (2003). Properties of the Temperament and Character Inventory in a Chinese sample. *Acta Psychiatrica Scandinavica, 108,* 367–378.

Parker, G., Cheah, Y. C., & Roy, K. (2001). Do the Chinese somatize depression? A cross-cultural study. *Social Psychiatry and Psychiatric Epidemiology, 36,* 287–293.

Parker, G., Gladstone, G., & Chee, K. T. (2001). Depression in the planet's largest ethnic group: The Chinese. *American Journal of Psychiatry, 158,* 857–864.

Peng, K., & Nisbett, R. E. (1999). Culture, dialectics, and reasoning about contradiction. *American Psychologist, 54,* 741–754.

Rector, N. A, Kocovski, N. L, & Ryder, A. G. (2006). Social anxiety and the fear of causing discomfort to others: Conceptualization and treatment. *Journal of Social and Clinical Psychology, 25,* 906–918.

Rocca, P., Marchiaro, L., Cocuzza, E., & Bogetto, F. (2002). Treatment of borderline personality disorder with risperidone. *Journal of Clinical Psychiatry, 63,* 241–244.

Ryder, A. G., Alden, L. E. & Paulhus, D. L. (2000). Is acculturation unidimensional or bidimensional? A head-to-head comparison in the prediction of personality, self-identity, and adjustment. *Journal of Personality and Social Psychology, 79,* 49–65.

Ryder, A.G., Bagby, R. M., & Schuller, D. R. (2002). The overlap of depressive personality disorder and dysthymia: A categorical problem with a dimensional solution. *Harvard Review of Psychiatry, 10,* 337–352.

Ryder, A. G., Yang, J., Zhu, X., Yao, S., Yi, J., Heine, S. J., et al. (2008) The cultural shaping of depression: Somatic symptoms in China, psychological symptoms in North America? *Journal of Abnormal Psychology, 117,* 300–313.

Sato, T., Sakado, K., & Sato, S. (1993). DSM-III-R personality disorders in outpatients with non-bipolar depression: The frequency in a sample of Japanese and the relationship to the 4-month outcome under adequate anti-depressant therapy. *European Archives of Psychiatry and Clinical Neuroscience, 242,* 273–278.

Sato, T., Sakado, K., Uehara, T., Sato, S., Nishioka, K., & Kasahara, Y. (1997). Personality disorder diagnoses using DSM-III-R in a Japanese clinical sample with major depression. *Acta Psychiatrica Scandinavica, 95,* 451–453.

Schneier, F. R., Luterek, J. A., Heimberg, R. G., & Leonardo, E. (2004). Social phobia. In D. J. Stein (Ed.), *Clinical manual of anxiety disorders* (pp. 63–86). Arlington, VA: American Psychiatric Publishing.

Seedat, S., & Stein, M. B. (2004). Double-blind, placebo-controlled assessment of combined clonazepam with paroxetine compared with paroxetine monotherapy for generalized social anxiety disorder. *Journal of Clinical Psychiatry, 65,* 244–248

Segal, Z. V., Williams, J. M. G., & Teasdale, J. D. (2002). *Mindfulness-based cognitive therapy for depression.* New York: Guilford.

Shen, E. K., Alden, L. E., Söchting, I., & Tsang, P. (2006). Clinical observations of a Cantonese cognitive-behavioral treatment program for Chinese immigrants. *Psychotherapy: Theory, Research, Practice, Training, 43,* 518–530.

Siever, L. J., & Davis, K. L. (1991). A psychological perspective on the personality disorder. *American Journal of Psychiatry, 148,* 1647–1658.

Skodol, A. E., Gunderson, J. G., Pfhol, B., Widiger, T. A., Livesley, W. J., & Siever, L. J. (2002). The borderline diagnosis: I. Psychopathology, comorbidity, and personality structure. *Biological Psychiatry, 51,* 936–950.

Spencer-Rodgers, J., Peng, K., Wang, L., & Hou, Y. (2004). Dialectical self-esteem and East-West differences in psychological well-being. *Personality and Social Psychology Bulletin, 30,* 1416–1432.

Spirrison, C. L., & Choi, S. (1998). Psychometric properties of a Korean version of the revised neo-personality inventory. *Psychological Reports, 83,* 262–274.

Sue, S. (1998). In search of cultural competence in psychotherapy and counseling. *American Psychologist, 53,* 440–448.

Suh, E. M. (2002). Culture, identity consistency, and subjective well-being. *Journal of Personality and Social Psychology, 83,* 1378–1391.

Taylor, C. T., Laposa, J. M., & Alden, L. E. (2004). Is avoidant personality disorder more than just social avoidance? *Journal of Personality Disorders, 18,* 571–594.

Terracciano, A., Abdel-Khalek, A. M., Ádám, N., Adamovová, L., Ahn, C.-K., Ahn, H.-N., et al. (2005). National character does not reflect mean personality trait levels in 49 cultures. *Science, 310,* 96–100.

Tomita, T., Aoyama, H., Kitamura, T., Sekiguchi, C., Murai, T., & Mutsuda, T. (2000). Factor structure of psychobiological seven-factor model of personality: A model revision. *Personality and Individual Differences, 29,* 709–727.

Torgersen, S. (1984). Genetic and nosological aspects of schizotypal and borderline personality disorders. *Archives of General Psychiatry, 41,* 546–554.

Torgersen, S., Lygren, S., Oien, P. A., et al. (2000). A twin study of personality disorders. *Comprehensive Psychiatry, 41,* 416–425.

Trull, T. J., Stepp, S. D., & Solhan, M. (2006). Borderline personality disorder. In M. Hersen & J. C. Thomas (Eds.), *Comprehensive handbook of personality and psychopathology* (pp. 299–315). New York: Wiley.

Tsai, J. L. (2007). Ideal affect: Cultural causes and behavioural consequences. *Perspectives on Psychological Science, 2,* 242–259.

Tseng, W.-S., Lee, S., & Lu, Q. (2005). The historical trends of psychotherapy in China: Cultural review. In W.-S. Tseng (Ed.), *Asian culture and psychotherapy: Implications for East and West* (pp. 249–264). Hong Kong: Oxford University Press.

Tweed, R. G., & Lehman, D. R. (2002). Learning considered within a cultural context. *American Psychologist, 57,* 89–99.

Tyrer, P., & Bateman, A. W. (2004). Drug treatment for personality disorders. *Advances in Psychiatric Treatment, 10,* 389–398.

Van de Vijver, F. J. K., & Leung, K. (1997). *Methods and data analysis for cross-cultural research.* Newbury Park, CA: Sage.

Wakefield, J. C. (2008). The perils of dimensionalization: Challenges in distinguishing negative traits from personality disorders. *Psychiatric Clinics of North America, 31,* 379–393.

Wang, D., Cui, H., & Zhou, F. (2005). Measuring the personality of Chinese: QZPS versus NEO PI-R. *Asian Journal of Social Psychology, 8,* 97–122.

Watts, J. (2002). Public health experts concerned about "hikikomori." *Lancet, 359,* 1131.

Westen, D., & Shedler, J. (1999). Revising and assessing Axis II: Part II. Toward an empirically based and clinically useful classification of personality disorders. *American Journal of Psychiatry, 156,* 273–285.

Widiger, T. A., Mangine, S., Corbitt, E. M., Ellis, C. G., & Thomas, G. V. (1995). *Personality Disorder Interview—IV: A semistructured interview for the assessment of personality disorders.* Odessa, FL: Psychological Assessment Resources.

Widiger, T. A., & Trull, T. J. (2007). Plate tectonics in the classification of personality disorder. *American Psychologist, 62,* 71–83.

Widiger, T. A., & Mullins-Sweatt, S. N. (2009). Five-factor model of personality disorder: A proposal for DSM-V. *Annual Review of Clinical Psychology, 5,* 197–220.

Wong, D. F. K. (2008). Cognitive behavioural treatment groups for people with chronic depression in Hong Kong: A randomized wait-list control design. *Depression and Anxiety, 25,* 142–148.

Wu, S., & Keysar, B. (2007). Cultural effects on perspective taking. *Psychological Science, 18,* 600–606.

Yang, K.-S., & Bond, M. H. (1990). Exploring implicit personality theories with indigenous or imported constructs: The Chinese case. *Journal of Personality and Social Psychology, 58,* 1087–1095.

Yang, J., McCrae, R. R., Costa, P. T., Jr., Dai, X., Yao, S., Gai, T., et al. (1999). Cross-cultural personality assessment in psychiatric populations: The NEO-PI-R in the People's Republic of China. *Psychological Assessment, 11,* 359–368.

Yang, J., McCrae, R. R., Costa, P. T., Yao, S., Dai, X., Cai, T., et al. (2000). The cross-cultural generalizability of Axis-II constructs: An evaluation of two personality disorder assessment instruments in the People's Republic of China. *Journal of Personality Disorders, 14,* 249–263.

Yik, M. S., & Bond, M. H. (1993). Exploring the dimensions of Chinese person perceptions with indigenous and imported constructs: Creating a culturally balanced scale. *International Journal of Psychology, 28,* 75–95.

Yik, M. S. M., Bond, M. H., & Paulhus, D. L. (1998). Do Chinese self-enhance or self-efface? It's a matter of domain. *Personality and Social Psychology Bulletin, 24,* 399–406.

Yik, M. S. M., Russell, J. A., Ahn, C., Fernandez-Dols, J. M., & Suzuki, N. (2002). Relating the five-factor model of personality to a circumplex model of affect: A five language study. In R. R. McCrae & J. Allik (Eds.), *The five-factor model of personality across cultures* (pp. 79–104). New York: Kluwer.

Yoshida, K., Tonai, E., Nagai, H., Matsushima, K., Matsushita, M., Tsukada, J., et al. (2006). Long-term follow-up study of borderline patients in Japan: A preliminary study. *Comprehensive Psychiatry, 47,* 426–432.

Young, J., Klosko, J., & Weishaar, M. (2003). Schema therapy for borderline personality disorder. In *Schema therapy: A practitioner's guide.* New York: Guilford.

Zanarini, M. C., & Frankenburg, F. R. (2001). Olanzapine treatment of female borderline personality disorder patients: A double-blind, placebo-controlled pilot study. *Journal of Clinical Psychiatry, 62,* 849–854.

Zhang, A. Y., Yu, L. C., Draguns, J. G., Zhang, J., & Tang, D. (2000). Sociocultural contexts of anthropophobia: A sample of Chinese youth. *Social Psychiatry and Psychiatric Epidemiology, 35,* 418–426.

Zhang, J., & Bond, M. H. (1998). Personality and filial piety among college students in two Chinese societies: The added value of indigenous constructs. *Journal of Cross-Cultural Psychology, 29,* 402–417.

Zhong, J., & Leung, F. (2007). Should borderline personality disorder be included in the fourth edition of the Chinese classification of mental disorders? *Chinese Medical Journal, 120,* 77–82.

PSYCHOPATHOLOGY AND TREATMENT MODELS INDIGENOUS TO ASIA

| 15 |

CULTURE-RELATED SPECIFIC PSYCHIATRIC SYNDROMES OBSERVED IN ASIA

Wen-Shing Tseng, Sung Kil Min, Kei Nakamura,
and Shuichi Katsuragawa

INTRODUCTION

Definition of the Term: Culture-Related Specific Psychiatric Syndromes

Culture-related specific psychiatric syndromes, also called culture-bound syndromes (Yap, 1967) or culture-specific disorders (Jilek & Jilek-Aall, 1985, 2001), refer to mental conditions or psychiatric syndromes whose occurrence or manifestations are closely related to cultural factors and thus warrant understanding and management primarily from a cultural perspective. A culture-related specific psychiatric syndrome is so called because it has a unique presentation, with special clinical manifestations (Tseng, 2001, pp. 211–263).

In the 1970s, a Chinese cultural psychiatrist from Hong Kong, P. M. Yap, after reviewing all the unique syndromes, suggested the term "culture-bound syndrome" to describe the various psycho-pathologies or atypical syndromes bound to certain cultures. Recently, however, cultural psychiatrists have realized that such psychiatric manifestations are not necessarily "bound" to particular ethnic-cultural groups. For instance, epidemic occurrences of *koro* (penis-shrinking panic) occur among Thai or Indian people, not only among the Southern Chinese, as previously believed; and sporadic occurrences of *amok* attacks (mass, indiscriminate homicidal acts) are observed in the Philippines, Thailand, Papua New Guinea, and in epidemic proportions in many places in South Asia, in addition to Malaysia, as originally described. Therefore, it was suggested that the incorrect term "culture-bound syndromes" be replaced with the term "culture-related specific psychiatric syndromes" (Tseng, 2001, pp. 211–263).

From a phenomenological and diagnostic point of view, such syndromes are not easily categorized according to existing psychiatric classifications, which are based on clinical experiences of commonly observed psychiatric disorders in Western societies, without adequate orientation toward less frequently encountered psychiatric conditions and diverse cultures worldwide. Furthermore, the current classification system of *DSM* used in the United States is descriptively oriented and not suitable to include disorders that need to be conceived etiologically and culturally.

In certain ways, all psychiatric disorders are more or less influenced by cultural factors in addition to biological and psychological factors for their occurrence and manifestations. Major psychiatric disorders (such as schizophrenia or bipolar disorders) are considered as determined more by biological factors and relatively less by psychological and cultural factors, but minor psychiatric disorders (such as anxiety disorders, conversion disorders, or situational adjustment disorder) are more subject to psychological causes as well as cultural factors. In addition to this, there are groups of psychiatric disorders that are heavily related to and influenced by cultural factors, and are therefore addressed as culture-related specific psychiatric syndromes (Tseng, 2001, 2008). Although the occurrence of culture-related specific syndromes is not very common, such syndromes provide the example and opportunity to examine how culture may impact on psychopathology, which in turn guides us to understand the nature of psychopathology.

Different Ways Culture Impacts on Psychopathology

It has been elaborated that, from a conceptual point of view, there are six different ways that culture can contribute to psychopathology (Tseng, 2001, pp. 178–183). They are:

a. Pathogenic Effects—Pathogenic effects refer to situations in which culture is a direct causative factor in forming or "generating" psychopathology. Cultural ideas and beliefs contribute to stress, which, in turn, produces psychopathology. Koro, Dhat syndrome, and frigophobia as described in this chapter are some examples. Koro, frequently observed among people in southeastern China, is induced by the cultural belief that excessive shrinking of the penis will cause death. Dhat syndrome, reported in India, is caused by the cultural belief that semen is an important body fluid and excessive loss of it will result in sickness. Frigophobia, reported in Taiwan and characterized by excessive fear of catching, or being exposed to, cold air, is based on the cultural belief in the importance of a balance between yin and yang, and catching cold air means excess intake of the yin element, resulting in weakness of the body.

b. Pathoselective Effects—Pathoselective effects refer to the tendency of some people in a society, when encountering stress, to select certain culturally influenced reaction patterns that result in the manifestation of certain psychopathologies. Family suicide, observed in Japan, hwabyung in Korea, as described in this chapter, or *amok*, which is observed to be prevalent in Malaysia, are some examples. In Japan, when parents encounter unresolvable difficulties in their lives, among various ways to cope they choose to commit suicide together with their children, with the cultural belief that it is better for children to die together with their parents than to be left as orphans and mistreated by other people. When Korean women encounter stress related to family members, in order to maintain the culturally emphasized value of harmony, they tend to react to their stress and feelings of resentment with a unique psychosomatic condition called *hwabyung* in Korean, meaning sickness of resentment with fire.

c. Pathoplastic Effects—Pathoplastic effects refer to the ways in which culture contributes to the modeling or "plastering" of the manifestations of psychopathology. Culture shapes symptom manifestations at the level of the content presented as well as the whole clinical picture. *Taijin-Kyofu-Sho* or brain fag syndromes are some of the examples. Taijin-Kyofu-Sho, described in this chapter, means fear of human interpersonal relationships, in Japanese. It refers to a situation in which young people who have been overprotected in childhood, with few socialization experiences, reach adolescence or young adulthood and begin to experience anxiety in social situations; the condition presents a unique clinical picture, including excessive concern with self-image and avoidance of social relations with acquaintances, manifesting a mixture of anxiety and social phobia.

d. Pathoelaborating Effects—While certain behavior reactions (either normal or pathological) may be universal, they may become exaggerated to the extreme in some cultures through cultural reinforcement. *Latah* observed in Malaysia is the example. It is human nature for a person, when suddenly startled, to react with anxiety, panic, or even dissociation. In Malaysia, however, the reaction to sudden startling is elaborated to such an extent that it has become a form of social entertainment to startle women, who become dissociated and exhibit uninhibited behavior, including saying sexually oriented, "dirty" words, which are normally strictly prohibited for women.

e. Pathofacilitative Effects—Pathofacilitative effects imply that, although cultural factors do not change the manifestation of the psychopathology too much—that is, the clinical picture can still be recognized and categorized without difficulty in the existing classification system—cultural factors do contribute significantly to the frequent occurrence of certain mental disorders in a society. Massive hysteria, drinking problems, or substance abuse are some of the examples.

f. Pathoreactive Effects—Pathoreactive effects indicate that, although cultural factors do not directly affect the manifestation or frequency of mental disorders, they influence people's beliefs and understanding of the disorders and mold their "reactions" toward them. Culture influences how people perceive pathologies and label disorders, and how they react to them emotionally, and then guides them in expressing their suffering. For example, in Latin America, when a person manifests an unusual mental condition, either anxiety, depression, or dissociation, the interpretation of the people surrounding him or her is that the person has lost his or her soul (*susto*, its local name), and needs to regain it in order to recover.

Any psychiatric syndrome can be influenced by culture in multiple aspects in different combination of ways as described above. The examples listed are merely to illustrate what is the most common modes of contribution from culture.

Clinical Implication of Studying Culture-Related Specific Syndromes

Many culture-related specific psychiatric syndromes, many of them from Asia, including South Asia, have been reported by scholars around the world. Some will be reviewed here briefly. It is important to be aware that the occurrence of culture-related specific psychiatric syndromes is relatively rare even in their home societies, and the syndromes discussed in this chapter would be extremely rare among Asian Americans. Yet, for clinicians, it is important to be aware of the existence of such specific syndromes and be prepared to understand their clients clinically when similar syndromes are presented by Asian patients. Most importantly, discussing the specific syndromes, from such extreme examples, will help the clinicians to be more sensitive toward the possible cultural impact toward any kind of psychopathology.

KORO (*SUOYANG,* GENITAL-RETRACTION ANXIETY DISORDER)

Definition of Koro Disease

Koro, in the Malay language, means the head of a turtle, symbolizing the male sexual organ. Among Malay people, koro refers to the clinical condition in which the patient is morbidly concerned that his penis is shrinking excessively and dangerous consequences (such as death) might occur. In Chinese, this condition is referred to as *suoyang* in traditional Chinese medicine documents, and known by ordinary people (Cheng, 1996). The term *suoyang* literally means "shrinking of yang organ (penis)."

The manifested symptoms may include simple anxiety, obsessive or hypochondriacal concern, and intense anxiety or a panic condition. Therefore, using existing *DSM* diagnostic categories, some clinicians have suggested categorizing the disorder as atypical anxiety disorder, or somatoform disorder. However, this is meaningless in terms of comprehending the nature of the disorder; nor is it useful for treating the disorder. Supportive therapy, with assurance, is usually the choice of treatment.

The majority of cases are young males. Besides the penis, the organ concerned may be any protruding part of the body, such as the nose or ear (particularly when patients are prepubertal children) or the nipples or labia for the females.

Koro often occurs as sporadic cases, but occasionally it may become epidemic. According to literature, koro epidemics have occurred in several areas in Asia, namely, Singapore (Ngui, 1969), Thailand (Suwanlert & Coates, 1979), India (Chakraborty, 1982), and China (Mo et al., 1987).

Sporadic Cases of Koro (Suoyang) Reported Among Chinese Patients

Chinese-Singaporean psychiatrist Gwee (1963) presented three Chinese-Singaporean cases he observed in Singapore. Cultural psychiatrist from Hong Kong, Yap (1965) reported that he was able to gather 19 cases in Hong Kong during his 15-year practice there. From Taiwan, Rin (1965) described two cases, both originally from central China. Recently, Tsai (1982), from Guangdong, China, reported five cases of *suoyang* that he observed over a period of four years. It is the general impression that *suoyang* cases are found more in southern China, particularly among the coastal provinces of Fujien and Guangdong including Hainan Island and Leizhou Peninsular, and is relatively rare in northern China.

Dynamic study of some cases shows that the male patients usually grew up without a father figure and lacked masculinity identity. Also, they strongly believed that there was a need to preserve vitality and not lose yang element in the body system by not indulging excessively in sexual activities (Rin, 1965, 1966). According to the yin-yang theory, protruding parts of the body, such as the ears, nose, feet, or penis, are considered yang organs, while concave areas, such as the mouth, nostrils, or vagina, are yin organs. Ginger, pepper, or any green vegetables are regarded as foods rich in the yang element, and are good remedies for yang-deficient physical conditions. Many patients tried to consume foods rich in the yang element to restore the yin-yang balance when they contracted *suoyang* condition.

Recurrent Koro (Suoyang) Epidemics in Southern China

The first Western report of a koro epidemic was published in a French medical journal in 1908, about 100 years ago. It described an endemic episode among school students in Sichuan province in central China with local diagnosis of suffering from *suo-yin-zheng* (meaning "shrinking of private part sickness").

Yet, the Chinese psychiatrists Mo and colleagues (1987), reviewing the local chronicle, reported that recurrent instances of *suoyang* epidemics had been noted on Hainan Island and the neighboring Leizhou Peninsula of Guangdong in South China about 145 years before.

No official record of a *suoyang* occurrence has been noted since then. Yet, Mo and his associates (1995) reported that five major epidemics were noted in Hainan, in 1952, 1962, 1966, 1974, and 1984. According to the recollections of old residents, the 1952 epidemic appeared during the period of land reform under the Communist regime, in which landlords' properties were distributed to the farmers—a time of severe social tension. The 1962 epidemic occurred after the Great Leap Forward movement, in which there was economic crisis throughout the country. The 1966 epidemic broke out at the beginning of the Cultural Revolution, when there was serious conflict and turmoil in the country. The 1974 epidemic started when there was an outbreak of encephalitis. The epidemic of 1984 occurred in an atmosphere of fear, when local fortune-tellers predicted a bad year for farmers. It seems that a specific social tension was related to the occurrence of each *suoyang* epidemic. Most of the people in the epidemic areas believed that all social disasters would ultimately result in a *suoyang* occurrence.

From a sociological point of view, it is noted that more than half the population of Hainan Island and Leizhou Peninsular are peasants and fishermen. Most of them live in remote village areas and have little formal education. People in Hainan and Leizhou are very religious. There are many temples, and people are still considerably influenced by supernatural beliefs of the past. Most of them still retain sex-related beliefs, such as the traditional medical concept of conserving semen to maintain the balance of yin and yang. They also believe that ghosts in hell are anxious to obtain human protruding body parts, particularly men's penises, which contain the rich yang force. The ghosts have lost their yang element, and are anxious to get yang force to enable them to return to the human world. Therefore, local people believe that a ghost disguised as a fair lady comes to collect men's penises. A ghost in the form of a female fox spirit is also thought to seduce a male victim in order to take away his yang force.

The last epidemic occurred in the summer of 1984, when the rice did not grow well in Hainan. Local fortune-tellers predicted it would be a troublesome year, in which the people would suffer from many disasters. It was in this uneasy atmosphere that the epidemic occurred (Tseng, et al., 1988). It usually involved a village for several days to a couple of weeks, with a dozen or more victims, then spread to a nearby village. In a period of six months, it was estimated that more than 3,000 people became victims of *suoyang*. All the victims were Han nationals. There were no cases in the central mountainous part of the island, inhabited by the minority groups of Li and Miao nationals, who did not share the concept of *suoyang*.

The research team conducted a questionnaire study of the koro group with comparison of clinical anxiety cases and non-koro, nonclinical cases as the control group (Tseng, Mo, et al, 1992). Results revealed that, as reflected by the symptom checklist, the symptom profile of the koro group was characterized by anxiety with phobic tendencies, but was not similar to that of the clinical anxiety group. A study of personality profiles showed that *suoyang* victims were different from usual anxiety disorder cases and, as a group, had lower intellectual endowments than the control group.

Since the *suoyang* epidemics tended to occur in the Guangdong area and not in other parts of China, a comparison of folk beliefs held in different regions in China was carried out in Jilin, northeastern China, and Taiwan, as well as in Guangdong (Tseng et al., 1993). The results revealed that there are different degrees of belief in and attitudes toward the *suoyang* folk concept among Chinese in different geographic areas and in different subcultures. The findings support the view that the belief in *suoyang* in Hainan and Leizhou of Guangdong is one of the major reasons for the recurrence of *suoyang* epidemics in those regions.

In summary, it can be said that koro is a culture-related specific psychiatric syndrome. It is based on the victim's strong cultural belief relating to sex and vitality, and it is developed through psychogenetic effects. It can occur as sporadic cases but also as collective cases in a contagious manner. Koro epidemics have been reported in South China, Singapore, Thailand, and India in the past, involving different ethnic and racial groups associated with the local social turmoil at the time of occurrence (Tseng, 2001, pp. 265–290).

DHAT SYNDROME (SEMEN-LOSS ANXIETY)

Very closely related to the genital-retraction anxiety disorder (koro) is the semen-loss or semen-leaking anxiety disorder, or spermatorrhea, also known by its Indian folk name, Dhat syndrome. According to Indian psychiatrists Bhatia and Malik (1991), the word *dhat* derives from the Sanskrit *Dhatu*, which refers to the elixir that constitutes the body. Of the seven types of *Dhatus* described, semen is considered the most important. In the Indian system of medicine, *Ayurveda*, it is suggested that disturbances in the *Dhatus* result in an increased susceptibility to physical and mental disease.

The term "Dhat syndrome" was first used by the Indian psychiatrist Wig in 1960, and by Neki in 1973. The syndrome refers to the clinical condition in which the patient is morbidly preoccupied with the excessive loss of semen from an "improper form of leaking," such as nocturnal emissions, masturbation, or urination. The underlying anxiety is based on the cultural belief that excessive semen loss will result in illness. Therefore, it is a pathogenically induced psychological disorder. The medical term "spermatorrhea" is a misnomer, as there is no actual problem of sperm leakage from a urological point of view.

From a clinical point of view, the patients are predominantly young males who present vague, multiple somatic symptoms such as fatigue, weakness, anxiety, loss of appetite, and feelings of guilt (about having indulged in sexual acts such as masturbation or having sex with prostitutes). Some also complain of sexual dysfunction (impotence or premature ejaculation). The chief complaint is often that the urine is opaque, which is attributed to the presence of semen (Paris, 1992). The patient attributes the passing of semen in the urine to his excessive indulgence in masturbation or other socially defined sexual improprieties (Bhatia & Malik, 1991). Clinically, the patient is characterized as anxious or hypochondriacal, and can be diagnosed according to the *DSM* system as atypical anxiety, hypocondriacal disorder, or somatoform disorder. However, these diagnostic categories do not help clinicians deal with clients regarding the underlying causes of their anxieties. As part of the illness behavior, the patient will ask the physician to examine his urine to determine whether there is leaking of semen or not. The patient also always asks for a tonic or other remedy to regain the vitality lost due to excess leakage of semen. In general, supportive psychotherapy, with medical explanations about the physiological phenomena of semen discharge, will be helpful to patients to some extent.

According to Bhatia and Malik (1991), the syndrome is also widespread in Nepal, Sri Lanka (where it is referred to as *prameha* disease), Bangladesh, and Pakistan. In Taiwan, Wen (1995) considers *shenkui* ("kidney deficiency," or insufficient vitality due to excessive loss of semen), prevalent among young Taiwanese men, as the counterpart of the Dhat syndrome observed among the Chinese. The *shenkui* disorder in traditional medical terminology is often considered equivalent to the neurasthenia referred to by modern Chinese psychiatrists.

No matter what term is used, Dhat syndrome in India, *prameha* in Sri Lanka, or *shenkui* in China, there is a common characteristic among these syndromes: they are based on folk beliefs that excessive loss of semen will result in illness. Akhtar (1988) pointed out that, according to the religious scriptures of the Hindus, "Forty meals produce one drop of blood, 40 drops of blood give rise to one drop of bone marrow, and 40 drops of marrow form one drop of semen." Variations on this saying are found in the other cultures where semen-loss anxiety disorder is observed. These cultural beliefs that conservation of vitality is important and loss of semen is harmful to the health create culture-genic stress and contribute to the formation of semen-loss anxiety.

FRIGOPHOBIA (MORBID FEAR OF CATCHING COLD AIR)

"Frigophobia," or "morbid fear of catching cold," is a clinical condition described by Chinese psychiatrists as a culture-related syndrome of the Chinese (Rin, 1966). In Chinese (Mandarin) it is called *pa-len* or *wei-han* (literally, fear of cold). Such a morbid condition is not very prevalent. Only sporadic cases have been reported since attention was given to the condition as a culture-related specific syndrome. Y. H. Chang and her colleagues reported five cases in Taiwan in 1975; N. M. Chiou and associates cited two cases in 1994. Among the five cases reported by Chang and her colleagues, four of the subjects were born in various parts of mainland China and migrated to Taiwan after the mainland was taken over by the communists. Up to now, few reports from mainland China have appeared in literature. Perhaps professional attention has not been paid to the disorder there as a culture-related specific disorder.

This unique disorder is characterized by the patient's excessive concern with and morbid fear of catching "cold" (from the point of temperature, such as cold air or cold wind). According to the Chinese traditional theory of yin and yang, an imbalance between yin and yang will result in disorders. Excessive yin, caused by cold air or excessive eating of cold food (such as watermelon) will result in weakness and sickness. The chilling sensation of cold sweat is interpreted as a sign of weakness due to excessive yin. Based on these folk concepts, even ordinary people will avoid cold air, cold rain, eating too much cold food, and will wear belly-bands around their abdomens to protect them from catching cold, particularly in cold whether.

At the extreme of this concern, a patient who develops frigophobia will overdress in warm clothes (even in hot weather), wearing a heavy hat to protect his head, surrounding his neck with a warm neckerchief, and wearing many layers of clothing to keep his body from catching cold air. In an extreme case, the patient will wrap himself up with a blanket or heavy quilt and stay in bed, afraid to go outside and be exposed to the cold air.

Clinical examination of patients often reveals psychiatric manifestations of depression, hypochondriasis, phobia, or anxiety with panic tendency, in addition to the morbid fear of catching cold air. In other words, the morbid fear of cold is a part of a compound clinical picture, rather than the total picture. However, because of the patient's excessive concern with and fear of catching cold air, many "odd" maneuvers for protecting the body from catching cold, including inappropriately heavy dress, become so obvious that frigophobia becomes a prominent part of the clinical condition, and warrants such a specific diagnosis. Based on the DSM system, some clinicians give a clinical diagnosis of anxiety, depression, hypochondriasis, or somatization disorder, depending on which symptom is most prominent, besides the illness-behavior of excessive fear and concern of catching cold air. Besides supportive psychotherapy, some patients respond well to antidepressants.

The personal histories in such cases often reveal that, during their early lives, the subjects were overprotected by their mothers and developed anxious or dependent personalities. The fear of catching cold air usually developed as a reaction to a crisis or a significant loss in the patient's life that provoked feelings of insecurity.

As pointed out by Chang and associates (1975), as well as Tseng and Hsu (1969/70), there is a common tendency for Chinese patients to manifest their psychological problems with somatized symptoms. However, in some cases, the somatization is not manifested merely as a somatic symptom, but as an elaborate way of being concerned and complaining about a morbid somatic condition. Fear of catching cold air is one such example. The disorder of frigophobia was based on the traditional concepts of hot and cold and folk beliefs about the importance of maintaining vitality, avoiding catching cold and keeping the body warm to preserve vitality. It may be said that instead of manifesting depression as reaction to loss, through the effects of culture, the patients may manifest their conditions as a unique and elaborate fear of cold syndrome.

HWABYUNG (FIRE SICKNESS)

Definition of the Clinical Condition

"Hwabyung" is a Korean term that literally means "fire-sickness." It is known as one kind of culture-related specific syndrome relating to anger or resentment, which is known as "anger disease" as well. In Korean, the word of *hwa* means fire and anger as well; *byung* means disease or sickness. Ordinary Koreans has used this folk term to address the emotional disorder relating to resentment or anger.

From epidemiological point of view, it has been reported that 4% to 5% of the general population in a rural area in Korea are reported as suffering from hwabyung (Min et al., 1990). The patients reported to suffering from hwabyung are frequently of middle-aged or older women of the lower social class (Min et al., 1987).

Patients suffering from hwabyung frequently relate their sickness with anger or resentment. They describe their anger in other terms as well, such as *uk-wool* and/or *boon*. "Uk-wool" is a term used to describe a feeling of depression-related anger that results from being a victim of unfair situation and wrong understanding; while "boon" a feeling of anger arising from a situation involving failure in spite of one's best effort due to indefensible external reasons beyond one's control. Accordingly, hwabyung is commonly a reactive response with anger to an unfair social situation. According to the culture, which emphasizes harmony, feelings of anger have to be suppressed so as not to jeopardize harmonious family or social relationships. However, if the unfair situations continue, the suppressed anger accumulates, becomes dense, and is finally manifested as the emotional sickness of hwabyung.

Clinically, most (Korean) patients know already that their hwabyung is a psychogenic disorder due to suppressed and accumulated anger that is reactive to unfair social violence or injustice (Min, 1989). A common case-scenario would be a middle-aged woman who developed hwabyung as a result of a conflict with her mother-in-law and/or husband, who instilled anger in her. Such women have to suppress their anger so as not to jeopardize harmonious family life. Suppression and control have been strong social codes of behavior in the traditionally familial, collective, and Confucian culture of Korea. Other anger-provoking situations are generally unfair social situations including social injustice, economic loss, failure in promotion, and being betrayed. Many patients also complain of feeling *haan* (resentment), another form of chronic anger.

Clinical Symptoms

The main symptoms of hwabyung are subjective feeling of fire-like emotion, that is, anger (described in Korean as: *uk-wool, boon,* and *haan*), anxiety state, panic attack, or depression, associated with anger-related somatization and behavioral symptoms (Min et al., 1987; Min & Kim, 1998). Somatic symptoms typically include heat/hot sensation in the body such as hot flushing, heat sensation on face or upper trunk, a hot mass in abdomen radiating heat upward, and intolerance of a hot environment. Other typical somatic symptoms are the feeling of something pushing up in the chest, mass sensation in the epigastrium or chest, chest oppression/stuffiness, heart-pounding, and dry mouth. Behaviorally patients show frequent talkativeness, sighing, going out of the house, or avoiding stuffy closed places. Also they complain of many thoughts. If given the chance, typical patients with hwabyung tend to talk for a long time with many tears and sighs, about how they have suffered from unfairness and how they have nevertheless controlled hatred and revengeful thoughts and will live sincerely. They used to say that their life was "a life full with resentment (*haan*)."

Recently Son and Min (2010) studied specific symptoms of hwabyung in 221 participants with depressive disorder, anxiety disorder, somatoform disorder, and adjustment disorder and patients who also complained of hwabyung. Instruments were SCID for *DSM-IV* diagnosis and a structured diagnostic interview schedule for hwabyung, which included the research diagnostic criteria for hwabyung. The predictability of hwabyung symptoms in research diagnostic criteria for hwabyung was assessed by using factor analysis, logistic regression sensitivity, specificity, and predictive values. As results, factor analysis yielded three symptom factors: hwabyung-unique symptoms, depressive symptoms, and other symptoms. Hwabyung-unique symptoms had high eigen values. Feeling of a mass in the epigastrium, heat sensation, feeling of something pushing-up in the chest, feelings of *uk-wool/boon* (being mortified), and feelings of *haan* had a relatively high odds ratio. Two symptoms (heat sensation and feeling *uk-wool/boon*, that is, being mortified) had high sensitivity and low positive predictive values. Three symptoms (feeling of a mass in the epigastrium, feeling of something pushing up in the chest, and feeling of *haan*) had high specificity and high positive predictive values; suggesting a hwabyung state. In conclusion, authors suggested that heat sensation and feeling of *uk-wool/boon* may be basic symptoms for diagnosis for hwabyung.

Clinical experiences show that hwabyung is a chronic form of anger syndrome with the mean duration of clinical course for about 12 years, ranging from 7 months to 46 years (Min & Hong, 2006).

Diagnostic Issues

Regarding diagnosis of hwabyung, there are two views held among Korean psychiatrists. One view is that hwabyung is a culture-related specific syndrome observed among Koreans (Min et al., 1989). The other view is that, hwabyung is merely a general folk term used by laypersons to describe a stressful or depressed state or psychological conflict.

The other issue is the question of how patients with hwabyung are diagnosed in the *DSM* or ICD system. Western psychiatrists considered that hwabyung is a kind of a variant of depression or somatization disorder (Prince, 1989; Lin et al., 1992). Diagnostically hwabyung shares many symptoms of depression but it seems to be different from depressive disorders by manifesting mainly subjective anger and anger-related somatic/behavioral symptoms. When most patients who identified themselves as suffering from hwabyung were diagnosed by psychiatrists according to *DSM-III-R*, they were found to have a combination of depressive and somatization disorders (Min et al., 1986, 1990). Recently a research conducted with a developed research criteria for hwabyung, found out that about 15% of the patients were diagnosed as having only hwabyung, not comorbid with any *DSM-IV* diagnosis (Kwon et al., 2005; Son, 2006, Min & Suh 2010).

For a diagnosis of hwabyung, Min and his colleagues (2009) suggested that heat sensation, subjective anger, the expression of anger, emotional complaints of *uk-woo/boon*, the sensation of having an epigastric mass, somatic complaints of feeling something pushing up in the chest, and the psychological sense of *haan* are the basic symptoms for the diagnosis of hwabyung. Recently, Min and his colleagues (2010) reported that, of 280 patients with depressive disorder, anxiety disorder, somatoform disorder, and adjustment disorder, and patients who also complained of hwabyung and were diagnosed with the research diagnostic criteria of hwabyung (Min et al. 2009) and SCID 1 for a *DSM-IV* diagnosis, 183 patients were diagnosed with hwabyung. Forty-seven of the patients had only hwabyung, and the rest had various comorbid *DSM-IV* diagnoses, with major depressive disorder and generalized anxiety disorder being the most frequent. The distributions of single diagnoses and comorbid diagnoses were similar for hwabyung, major depressive disorder, and generalized anxiety disorder. These results suggest that hwabyung, which comprises unique anger-related symptoms, is comparable to major depressive disorder or generalized anxiety disorder in a comorbidity profile.

Treatment

Before seeing a psychiatrist, many hwabyung patients have already sought help from various treatment modalities (Min et al., 1987), including traditional herb remedies and even Christian faith healing (confirming prayer) or shaman rituals.

Most Korean psychiatrists recommend integrated treatment combining psychosocial therapy, including psychoanalytic-oriented therapy, cognitive-behavioral therapy, religious therapy, and drug therapy (Min et al., 1989). It is also necessary for psychiatrists to enrich their treatment strategies with some of the wisdom and techniques derived from culture including traditional medicine and religions. In drug treatment, most psychiatrists (78.5%) suggested the combined use of antidepressants and antianxiety drugs (Min et al., 1989).

Cultural Comments

Hwabyung has been suggested as a culture-related specific syndrome of Korea because it is closely related to Korean culture. From macroscopic view, at national level, it can be pointed out that the feeling of resentment (*haan*) is a unique traditional collective sentiment of Koreans, which may be defined as a pathos, a chronic mixed mood of missing, sadness, and suppressed anger (*uk-wool* and *boon*). Historically, through their long period of endurance and forbearance of a hard life from generation to generation due to unfair external invasion and treatment, and violence against them, by repeated invasions and exploitations of aggressive neighboring countries (namely Japan and China), Koreans have suffered. Koreans, as a group of national people, have suppressed and accumulated anger (*uk-wool* or *boon*), which, in turn, have been transformed into a collective and/or personal feeling of resentment (*haan*). This is particularly true for Koreans who have been victims of exploitation, poverty, and war. Accordingly, many Korean intellectuals have discussed the history of *haan*, the *haan* of nation, and the culture of *haan*.

In Korean language, many terms are used in their daily life to express the feeling of resentment, such as "affectionate resentment" (*jeong-haan*, the longing for or missing of a loved one who has left), "regretful resentment" (*hoe-haan*, regret for not having done one's best), "hateful resentment" (*won-haan*, harboring of revenge), and "painful resentment" (*tong-haan*, emotionally painful resentment), reflecting that resentment is a collective sentiment of Korean.

Microscopically, at the individual level, resentment (*haan*) is usually related broadly to a failed love affair or separation from lover, unmarried state, a bad spouse, sexual frustration, domestic violence, having no child, early separation from or death of parents, poverty, hardship in life, lower family class, low education level, having no chance to show one's filial piety before parents' death, disease, handicap, being crippled, deformity, having problem children, an unfair trial, a swindle, betrayal, being harmed, and miserable fate. But typically, resentment (*haan*) has been associated with being women, who have been considered the weaker gender, often mistreated harshly by mothers-in-law or husbands. Another group is the so-called *sang-nom* (lower-class people), which include maids, servants, roaming entertainers, and butchers.

Defense style and coping strategies related to the feeling of resentment (*haan*) are reported to be: somatization, suppression-inhibition-withdrawal, splitting-projection, passive-aggressiveness, oral consumption, primitive idealization, stimulus reduction, self-pity, shared-concerns, and dependency (Min et al., 1997). It can be said that a feeling of resentment (*haan*) is described by patients with hwabyung as one of their symptoms as well as one of the etiologies of their problem (Min, 1991). The etiological emotions (anger, *uk-wool*, and *boon*) and the explanation for the formation of syndrome (repeating and accumulating) are common in both conditions.

For the Chinese traditional medicine observed in Korea, it considered that a health state is restored by harmonious interaction between yin and yang, and among five elements (*qi*), namely: fire, water, wood, metal, and earth, in various body organs. Fire is the symbol of anger. The concept of hwabyung seems rooted in the traditional medical concept. If fire-element becomes excessive, various diseases may develop depending on the organs affected. Consequently, this kind of fire-elevated disease may be controlled by opposite element, namely, water. Practically, traditional herb doctors in Korea try to treat hwabyung based on these concepts.

Finally, it needs to be pointed out that Korean culture emphasizes harmonious, family-oriented, interdependent, collectivism. Within this culture, one tries to control oneself and avoid aggression toward others. Suppression and endurance are considered virtues. This culture of "relationship" for the collective society seems to be intensified by Confucian teachings, which are still prevalent in Korea. Hwabyung seems to be the result of efforts of the victim not to jeopardize harmonious relationship with others. Therefore hwabyung frequently develops under pressure in the family relationship.

TAIJIN-KYOFU-SHO (ANTHROPOPHOBIA, INTERPERSONAL RELATION PHOBIA)

Definition and Nature of the Disorder

"Anthropophobia" is the English-translation for the Japanese term Taijin-Kyofu-Sho (the disorder with fear of interpersonal relation), a psychiatric diagnostic term invented by Japanese psychiatrists to address a special type of social phobia commonly observed among Japanese patients.

Taijin-Kyofu-Sho was said to be prevalent among Japanese and is considered a culture-related specific psychiatric disorder. According to Iwai (1982), among outpatients with minor psychiatric disorders (such as anxiety, and obsessive or hypochondriac disorders) who visited one of the metropolitan psychiatric hospitals in Tokyo, 11% were diagnosed as anthropophobic. Yamashita (1977/93) reported that, among the outpatients who visited the university psychiatric clinic in Hokkaido, 7.8% were given this diagnosis. Kasahara (1974) reported that, among 430 college students who received mental health services at the student health service of Kyoto University in 1968, one-half were neurotic and, among them, 18.6% could be classified as Taijin-Kyofu-Sho cases (of the rest, 24% were depression and 20% were psychosomatic disorders). According to Mori and Kitanishi (1984), at the Morita Clinic set up in Jikei University in Tokyo, specializing in residential treatment for *shinkeishitsu* (neurotic patients), 34.2% of the total population were diagnosed as Taijin-Kyofu-Sho cases, 35.3% as obsessive-compulsive, and 20.2% as having anxiety disorders.

However, it is Japanese psychiatrists' general impression that this disorder has gradually been declining over the past several decades. It is not clear whether it is due to the change of classification system or actual decrease of this special social phobia associated with sociocultural change and socialization pattern among the youngsters.

Major Clinical Picture

Several clinical studies reported by Japanese psychiatrists provide overviews of the clinical picture of the disorder. Yamashita (1977/93) reviewed 100 consecutive cases of Taijin-Kyofu-Sho under his care at the university clinic. According to the data, patients experienced onset of the illness as early as 10–14 years old (18%), most between 15–19 years (44%), some at 20–24 years (26%), and a few after 25 years (12%). In his series of cases, there were 76 males and 24 females, showing that the disorder is more prevalent among males, with a ratio of roughly 3:1. The cardinal symptoms manifested by the patients are: fear of one's bodily odors (28%), fear of flushing (22%), fear of showing odd attitudes toward others (18%), fear of eye contact with others (15%), concern about others' attitudes toward oneself (9%), and fear of body dysmorphia (5%).

Kato (1977, p. 30) reviewed the medical charts of 560 cases of Taijin-Kyofu-Sho who visited one of the mental hospitals specializing in the treatment of Taijin-Kyofu-Sho in Tokyo during the years 1953 to 1955 and 1962. The age distribution was concentrated at 15–19 years (33%) and 20–24 years (46%). The chief complaints, allowing for multiple calculations, were fear of flushing (50%), fear of crowds (45%), fear of making a public speech (36%), fear of interacting with the opposite sex (35%), fear of carrying on a conversation with others (34%), fear of eye contact with others (31%), feeling inferior (31%), fear of socialization (26%), and fear of relating with authority (24%). The sex ratio was also 3:1, but, based on Kato's clinical experience, it was his impression that female cases were increasing slightly after the war.

In summary, the majority of the patients suffering from Taijin-Kyofu-Sho were teenagers or young adults. Males were three times more likely than females to suffer from this disorder.

Dynamic Interpretation and Culture Formulation

Regarding the nature of Taijin-Kyofu-Sho, the Japanese psychiatrist Kasahara (1974) brought out an important point about the nature of such disorder, namely, the characteristic of Taijin-Kyofu-Sho is that the fear is induced in the presence of classmates, colleagues, or friends—those who are neither particularly close (such as family members) nor totally strange (such as people in the street). In other words, subjects are concerned with how to relate to people of intermediate familiarity. It is toward these people that a person must exercise delicate social etiquette.

Kasahara explained further that Japan is a situation-oriented society, very much concerned with how others see your behavior. Japanese parents often discipline their children by saying, "Neighbors are watching whatever you do." Also, the act of staring at the person to whom one is talking is considered quite extraordinary and rude. Thus, there are cultural characteristics that cause Japanese to be hypersensitive about "looking at" and "being looked at."

Kimura (1982) pointed out that patients who were suffering from Taijin-Kyofu-Sho were not phobic toward human subjects. On the contrary, they were eager to socialize with others. However, because they were concerned with how they were perceived by others, particularly their friends, they became embarrassed and nervous when relating to them. They were not so concerned about strangers or close family members, just semiclose friends. Within Japanese society, there is such a strong demand to be sensitive to interpersonal interactions that sensitivity is heightened.

From a dynamic point of view, Yamashita (1977/93) clarified that, although sufferers of both hypochondriasis and Taijin-Kyofu-Sho complained about their physical conditions, the symptoms of the former were related to the physical self and of the latter to the social self—that is the basic difference between them.

Taijin-Kyofu-Sho is a psychological disorder of the adolescent. It is closely related to the problems associated with psychological development in the area of socialization. The Japanese child is raised in an atmosphere of indulgence and trust. However, when this protected child enters the wider world of junior high school, he or she faces multiple tasks—coping with conflict between biological needs and social restrictions, personal identity problems, and an increasing need for acceptance and love by others in social settings. This intensifies a feeling of unworthiness, making him or her more concerned about other's sensibilities and reactions (Yamashita, 1977/93).

Diagnostic Considerations

There has been controversial argument among scholars and clinicians that whether Taijin-Kyofu-Sho is a culture-related special psychiatric syndrome or merely a cultural variation of social phobia. In other words, whether it is the matter of classification criteria or diagnostic pattern.

In order to test the way in which American mental health professionals diagnosed Japanese anthropophobia, Tanaka-Matsumi (1979) gave six Japanese case descriptions of Taijin-Kyofu-Sho to American clinical psychologists and psychiatric residents for their diagnostic impressions. It was found that American mental health professionals grouped the Japanese cases of Taijin-Kyofu-Sho into a number of heterogeneous categories, including schizophrenia, paranoid personality, anxiety neurosis, phobic neurosis, and others.

As a follow-up to this, a comparison study was made between the diagnoses of social phobia by Japanese psychiatrists in Tokyo and American psychiatrists in Hawaii (Tseng, Asai, et al., 1992). A brief segment of videotaped interviews and written case histories of Japanese patients from Tokyo and Japanese-American patients from Hawaii, who were clinically confirmed as social phobic cases by their psychiatrists, was blindly presented to the clinicians for their diagnoses. It was found that Japanese psychiatrists tended to diagnose social phobia congruently in the Japanese cases but not in the Japanese American cases (from Hawaii). The American psychiatrists tended to diagnose incongruently in various categories (including anxiety disorder and avoidant personality disorder, in addition to social phobia) for patients from both Tokyo and Hawaii. This study illustrated that the diagnostic patterns for social phobia varied considerably between the psychiatrists of these two countries. In addition to the unique nature of the psychopathology and the patients' stylized patterns of presenting problems, the clinicians' professional orientations and familiarity with the disorder had a strong impact on the results.

In the latest American classification system of *DMS-IV*, Taijin-Kyofu-Sho is introduced in the "Glossary of Culture-Bound Syndromes" as "a culturally distinctive phobia in Japan," while at the same time, it is mentioned in the section on social phobia or social anxiety disorder that "In certain cultures (e.g., Japan and Korea), individuals with social phobia may develop persistent and excessive fears of giving offense to others in social situations, instead of being embarrassed." Therefore, there still remains some ambiguity as to whether Taijin-Kyofu-Sho is an independent culture-related specific psychiatric syndrome or a type of social anxiety disorder.

Regarding the extent to which Taijin-Kyofu-Sho and social anxiety disorders as defined in *DSM* system overlap or differ, very few empirical studies have been conducted. Recently, Nakamura and colleagues (2002) carried out such a study. A total of 38 cases of patient who visited the Department of Psychiatry, Jikei University, Daisan Hospital, in Tokyo, Japan, and were given the clinical diagnosis of Taijin-Kyofu-Sho, were identified as study subjects. This group included 27 cases of the neurotic subtype of Taijin-Kyofu-Sho (71.1%) and 11 cases of the delusional subtype (the offensive or severe type) of Taijin-Kyofu-Sho (28.9%). The rediagnosis was made by the research team using the structured clinical interview, SCID (Japanese version) for *DSM-III-R*. In this study, 25 of the total 38 cases (65.8%) were rediagnosable as social anxiety disorder according to *DSM-III-R*. Furthermore, it was found that, for the neurotic Taijin-Kyofu-Sho cases, the percentage was high at 81.5%; while among the delusional Taijin-Kyofu-Sho cases, it was only 27.3%.

Anthropophobia in Other Areas of Asia

For many years, Japanese psychiatrists held the view that Taijin-Kyofu-Sho (anthropophobia) was a culture-related specific psychiatric disorder especially related to Japanese culture. This view was challenged when the Korean psychiatrist Lee (1987) reported that anthropophobia is found to be prevalent in Korea, as well. Later, a similar view was expressed by psychiatrists from mainland China (Y. H. Cui, 1996, personal communication; H. Lin, 2008, personal communication). Based on this new information, it may be said that Taijin-Kyofu-Sho is not a psychiatric condition "bound" to Japanese society (or culture). It is a psychiatric problem that can be observed in various societies in Asia in which there are certain cultural traits, that is, where there is overconcern about interpersonal relations with intermediately surrounding persons and a child-development pattern that tends to make it difficult for adolescents, who were overprotected in childhood, to deal with delicate social relations after entering young adulthood.

FAMILY SUICIDE AND GROUP SUICIDE

Although suicide, ending of life by oneself, is a common phenomena observed across cultures, such behavior tends to occur more in certain societies. For example, the Japanese have a relatively high rate of suicide. Not only is the prevalence high but also the culture itself is very much elaborated on the terms of suicide. In the language of daily life, the terms *jio-shi* (suicide due to love affair), *fen-shi* (suicide due to resentment), and *kan-shi* (suicide to indicate advice to one's superior) indicate different types of suicide.

In the past, *seppuku* was considered and practiced by the *samurai* (warrior) as an honorable way to end their lives if necessary. Japan is known also for using suicide as a means to deal with war situations. The famous *Kamikaze* suicide attacks in the Okinawa battle (air pilots were ordered to attack the enemy ships by crashing the airplane with bombs) or *Banzai* suicide in Saipan Island (many hundreds of civilians were ordered to jump from the high cliff shouting *banzai* to the Japanese emperor to end their lives rather surrendering to the enemy) at the end of the World War II, are well-known episodes.

Furthermore, in daily life, two unique types of suicide are observed and reported in Japan, namely, family suicide and group suicide, which are closely related to the culture.

Family Suicide

When parents encounter severe difficulty (such as financial debt or a disgraceful event), they may decide to commit suicide together with their young children. This stress-coping method is based on the cultural belief that it would be disgraceful to live after a shameful thing had happened, and that the shame would be relieved by ending one's life. This is coupled with the belief that the children, if left as orphans, would be mistreated by others. Therefore, it would be better for them to die with their parents. Thus the situation actually involves couple suicide and the homicide of children. This unique way of solving problems by dying together as a family was often observed in Japan in the past, even though it is becoming less common (Tseng, 2001, p. 234).

Some case scenarios will help us to understand the uniqueness of the family suicide observed in Japan (Tseng, 2001, pp. 234–235). Case A—Mr. A borrowed some money from friends for investments, hoping that he would be able to return it soon. However, his investments failed, and there was no way to return the money. He tried to get help from his relatives, but was refused. He decided to commit suicide to pay for his mistake. When he explained the situation to his wife, she indicated her wish to die with him. As a result, they planned a family suicide, asking their 14-year-old son and 7-year-old daughter to sit with them in their car, where they would die together from exhaust fumes. Case B—In order to buy a house, Mr. and Mrs. B borrowed money from a loan shark because the mortgage they obtained from the bank was not enough. Their financial situation became worse, and the loan shark came after them to repay the debt. They asked for help from relatives, but were politely refused. They planned a family suicide to deal with the embarrassing situation. With their two daughters (11 and 10 years old), they drove their car over a cliff into the sea. The event was reported in the newspaper, with the headline: "Another Family Suicidal Event."

These case examples clearly illustrate that the parents agreed to commit double suicide as one way to resolve the difficult, shameful, and seemingly unresolvable crisis in their lives. They persuaded their young children to die together with them, rather than being left as miserable orphans without biological parents. Thus, the family group decided to die together. From a cultural point of view, their action received a sympathetic reaction from the general society even though, legally, double suicide by adult parents and the murder of their young children has been forbidden. This phenomenon occurs relatively frequently in Japan (at least until the recent past), but it is quite different from the phenomenon usually observed in other societies, in which a family member is murdered by another adult member, often associated with resentment or hatred toward the other family member.

Group Suicide or Internet Suicide

A new phenomenon, observed in Japan recently, involves groups of people, strangers to each other, who learn through the Internet about their intent to end life, and get together at certain places to commit suicide collectively. This is called *net-shinjyu* (Internet group-suicide) (Katsuragawa, 2007/2009). This kind of group suicide was reported for the first time in media in the fall of 2000. According the police department's report in February 2006, there were 19 events in 2004 (resulting in 55 persons who successfully committed suicide collectively), and 34 events in 2005 (resulting in 91 persons who successfully committed suicide collectively).

It is difficult to study retrospectively why persons take part in this kind of group suicide. However, the demographic information shows that many of them are young people, of both genders, but some are middle-aged persons. The most important fact is that they are not related to each other before the suicide-event, only connected by the Internet. They all feel hopeless in life, and are feeling lonely, or tired of living, considering suicide as the way to deal with their situation. After they find others facing similar circumstances, through Internet communication they, as a small group, decide the place to get together and to die together. The method of suicide can be taking sleeping pills or intoxication by automobile gas. It is the phenomenon of wanting to die together with accompanying persons. It is speculated that when some young people, depressed with helpless ideas, see the advertisement to die together, they are activated in their suicidal intent and action, reflecting the fact that they feel lonely in the present life, without relating to their own family members or any close friends. This is a reflection of the modernized society, which is associated with the broken family systems, losing the close, interconnected, interpersonal life that was observed in the traditional society in the past. In this regard, *net-sinjyu* can be said the product of the new culture.

This type of *net-sinjyu* is quite different from the group suicide that has been observed in other societies. In Japan or India, a group of people may undertake group suicide when they face the loss of a war, not wanting to be taken prisoner and be humiliated by the enemy. Also, collective suicides have been reported among cult members who have committed suicide because of their religious beliefs (Tseng, 2001, pp. 282–283).

FINAL COMMENTS RELATING TO ASIAN AMERICANS

It has been said in the beginning that, those culture-related specific psychiatric syndromes observed in Asia are not to be observed often among Asian people in the United States, particularly among Asian Americans of several generations. For example, family suicide is never reported among Japanese American in Hawaii or other places in the United States. The only case found in the newspaper more than one decade ago was a Japanese national. A Japanese woman, living in California, when she discovered that her husband had been cheating on her for many years, tried to drown herself together with her two small children.

In the literature, koro symptoms (concern over the penis shrinking) have been reported around the world, including United States, of various ethnic/racial group, but usually as a "symptom" of (ordinary) psychiatric disorders (such as psychoses of different nature, including severe depression), not as koro syndrome. It is important to distinguish among koro "symptom," koro "syndrome," and koro "epidemic." Koro epidemic has not been reported from regions outside of Asia or South Asia in the past. No literature has been found about the occurrence of koro syndrome among Chinese Americans.

According to a community study (Lin et al., 1992), the folk term hwabyung is frequently used by Koran Americans to describe their illnesses. Therefore, it is important for clinicians to understand what it means psychologically and culturally for the Korean American patients and to provide relevant family-stress-focused therapy.

In contrast to this, the term *Taijin-Kyofu-Sho* is seldom used by Japanese American patients to present their problems or by clinicians to make clinical diagnoses. There are several speculative explanations for this phenomenon. Most Japanese Americans, whose families originally migrated from rural areas in the south of Japan, are third- or fourth-generation Americans, and may not be familiar with the term. The other explanation is that the young children of Japanese Americans are not overprotected in the host society of America; there are ample opportunities and experiences for early socialization, and they do not face the developmental crisis of becoming socially phobic when they reach the stage of adolescence, as might have happened in their homeland of Japan in the past.

From the above discussion, it may be said that unique syndromes are not necessarily bound to people. If the social environment has changed, the lifestyle modified, and the cultural concept weakened, the culture-related specific psychiatric syndromes may become less frequent or even disappear. This is another way to support the view that they are, after all, culture-related but not bound to any specific ethnic or cultural group.

As a summary, it can be said that, even though the disorder is not very prevalent, and only a handful of cases have been collected even in the societies at where the cases are reported in Asia, these few cases, like the tip of an iceberg above the sea, illustrate how basic folk beliefs and cultural value systems can model unusual clinical manifestations. It will highlight the need for clinicians to be aware in which way culture will impact psychopathology, for any particular group of psychopathology, and how that will impact on clinical assessment and management. This sensitivity is needed for patients of any cultural background, no matter whether they are minority or majority, migrant or local residents of any society.

It is important for clinicians to be aware that American classification system (*DSM*) is merely a product of the clinical experiences of American psychiatrists for treating American patients of majority group. Furthermore, it is based on a descriptive approach with diagnostic criteria. Cultural consideration is minimal. Therefore, the clinical application is sometimes limited for patients of other ethnic/cultural groups. It is a culture-bound classification system that should not be used rigidly for people from other society or culture.

In dealing with patients of Asian background, whether recent immigrants or Asian Americans for generations; their family culture, way of psychosexual development, and culture-patterned management of emotion and coping style all need to be taken into consideration any time in clinical work, as for any other patients of other cultural backgrounds.

REFERENCES

Akhtar, S. (1988). Four culture-bound psychiatric syndromes in India. *International Journal of Social Psychiatry, 34*, 70–74.

Bhatia, M. S. & Malik, S. C. (1991). Dhat syndrome—A useful diagnostic entity in Indian culture. *British Journal of Psychiatry, 159*, 691–695.

Chakraborty, A. (1982). *Koro* makes an epidemic appearance in India. *Transcultural Psychiatric Newsletter, 3*(No. 3 & 4, December).

Chang, Y. H., Rin, H. & Chen, C. C. (1975). Frigophobia: A report of five cases [In Chinese]. *Bulletin Chinese Society of Neurology and Psychiatry, 1*(2), 9–13.

Cheng, S. T. (1996). A critical review of Chinese *koro. Culture, Medicine, and Psychiatry, 20*, 67–82.

Chiou, N. M., Liu, C. Y., Chen, C. C. & Yang, Y. Y. (1994). Frigophobia: Report of two cases [in Chinese]. *Chinese Psychiatry, 8*(4), 297–302.

Gwee, A. L. (1963). Koro: A cultural disease. *Singapore Medical Journal, 4*, 119–122.

Iwai, H. (1982). *Shinkeisho* (Neuroses). Tokyo: Nihonbunka Kagakusha.

Jilek, W. G., & Jilek-Aall, L. (1985). The metamorphosis of "culture-bound" syndromes. *Social Science Medicine, 21*(2), 205–210.

Jilek, W. G., & Jilek-Aall, L. (2001). Culture-specific mental disorders. In F. Henn, N. Sartorius, H. Helmchen, & H. Lauter (Eds.), *Contemporary psychiatry: Vol. 2. Psychiatry in special situations* (pp. 219–245). Berlin: Springer.

Kasahara, Y. (1974). Fear of eye-to-eye confrontation among neurotic patients in Japan. In T. S. Lebra & P. L. Lebra (Eds.), *Japanese culture and behavior.* Honolulu: University Press of Hawaii.

Kato, M. (1977). Japanese characteristics of neurosis. In *Shakai to Seishinbyori* (Society and Psychopathology) [in Japanese]. Tokyo: Kobundo.

Katsuragawa, S. (2007). Family and group suicide in Japan: Cultural analysis. Presented at the Cultural Psychiatry Conference, Kamakura, Japan, and published in the *World Cultural Psychiatry Research Review, 4*, 28–32 (2009).

Kimura, S. (1982). *Nihonjin no taijinkyofushio* (Japanese anthrophobia) [in Japanese]. Tokyo: Keso Shobo.

Kwon, J. H., Min, S. K., & Kim, J. W.(2005). A diagnostic study of hwabyung. Presented at 2005 Annual Meeting of the Korean Neuropsychiatric Association. October 21–22, 2005, Seoul.

Lee, S. H. (1987). Social phobia in Korea. In *Social phobia in Japan and Korea, Proceedings of the First Cultural Psychiatry Symposium between Japan and Korea.* Seoul: East Asian Academy of Cultural Psychiatry.

Lin, K-M., Lau, J. K. C., Yamamoto, J., Zheng, Y-P., Kim, H-S., Cho, K-H., et al. (1992). Hwa-byung. A community study of Korean Americans. *Journal of Nervous and Mental Disorder, 180*, 386–391.

Min, S. K. (1989). A study on the concept of hwabyung [in Korean]. *Journal of Korean Neuropsychiatric Association, 28,* 604–615.

Min, S. K. (1991). Hwabyung and the psychology of haan [in Korean]. *Journal of Korean Medical Association, 34,* 1189–1198.

Min, S. K. & Hong, H. J. (2006). Prognosis of hwabyung [in Korean]. *Behavioral Science in Medicine, 5,* 93–99.

Min, S. K., & Kim, K. H.(1998). Symptoms of hwabyung [in Korean]. *Journal of Korean Neuropsychiatric Association, 37,* 1138–1145.

Min, S. K., Lee, J. S., & Hahn, J. O.(1997). A psychiatric study on haan [in Korean]. *Journal of Korean Neuropsychiatric Association, 36,* 603–611.

Min, S. K., Lee, M. H., Kang, H. C., & Lee, H. Y.(1987). A clinical study of hwabyung [in Korean]. *Journal of Korean Medical Association, 30,* 187–197.

Min, S. K., Lee, M. H., Shin, J. H., Park, M. H., & Lee, H. Y. (1986). A diagnostic study on hwabyung [in Korean]. *Journal of Korean Medical Association, 29,* 653–661.

Min, S. K., Namkoong, K., & Lee, H. Y.(1990). An epidemiological study of hwabyung [in Korean]. *Journal of Korean Neuropsychiatric Association, 29,* 867–874.

Min, S. K., Soh, E. H., & Pyohn, Y. W. (1989). The concept of hwabyung of Korean psychiatrists and herb physicians [in Korean]. *Journal of Korean Neuropsychiatric Association, 28,* 146–154.

Min, S. K., & Suh, S. Y. (2010): Anger syndrome, hwa-byung, and its co-morbidity. *Journal of Affective Disorders, 124,* 211–214.

Min, S. K., Suh, S. Y., Cho, Y. K., Hur J. S., & Song K. J. (2009). The development of the Hwa-byung Scale and the research diagnostic criteria of hwa-byung [in Korean]. *Journal of Korean Neuropsychiatry Association, 48,* 77–85.

Mo, G. M., Chen, G. Q., Li, L. X., & Tseng, W. S. (1995). *Koro* epidemic in Southern China. In T. Y. Lin, W. S. Tseng, & E. K. Yeh (Eds.), *Chinese societies and mental health.* Hong Kong: Oxford University Press.

Mo, K. M., Li, L. S., & Ou, L. W. (1987). Report of koro epidemic in Leizhou Peninsula, Hainan Island [in Chinese]. *Chinese Journal of Neuropsychiatry, 20,* 232–234.

Mori, W. & Kitanishi, K. (1984). Morita-shinkeishitsu to DSM-III [Morita nervous temperament disorders and DSM-III] [in Japanese]. *Rhinsho-seishin-igaku* (Clinical psychiatry), *13,* 911–920.

Nakamura, K., Kitanishi, K., Miyake, Y., Hashimoto, K., & Kibpta, M. (2002). The neurotic versus delusional subtype of tajin-kyofu-sho: Their DSM diagnoses. *Psychiatry and Clinical Neurosciences, 56,* 595–601.

Neki, J. S. (1973). Psychiatry in South-east Asia. *British Journal of Psychiatry, 123,* 256–269.

Ngui, P. W. (1969). The koro epidemic in Singapore. *Australian New Zealand Journal of Psychiatry, 3,* 263–266.

Paris, J. (1992). Dhat: The semen loss anxiety syndrome. *Transcultural Psychiatric Research Review, 29*(2), 109–118.

Prince, R. H. (1989). Reviews on a clinical study of hwabyung by Sung Kil Min and Ho Young Lee. *Transcultural Psychiatry Research, 26,* 137–147

Rin, H. (1965). A study of the aetiology of *koro* in respect to the Chinese concept of illness. *International Journal of Social Psychiatry, 11,* 7–13.

Rin, H. (1966). Two forms of vital deficiency syndrome among Chinese male mental patients. *Transcultural Psychiatric Research Review, 3,* 19–21.

Son, S. J., & Min S. K. (2010). A study on the diagnosis of hwabyung: Discrimination of distinctive symptoms of hwabyung [in Korean]. *Journal of Korean Neuropsychiatry Association, 49,* 171–177.

Suwanlert, S., & Coates, D. (1979). Epidemic koro in Thailand—Clinical and social aspects. *Transcultural Psychiatric Research Review, 15,* 64–66.

Tanaka-Matsumi, J. (1979). Taijin kyofusho: Diagnostic and cultural issues in Japanese psychiatry. *Culture, Medicine, and Psychiatry, 3*(3), 231–245.

Tsai, J. B. (1982). *Suoyang* disorder: Five cases report [in Chinese]. *Zhunguo Senjing Jjingsenbin Zazhi* [Chinese journal of neuro-psychiatry], *4,* 206.

Tseng, W. S. (2001). *Handbook of cultural psychiatry.* San Diego: Academic.

Tseng, W. S. (2008). Culture-related specific psychiatric syndromes. In M. Gelder, J. J. Lopez-Ibor, Jr., N. C. Andersen, & J. Geddes (Eds.), *New Oxford textbook of psychiatry* (2nd ed., ch. 4.16). Oxford: Oxford University Press.

Tseng, W. S., Asai, M., Kitanish, K., McLaughlin, D. G. & Kyomen, H. (1992). Diagnostic patterns of social phobia: Comparison in Tokyo and Hawaii. *Journal of Nervous and Mental Disease, 180,* 380–385.

Tseng, W. S., & Hsu, J. (1969/70). Chinese culture, personality formation and mental illness. *International Journal of Social Psychiatry, 16*(1), 5–14.

Tseng, W. S., Mo, K. M., Hsu, J., Li, L. S., Ou, L. W., Chen, G. Q., et al. (1988). A sociocultural study of koro epidemics in Guandong, China. *American Journal of Psychiatry,145*(12), 1538–1543.

Tseng, W. S., Mo, K. M., Hsu, J., Li, L. S., Chen, G. Q., Ou, L. W., et al. (1992). Koro epidemics in Guandong, China: A questionnaire survey. *Journal of Nervous and Mental Disease, 180*(2), 117–123

Tseng, W. S., Mo, G. M., Chen, K. C., Li, L. S., Wen, J. K., & Liu, T. S. (1993). Social psychiatry and *koro* epidemic: (4). Regional comparison of *SuoYang* belief [in Chinese]. *Chinese Mental Health Journal, 7,* 38–40.

Wen, J. K. (1995). Sexual beliefs and problems in contemporary Taiwan. In T. Y. Lin, W. S. Tseng, & E. K. Yeh (Eds.), *Chinese societies and mental health.* Hong Kong: Oxford University Press.

Wig, N. N. (1960). Problem of mental health in India. *Journal of Clinical and Social Psychiatry* (College of Lucknow, India), 17(2), 48–53.

Yamashita, I. (1977/93). *Taijin-kyofu or delusional social phobia.* Sapporo: Hokkaido University Press. (English translation of Japanese book originally published in 1977, Tokyo: Kanehara) [Reviewed in *TPRR, 2,* 283–288, 1984 by S. C. Chang].

Yap, P. M. (1965). Koro—A culture-bound depersonalization syndrome. *British Journal of Psychiatry, 111,* 43–50.

Yap, P. M. (1967). Classification of the culture-bound reactive syndromes. *Australia and New Zealand Journal of Psychiatry, 1,* 172–179.

GLOSSARY

([C]: Chinese words; [J]: Japanese words: [K]: Korean words)

banzai [J] 萬歲

boon [k] 憤

fen-shi [J] 憤死

haan [k] 恨

hoe-haan [k] 悔恨

hwabyung [k] 火病

jeong-haan [k] 情恨

jio-shi [J] 情死

kamikaze [J] 神風

kan-shi [J] 諫死

net-shinjyu [J] (inter)net心中

pa-len [C] 怕冷

seppuku [J] 切腹

suoyang [C] 縮陽

Taijin-Kyofu-Sho [J] 對人恐怖症

tong-haan [k] 痛恨

uk-wool [k] 抑鬱

wei-han [C] 畏寒

won-haan [k] 怨恨

yin [C] 陰

yang [C] 陽

| 16 |

UNIQUE PSYCHOTHERAPIES DEVELOPED IN ASIA

Wen-Shing Tseng, Kenji Kitanishi, Teruaki Maeshiro, and Jinfu Zhu

INTRODUCTION

It is a salient fact that performance of counseling or psychotherapy will be subject significantly to cultural factors (Tseng, 2001, pp. 515–610). Therefore, culture-sensitive, -relevant, or -competent psychotherapy is warranted for care of patients of any ethnic/cultural background, either minority or majority, immigrant or local residents, because every person's emotions, psychology, and behavior are based heavily on culture (Tseng & Streltzer, 2001). This applies not only to the culture of patients but also to that of the therapists. This is no less true for situations in which patients of Asian background or heritage are treated by either Asian therapists or non-Asian therapists (Sue & Morishima, 1982).

There are several approaches to reviewing and understanding cultural aspects of psychotherapy. One approach is to examine intensively the circumstance of intercultural psychotherapy, when the patient and therapist have divergent cultural backgrounds and the interactional impact of cultures between them in the process of therapy become significant (Hsu and Tseng, 1972). If a broad definition of psychotherapy is used, various forms of psychological therapy can be subdivided into three major groups, namely, culture-embedded "indigenous" healing practices, culture-influenced "unique" psychotherapy, and culture-related "common" psychotherapies (Tseng, 2001, pp. 515–561). Examining these different modes of psychotherapy regarding cultural input for therapy is another approach.

Culture-embedded indigenous healing practices, such as shamanism, Zar cult, divination, or fortune-telling, usually with a supernatural orientation and an unorthodox approach, are developed in any society to help clients. They rely on the strong beliefs held by the members of the society and are, thus, embedded in the culture and are difficult to apply to other societies as they are.

Culture-influenced unique psychotherapies are therapeutic modes that are very much culture flavored and characteristically unique, different from the common or mainstream modes of psychotherapy that are currently practiced around the world. Theoretically, any form of psychotherapy is more or less influenced by culture; even the so-called mainstream psychotherapies, such as psychoanalysis, cognitive behavioral therapy, marital or family therapy, and group therapy, which originally developed in the West, are considered "culture-related" (Tseng, 2009, 2010).

The term "culture-influenced unique psychotherapies" is used here to indicate therapies that are strongly colored by the philosophical concepts or value systems of the non-Western societies in which they were invented, mainly in the East. Morita therapy, Naikan therapy, and Daoistic cognitive therapy, which will be elaborated in this chapter, are primary examples. Because these therapies are based in Eastern philosophy, and are characteristically different from Western therapies, they provide an opportunity for us to review the ways culture impacts the theory and practice of psychotherapy. This, in turn, will guide clinicians in carrying out culturally appropriate therapy for patients with considerations of his/her cultural backgrounds.

In this chapter, the unique psychotherapies that have been invented and developed in Asia will be reviewed, with particular emphasis on the philosophical thought and value system behind such practice of therapy. This will include the discussion of Morita therapy and Naikan therapy invented in Japan, and Daoistic cognitive therapy in China.

Associated with the promotion of cultural psychiatry, minority movements, and concern for mental-health-care delivery for minorities and immigrants, there is an increased tendency to promote indigenous psychology and psychotherapy. The study of culture-influenced unique psychotherapy is a part of this larger movement. However, a caution and clarification are needed. Paying attention to culture-unique or indigenous psychotherapy is not solely for the promotion of culture-relevant psychotherapy. It merely helps us to increase cultural awareness and to examine how culture influences the background philosophy and technique of psychotherapy. In other words, the development and promotion of culturally unique psychotherapy alone is not enough to improve culture-relevant psychotherapy. Achieving culture-competent psychotherapy requires attention to clinical, theoretical, and philosophical aspects in any forms of therapy applied (Tseng, 2010).

MORITA THERAPY

Brief Introduction and History

Morita therapy is a unique psychotherapeutic approach that was established in Japan by Shōma Morita, a professor of psychiatry at Jikei University in Tokyo in the early 1920s (Kondo, 1976). Originally the therapy was called "personal-experience therapy" by Morita himself to indicate the basic nature of the therapy. But it was later named after him by his followers (Chang, 1974).

According to Morita (1922/1974), he studied and examined Western psychotherapeutic techniques that were introduced during that period in Japan in the 1920s. Morita was extremely critical of Freud's theory of psychoanalysis attempting to control anxiety by examining and recognizing the causes of anxiety. He asserted that repression is a natural phenomenon, and that many people experience psychological trauma. Morita's criticisms were also directed at Dubois's "persuasion method." He criticized Dubois's argument that neurosis was caused by false thought processes, and that it could be cured through rational persuasion and correct educational methods. Morita asserted that experience is what is important (not reasoning).

Morita viewed human suffering and anxiety from the perspective of the "circular theory" rather than linear causality. He placed "nature" at the foundation of his psychotherapy. This is an Eastern criticism of Western psychotherapy that centers on logical reasoning. Morita proposed a psychotherapy modality that is based on Eastern ideology.

As a procedure, it was originally characterized as a treatment that took place in a residential setting, with an initial stage of absolute bed rest and isolation (for about one week), followed by a stage of gradual restoration and experience of normal life, with instructions given through a diary to produce changes in philosophical attitude (with an emphasis on accepting things as they are).

Morita therapy helps people explore their unnatural and unbalanced way of living. With the assistance of a therapist, they try to modify their way of living and seek a more unique and natural way of being. This task in and of itself is a transformation from the attachment to egocentrism and narcissism to living with love or living naturally according to one's individuality (real self).

In contrast to the traditional view of Morita therapy, to be carried out in an inpatient setting, Kitanishi (2005) indicates that, at its core, it is a therapeutic method that resolves egocentric love and suffering caused by desires. It can be performed in an outpatient setting. This is the new trend of Morita therapy, called Neo-Morita therapy. It is based on clinical experiences of Morita therapy with Japanese outpatients suffering from modern daily problems. Morita therapy seeks to resolve suffering by focusing on the love and desire that cause it.

Neo-Morita therapy views the cause of human suffering as excessive self-centered love and desire. It centers on each person's "living," and is based on the core East Asian understanding of humanity. The therapy incorporates the ideas of egolessness (not having a mind of self) and mind-body unity (not separating mind and body and their relations with nature), which are based on East Asian naturalism (which views nature as having the power to guide humans in the way they are supposed to live). The totality of these ideas points to a natural and unique way of living. The various theories that explain the nature of suffering will be elaborated in the following section (Kitanishi, 2005).

Various Theories of Morita Therapy

The Circular Theory

Circular understanding is a basic epistemology in Morita therapy. It recognizes the Buddhist's concept of *in-nen*, (in Japanese, *in* means cause, and *en* relation or connection). Buddhism teaches that there cannot be a sole cause to phenomenon even though there may be a major cause behind an event. In order for the major event to actualize, other supportive causes must exist, and these are called *en* relation. In other words, phenomenon is caused by *in-nen* (cause and relational connection). Events that occur in the body and the mind are understood in relation to other things.

This is the basic epistemology behind Morita's understanding of mental phenomena. In Morita therapy, the first goal of treatment is to break away from the negative circularity, that is, a simple, linear causality.

The circular theory holds the following therapeutic significance for Morita therapy:

1) It is natural for people to want to know the reasons for their suffering, anxieties, and fears. However, they must change this attitude simply because seeking the causes will destroy or damage their power to live. For example, in the course of therapy, patients may discover how they were wounded from their relationships with their parents. However, it is extremely important for them to recognize that this awareness is on a different dimension than healing the suffering, discovering a new self, and moving forward with their lives.

There was a difference between understanding the painful events of the past and finding a way to live. It is too simplistic to think that a patient's suffering can be helped by searching for and finding its cause. Suffering is not caused by one thing. Suffering is constantly activated and strengthened in relationships.

The resolution for suffering is not to find its cause. Searching for the cause often reinforces one's suffering. Patients must free themselves from this process, and instead examine their interaction with the surrounding world in the here and now and try to break away from the negative cycle. They must also work toward claiming back their sense of living.

This recognition is important for the therapist, as well. If the therapist is obsessed with the past and with anxiety and does not pay attention to the patient's suffering in "living" in reality, the patient will also end up focusing on the past. This will destroy or damage the patient's power to "live" in the present.

2) Breaking the negative cycle by bringing about changes in life. The Morita therapist is first and foremost a specialist who identifies and eliminates the negative cycle. It is important to recognize the negative cycle in which the patient is trapped, and to work with the patient to enable him to break away from this pattern. The therapist believes that destroying the negative cycle will activate the patient's hidden abilities and natural healing power. In fact, with patients who are not severely obsessed, breaking the negative cycle is often all that is necessary in therapy.

3) Establishing a new social relationship with others. Suffering is not equal to being obsessed with anxiety. Those who are obsessed with their internal pain often sever their relationships with significant family members and other social relationships. They suffer in isolation or in a closed world with their family, which increases and deepens their suffering. The therapist assists patients to establish new familial and social relationships, and helps the patient break away from a negative cycle with these relationships at the core.

The notion of "leaving things unquestioned" in Morita therapy signifies a passive approach in which the therapist does not question the past, the symptoms, or the therapeutic relationship. Morita therapy actively explores the patient's relationship with the world, and assists in establishing new relationships.

Conflict Between the "Ideal" and "Reality"

What is human suffering and conflict? In the original concept from Buddhism, suffering is understood as "not being able to control things according to our will," or "things that do not go according to our wish." We suffer because we think that our body and mind and all other phenomena belong to us, and we try to control them according to our will.

Morita (1926/1974) also tried to explain neurosis and general human suffering by using the concepts of desire and fear. Morita, in line with the Buddhist understanding of suffering, thinks that desire causes fear. In other words, the desire to live produces the fear of death, that is, suffering. The desire to live contains the fear of death, and Morita thought that the harmony of desire and fear (suffering) was important. Thus, for Morita, desire and fear were natural phenomena that were "real." Morita viewed the basic organization of human conflict as an opposing structure to nature, that is, the "real" and the "ideal."

The natural or "real" as espoused by Morita (1922/1974, 1926/1974) includes: (a) physicality, senses, emotions; (b) desire and fear (emotions in general); and (c) general activities of the mind. The "ideal" is the narcissism of the ego or an attachment to the self that opposes the existence of the natural (real), and tries to gain control through thought. Thought is a medium of language. This "ideal" is characterized by: (a) thinking of the self and the world as "one's own," (b) logic that is formulated on this thinking, (c) an enlarged sense of ego, and (d) the superiority of logic and the inferiority of the body (or emotions) that are supported by language. In Morita therapy, this type of ego or sense of ego must be destroyed or eliminated. Morita therapy is a psychotherapy that treats the pathology of narcissism by bringing it to the fore according to a unique way of thinking.

Unlike the denial of desire in Buddhism, Morita therapy employs paradoxical treatment strategies. The ego (narcissistic ego) that clings to possessing the self and tries to manipulate it according to one's will must be broken down. In addition, desire must be experienced as desire, and fear must be experienced as fear. This is the harmony between desire and fear that is considered the natural way of human beings.

Desire and Fear

Desire itself is a paradox in nature. As with narcissism, we cannot exist without it, but, at the same time, it creates suffering when it becomes pathological. The desire to live later became one of the key concepts of Morita therapy. This concept, like desire, has two contrasting characteristics. On the one hand, it promotes the act of living itself, but, on the other, it brings about suffering. Desire makes us attempt to rebel or fight against suffering, which in turn brings about *toraware* (obsessive preoccupation). This understanding of desire and fear is what makes Morita therapy effective in resolving modern-day suffering as well as the suffering of the future. Morita (1926/1974) is not only unique because he developed his treatment method in a home environment, but also because he discovered the meaning of desire in an Eastern context and placed it at the core of his treatment. This places the focus of Morita therapy on living and on the discovery of desire.

Morita (1921/1974) identified the hypochondriac temperament (tendency to become anxious) as the basis of Morita *shinkeishitsu* (literally, "nervous temperament" in Japanese), and psychic interaction as the mechanism that strengthens and fixates anxiety, which is a natural human reaction. A hypochondriac temperament is a psychic reaction toward incidents that is regulated by temperament. We can speculate that in naming this term Morita had thought of the fear of death and the fear of illness as the bases of suffering. Making the fear of death the basis of human fear came to hold two meanings. One was to see the fear of death from the perspective of living. Fear comes about because we try to live. We cannot eradicate this fear. To eliminate this fear is to deny "living." In other words, humans live with this basic paradox. The pathology of narcissism is not being able to accept this paradox and to pursue a perfect, secure, and self-centered life. Pathological narcissism is a state of mind in which one tries to control things that do not exist in reality, things that are temporary or that one cannot control. Morita considers a person with a hypochondriac temperament as one who experiences the suffering of living more than others. In other words, he has a stronger experience of the suffering of being born, of illness, of aging, and of death. He is clumsy at living, is intense, and easily experiences difficulties. It is at times difficult for him to accept and love himself.

However, pathological narcissism itself is a paradox. Pathological narcissism, on the one hand, causes obsession (*toraware*) of fear. On the other hand, it promotes a natural and unique way of living that leads to creativity. It is desire that exists behind the fear, and the uniqueness of a person lies in the way he looks at this desire and actualizes it. This phenomenon can be found among people with social phobias, who have succeeded at occupations such as acting. Despite their social phobias, they are in a profession that requires expressing themselves in front of others.

In other words, we all live with problems. Is there a person who is perfectly healthy with no problems? To suffer over living and to overcome this suffering is the beginning of living. At the point where we think we have overcome suffering, we face suffering again. We then overcome it again. It is in this process that our mental capacity to contain this suffering becomes larger. This is what it means to live and to grow. Through failures and disappointments, we are able to modify our excessive unrealistic narcissism, which lacks flexibility and needs omnipotent control. This, in turn, enriches our process of living.

Pathological Narcissism: Self-Centered Excessive Love and Desire

To be fixated on the self signifies a life that is full of suffering, which comes from trying to control the self, others, and the surroundings, because of the inability to love one's self adequately. Alternatively, it is the story of love that is filled with suffering because the self has to continuously seek love and validation from others. This desire and love create suffering such as anxiety, fear, and depression, and become the sources of obsession (*toraware*). Neo-Morita therapy resolves this suffering of desire and love based on Eastern philosophy. Pathological narcissism includes pathology with which Eastern psychology, religion, and philosophy have dealt. It is the extreme desire that tries to control the ever-changing nature of things or relationships according to one's desires. This desire creates suffering, fear and pathological narcissism, and obsession (*toraware*) toward this suffering. When searching behind this suffering, we find the minimization of this natural and unique way of living and the inability to love one's self. This is an extreme form of perfectionism and behind it we find a strong desire for control. This creates our suffering and our obsession (*toraware*) toward our suffering. Other issues are closely related to this pathological narcissism.

In the United States, the problem of narcissism and how to love one's self has received much attention since the 1970s (Kohut, 1971). At the focus is the suffering of the person who excessively seeks the love and validation of others. This desperation for attention, notice, and love leads to feelings of inferiority, depression, and interpersonal anxieties. Moreover, one cannot acknowledge this self. This, in turn, is the pathology of excessive self-consciousness and narcissism. Even here, it is found that self-centered and excessive love and desire create fear.

Eastern Naturalism and Egolessness

For Morita (1922/1974), body, emotions, and desires are a natural part of human being. Human contradictions and conflicts are caused by the attempt to control them with thought and knowledge, which Morita considered the ego. Furthermore, self-actualization comes from becoming aware that nature exists within one's self, and by acting according to the laws of nature. This type of thinking about nature is not unique to Japan.

As indicated by Mori (1994), the Chinese philosopher Lao-zi points out that the moment humans discard intentionality; nature starts to exert its function. In other words, in order for people to survive and develop, humans must adapt to nature, and learn from it. In nature there is an order that cannot be comprehended by human intellect, rather, it becomes apparent in the conditions of selflessness or egolessness. This is what Morita therapy considers following nature or being *arugamama*, which means "accepting reality as it is."

Zhuang-zi, the follower of Lao-zi (also known previously as Lau-tzu by Webster spelling system), stated that truth cannot be transmitted to others through writing or words, and that one cannot transmit truth through teaching. He stated that truth can only be understood through direct experiential intuition. Morita's thinking about the importance of experience and the limitations and distrust toward language and the logic that is behind words can be seen in the Eastern view of nature and egolessness; the ideology of egolessness is interwoven in forming the philosophical background of Morita therapy. Furthermore, the ideology of the Eastern view of nature and egolessness also illustrates the way of the self in addition to the awareness of nature in the East and the relationship between humans and nature. This basic philosophy of Morita therapy rests on the same foundation as the ideologies of: Lao-zi and Zhuang-zi, the original Buddhism of India, and the ideologies of Mahayana Buddhism (Kitanishi, 1999).

Egolessness and Arugamama

Naikan therapy (another unique Japanese psychotherapy, which is carried out through self-inspection, to be discuss later in the following section) and Morita therapy shared the same view, that individual unhappiness and maladjustment were caused by a self-centered way of life, and that both therapies aimed at improving this (Murase, 1976, 1977). To state this in Japanese terms, the treatment goals are to "get rid of the ego and to become *sunao* (plainly mind of self)." This means that the treatment goals of both Naikan and Morita therapy are to treat this pathological narcissism and to get rid of the ego, which means reaching a state of egolessness. Morita referred to this state as "pure mind." Morita also states, "this is first experienced when a person becomes free from the belief that things should be a certain way, or free from concern about those around us." He notes that this is a state that is learned in the process of treatment.

People can experience two states of mind when they overcome this pathological narcissism. One is to actualize one's feelings and instinct, the other is to do things reluctantly while making an effort to master the feelings of reluctance. In other words, in the latter state of mind they contain what they don't like, while continuing to move forward and tackle issues. When we are internally able to take care of the pathological narcissism that is at the root of obsession (*toraware*), then we can experience a pure mind, sincere mind. This, in turn, enables us to be in harmony with our surroundings. There is no doubt that it is this state of mind for which Morita therapy and Naikan therapy aim. How does one reach this state of mind? Kora (1965) called it *arugamama* (being as it is) and defined it as follows: The first point of *arugamama* is to genuinely recognize one's symptoms and accompanying suffering and anxiety, and to accept them. Morita calls this "notion of acceptance." This is the key to preparing one's mind to accept one's emotions. The second point is to accept the symptoms as they are while behaving constructively according to one's original desire to live. In other words, eliminating pathological narcissism (accepting symptoms as they are) and exerting narcissism (actualizing the desire to live) must progress simultaneously. This psychological process will be discussed in the following.

1) Narcissism, which must be destroyed or discarded. Here the ego signifies the way of being, which, according to Kora, resists, denies, cheats, avoids, and is unable to recognize one's symptoms. In order to discard narcissism, a person needs to know oneself and to know one's limitations.

Knowing oneself—We suffer when we encounter difficulties in life and become stuck. This is an opportune time for us to search for ourselves, to modify the way we are, and to grow. However, for many, their pathological narcissism, in other words, their perfectionism and excessive self-consciousness, comes to the fore. Thus, the first step in overcoming the self is to know one's self. It is important to recognize that people become more perfectionist or excessively self-conscious when trying to overcome their problems. We understand this to mean that people do not become stuck because something is lacking, but rather, they suffer due to excessiveness.

Knowing one's limitations (actualizing one's self)—It is difficult for those who are suffering to know their own limitations. They may object, stating, "I am suffering because I have been confronted so much by my own limitations." However, when people become stuck, they easily become extreme perfectionists. In other words, they fall into a limbo between the self that is a total failure and the self that dreams of becoming a superman. Knowing the limitations of a perfectionist or excessive self-consciousness enables one to modify the self. Modifying the excessive self and excessive way of living is what it means to live according to one's individuality and in a natural way. On the one hand, one discards pathological narcissism, while, on the other, one activates one's strength.

2) Sense of helplessness. A sense of helplessness is the most important experience in giving up pathological narcissism. It is the most important element in the task of living, as well. Quite often, patients experience a sense of helplessness with elation, in which they state, "I had been trying to control everything" or "I was a self-centered person" at a turning point in therapy. There is a sense of giving up, which also connotes a sense that "it is only me, but it is me." To give up not only

means giving things up, it also means gaining more clarity about a situation. What is given up is a way of living that is attached to the ego. Also included in this task is the giving up of pathological narcissism and the process of clarifying a way of living that is natural and according to one's individuality. This naturally has to be accompanied with a transformation toward a new way of living. This is what Kora (1965) calls the actualization of the desire to live. The author believes that the "sense of helplessness" and "giving up" that occurs during treatment serve as the key impetus for the experience of egolessness.

3) Toward a new self: Living according to one's individuality. Treatment does not end when a person is able to discard his ego. A person must also discover a natural way of living according to his individuality in order to discard his ego. What is this like? The author believes that there are other aspects besides actualizing the desire to live. They include:

Strengths of recognizing one's weakness — The image of the new self is one in which a person lives actively according to one's desires. However, this means that one recognizes one's emotions, pain, and state of mind and body, and is able to express them. This is understood as real strength and the natural and way of living according to one's individuality. When one has attachment toward one's self, he seeks strengths and perfection in himself. He cannot accept his weakness and he fears that others will discover his weakness. This is what creates suffering. *Arugamama* means to recognize and accept one's weakness. It also means to reawaken from narcissistic, perfectionist illusions about one's self, and to find one's natural self.

Strengthening one's foundation — This weakness, however, indicates a person's imperfections and ambiguities, that is, his natural aspects. In order for people to acknowledge this weakness, they must have a foundation in real life. It is important for people to experience a sense that they are actively involved with their families and society. The Morita therapist always encourages the patient to face the reality of the "here and now." This is because a patient's sense of being grounded is strengthened through active involvement with reality, failures, and the correction of failure. The experience of *arugamama* cannot exist without the task of grounding one's self in a life that is based on reality.

4) *Arugamama* and Disillusion. *Arugamama* (accepting things as they are) means to accept one's anxieties internally, and to recognize and exert one's natural desires. However, this is not all there is. It is also important to get out of one's pathological narcissism toward one's self and the surrounding world, and to change it to a more realistic understanding. A person must see things as they are and accept them. He is then able to behave according to his inner natural desire. By awakening from such pathological narcissism, for the first time he is able to accept anxiety as his own, become aware of his desires, and actualize them. This is not only unique to neurotic patients. When we face psychological crisis, we are influenced by pathological narcissism. In other words, in the process of living, we all fall into this sort of pathological narcissism, and then go through the process of awakening from it. In order to awaken from this pathological narcissism, one needs to interact with therapists and significant others to examine the illusions in real-life situations. This requires a therapist's assistance. Naturally, there are areas in which people will fail. However, it is important to incorporate this failure and disappointment for a person to be able to modify pathological narcissism. Perfectionists and people who are excessively self-conscious

become stuck because they have failed to fail appropriately. This, in fact, is paradoxical. In addition, these people view little failures as signs of total failure on their part, and do not learn to modify their illusions from these failures. To be *arugamama* means that people live according to their individuality. This means that people become free from "pathological narcissism," which dictates how a person should be. This means achieving the developmental tasks of adolescence and young adulthood of becoming autonomous from one's parents and becoming involved with society. In middle adulthood, this means psychological separation from one's parents and living one's life according to one's individuality. In late adulthood, this means accepting the aged self, and actualizing one's potential.

Body-Mind-Nature Monism

Morita (1922/1974) takes the position of returning all body and emotional phenomena to nature. There is absolute affirmation of nature and a latent optimistic affirmation of humans, which include desire. This view of nature opposes Western dualism, and tries to see mind and body as one. As stated, these are traditional Eastern ways of understanding, and, at the same time, an antithesis to the logos-centered ideology that was introduced from the West. In concrete terms, it is a recognition that physical activities must be included if changes are to be brought about in the mind. In addition, according to traditional Japanese thinking, mastering physical forms is very important in the process of acquiring or learning a skill or achieving enlightenment. For example, when craftsmen learn their trade, they learn the form of their work before learning the content. The form of sitting is emphasized when sitting in meditation (*zazen*). This is the logical foundation for the sequence of bed rest in the treatment system of Morita therapy. In addition, this type of understanding of the mind and body naturally leads to the importance of physical activity and a concept of self that includes the body.

Morita therapy emphasizes consciousness. A narcissistic ego that eliminates nature, such as body, action, and emotions must be broken up. The goal of treatment is the development of a self that incorporates nature. This is the state of "accepting reality as it is (*arugamama*)." Wisdom in this case is knowledge that is based on nature, that is, facts, and is always in harmony with nature. People in this condition can experience and express nature, and express the way of the open self.

Effectiveness of the Therapy

After reviewing treatment outcomes of different Morita therapy institutions, Kitanishi (2005) indicated that Morita therapy has been effective continuously for Morita *Shinkeishitsu* from the 1920s, when it was first developed, to the present day. Although there are some variations in the criteria for improvement, and caution is needed in evaluating the data, because the evaluations were made by the therapists themselves, the therapy was found to have a high rate of effectiveness when suitable members of the population were selected for treatment. The improvement rates from Morita therapy for Morita *Shinkeishitsu* have been reported, in chronological order, as 93.3 % for the period 1919–1929; 92.9% for 1929–1937; 92.7% for 1963–1974; and 77.6% for

1972–1991. The rate for the last period is lower because it represents findings from a study conducted at the Jikei University, where the treatment of atypical cases other than Morita *Shinkeishitsu* was included.

According to clinical experiences (Kitanishi, 2005), the treatment effectiveness was found to be better among male patients who were in their 20s and 30s, who had typical *shinkeishitsu* symptoms, adequate time for treatment, and voluntarily sought Morita therapy. Treatment was not found to be as effective among patients who had social phobia, were of the delusional type, and had an obsessive-compulsive disorder, including compulsive behaviors irrespective of age at the time of admission for treatment.

Neo-Morita Therapy

As a summary, the traditional Morita therapy has evolved into contemporary Neo-Morita therapy, which focuses on the basic concept and theories of human nature, with broad application to the client who suffers from contemporary daily problems. It has been elaborated that the core of Neo-Morita therapy is helping clients resolve basic philosophical attitudes toward living.

The therapy is based on the circular theory, according to which things are influenced by cause and relation with endless, multiple, interactional factors, rather than by lineal cause. As a therapeutic approach, it emphasizes discovering a new self and moving forward in life, rather than searching for the reasons for suffering, anxieties, or fears.

The circular theory takes the view that people who suffer tend to be preoccupied with self-centered excessive love and desire. The Eastern view of nature and egolessness, or the attitude of accepting things as they are (*arugamama*), is used to correct pathological narcissism. The therapy focuses on the development of a self that incorporates nature. Thus, Morita therapy is not as concerned with technique or procedure as it is with the enhancement of a philosophical view that is strongly rooted in Asian culture and the Buddhist and Daoist views of life and its relationship with nature.

NAIKAN THERAPY

Naikan therapy was invented by a Japanese ordinary person and a Buddhist believer, Yoshimoto Ishin, in Japan five decades ago initially for the purpose of treating juvenile delinquency and other problems (Kawahara, 2005). The Japanese Zen Buddhism used the term *mishirabe* to describe the practice of one's own personal inspection. Ishin used the term *naikan* (literally, "intrainspection" in Japanese) to address the practice of internal inspection that he advocated for therapy of psychological problems (Maeshiro, 2005).

According to Reynolds (1977), the roots of Naikan lie in one sect of Japanese Buddhism, the Jodo Shinsu sect. The founder of the sect, Shinran, promised ten kinds of profit to those who believed—among them: Joyful acceptance of any hardship and the desire to repay others with a joyful heart. These two benefits are common results of Naikan meditation. Yoshimoto discovered the usefulness of Naikan during his own search for enlightenment. He eased the physical restrictions and modified the procedure somewhat for laymen. Interestingly, as noted by Reynolds, the founder, Yoshimoto, maintained that there is no real relationship between Naikan therapy and the Jodo's religious concepts, other than a historical one.

The core of the Naikan practice is the client carrying out self-inspection about his own life in the past, with a particular focus on the kind of relationships he or she has had with significant persons—usually his parents. The client is instructed to review the kinds of things his parents did for him, and what he did in return. Through the process of self-inspection, the client may obtain insight about his attitudes and learn not to complain and cause trouble for others, but to repay others with appreciation and a joyful heart. The change in the patient's attitude toward others and his view of life are the core of the therapy.

Although Naikan therapy was invented by a Buddhist believer, the Japanese cultural psychologist Murase (1976) commented that the goal of Naikan therapy is to assist the client to obtain the psychological state of *sunao*, a unique Japanese term and value system. *Sunao* is derived from the Japanese character meaning things in their original state without any transformation. It implies the harmonious and natural state of mind directly associated with honesty, humility, docility, and simplicity. Murase pointed out that the concept of *sunao* does not belong to the imported religions of Buddha, but is essentially derived from ancient Shintoism—a value system that remains a strong undercurrent of Japanese culture. Thus, in his analysis, the emphasis of Naikan therapy is to search for the culturally sanctioned state of mind of *sunao*—a mind of simplicity.

From psychotherapeutic point of view, Naikan therapy is oriented to philosophical and psychological perspectives of life. Under the therapist's formal but simple guidance to perform preprogrammed self-examination is the therapeutic operation. Reappraising the primary interpersonal relationships within the family, and discouraging a narcissistic view of the world by learning to appreciate others, rather than making demands for the others, are the basic therapeutic mechanism utilized. Making use of culture-sanctioned value systems relating to parent-child relationships to restore family or group relations is the aim of the practice.

In the very beginning, the spread of the practice of Naikan therapy was supported by a millionaire who offered its benefits to prisoners (Kawahara, 2005). Other than a major center in Nara, there are only a few religious institutions that offer this therapy. The practice is gradually fading away, but it is gaining its attention internationally, particularly in China. Due to its uniqueness, it has historically attracted scholars' attention. It has also attracted the interest of some Westerners.

An American psychologist, Reynolds, who himself participated in a Naikan therapy experience in Japan, has reported that the few Americans who tried Naikan therapy in Japan shared some common difficulties. According to Reynolds (1980), culturally, the Japanese tend to believe that if they receive some kind of benefit or favor from others, it is their moral duty to repay at least as much as they received. However, Americans tend to see social relations as relations among equals, with shared responsibilities and faults. Thus, because of its culturally patterned view of the world and interpersonal relationships, it is difficult for American people to receive and benefit from Naikan therapy. This illustrates that the transcultural application of certain healing practices is limited if those practices are particularly culturally flavored.

DAOISTIC COGNITIVE PSYCHOTHERAPY

Introduction

Led by Deseng Young, professor of psychiatry of Xiang-Ya Medical College, Central South University, and a group of his followers, the Chinese Daoistic cognitive psychotherapy has been developed in China for the past decades. The therapy is conceptually based on Daoism philosophy and practically carried out in the form of cognitive psychotherapy plus supplemental behavioral exercise (Xiao et al., 1998; Young, 1997, 2005; Zhu, 2007a).

Daoist philosophy was developed originally by the Chinese ancient scholar Lao-zi, about 25 centuries ago, with its unique view of life and value system as well as how to deal with stress in life and to facilitate the solution of mental suffering. It interprets that humans' anxiety, depression, and behavior problems are caused not only by the dysfunctional responses to the external stimuli, but also by the ill-cognition that is often shaped by cultural values of the society.

With this understanding, Daoistic cognitive psychotherapy has been developed with multiple references to: Daoistic philosophy, Chinese ancient practice of *qigong* (deep breathing therapy) and *taijiquan* (shadow boxing), Japanese Morita therapy, and Western-derived ordinary cognitive therapy. The therapy is used for the treatment of patients with neurotic and psychosomatic disorders, and it has been found useful to the patients, particularly for aged persons suffering from obsessive desire for achievement (Zhu, 2007a).

The Core Value System Applied in Daoistic Cognitive Psychotherapy

The following eight principles (and slogans) of Daoistic thought are used in the clinical application for psychological consultation. They are:

a. Benefit without harm to yourself as well as to others—Only do things beneficial to yourself and others, help others as a pleasure, don't be jealous to the success of others, never take pleasure at the misfortune of others; don't make trouble with yourself, your family members, and others. Don't hate others, don't make enemies, don't retaliate against others, don't expect others to be perfect.

b. Do your best without competition with others—Do your best and according to your capacity, without competition with others. In front of reward, financial gain, position, good opportunity, don't impose to get, don't implicate and compare with who won it justly. Don't strive to outshine others. Too clean a clothes is easily to be dirtied, too tall a tree is easily crashed by wind or thunder. Just due to your un-competition, so that nobody around would be able to compete with you.

c. Moderate desire and limit selfishness—A vigorous spirit by limitation of desires, don't bother so much as to cause mental exhaustion. The most ambitious and aggressive person always lets his/her body be driven by others, lets his mind be ruled by others, being busy for his/her entire life and never aware of the purpose of life is for what. The most selfish and competitively driven person always meets rejection by society, and it becomes harmful to personal well-being and induces problems for social adaptation.

d. Know when to stop and learn how to be satisfied—Human desire may be higher even than heaven, so that there is no enduring satisfaction. The fortune of the majority layman is thinner than slim paper, so there is only consistent sorrow and suffering. A person who is easily contented and satisfied, always enjoys him/herself. A person who learned when to stop never met humiliation from others.

e. Know harmony and put one's self on a humble position—Be simple and easy to approach, treat others kindly, treat others with love even though you're treated with misunderstanding and even hate. Keep harmony with others in your full effort. Don't behave arrogantly, don't look down on others, don't consider oneself always in the right, don't try to manipulate others.

f. Hold softness to defeat hardness—Take drawing back as advancing, take defense as offense. Knowing brightness but remain in darkness, knowing masculine attitude but keep one's self on feminine style. Tolerance to injustice and grievance, resistance to attack and maltreatment. Prepare in advance the worst result and strive for the best outcome.

g. Return to the initial purity and back to the original innocence—To be an honest person, always speak and behave honestly. Knowing others is wise; knowing one's self is a clear-minded person. Don't behave factiously and pretentious, don't comport yourself sentimentally and nervously, don't feel inferior, unworthy and pitiful, don't blame everything and everybody without excuse.

h. Following the rule of nature—Do things according to natural rules. Select your life style following healthy principles. Recognize there is some inevitable certainty and then you may act freely. Never fight with compulsive or obsessive symptoms, coexist with them peacefully. At the same time transfer your attention to other things that you enjoy the most to find some moments of quietness and happiness.

Practical Aspects of Daoistic Cognitive Psychotherapy

The treatment program is applied to a group of patients for the short period of course (about one to three months). The therapeutic procedure is easily carried out. From a technical point of view, the therapy is applied practically with the following four components of therapy:

a. Cognitive therapy by group discussion—The discussion and analysis of the possible cause of their neurosis or psychosomatic disease. The purpose of the discussion is to let the patients find out the causes of their diseases, the vulnerable personality traits they have, and the life events they encountered. What is most important is to help the patients learn how to adjust their thinking style, and emotional and behavioral reaction according to the eight principles of Daoistic thought and health keeping rules. It is encouraged to apply these principles in their daily life to reduce their anxiety and depression, to improve their social adaptation efficiently and to obtain life tranquility. It has been found that many patients are always oversensitive to trivial things occurring in their environment including home, and even some uncomfortable words said by other people. After several sessions, most patients will learn how to modify their life coping skills, and be psychologically adaptive to their environment, and, most importantly, to understand the necessity of change in their understanding and attitude toward a better life.

b. Writing of personal reflection for supervision—The patient is asked to write notes about their understanding and experience during the treatment period, in the form of a diary. The notes will be reviewed weekly by the therapist with comments to assist the communication with the patient individually for concrete suggestions, direction, and encouragement.

c. The indigenous technique of relaxation and meditation—This technique attempts to teach the patients how to relax the muscles of the whole body and to keep the mind peaceful to get rid of all kinds of distracting thoughts. After they have mastered this technique, patients are recommended to practice one to two times per day regularly, with 15 minutes each time.

d. The practice of "soft and slow" whole body movements—Following the principle of the Chinese *taijiquan* (shadow boxing) and *qigong* (breathing therapy), the patient was instructed to practice soft and slow whole body movement for 15 minutes each time and four times a day. Before the practice, the patients are asked to read silently the eight principles of Daoistic thought to remember the basic philosophy emphasized. In particular, they are reminded to perform the exercise according to the rule of "do without competition with others" and "follow the role of nature." In practice, the technique of the soft and slow whole body movement is not the only way for the patients to practice, but other forms of exercise such as shadow sword-waving and jogging can be applied.

Effectiveness of the Therapy

The therapy has been performed for various kinds of disorders, including anxiety and depression, and the effectiveness of the therapy were examined by the team. The results indicated that, in general, the therapy was not useful for anxiety disorder, particularly for young patients who were eager to improve their academic or occupational performances. Neither was it helpful for depressive patients. However, the therapy was very effective for older patients who had obsessive, or so-called type-A personalities and had suffered from coronary heart disease. Those patients were characterized as working very hard in their lives to achieve all they could. The therapy was very useful for this group, changing the patients' cognition and attitudes toward their lives, and learning to live in accordance with nature, rather than being overambitious. The carefully designed study, including the control group, demonstrated that the effectiveness of the therapy lasted more than three years after the therapy was terminated (Zhu, 2010).

Cultural Comments

Chinese Daoistic cognitive psychotherapy is a therapy that utilizes the indigenous Daoism philosophy for the improvement of self-awareness, social coping style, and health keeping strategy. Traditionally Confucianism has exerted wide and deep influences in Chinese people for the formation of national characteristics and value orientation. Confucian scholars emphasize that a person needs to conduct oneself so as to be accepted by the society, to serve the people, to be active and promising, and to emphasize ethic morality. On the other hand, Chinese Daoistic cognitive therapy emphasizes the quality of inner emotional well-being and psychic detachment, with spiritual freedom and natural growing up as the high points (Young et al., 2005). The philosophical concept and practice is indigenous in nature, and patients are familiar with them. It is relatively easily accepted and practiced by patients. Clinical experience has shown that it is particularly helpful to patients who are overanxious for success, too eager for improvement, and who manifest psychosomatic problems (Zhu, 2007b).

COMPARISON OF PSYCHOTHERAPY: EAST AND WEST

From the discussion above of various unique psychotherapies that have evolved in the East, it can be summarized that there are different emphases that exist in the East and West regarding the fundamental approaches to psychotherapy (Tseng, 2010), as in Table 16.1.

FINAL COMMENTS: APPLICATION FOR ASIAN AMERICANS

The unique psychotherapies that have been invented in Asia are reviewed in this chapter with particular focus on the philosophical background behind these culture-influenced unique therapies. Besides the society where it was invented, Morita therapy has spread to China (Cui, 1997), with some practices in the United States and Australia (LeVine, 2008). Naikan therapy has spread to China as well. There has been no attempt to spread the practice of Daoist cognitive therapy outside of China yet. In other words, there is almost no active practice of these culture-influenced unique therapies to be observed in the United States for Asian patients nor other non-Asian patients.

However, the contribution of these culture-influenced unique psychotherapies is at the theoretical level. The review of these culture-influenced unique psychotherapies observed in Asia hopefully will stimulate scholars and clinicians to consider what kind of modifications or considerations are needed for understanding the nature of psychological problems and psychopathology, and psychotherapy at a philosophical level. This includes how to understand the nature of mental suffering and what are suitable ways to deal with such suffering.

TABLE 16.1: Fundamental approaches to psychotherapy

Eastern Approach	Western Approach
Suppression of complex	Uncovering of complex
Focus on interpersonal adjustment	Focus on individual adjustment
Harmonious resolution	Confrontation, challenge
Intuitional enlightenment	Logical solution
Actual experience	Cognitive insight
Philosophical acceptance of problems	Active resolution of problems

Cultural adjustment is needed for psychotherapy at practical, theoretical, and philosophical levels (Tseng, 1995, 1999). There are numerous publications concerned with the practical aspects for culture-relevant psychotherapy. Yet, few address the theoretical adjustment needed for therapy of patients from different cultural backgrounds. There are almost none that examine the philosophical perspectives.

The review of unique psychotherapies that were invented originally in Asia illustrated that these Eastern therapies, in contrast to Western psychotherapies that were invented and conducted in Western societies, are characterized by radically different approaches. Namely, instead of focusing on how to help patients outwardly to deal with, cope with, and conquer the problems encountered in his/her immediate surrounding reality, the Eastern therapy help patients to adjust inwardly his/her own philosophical view and attitude toward life, with emphasis on harmony with nature. Instead of focusing on cognitive awareness and insight about the problems and reasoning the ways to solve the challenge, Eastern therapy values more actual experience and philosophical enlightenment.

This provides the opportunity to expand the scope of knowledge and method of mind healing, and to help clinicians and scholars to know that there are more different and divergent ways to work with the patients, not only for Asian American patients but patients of any cultural background.

REFERENCES

Chang, S. C. (1974). Morita therapy. *American Journal of Psychotherapy, 28,* 208–221.

Cui, Y. H. (1997): The examination and experiences of Japanese Morita therapy practiced in China [in Chinese]. In W. S. Tseng (Ed.), *Chinese mind and therapy.* Beijing: Beijing Medical University & China Xie-He Medical Joint Publisher.

Hsu, J., & Tseng, W. S. (1972). Intercultural psychotherapy. *Archives of General Psychiatry, 27,* 700–705.

Kawahara, R. (2005). Japanese Buddhist thought and Naikan therapy. In W. S. Tseng, S. C. Chang, & M. Nishizono (Eds.), *Asian culture and psychotherapy: Implications for East and West* (pp. 186–198). Honolulu: University of Hawaii Press.

Kitanishi, K. (1999). Tōyōteki tetsugaku to morita ryōhō to naikan ryōhō (Asian philosophy and Morita therapy and Naikan therapy) [in Japanese]. *Seishin Igakushi Kenkyu* (Psychiatric Research), 2, 60–65.

Kitanishi, K. (2005). The philosophical background of Morita therapy: Its application to therapy. In W. S. Tseng, S. C. Chang, & M. Nishizono (Eds.), *Asian culture and psychotherapy: Implications for East and West* (pp. 169–185). Honolulu: University of Hawaii Press.

Kohut, H. (1971). *The analysis of self.* Madison, CT: International University Press.

Kondo, K. (1976). The origin of Morita therapy. In W. Lebra (Ed.), *Culture-bound syndromes, ethnopsychiatry, and alternate therapies* (pp. 250–258). Honolulu: University Press of Hawaii.

Kora, T. (1965). Morita therapy. *International Journal of Psychiatry, 1,* 611–640.

LeVine, P. (2008, September). Use of Morita therapy for treatment of trauma across the four stages. Presented in 5th World Congress for Psychotherapy, Beijing, China.

Maeshiro, T. (2005). *Shinriryoho toshite no naikai* (*Naikan* as a psychotherapy) [in Japanese]. Osaka: Toki Shobo.

Mori, M. (1994). *Lo-shi to Sou-shi* (Lao-zi and Zhuang-zi) [in Japanese]. Tokyo: Kodansha.

Morita, S. (1921/1974). Shinkeishitus oyobi shinkeisuijaku-sho no ryōhō (The treatment of shinkeishitus and neurasthenia) [in Japanese]. In T. Kora (Ed.), *Morita Shoma Zenshiu* (Shoma Morita's collection of essays) (Vol. 1, pp 231–506). Tokyo: Hakuyosha.

Morita, S. (1922/1974). Seishinryohou kogi (Psychotherapy lecture) [in Japanese]. In T. Kora (Ed.), *Morita Shoma Zenshiu* (Shoma Morita's collection of essays) (Vol. 1, pp. 509–638). Tokyo: Hakuyosha.

Morita, S. (1926/1974). Sinkeisuijaku-shō oyobi kyohaku-kannen no konchihō (The treatment of neurasthenia and obsession) [in Japanese]. In T. Kora (Ed.), *Morita Shoma Zenshiu* (Shoma Morita's collection of essays) (Vol. 2, pp. 71–282). Tokyo: Hakuyosha.

Murase, T. (1976). Naikan therapy. In W. Lebra (Ed.), *Culture-bound syndromes, ethnopsychiatry, and alternate therapies* (pp 259–269). Honolulu: University Press of Hawaii.

Murase, T. (1977). Naikan tshirio to Morita tsirio (Naikan therapy and Morita therapy). In K. Ohara (Ed.), *Gendai no Morita rhyoho* (Modern Ogawa, B. [2008, September]). Morita therapy in higher education in the USA: A human services model. Presented in 5th World Congress for Psychotherapy, Beijing, China.

Reynolds, D. K. (1977). Naikan therapy: An experiential view. *International Journal of Social Psychiatry, 23,* 252–263.

Reynolds, D. K. (1980). *The quiet therapies: Japanese pathways to personal growth.* Honolulu: University Press of Hawaii.

Sue, S., & Morishima, J. K. (1982). *The mental health of Asian Americans: Contemporary issues in identifying and treating mental problems.* San Francisco: Jossey-Bass.

Tseng, W. S. (1995). Psychotherapy for the Chinese: Cultural adjustments. In, L. Y. C. Cheng, H. Baxter, & F. M. C. Cheung, (Eds.), *Psychotherapy for the Chinese* (Vol. 2). Hong Kong: Department of Psychiatry, Chinese University of Hong Kong.

Tseng, W. S. (1999): Culture and psychotherapy: Review and practical guidelines. *Transcultural Psychiatry, 36,* 1331–1179.

Tseng, W. S. (2001). *Handbook of cultural psychiatry.* San Diego, CA: Academic.

Tseng, W. S. (2010): Culture and psychotherapy: Clinical, theoretical, and philosophical explorations from a worldwide perspective. Keynote presentation for 20th World Congress of Psychotherapy, Lucerne, Switzerland (June). To appear in: *Professor Wen-Shing Tseng's Collected Work.* Beijing: Beijing University Medical Publisher (in preparation).

Tseng, W. S., & Streltzer, J. (Eds.). (2001). *Culture and psychotherapy: A guide for clinical practice.* Washington, DC: American Psychiatric Press.

Young, D. S. (1997). Zhongguoren de xinli yu zhongguo tese de xinlizhiliao (Chinese mind and Chinese unique therapy) [in Chinese]. In W. S. Tseng (Ed.), *Huaren de xinli yu zhiliao* (Chinese mind and therapy) (pp. 22–38). Beijing: Beijing Medical University and Chinese Xiehe Medical University Joint Publisher.

Young, D., Tseng, W. S., & Zhou, L. (2005). Daoist philosophy: Application in psychotherapy. In W. S. Tseng, S. C. Chang, & M. Nishizono (Eds.), *Asian culture and psychotherapy: Implications for East and West* (pp. 142–155). Honolulu: University of Hawaii Press.

Xiao, S. Y., Young, D. S., & Zhang, H. G. (1998). Taoistic cognitive psychotherapy for neurotic patients: A preliminary clinical trial. *Psychiatry and Clinical Neurosciences, 52* (Suppl), S238–S241.

Zhu, J. F. (2007a, April). Daoistic cognitive therapy developed in China. Presented at Cultural Psychiatry Conference. Kamakura, Japan.

Zhu, J. F. (2007b, September). Daoistic cognitive psychotherapy: Clinical application. Presented at Regional Congress of World Psychiatric Association. Shanghai, China.

Zhu, J. F. (2010). Daoistic cognitive therapy: Clinical effectiveness [in Chinese]. Presented at International Transcultural Psychiatry Congress, Shanghai, China (April).

| SECTION IV |

CONCLUSION

| 17 |

WHERE DO WE GO FROM HERE? FUTURE DIRECTIONS, CHALLENGES, AND CONSIDERATIONS

Cathryn G. Fabian and Edward C. Chang

Throughout this volume, we have sought to consolidate the knowledge base for psychiatric disorders in Asians into one cohesive resource for both clinicians and researchers. In doing so, we hope that we have highlighted challenges in applying conventional Western notions of psychopathology to Asians, and have identified several areas of potential future inquiry and innovation. The emergence and development of cultural psychopathology as a distinct field of inquiry in the past 20 years has had a profound impact on our understanding of the social context of mental illness (Lopez & Guarnaccia, 2000). Thus, the study of psychopathology in Asians is grounded in an awareness of the interrelationship between individuals and the values, beliefs, and behaviors that are particular to their ethnocultural group. We would like to conclude this handbook by identifying potential directions, challenges, and considerations for future work in this area.

BROADENING THE SCOPE OF ASIAN CULTURAL PSYCHOPATHOLOGY

Asians comprise a heterogeneous racial category that is distinguished by significant diversity in ethnicity, language, culture, values, and histories. The term "Asian" itself refers people who have origins in indigenous peoples of East Asia, Southeast Asia, or the Indian subcontinent; consequently, Asians represent over 50 different ethnic and national subgroups, and speak over 100 languages and dialects. However, this diversity has yet to be fully embraced by mental health researchers. Comparative data from epidemiological studies of mental disorders in less-developed Asian nations is scant, and much of what is know about the prevalence of mental disorders in

Asia is extrapolated from what data can be collected from more economically advanced nations that have established mental health care systems. Even within the United States, many studies that seek to compare prevalence in mental disorders across racial groups do not include Asians. When Asians are included in such studies, they are usually addressed as one culturally monolithic group. This inattention to the diversity of Asians, while helpful for establishing a starting point for research, is ultimately detrimental to the advancement of the field. Thus, future epidemiological research into the prevalence of psychopathology must strive to be more globally representative, and be proactive in sampling understudied cultural and ethnic groups, particularly South and Southeast Asians (Chang & Yeh, 2003; Haque, 2010). Rapid economic development, coupled with histories of war and colonialism, has brought to light mental health issues that require a much more nuanced cultural understanding of sociopolitical context. Increased emigration from Asia to different parts of the globe has also brought greater attention to how to effectively address mental health issues within a larger transnational context. Field studies that include large and culturally diverse samples would give researchers the ability to assess the generalizability of our current diagnostic classification of mental disorders across cultures, and the ability to identify culturally specific phenomena that may influence prevalence rates. Not acknowledging such significant cultural differences among Asians inadvertently promulgates the use of the "one-size-fits-all" approach frequently derided in criticisms of our current diagnostic system for psychiatric disorders.

The integration of a cultural perspective into the *DSM-IV* in 1994 represented a major step forward toward the acknowledgment of the role of culture in psychopathology (Lopez & Guarnicca, 2000). For the first time, there was discussion of how cultural factors could influence the expression, assessment, and prevalence of certain disorders. The *DSM-IV* also provided an outline for cultural formulation for clinicians to use as a framework to assess the impact of culture on psychiatric disorders. The outline for cultural formulation provides a systematic means to elicit and evaluate cultural issues as part of the diagnostic process. The cultural formulation includes the following five components of assessment:

1. Cultural identity of the individual
2. Cultural explanations of the individual's illness
3. Cultural factors related to psychosocial environment and levels of functioning
4. Cultural elements of the relationship between the individual and the clinician
5. Overall cultural assessment for diagnosis and care.

The outline for cultural formulation allows the clinician to diagnose culturally patterned experiences of mental distress that fall outside mainstream diagnostic criteria. It can be a useful tool in instances where the clinician and the patient are of different cultural backgrounds, as it can call attention to cultural features that can be used to guide treatment. Use of the outline for cultural formulation can also be useful when there is no apparent cultural mismatch, as it can bring forth information about cultural values, norms, and behaviors (such as health practices, physiological attributions, and religious beliefs) that may differ between the clinician and the patient (Lewis-Fernandez & Diaz, 2002).

While compared to previous versions, the *DSM-IV* provided more guidance to clinicians to make culturally informed diagnoses, its cross-cultural validity has been criticized for its lack of attention to cultural variations in phenomenology, risk and protective factors, and course based on its reliance on epidemiological data that is removed from its social context (Gold & Kirmayer, 2007). Furthermore, critics contended that the *DSM-IV* oversimplified the integration of data from sociocultural context in diagnosis, reifying essentialist views that preclude more intensive exploration into how culture itself shapes the etiology of mental disorders (Alcarón et al., 2002). There are calls for the forthcoming *DSM-5* to build on the progress brought forth by its predecessor to elaborate on the existing *DSM* cultural formulation as a means to facilitate the integration of sociocultural contextual data into the diagnostic process (Alcarón et al., 2009). Giving the outline for cultural formulation a more prominent position in the main text of the *DSM-5*, as opposed to an appendix, as in the *DSM-IV-TR*, would call attention to the importance of the cultural context in shaping psychopathology. In doing so, the clinical validity of the *DSM-5* would be greatly enhanced, and clinicians would be able to make more comprehensive diagnoses that recognize the influence of sociocultural factors.

Treating Mental Disorders in Asians

Research on treatment methods for Asians is also limited in scope; even when racial and ethnic minority groups are included in clinical efficacy studies, Asians are rarely included as a distinct comparison group, and even fewer studies focus exclusively on Asian populations. A particular treatment modality (with appropriate cultural adaptations) may be effective in one culture, but that same treatment may be ineffective or even harmful in another. The contributors to this volume have each discussed at length evidence-based treatments for psychiatric disorders among Asians, but the knowledge base on treatment outcomes as a whole is still limited (Leong & Lau, 2001). Most, if not all, existing treatments have been manualized with European American samples, which may fail to take into account or even contradict cultural factors that may influence the psychotherapeutic process. This cultural mismatch may undermine the effectiveness of these treatments in their application to racial and ethnic minority groups. The incorporation of culture into existing models of psychotherapy is a commonly suggested method of adapting existing treatment methods for use with non-European American samples (Hall, 2001; Hwang, 2006). However, Kazdin (1993) contended that the cost of developing and training mental health providers to provide culturally adapted treatments was not justified given the lack of convincing empirical support for their efficacy. Meta-analytic research has since suggested a modest beneficial effect for culturally adapted psychotherapy (Griner & Smith; 2006; Huey & Polo, 2008), although there is no consensus framework about how to adapt interventions within a given cultural context. Furthermore, the literature on culturally adapted interventions is even more limited in identifying the ways in which these specific adaptations are beneficial to the patients, and in testing potential moderators or mediators through which these cultural adaptations enhance treatment outcomes (Pan, Huey, & Hernandez, 2011).

In a similar vein, there is also a growing call for increased research into the use of psychotropic medications in Asian populations. For similar psychiatric conditions, Asian patients typically respond to significantly lower doses of psychotropic medications than Caucasian patients receiving the same treatment (Ng et al., 2005; Ng et al., 2006). When starting an Asian patient on a new psychotropic medication, Lin and Cheung (1999) recommended a dosage level of half of that which would normally be prescribed to Caucasians, while allowing for substantial in-group variability. Asians are also more susceptible to severe or more frequent side effects when treated with the same dosages as Caucasians (Lin & Cheung, 1999). These findings are most likely the result of genetic differences in the activity of enzymes that metabolize psychotropic medications and allow for their removal from the body. However, the activity of these enzymes is also highly susceptible to environmental influences, such as diet. Thus, future research into the use of psychotropic medications in Asians must (1) further elucidate the ways in which genetic differences between Asians and other groups affect the effectiveness across varying dosage levels; and (2) identify social and lifestyle conditions that can impinge on or promote a desired individual response to psychotropic medications.

The limitations of the effectiveness of conventional models of Western mental health treatment may necessitate the innovation of new treatment paradigms that incorporate more indigenous understandings of health and healing. In Asia, mental health services are marginalized among the health services, and there is much variation between countries as to the development of service infrastructure for the mentally ill (Deva, 2008). Consequently, medication is the most favored treatment method in Asia, as counseling, psychotherapy, and rehabilitation services have yet to be embraced to the extent they are in Western nations (Deva, 2008; Watters, 2010). As Tseng and colleagues discussed in Chapter 16, some scholars have attempted to address this need by developing treatment modalities based on the values and traditions of a particular culture. The advancement of Asian indigenous psychologies, as described by Saw and Okazaki in Chapter 2, will only further inform our knowledge of how to effectively treat psychiatric disorders in Asians by grounding such treatments within the cultural frameworks of specific ethnic groups.

The incorporation of indigenous lay theories of health into nosological and treatment paradigms for mental illness in Asians also holds great potential for the development of culturally sensitive assessment and intervention methods. Lay theories of health involve unarticulated beliefs by nonexperts about what it means to be healthy (Downey & Chang, 2011). Such an approach resounds with the notion that health is more than the absence of illness (World Health Organization, 1948), and moves us toward a more biopsychosocial model of health and well-being (Engel, 1977). Among Asians, the common cultural belief that the mind and body are one integrated entity leads to somatized symptoms of emotional issues in clinical settings (Lin, 1980). Thus, psychological distress may take the form of physical complaints, such as insomnia, loss of appetite, and headaches (Sue & Sue, 1987). Treating the physical issues before the underlying psychological issues can be more effective in that it establishes trust in the therapeutic process (Paniagua, 1998). As another example of a lay theory, traditional Chinese cultural beliefs about mental illness hold that psychosis is the only type of mental illness, and that any other type of illness is physical in nature (Hsiao, Klimidis, Minas, & Tan, 2006). In this particular case, appropriate treatment for mental health issues may be delayed due to the attribution of symptoms to physical causes. Educating patients about Western conceptualizations of mental health, and the distinction between mental and physical illness, can help them to better understand the causes of their distress. Employing methods such as these recognizes the cultural dimensions of the definitions of well-being for a particular group, and moves us one step closer to the culturally situated contextual perspective on mental health and illness.

The significance of religion and spirituality as they pertain to well-being among Asians cannot be underscored enough, as they are intertwined with many cultures' beliefs about health, mental health, and health practices. Asians themselves as a whole encompass a wide variety of religious affiliations, including but not limited to Buddhism, Hinduism, Christianity, and Islam, as well as animism and ancestor worship. While a survey of the vast religious diversity among Asians is beyond the scope of the present work, it is important to note that religion also can powerfully influence worldviews, behaviors, and patterns of social interactions, and is another aspect of an individual's sociocultural context to be considered when applying the cultural formulation to Asian patients. Research on religion and spirituality among Asians is fairly limited, but there is some evidence to suggest that Asian Americans tend to rely more on spirituality as a form of coping than Caucasian Americans (Bjorck, Cuthbertson, Thurman, & Lee, 2001). Given the general positive relationship between spirituality and health outcomes (Richards & Bergin, 2000), the role of religion and mental health serves as a potential area for future inquiry into the innovation of prevention and intervention methods for mental disorders among Asians.

The intersection of culture, religion, and spirituality can also profoundly affect help-seeking behaviors among Asians for mental illnesses. For some cultures, religious beliefs dictate that indigenous healing methods may be more highly regarded than those of mainstream Western medicine, as these methods are in greater concordance with their notions of health and illness. Many Asians and Asian Americans may prefer to seek help for mental health issues from traditional healers, or seek informal support from within their immediate social network, such as from friends, family members, or the clergy (Sue & Morishima, 1982; Zhang, Snowden, & Sue, 1998). Thus, the reliance of many cultures on complementary and alternative medicine as another means of achieving mental health must also be taken into account by clinicians and researchers who work with Asians. These indigenous methods differ from Western psychotherapy in that they: (1) emphasize interdependence and the interconnectedness between the mind, body, and spirit; (2) value a circular perspective, which emphasizes intuitive reasoning and qualitative understanding, over a more Western linear (cause-and-effect) perspective of healing; (3) allow for intervention at a spiritual level, rather than a cognitive or affective level; and (4) view the role of the healer as an active agent in bringing about change in the person, rather than as a passive facilitator (Yeh, Hunter, Madan-Bahel, Chiang, & Ahora, 2004).

A pertinent question for future work would be to examine the extent to which complementary and alternative medicines can be used to complement traditional or conventional treatments for mental health issues, and what factors may predict use of one treatment method over another. Yang, Phelan, and Link (2008) found that Chinese Americans actually perceived Western psychiatric services as being more effective in treating mental illness than traditional Chinese medicine, but also considered seeing a Western doctor for mental health issues as more shameful than seeing a practitioner of Chinese medicine, such as an herbalist or acupuncturist. Using a national sample, Asian Americans with a probable *DSM-IV* diagnosis of any mental disorder were much more likely to use complementary and alternative medicine than either traditional mental health care, or a combination of the two (45.2%, 28.7%, and 26.1%, respectively; Choi & Kim, 2010). The same study found that use of traditional healers and informal services is also associated with education level, English proficiency, and education level. Research on acculturation and the use of complementary and alternative medicines has yet to establish a definitive directional relationship;

in concordance with findings from the aforementioned study by Choi & Kim (2010), results from a telephone study of Chinese Americans found that U.S.-born respondents were less likely to endorse the use of traditional medicine for psychiatric disorders than their foreign-born counterparts (Yang, Corsini-Munt, Link, & Phelan, 2009). However, another study of Asian Americans in California found no relationship between immigration status and English-language preference on the use of complementary and alternative medicines (Hsiao et al., 2006). While acculturation may not be as pertinent to the study of Asians in Asia, it may nonetheless be relevant to examine how the greater adoption of Western medicine, and increased access to medical and mental health services, may change these attitudes toward complementary and alternative medicines over time.

FUTURE CONSIDERATIONS

Stigma

As many of the contributors have noted in preceding chapters, the stigma of mental illness continues to be the most significant barrier in addressing mental health issues among Asians. Stigmatization and discriminatory attitudes about mental illness are widespread in Asia, marked by a general fear of people with mental illness, and a sentiment that some social distance should be made between people with mental illness and the general community (Ng, 1997). Attitudes about mental disorders, such as the perception that mental disorders are the result of moral weakness and poor upbringing, continue to influence the ways in which Asians express symptomatology, engage in help-seeking behaviors, and relate to those suffering from mental illness. Despite the vast cultural heterogeneity among Asians, mental illness stigma in Asian cultures still share some common features. Fabrega (1991) identified common themes of stigma in non-Western societies: (1) the belief that the mind and body are inextricable from one another; (2) somatization of symptoms and the medicalization of mental illness; (3) supernatural, religious, moralistic, and magical approaches to illness and behavior; and (4) the belief that mental illnesses are chronic, irreversible, and relapsing. In addition, the interdependent nature of Asian cultures places emphasis on the family as the primary social unit. In cultures such as these, where a person is viewed in terms of their family, the stigma of mental illness may be more severe because it affects the entire family unit, and requires a collective response (Kirmayer, 1989).

Mental illness stigma is prevalent throughout Asia, but this is far from a commonly held sentiment among all Asian cultures. In fact, some cultures respond to mental illness quite differently. For example, in India, Ayurvedic medical practitioners who treat the mentally ill do not regard mental illness as stigmatizing (Fabrega, 1991). In Sri Lanka, mental illness is seen as transient and treatable, and the person is not viewed as being responsible for his or her illness (Waxler, 1974). In both these cultures, the conceptualization and labeling of mental illness contribute to a sociocultural environment that is less stigmatizing toward those with mental illness. Thus, mental illness stigma must be studied with consideration of its origins, definitions, and ramifications within a specific culture.

Attitudes toward mental illness and people with mental illness are likely to evolve in the coming years with the rapid social and economic changes in Asia. While these developments have done much to improve the standard of living for many Asians, lack of access to mental health services can further exacerbate mental illness stigma. As mentioned in Chapter 1, mental health professionals are scarce throughout much of Asia. Psychiatrists and psychologists are more likely to be located in urban areas, and people with mental illness without the financial means to travel may not be able to access the help they need (Lauber & Rossler, 2007). Mental health professionals themselves may possess stigmatizing attitudes toward people with mental illness, as psychiatric education and training in Asia widely varies in quantity and quality (Singh & Ng, 2008). These factors consequently create barriers to seeking help, and further contribute to the stigmatization and marginalization of people with mental illness.

While mental illness stigma persists even in the context of immigration and resettlement, there is still potential to develop interventions that employ a public health perspective to address the stigma of mental illness. Multiple studies have correlated mental illness stigma among Asian Americans with increased reluctance to use formal mental health services (e.g., Loya, Reddy, & Hinshaw, 2010; Miville & Constantine, 2007; Shea & Yeh, 2008; Ting & Hwang, 2009). A study of undergraduates in the United States found that Asian American perceived people with mental illness as more dangerous, and expressed more desire to be segregated from the mentally ill (Rao, Feinglass, & Corrigan, 2007). However, results from an intervention conducted as part of the aforementioned study also found that after having contact with a person with a person with mental illness, the perception of people with mental illness as being dangerous had changed the most among Asians compared to Caucasians, African Americans, and Latinos. This suggests that Asians are amenable to interventions to reduce mental illness stigma, and such interventions should be targeted toward the cultural background of its participants.

Clinical Bias in Diagnosis

Another major barrier pertaining to the effective treatment of mental disorders for Asians is the potential for therapist bias. Akutsu and Chu in Chapter 2 described how current assessment methods based on Western nosological systems are limited in their ability to evaluate individuals from non-Western ethnic and cultural backgrounds. This lack of culturally appropriate assessment tools, coupled with the perception of Asians as being docile and less susceptible to mental illness (Sue, Sue, Sue, & Takeuchi, 1995), may lead to misdiagnosis or inaccurate appraisal of the severity of mental illness. Since these diagnoses are used to inform treatment plans, any misdiagnosis due either to cultural biases in our current nosological system or cultural biases of the therapist would result in inappropriate or ineffective courses of treatment. Lopez (1989) identified two broad types of biases in clinical evaluations: biases in the diagnosis, and biases in the severity of symptoms. Two types of errors can be made in diagnostic assessment: Overdiagnosis occurs when clinicians favor one diagnosis over another due to the patient's gender, race, or age. In contrast, underdiagnosis occurs when a disorder is thought to be less likely to occur in certain groups. Clinicians also need to be aware of biases in the assessing the severity of symptoms, and take care to avoid overpathologizing, (i.e., misinterpreting culturally prescribed behavior as symptoms of psychopathology), and underpathologizing, (i.e., minimizing nonnormative behavior and attributing psychiatric symptoms to the patient's culture) (Lopez, 1989; Okazaki & Sue, 1995).

Studies of interpretive bias among clinicians have found support that Asians are susceptible to such biases. In a study comparing clinical judgments of Chinese American and Caucasian therapists, Li-Repac (1980) found that clinical assessments varied as a function of an interaction of the therapist's and patient's ethnicity. Each group assessed the patients from their own ethnic group more positively than patients from the other ethnic group. Another study of Asian American and non–Asian American clinical social workers found that when presented with a hypothetical Asian client, non–Asian American clinicians assessed the case as being more severe, and predicted poorer outcomes. Compared to non-Asian Americans, Asian American clinicians placed more emphasis on the need to build rapport with the client, and on acculturation and family dynamics (Lu, 1996). While ethnic matching between the therapist and the client is generally desirable, it is not a panacea to solving these issues of clinician bias. The continued implementation and evolution of the cultural formulation, as well as enhanced training in cultural competence for clinicians, is a promising initial step into better serving the mental health needs of Asians and Asian Americans.

Globalization, Migration, and Mental Health

Globalization has brought about rapid economic development and changes in social values, norms, and values throughout Asia. While globalization is generally thought of as an economic process, it is becoming increasingly perceived as a more complex phenomenon that ultimately shapes the health and well-being of individuals. Huynen, Martens, and Hilderink (2005) proposed a model which posited that globalization impacts health by changing conditions at the institutional, economic, sociocultural, and ecological levels, which in turn shape direct and indirect determinants of population health. Evidence for the direct effect of globalization on specific health outcomes is still lacking (Lee & Collin, 2001), but cross-national research on the link between poverty and mental disorders in developing nations suggests that economic conditions, such as the availability of health, economic, social programs have unanticipated indirect benefits on mental health (Patel & Kleinman, 2003). Economic development can also provide for greater access to mental health care, as more funds become allocated for the training of mental health professionals, and improved standards of living may lead more individuals to seek treatment for conditions that otherwise may have gone undiagnosed. However, despite these benefits, globalization, and more specifically, the export of Western culture to Asia has also created new deleterious social conditions which affect mental health. The rigorous methodological standards for research on models of evidence-based practice that inform intervention in Western medicine are difficult to replicate using local knowledge, beliefs, and resources (Kirmayer, 2006). In addition, the prevalence of certain psychiatric disorders in some countries has increased as a direct result of aggressive marketing campaigns of psychotropic medications by pharmaceutical companies, who publicize disorders alongside with their products (Kirmayer, 2002; Watters, 2010). Thus, globalization presents a double-edged sword of sorts for psychopathology among Asians; while it presents greater opportunities for access to care, it also services a vehicle for cultural imperialism, through its wholesale imposition of Western conceptualizations of mental health and illness.

The migration of individuals from rural to urban centers, and from developing nations to more prosperous nations, also has implications for mental health. As Chun and Hsu noted in Chapter 14, the transition from one culture to another can precipitate the development of psychiatric disorders, as the negotiation of two distinct cultures can create much distress for an individual. Migration also places individuals at greater vulnerability since it removes them from existing social support networks, which can buffer against mental illness (Bhugra, 2005; Taylor et al., 2004). Migration also allows for the development of hybridized cultures and multicultural identities, in which individuals may develop more complex understandings of their cultural backgrounds. Therefore, over the course of time, it may be more appropriate to treat culture as a fluid, subjective experience, rather than as a static entity. While an individual may be of a particular cultural background, it may be just as relevant to study cultural variables related to the cognitive and behavioral aspects of culture. For example, Barry and Beitel (2009) proposed a three-factor approach that employs acculturation, self-construal, and ethnic identity as proxy variables for culture. This more multi-dimensional view of culture allows both clinicians and researchers to consider how individuals orient themselves toward culture, and allows for the further development of more appropriate diagnostic and treatment methods.

CONCLUDING THOUGHTS

In closing, it is clear to us that the study and treatment of mental disorders in Asians require greater attention than ever before as this diverse population continues to grow and impact, as well as be impacted by, both the local and global communities Asians participate in. We believe that the present volume makes an important contribution to the study and treatment of psychopathology in Asian adults but, as we have noted in this chapter, much more work needs to be done here in appreciating the complexities of working with Asians. Alternatively, we believe that more work is also needed to understand the developmental and interpersonal context of mental health in Asians. For example, little work has been done focusing on the developmental psychopathology of Asian children. Similarly, we believe that more research is needed that looks at the interpersonal and familial context of psychopathology in Asians. Going forward, we believe that by focusing on more studies that examine the complex interplay between culturally situated antecedents, consequences, and concomitants involved in the experience of psychopathology in Asians across the life span, it can eventually lead to the development of more useful clinical models and better diagnostic, assessment, and treatment options that we hope will be of benefit to all Asian patients in the future.

REFERENCES

Alcarón, R. D., Bell, C. C., Kirmayer, J., Lin, K. M., Lopez, S., Ustun, B., et al. (2002). Beyond the funhouse mirrors: research agenda on culture and psychiatric diagnosis. In D. J. Kupfer, M. B., First, & D. A. Regler (Eds.), *A research agenda for DSM-V* (pp. 219–281). Washington, DC: American Psychiatric Association.

Alcarón, R. D., Becker, A. E., Lewis-Fernández, R., Like, R. C., Desai, P., Fouks, E., et al. (2009). Issues for DSM-V: The role of culture in psychiatric diagnosis. *Journal of Nervous and Mental Disease, 197,* 559–560.

Barry, D. T., & Beitel, M. (2009). Cultural considerations regarding perspectives on mental illness and healing. In S. Loue & M. Sajatovic (Eds.), *Determinants of minority mental health* (pp. 175–191). New York: Springer.

Bhugra, D. (2005). Cultural identities and cultural congruency: A new model for evaluating mental distress in immigrants. *Acta Psychologica Scandinavica, 112*, 84–93.

Bjorck, J. P., Cutherbertson, W., Thurman, J. W., & Lee, S. J. (2001). Ethnicity, coping, and distress among Korean Americans, Filipino Americans, and Caucasian Americans. *Journal of Social Psychology, 141*, 421–442.

Chang, T., & Yeh, C. J. (2003). Using on-line groups to provide support to Asian American men: Racial, cultural, gender, and treatment issues. *Professional Psychology: Research and Practice, 34*, 634–643.

Choi, N. G., & Kim, J. (2010). Utilization of complementary and alterative medicines for the use of mental heath problems among Asian Americans. *Community Mental Health Journal, 46*, 570–578.

Deva, M. P. (2008). Bringing changes to Asian mental health. *International Review of Psychiatry, 20*, 484–487.

Downey, C. A., & Chang, E. C. (2011). Assessment of everyday concepts of health: The Lay Theories of Health Inventory. Manuscript submitted for publication.

Engel, G. L. (1977). The need for a new medical model: A challenge for biomedicine. *Science, 196*, 129–136.

Fabrega, H. (1991). Psychiatric stigma in non-Western societies. *Comprehensive Psychiatry, 32*, 534–551.

Gold, I., & Kirmayer, L. J. (2007). Cultural psychiatry on Wakefield's procrustean bed. *World Psychiatry, 6*, 165–166.

Griner, D., & Smith, T. B. (2006). Culturally adapted mental health interventions: A meta-analytic review. *Psychotherapy: Theory, Research, Practice, Training, 43*, 531–548.

Hall, G. C. N. (2001). Psychotherapy research with ethnic minorities: Empirical, ethical, and conceptual issues. *Journal of Consulting and Clinical Psychology, 69*, 502–510.

Haque, A. (2010). Mental health concepts in Southeast Asia: Diagnostic considerations and treatment implications. *Psychology, Health, and Medicine, 15*, 127–134.

Hsiao, A.-F., Wong, M. D., Goldstein, M. S., Becerra, L. S., Cheng, E. M., & Wenger, N. S. (2006). Complementary and alternative medicine use among Asian-American subgroups: Prevalence, predictors, and lack of relationship to acculturation and access to conventional health care. *Journal of Alternative and Complementary Medicine, 12*, 1003–1010.

Hsiao, F. H., Klimidis, S., Minas, H. I., & Tan, E. S. (2006). Folk concepts of mental disorders among Chinese-Australian patients and their caregivers. *Journal of Advanced Nursing, 55*, 58–67.

Huey, S. J., Jr., & Polo, A. J. (2008). Evidence-based psychosocial treatments for ethnic minority youth. *Journal of Clinical Child and Adolescent Psychology, 37*, 262–301.

Huynen, M. M. T. E., Martens, P., & Hilderink, H. H. M. (2005). The health impacts of globalization: a conceptual framework. *Globalization and Health, 1*, 14.

Hwang, W.-C. (2006). The psychotherapy adaptation and modification framework: Application to Asian Americans. *American Psychologist, 61*, 702–715.

Kazdin, A. E. (1993). Adolescent mental health: Prevention and treatment programs. *American Psychologist, 48*, 127–141.

Kirmayer, L. J. (1989). Cultural variations in the response to psychiatric disorder and emotional distress. *Social Science and Medicine, 29*, 327–329.

Kirmayer, L. J. (2002). Psychopharmacology in a globalizing world: The use of antidepressants in Japan. *Transcultural Psychiatry, 39*, 295–312.

Kirmayer, L. J. (2006). Beyond the "new cross-cultural psychiatry": cultural biology, discursive psychology, and the ironies of globalization. *Transcultural Psychiatry, 43*(1), 126–144.

Lauber, C., & Rossler, W. (2007). Stigma toward people with mental illness in developing countries in Asia. *International Review of Psychiatry, 19*, 157–178.

Lee, K., & Collin, J. (2001). *Review of existing empirical research on globalization and health.* Geneva: World Health Organization.

Leong, F. T. L., & Lau, A. S. L. (2001). Barriers to providing effective mental health services to Asian Americans. *Mental Health Services Research, 3*, 201–214.

Lewis-Fernandez, R., & Diaz, N. (2002). The cultural formulation: a method for assessing cultural factors affecting the clinical encounter. *Psychiatric Quarterly, 73*, 271–295.

Li-Repac, D. (1980). The effects of therapist-client ethnic match in the assessment of mental health functioning. *Journal of Cross-Cultural Psychology, 27*, 598–615.

Lin, K. M. (1980). Traditional Chinese medical beliefs and their relevance for mental illness and psychiatry. In A. Kleinman & T. Y. Lin (Eds.), *Normal and abnormal behavior in Chinese culture* (pp. 95–111). Boston: Reidel.

Lin, K. H., & Cheung, F. (1999). Mental health issues for Asian Americans. *Psychiatric Services, 50,* 774–780.

Lopez, S. R. (1989). Patient variable biases in clinical judgment: Conceptual overview and methodological considerations. *Psychological Bulletin, 106,* 184–203.

Lopez, S. R., & Guarnaccia, P. J. J. (2000). Cultural psychopathology: Uncovering the social world of mental illness. *Annual Review of Psychology, 51,* 571–598.

Loya, F., Reddy, R., & Hinshaw, S. P. (2010). Mental illness stigma as a mediator of differences in Caucasian and South Asian college students' attitudes toward psychological counseling. *Journal of Counseling Psychology, 57,* 484–490.

Lu, Y. E. (1996). Underutilization of mental health services by Asian American patients: The impact of language and culture in clinical assessment and intervention. *Psychotherapy in Private Practice, 15,* 43–61.

Miville, M. L., & Constantine, M. G. (2007). Cultural values, counseling stigma, and intentions to seek counseling among Asian American college women. *Counseling and Values, 52,* 2–11.

Ng, C. H. (1997). The stigma of mental illness in Asian culture. *Australian and New Zealand Journal of Psychiatry, 31,* 382–390.

Ng, C. H., Chong, S. A., Lambert, T., Fan, A., Hackett, L. P., Mahendran, R., et al. (2005). An inter-ethnic comparison study of clozapine dosage, clinical response and plasma levels. *International Clinical Psychopharmacology, 20,* 163–168.

Ng, C. H., Easteal, S., Tan, S., Schweitzer, I., Ho, B. K., & Aziz, S. (2006). Serotonin transporter polymorphisms and clinical response to sertraline across ethnicities. *Progress in Neuro-Psychopharmacology and Biological Psychiatry, 30,* 953–957.

Okazaki, S., & Sue, S. (1995). Methodological issues in assessment research with ethnic minorities. *Psychological Assessment, 7,* 367–375.

Pan, D., Huey, S. J., Jr., & Hernandez, D. (2011). Culturally adapted versus standard exposure treatment for phobic Asian Americans: Treatment efficacy, moderators, and predictors. *Cultural Diversity and Ethnic Minority Psychology, 17,* 11–22.

Paniagua, F. A. (1998). *Assessing and treating culturally diverse patients* (2nd ed.). Thousand Oaks, CA: Sage.

Patel, V., & Kleinman, A. (2003). Poverty and common mental disorders in developing countries. *Bulletin of the World Health Organization, 81,* 609–615.

Rao, D., Feinglass, J., & Corrigan, P. (2007). Racial and ethnic disparities in mental illness stigma. *Journal of Nervous and Mental Disease, 195,* 1020–1023.

Richards, P. S., & Bergin, A. E. (2000). *Handbook of psychotherapy and religious diversity.* Washington, DC: American Psychological Association.

Shea, M., & Yeh, C. J. (2008). Asian American students' cultural values, stigma, and relational self-construal: Correlates and attitudes toward professional help seeking. *Journal of Mental Health Counseling, 30,* 157–172.

Singh, B., & Ng, C. H. (2008). Psychiatric education and training in Asia. *International Review of Psychiatry, 20,* 413–418.

Sue, S., & Morishima, J. K. (1982). *The mental health of Asian Americans.* San Francisco: Jossey-Bass.

Sue, D., & Sue, S. (1987). Cultural factors in the clinical assessment of Asian Americans. *Journal of Consulting and Clinical Psychology, 55,* 479–487.

Sue, S., Sue, D. W., Sue, L., & Takeuchi, D. T. (1995). Psychopathology among Asian Americans: A model minority? *Cultural Diversity and Mental Health, 1,* 39–51.

Taylor, S. E., Sherman, D. K., Kim, H. S, Jarcho, J., Takagi, K., & Dunagan, M. S. (2004). Culture and social support: Who seeks it and why? *Journal of Personality and Social Psychology, 87,* 354–362.

Ting, J. Y., & Hwang, W. (2009). Cultural influences on help-seeking attitudes in Asian American students. *American Journal of Orthopsychiatry, 79,* 125–132.

Watters, E. (2010). *Crazy like us: The globalization of the American psyche.* New York: Simon & Schuster.

Waxler, N. E. (1974). Culture and mental illness. *Journal of Nervous and Mental Disease, 159,* 379–395.

World Health Organization. (1948). *Constitution of the World Health Organization.* Geneva, Switzerland: World Health Organization Basic Documents.

Yang, L. H., Corsini-Munt, S., Link, B., & Phelan, J. (2009). Beliefs in traditional Chinese medicine efficacy among Chinese Americans: Implications for mental health service utilization. *Journal of Nervous and Mental Disease, 97,* 207–210.

Yang, L. H., Phelan, J. C., & Link, B. G. (2008). Stigma towards traditional Chinese medicine and psychiatric treatment among Chinese-Americans. *Cultural Diversity and Ethnic Minority Psychology, 14,* 10–18.

Yeh. C. J., Hunter, C. D., Madan-Bahel, A., Chiang, L., & Arora, A. K. (2004). Indigenous and interdependent perspectives of healing: Implications for counseling research. *Journal of Counseling and Development, 82,* 410–419.

Zhang, A. Y., Snowden, L. R., & Sue S. (1998). Differences between Asian and white Americans' help seeking and utilization patterns in the Los Angeles Area. *Journal of Community Psychology, 26,* 317–326.

INDEX

somatization disorder, 180–181
  diagnostic criteria for, 180
  economic factors for, 181
  prevalence of, 180–181
  symptoms of, 180
somatization tendencies, in Asians, 185–186
  in China, 185–186
  in cultural models, for somatoform disorders,
    192–193
  personality characteristics as influence on, 193
somatoform disorders
  in Asians, 185–186
    in China, 185–186
  body dysmorphic disorder, 184
  conversion disorder, 182–183
    diagnostic criteria for, 182
    economic factors for, 182–183
    prevalence rates for, 182
  DSM criteria for, 180–189
    diagnostic limitations in, 186–189
  etiological models of, 189–194
    cultural, 192–194
    psychobiological, 189–190
    psychological, 190–191
    social, 191–192
  hypochondriasis, 184
  ICD classification of, 186–187
  identification of, 179
  neurasthenia and, in Asians, 187–189
    in China, 187
    prevalence of, 188–189
  not otherwise specified, 184
  pain disorder, 183
    prevalence of, 183
    symptoms for, 183
  somatization disorder, 180–181
    diagnostic criteria for, 180
    economic factors for, 181
    prevalence of, 180–181
    symptoms of, 180
  treatment strategies, 194–196
    biological approaches, 195
    with CBT, 196
    psychological approaches, 196
    through reattribution technique, 196
    with SSRIs, 195
  undifferentiated, 182
specific phobias, 144
  prevalence rates for, 144
    in NESARC, 144
SRBDs. See sleep-related breathing disorders
SSRIs. See selective serotonin reuptake inhibitors
STAI. See State Trait Anxiety Inventory

Standard Nomenclature of Diseases and
  Operations, 2
State Trait Anxiety Inventory (STAI), 33
Strengthening of Intergenerational/Intercultural
  Ties in Immigrant Chinese American
  Families (SITICAF), 348
stress. See acculturation stressors; bicultural stress
stress-diathesis model, 93
Structured Clinical Interview for DSM-IV Diagnoses
  (SCID), 37
substance use disorders (SUDs)
  in Asia
    with ASTs, 62
    prevalence rates, 62
  as continuum, 59–61
  criteria, 59
    in DSM-IV, 60
  etiology of, 62–70
    age at immigration and, 68–69
    availability of access in, 67
    biological factors in, 63–64
    cultural factors in, 68–70
    cultural norms as influence on, 69–70
    ethnic identity and, 69
    family influences in, 64–66
    genetic research for, 63–64
    nativity status and, 68–69
    peer influences in, 66–67
    psychological factors in, 68
    research limitations for, 70
    self-reported unfair treatment in, 67
    social factors in, 64–67
  prevalence rates, 61–62
    among AAPIs, 61–62, 68–69
    in Asia, 62
    in Cambodian Americans, 62
    in Canada, 62
  self-esteem and, 68
  treatment for, 71–76
    among AAPIs, 71–72
    Alcoholics Anonymous and, 74
    barriers to, 72–74
    cultural credibility of, 73–74
    EBPs in, 75–76
    recognition of problem and, 72–73
    social stigma and, 73
    utilization of services in, 71–72
suicide
  for Asians, 6
  in China, for females, MDD and, 123–124
  family, 408–409
  net-shinjyu, 409–410
  seppuku, 408